Developmental Psychology

AN INTRODUCTION

Developmental Psychopathology

AN INTRODUCTION

Fred R. Volkmar, MD

Irving B. Harris Professor, Child Psychiatry, Pediatrics and Psychology
Child Study Center
Yale University School of Medicine
Dorothy B. Goodwin Family Endowed Chair of Special Education
Southern Connecticut State University
New Haven, Connecticut

Eli R. Lebowitz, PhD

Associate Professor
Child Study Center
Yale University School of Medicine
New Haven, Connecticut

Denis G. Sukhodolsky, PhD

Associate Professor
Child Study Center
Yale University School of Medicine
New Haven, Connecticut

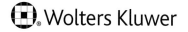
Wolters Kluwer

Philadelphia • Baltimore • New York • London
Buenos Aires • Hong Kong • Sydney • Tokyo

Acquisitions Editor: Chris Teja
Development Editor: Ariel S. Winter
Editorial Coordinator: Oliver Raj
Marketing Manager: Kirsten Watrud
Production Project Manager: Kim Cox/Kirstin Johnson
Design Coordinator: Stephen Druding
Manufacturing Coordinator: Beth Welsh
Prepress Vendor: S4Carlisle Publishing Services

First Edition

Library of Congress Cataloging-in-Publication Data

ISBN-13: 978-1-975149-64-2
ISBN-10: 1-975149-64-5

Library of Congress Control Number: 2021907773

shop.lww.com

To our wives, Lisa, Mira, and Miyun

And our children, Lucy, Emily, Itamar, Michael, Ben, Alex, and Andrew

And grandchild Henry

■ PREFACE

This book comes from the three of us collaborating for a number of years now on a course we have taught on *Developmental Psychopathology*. As part of this course, advanced undergraduate students and some graduate students have a weekly supervised experience working with children or adolescents in some clinical setting—outpatient, inpatient, or one of several local school settings. Over the years that we have taught the course, we have had more and more graduate and professional students from a range of disciplines—nursing, public health and epidemiology, cognitive science, law, and linguistics. Through them, we have become aware of the interest and need that students from various helping professions have for an introduction to the field of developmental psychopathology.

In doing this course, we have been somewhat stymied in the search for a good textbook. There are a number of textbooks on developmental psychopathology that are aimed essentially at graduate students in psychology. These books are excellent, but are both a bit above the level we seek and also not quite so clinically oriented as we might like. On the other hand, we also know of a number of major textbooks in the field of child and adolescent psychiatry—including *Lewis's Child and Adolescent Psychiatry* that one of us (F.V.) has been an editor of for several editions. The problem with these books is that although the information is very good—indeed there is *a lot of it*—it is really intended for specialists in the field. Hence, our awareness of a need for a book such as this one, one that tries to strike a balance between providing up-to-date theory, research, and clinical information without overloading and overwhelming the beginning reader.

In assigning reading for our class, we found some chapters from the 2011 condensed version of the Lewis's textbook helpful. They were highly readable, but by now many were out of date and had to be supplemented by new material—hence our proposal to Wolters Kluwer to develop this book. We have used, when we can, material from the *Essentials of Lewis's Child and Adolescent Psychiatry* (2011), but have updated it with tables and figures and new information relying whenever possible on the latest edition of *Lewis's Child and Adolescent Psychiatry: A Comprehensive Textbook* (2018). Our aim is to provide a readable volume that will be of interest to students in a range of disciplines—psychiatry, pediatrics and general medicine, nursing, social work, speech-language pathology, occupational and physical therapy, the law, and other disciplines—who wish to obtain a focused and relatively short introduction to developmental psychopathology.

We are deeply gratefully to our publisher, Wolters Kluwer, for their permission to use materials from our earlier book as well as from the fifth edition of *Lewis's Child and Adolescent Psychiatry*. Our thanks to the editors of the latter and to the authors. We also wish to thank Chris Teja and Ariel S. Winter and the Wolters Kluwer production team who have worked so patiently with us. In addition to our families, our local assistants and supporters have included Monica Podles and Lori Klein at Yale.

Fred R. Volkmar, MD
Eli R. Lebowitz, PhD
Denis G. Sukhodolsky, PhD

Martin, A., Bloch, M., & Volkmar, F. R. (2018). *Lewis's child and adolescent psychiatry* (5th ed.). Wolters Kluwer.
Volkmar, F. R., & Martin, A. (2011). *Essentials of Lewis's child and adolescent psychiatry.* Lippincott Williams & Wilkins.

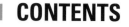

CONTENTS

CHAPTER 1 ■ AN INTRODUCTION TO DEVELOPMENTAL PSYCHOPATHOLOGY: HISTORY, THEORY, AND METHODS

■ HISTORICAL PERSPECTIVES

The field of child mental health in general and developmental psychopathology in particular is a relatively recent one. Work in the area increased dramatically in the 20th century with an explosion of knowledge over the last several decades in particular. This body of work draws on various, sometimes distinctive and sometimes overlapping, historical and professional traditions and disciplines. It includes expanding knowledge about both normative/typical child development and developmental processes as well as about the origins, expression, and treatment of psychopathology. Parts of the field have their origins in the social welfare movement and the concern for better approaches to juvenile justice. Another contribution stems from the long-standing concerns for children with significant intellectual deficiency (mental retardation). Another line of work relates to mental illness originating in childhood or having precursors in childhood. All these efforts had their origins in an interest in children and their development that had begun to increase in the 1700s and also was fueled by concerns for the education of future citizens. This area of work and the overlap of educational and child developmental and mental health concerns remain an important issue for schools and mental health professionals to this day.

Interest in understanding children's development can be traced to ancient times. Several different models of development were proposed. The preformationists included individuals like Hippocrates who assumed that body structures in the embryo were formed simultaneously, whereas others like Aristotle suggested that development was more dynamic with the embryo formed by a series of transformations and differentiations (Hunt, 1961). Preformationist thought continued well into the 1600s when, with the development of the microscope, small humans were initially seen in views of human sperm (see Figure 1.1)!

Consistent with this view was the notion that children could survive on their own without considerable parental support. The story of Romulus and Remus (see Figure 1.2) reflects this view. In reality, of course, for birds and mammals, a considerable dependence on an adult caregiver(s) is required. This fantasy does, however, persist into the present with periodic reports in the popular press of children being cared for by animals (see Candland, 1993).

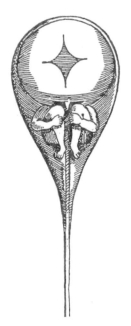

FIGURE 1.1. Hartsoeker's drawing of a human sperm (1694) reflected "preformationist" ideas about embryologic development. The increased awareness of the complexity of development during the embryonic period paralleled an increased interest in the ways in which children's psychological development changed and reorganized over time. From Hartsoeker, N. (1694). *Essay de dioptrique.* Chez Jean Anisson. Courtesy of Harvey Cushing, John J. Whitney Medical Library, Yale University School of Medicine.

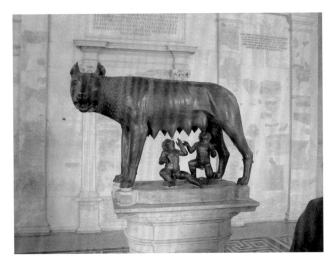

FIGURE 1.2. Romulus and Remus and their she-wolf mother. Sculpture in Vatican Museum. Photo by F. R. Volkmar.

Children were typically viewed as "chattels" (moveable property) with limited rights, and high rates of child mortality (particularly infant mortality) were observed.

Views of children, their development, and education began to change during the 18th century in a time that has come to be called the "Enlightenment." The nature of child development and needs for education became much discussed. In countries like the newly independent United States, there were particularly important issues for having an educated electorate. And, in the expansion of the United States, provision was made for country schools to serve this need.

The Enlightenment was not a single movement and indeed many of the philosophers central in it had divergent and sometimes contradictory views. For example, John Locke, the Scotch physician and philosopher, was interested in education and psychological development. He suggested that babies are born with a mind that is a blank slate (*tabula rasa*), on which experience and growing conscious awareness shape the developing child. For him, education was therefore essential. Although agreeing with Locke on the importance of education, in contrast to him, the philosopher Jean-Jacques Rousseau believed that children were innately good and that a corrupt society contributed to their difficulties.

In the 19th century, the growing emphasis on education, attempts to reform child labor laws (not to mention concerns about slavery), and an expanding interest in women's rights (including the right to an education) had a major impact. Darwin's work on evolution revolutionized psychology as well as biology (see Figures 1.3 and 1.4).

Darwin was interested in psychological development in men and animals (and published a book on facial expressions in man and animals—1871) to clarify potential biologic relationships and similarities in emotional expression. His interest in children also reflected an awareness that, to some extent, children's development has important similarities, particularly at the embryologic level, to evolutionary development (Darwin, 1859). Darwin (1877) also kept a detailed diary of one of his children's development. His work inspired subsequent psychologists, including Freud as well as individuals like G. Stanley Hall, who tried to

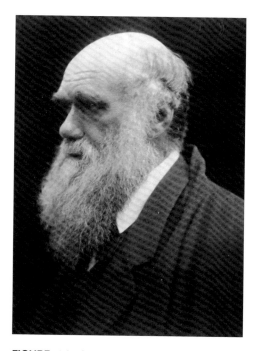

FIGURE 1.3. Charles Darwin *c.* 1860 by Julia Margaret Cameron.

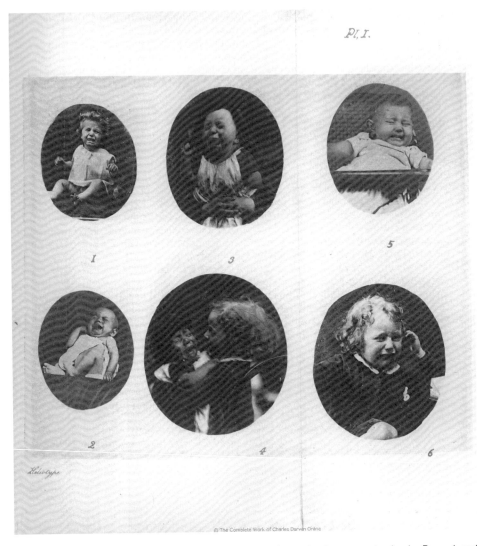

FIGURE 1.4. From Charles Darwin: Plate I. Expression of emotion in man and animals. Reproduced with permission from Darwin Online.

understand child development in an evolutionary context. Darwin's book on the *Expression of Emotion in Man and Animals* marks the beginning of comparative psychology, and along with his baby diary of his developing child, the beginning of the field of child psychology.

Reduced rates of infant and child mortality also meant that more children survived to need educational and other services. Beginning in the 19th century, several factors contributed to reducing mortality rates (see Box 1.1). These included better nutrition, housing, sanitation, various public health efforts (e.g., as the mechanisms of disease pathogenesis became clear), the development of immunizations to prevent the frequent, serious childhood infections, and, finally, the development of antibiotics. Before the 1800s, child mortality in general and infant mortality in particular was high with considerable fluctuation reflecting epidemics, famine, conflict, and other factors. Probably, at least one-third of infants succumbed to illness on average.

BOX 1.1　　**Infant Mortality**

Historically, human population growth was very slow because of high rates of infant and child mortality: in ancient Rome, probably 30% died before their first birthday and only about 50% survived to puberty. These numbers changed only relatively recently. Congregate facilities (orphanages) were associated with very high mortality rates. With advances in hygiene and science, these numbers began to slowly change and the advent of immunizations and better medical care gradually led to a marked improvement so that by 1900, the rate was <1% and by 1997 <0.01%. Measles, pertussis, smallpox, and other infectious (and now preventable) diseases were major causes of death. Birth control was, of course, nonexistent until recently, and child abandonment and infanticide were also relatively frequent (Boswell, 1989; Volk & Atkinson, 2013).

Pediatrics began to develop as a specialty with the growing awareness of differences in medical care in younger patients reflecting differences in physiology and drug metabolism. Hospitals for the care of sick children began to be established in Europe and the United States. These medical specialists also were increasingly concerned with fostering children's healthy development and providing practical guidance to parents.

Interest in intellectual deficiency/mental retardation also contributed to the development of the various child specialists. Although recognized since antiquity, scientific interest increased as attempts were made to understand the underlying brain basis of severe cognitive impairment, for example, the English anatomist Thomas Willis related intellectual deficiency to small brain size, and by 1866 John Down suggested that the syndrome that now carries his name (Trisomy 21) reflected an evolutionary throwback in development. Inspired by Darwin, individuals in the eugenics movement suggested the idea of improving society through selective breeding. (See Gould, 1996 for an excellent discussion.)

A different, and more optimistic, approach to the care of the mentally retarded arose in France where work by Itard on the so-called feral child, Victor (see Figure 1.5), stimulated his interest in the remediation of significant developmental difficulty. His inspiration of the French physician Édouard Séguin led to a new approach in classifications and attempts to improve functional outcome. Séguin immigrated to the United States and had a profound influence on the development of intervention programs. In the United States, a series of special institutions, originally focused on rehabilitation of developmentally disabled children, were created. Other such institutions were established to care for children with blindness or deafness. A professional organization was established in 1876 that became what would be the American Association on Mental Retardation. The development of the first reliable tests of intelligence by Binet and Simon (see Chapter 6) also contributed to earlier identification of less severely impaired children with developmental delays. Clinics for the care of children with developmental difficulties began to be established in the late 19th century.

Although the development of institutions and better approaches to assessment were positively intended, both led to abuses. Intelligence tests were used, sometimes highly inappropriately, to bolster the efforts of the eugenics movement, and, over time, the many negative effects of institutionalization also became apparent. In the United States, G. Stanley Hall, a pioneer psychologist and educator, began to use new approaches to study normative development. He used questionnaires to assess what children had learned and to document their interests and activities. He used this information in helping teachers understand development. The growing child study movement led to the establishment, in the early 20th century of a number of research centers around the country. Around this time, the length of children's years of education began to increase as increase in technology required a more educated workforce. Hall's work influenced many in the next generation of researchers including Arnold Gesell, and Gesell's student, Benjamin Spock.

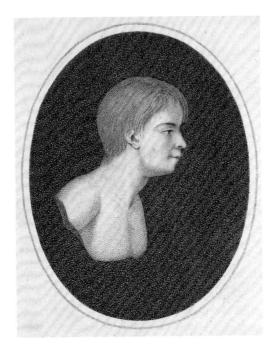

FIGURE 1.5. Victor the "wild boy" of Aveyron was reported to be a feral child who had lived alone in the woods prior to his eventual capture. Although reports of wild or "feral" children abound in mythology, we usually see reports relate either to children raised in profound isolation (but NOT by animals) or with serious developmental problems like autism. From Itard, E. M. (1802). *An historical account of the discovery and education of a savage man, or of the first developments, physical and moral, of the young savage caught in the woods near Aveyron, in the year 1798.* London: Richard Phillips.

Children who had difficulties with the law became a focus of increased concern. In the early 1900s, Healy established a clinic that advised the juvenile court regarding children. Healy's psychologically informed approach proved influential. He collaborated with a number of individuals including Jane Adams, whose work at Hull House in Chicago served as a base for the development of social work as a discipline. Healy eventually moved to Boston where he and a colleague founded the clinic supported by the Judge Baker Foundation. Around the same time, Arnold Gesell, one of the first PhDs in developmental psychology, moved to Yale where he completed medical and pediatric training and founded what would become the Yale Child Study Center. In contrast to Healey's work, Gesell strongly emphasized the recognition of innate factors in development. Gesell conducted innovative work in charting normal development in infants and younger children using techniques like still-frame movie cameras to examine more precisely the aspects of infant motor development (Gesell et al., 1938).

Gesell's work had a profound influence on pediatrics, education, and child rearing practices. The contrasting views of various individuals, each emphasizing either biologic or environmental factors, paralleled earlier debates on the relative contributions of nature versus nurture (see Chapter 2). These tensions continued theoretically, for example, in the tensions between theories of development grounded in behaviorism and psychoanalysis.

The increased interest in children with developmental, mental health, and legal issues led to the establishment of the American Orthopsychiatric Association in the 1920s. This organization strongly supported the importance of interdisciplinary collaboration in child mental health work. The interface of mental health issues with pediatrics led to the formal establishment of child psychiatry as a discipline. Although psychiatrists like Maudsley in the 1800s had recognized the childhood onset of major psychiatric difficulties, it was only in 1930 that Leo Kanner was recruited to Johns Hopkins to serve as a liaison between pediatrics and psychiatry there and wrote the first textbook of psychiatry devoted to children (1935). Among his many accomplishments was his pioneering work in pediatric consultation–liaison psychiatry (see Chapter 27) and the recognition of autism as a distinctive condition (see Chapter 7). Before World War II, pediatricians were beginning to spend time training in child psychiatry as fellows in various sites around the country. At this time, psychoanalytic influences also became strong, and were further strengthened by an influx of European psychoanalysts before and subsequent to the war. The federal government established the first training grants shortly after the war. As the Child Guidance clinics increased, so did the need for psychiatrists with specialized child training. The American Academy of Child Psychiatry was established in 1953, and by 1957 the field was recognized as a subspecialty of psychiatry with standards for training and board examinations and its own journal.

THEORIES OF DEVELOPMENT

Over the past century, a number of attempts have been made to provide broad, overarching theories of development. Typically, these approaches draw on one or more perspectives in their attempt to account for the complex interplay of biologic and experiential/psychological factors that play a role as children grow and develop. These approaches vary in a number of respects. Some focus more on one aspect of development (emotional or cognitive), whereas others are more concerned with mechanisms (e.g., of learning). Although many early theories, like Freud's, were concerned with early development, subsequent work has often extended these theories to other aspects of the life cycle, for example, Erik Ericson was inspired by psychoanalytic theory and provided an overarching model for development from infancy to old age (see Table 1.1).

TABLE 1.1

Eric Erickson's Stages of Development

Stage of Development	Approximate Age Range	Brief Summary
Trust vs. Mistrust	0–18 months	Depending on task: with consistent caretaking environment, infant develops a sense of trust in the social world.
Autonomy vs. Shame and Doubt	18 months to 3 years	Young child develops a sense of their control and independence.
Initiative vs. Guilt	3–5 years	The child becomes more assertive and interactive in play and interaction.
Industry vs. Inferiority	5–12 years	Peers and the ability to work and learn become important.
Identity vs. Role Confusion	12–18 years	Major focus on development of sense of self and personal values
Intimacy vs. Isolation	18–40 years	Development of capacities for intimacy, family connectedness
Generativity vs. Stagnation	40–65 years	Nurturing of others and sense of contribution to others and society
Ego Integrity vs. Despair	65 years to death	Appreciation of personal accomplishments and sense of having led a successful life

An increased awareness of the complexity of both genetic and experiential mechanisms and their interaction has also clarified important issues in development. For example, genes may change in their function over time. Specific environmental factors may have more effects at some points than at others. For example, early exposure may predispose some children to develop allergic responses. Another complexity arises because some traits, behaviors, and features may reflect a stronger genetic or psychological component. Environmental factors, including both endogenous and exogenous, may contribute, in varying degrees, to development. The idea of experience-dependent plasticity has been used when there are strong effects of experience at certain points in development. A child deprived of vision early in life may later have trouble if sight is restored in coordinated use of the eyes and perception of depth and three dimensions. Finally, of course, development occurs in a family-societal context. The environment that children experience is itself partly shaped by the parents' experience and endowment.

All theories of development face several important challenges. How is the interplay between endowment (nature) and experience (nurture) to be understood? How and why does change happen? Is development continuous or discontinuous? For example, for a theorist like Piaget who proposes rather major changes in cognitive functioning over childhood, what accounts for these changes? Relating theories to age and normative expectations presents another challenge. Early studies of child development were initially concerned with documenting normative processes. It became possible to describe typical behavior of a 1-year-old simply by evoking age as an explanation. Given major changes and developmental accomplishments, it is typical for presentations on children's development to be constructed around intervals that are roughly age defined, for example, infancy, toddler, preschool, school age, and adolescence. Although understandable, this type of exposition tends to perpetuate the notion that somehow developmental change is caused by age alone. Over time, the field has moved from an initial focus on simple measures and age-related correlation to more sophisticated approaches. Although many broad theories of development have been postulated, a recent trend has been the focus on very specific aspects of development. In this chapter, we briefly summarize three major theories of development that have had a major impact on the field: psychoanalysis, Piaget's cognitive theory, and learning theory.

Psychoanalytic Theory

This approach to understanding children's development is based on the work of Sigmund Freud (Figure 1.6) and others. Trained as a neurologist but also with a strong interest in embryology and Darwinian thought, Freud actually developed several different, often overlapping, theories. His work includes a general theory attempting to understand the mind and behavior as well as mental illness. Although he only rarely worked with children, he had a strong interest in child development and had a profound influence on the development of early psychotherapeutic work with children and adults (see Chapter 28 and S. Freud, 1955 [originally published 1909]).

Freud's early work focused on distinctions between conscious and unconscious thinking and the impact of trauma in causing mental illness. His early work with women who had hysteria led him to assume, based on their reports, that trauma, particularly of a sexual nature, contributed to their difficulties. Although his subsequent theoretical model continued to emphasize the importance of sexual factors (including from very early in life), he became aware that the early reports could not be taken at face value and rather reflected the complicated interaction of wishes, cultural values and norms, and difficulties in coping with sexual thoughts, impulses, and feelings. His work led him to speculate that a significant contribution came from factors that were in the unconscious part of the mind. This, in turn, led him to think about other processes like dreams, slips of the tongue, and mistakes of various types as having psychological meaning. His theory developed a distinction between the conscious and unconscious mind, the latter being characterized by what he termed *primary process*, whose contents could be inferred from dreams, behavior, slips, and, eventually, through his method of treatment called "free association."

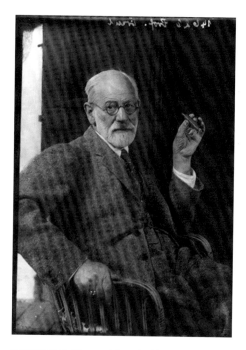

FIGURE 1.6. Sigmund Freud with cigar in a wicker chair, around 1929. © Sigmund Freud Foundation, Vienna. Photographer: Max Halberstadt.

Over the course of his professional work, Freud developed three different theories. The initial "topographic" model posited that the mind was divided into conscious, preconscious, and unconscious systems of thought. To put it another way, some things are easy for us to think about, others are deeply hidden, whereas some sit at the edge of being conscious. His growing interest in sexuality and gender identity led him to develop a model with a very developmental focus. He proposed this model in (1962/1905) in his book *Three Essays on the Theory of Sexuality*, where he described various phases of psychosexual development: an oral phase (from birth to early toddlerhood), an anal phase (roughly ages 2–4 or so), and oedipal phase (after the anal phase and up to about age 5). After the oedipal phase, he suggested there was a period of psychosexual latency (roughly school age) that lasted until puberty when sexual feelings strongly resurfaced. In his view, fixations (developmental arrests) could occur at these various phases and result in characteristic psychiatric problems.

Over time, he became increasingly concerned with understanding phenomena like depression, suicide, and the effects of trauma and his thinking began to include an emphasis on understanding aggressive as well as sexual feelings. As a result, he developed a second model in which he postulated the existence of an id, ego, and superego that coexisted, in some ways, with his first model. The id is presumed to be the place where basic impulses and instincts arise with little organization and outside immediate awareness, that is, largely unconscious. The ego is the part of the mind that develops as the infant struggles as they operate in the world and the basic impulses of the id must cope with the various reality constraints all of us experience. In contrast to the id (which operates on the pleasure principle), the ego operates based on the reality principle. In Freud's model, the superego is that part of the ego that develops a capacity for self-reflection and judgment. While the id is outside consciousness, both the ego and the superego have conscious as well as partly conscious aspects. He also focused on ways in which these structures coped with anxiety and the ways the mind defends against it.

One of the most famous of Freud's ideas was the importance of what he termed the *Oedipus complex* in children's development. This idea refers to the mechanisms, early in life, in which the child's sexual feelings for the opposite-sex parent become transformed into an identification with the same-sex parent resulting in a consolidation of gender identity formation.

In the final major revision of his theory, he proposed a model that included aggression and the death instinct. In some important ways, this last revision of his views reflected an awareness of the persistent nature of traumatic events for soldiers from World War I, which, in his earlier theories, ought to be forgetting (rather than remembering) the traumas they had experienced. This interest in trauma was carried forward by Freud's daughter, Anna, in her work with Londoners experiencing the blitz in World War II (A. Freud, 1946).

Although not directly treating children himself, Freud did publish some of the earliest work on childhood phobia (the treatment actually conducted by the child's father, see S. Freud, 1955 [originally published 1909]). After his death, Anna made important contributions to child development and more general psychoanalytic theory, particularly around understanding the work of the conscious mind and defense mechanism (A. Freud, 1936). This work was also carried on in the United States by a group of psychoanalysts who focused on what was termed *ego psychology*. Developmental considerations continued to be highly important theoretically and clinically.

Another prominent British psychoanalyst, Melanie Klein (1932), focused more on the interpersonal aspects of development and the ways a person developed representations of themselves or others. This approach, termed *object relations theory*, also is highly developmental but, if anything, moved critical issues and conflicts to very early in life. This model attracted a number of proponents in Great Britain and has been applied in the study of more severe psychiatric disturbances in children and adults. It focuses, in many ways, more on the final phase of Freud's model around issues of trauma and aggression.

Other aspects of psychoanalysis were incorporated in other theories including attachment theory, and many of the current "talking therapies" owe a great deal to Freud's attempt to understand human behavior and help patients struggling with psychiatric difficulties. Although classic psychoanalysis is now less common, an increasing body of work has attempted to clarify the situations in which it is useful. Cognitive behavior therapy (see Chapter 28) along with family interventions (see Chapter 30) also has important roots in the early developments of psychoanalytic theory and practice.

Freud's influence also had a profound impact on a number of students, some of whom developed their own approaches to understanding development. For example, Erik Erickson (1997) was a teacher enrolled in the Vienna Psychoanalytic Institute who relocated to Boston and then to New Haven. He was interested in understanding cultural influences on development and worked with children of the Sioux. After some years in California, he returned to Massachusetts to work at the Austin Riggs Center. He developed a lifetime model of development characterized by a series of stages not just limited to the first years of life. His approach focused around a series of tensions, for example, initially over trust versus mistrust. These are summarized in Table 1.1. Erikson also made major contributions to the growing field of ego psychology. His interest in cultural factors in a life-span approach was also reflected in a series of psychologically informed biographies of Martin Luther and Gandhi. His interest in continued development, particularly in adolescence, also contributed to renewed interest in clinical work with this age group. His work is probably underappreciated today, but it offers a very helpful life-span perspective on development noting the tensions inherent in each developmental period of life.

Piaget's Theory

In contrast to Freud, the Swiss psychologist Jean Piaget (1896–1980) (Figure 1.7) was more concerned with children's cognitive development. He had an early interest in teaching, worked briefly on the early tests of intelligence, and became intrigued by the issue of why children

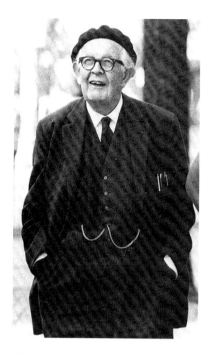

FIGURE 1.7. Photograph of Jean Piaget at the University of Michigan campus in Ann Arbor.

made certain kinds of mistakes. Eventually, Piaget (1932, 1952, 1955, 1962) developed a comprehensive model for cognitive development that was not, however, widely appreciated in the United States until the 1960s—in large part because his methods (direct discussion with children, including his own) were so antithetical to the research approach employed in American psychological research. In addition, he wrote in French and his language was somewhat difficult to translate. Despite the early lack of interest, his work has now become widely appreciated. (See Hunt, 1961 for a discussion.)

Piaget was interested in both the content and process of children's thinking and problem solving. Like Freud, he made various modifications to this theory over time. He discovered early on in his career, in talking with children, that over time they moved from a highly self-centered, egocentric world view to one that was much more able to appreciate other people and their views. His method started with a set of standard questions and he would then ask other questions, remaining very alert to the meaning of children's answers—including their mistakes, indeed finding those as intriguing as successes. He began his consideration of development by believing that the ways in which children think and learn are an important extension of biologic adaptation. He developed several key concepts regarding this process: assimilation, accommodation, and schemas.

A **schema** is a way of relating to the world, for example, an infant exploring an object with its mouth. In **assimilation**, the child uses an existing **schema**, for example, the baby that has been breast feeding discovers they can also suck their thumb. On the other hand, if the new experience, material, or event is so different that it cannot be assimilated, the child is then forced to **accommodate** or modify the schema. For example, if you are learning a new language, you initially will try to pronounce words using the patterns you are familiar with in your native language; if the new language has very different sounds, you will, over time, accommodate so that you can differentiate what was not heard before. Similarly, a child learning a new word like "horsey" may initially apply that label to all animals, but, over time, the concept will become refined and much more specific.

In Piaget's view, some of the early reflexive behaviors, like sucking, become modified over time by this process so that, for example, the infant moves away from exploring things with mouth, taste, and smell and more to visual inspection. It is important to emphasize that Piaget's theory is not simply one of innate maturation—rather he sees an active process depending on the individual child and their environment. As he considered children's development using this idea, and with a strong awareness of some of the unusual aspects of children's thinking, he developed a model with a series of progressive stages that elaborate the child's growing appreciation of reality and their increasingly sophisticated cognitive ability. Toward the end of his life, he also became interested in other processes like perception and memory.

The **sensorimotor period** lasts from birth to roughly 18–24 months of age. Initially, the infant has reflexes but behavior is poorly coordinated. The initial phase of this period (what Piaget termed the *stage of simple reflexes*) involves the baby's use of basic reflexes in relating to the world. As the process of assimilation and accommodation occur, the infant begins to coordinate processes; between the first and fourth months (roughly), the infant develops progressively more motor control and also is able to experience pleasure and can discover ways to maintain this, for example, by repeating an activity. This repetition is what Piaget termed a **primary circular reaction** (the name for this phase) (Piaget, 1952) and underscores the importance of both sensation and motor coordination at this point in development. This third stage (of **secondary circular reactions**) typically occurs between the fourth and eighth months. During this time, the infant becomes more oriented to the world and objects and may, for example, discover that shaking a rattle produces a noise and that this action can be repeated. This phase is followed by a period of **coordination of secondary circular reactions** (roughly 8 months to 1 year) when intentionality becomes more obvious. Behavior is now more goal directed, for example, use of a tool to get a desired object. At this time, objects start to acquire meaning and the child will search for objects that have vanished from sight (object permanence). As Piaget noted, this implies a capacity for symbolic thinking that, for humans, becomes critical for language and subsequent cognitive development. For the first time, the baby realizes things exist even if they are not visible. The fifth period is one of **active experimentation** on the part of the infant. During this phase (of what Piaget termed *tertiary circular reactions* roughly 12–18 months), there is a strong interest in new objects and a willingness to try new things. During the final phase of the sensorimotor period (internalization of schemas period roughly 18–24 months), symbolic thinking begins to dominate as mental representations begin to endure. The child now starts to develop a whole new way of viewing the world.

The **preoperational stage** (roughly ages 2–6 or 7 years) is heralded by this shift to more symbolic modes of thinking. During this time, the child is able to engage in verbal reasoning and the beginnings of make-believe play are observed. On the other hand, the child's view of the world continues to be constrained in some ways so that, for example, inanimate objects are believed to have feelings or life (animism). Similarly, the child's perception of life and death has to do with movement or whether something is alive (e.g., a potential complication in toileting if the child assumes that their feces are alive, only to see them flushed away!). Similarly, a fall over a toy may result in the child being angry at the toy for tripping them! Temporal or spatial relationships may be assumed to reflect some aspect of causality. Although the child has great capacities for symbolic thinking, these are not yet as flexible as they will be somewhat later. Animistic thinking is common, as Piaget noted children may exhibit animism in describing the movement of sun or moon.

During this time, language has an increasingly important role in mediating experience and the child's behavior and thought become more complex and less limited to concrete goals. During this time, however, thought remains limited in important ways. Perception tends to dominate and even here the child has difficulty if they need to attend to more than one perceptual dimension at a time. Thought remains very egocentric and the child has trouble differentiating thoughts/feelings and objective reality (one of the reasons dreams and nightmares at this period can be very frightening). Nonlogical relationships are assumed based on continuity in space or time rather than on cause and effect, and the child is relatively unconcerned about the inconsistencies that emerge from this point of view. This is also often reflected in children's drawing various parts of an object but being unaware of important interrelationships to produce a drawing that reflects a coherent, integrated view of the object.

These difficulties are also reflected in ways children at this age deal with concepts like numbers. If, for example, you arrange a row of candies in front of the child and then arrange a second row with exactly the same number of candies behind the first but make it longer, the 4-year-old may say that there are "more" candies in the longer row. Thus, the child focuses on the length of the row rather than number. Piaget termed this difficulty *static representation*. He also noted that thought remained egocentric at this age, for example, a child might use a made-up word not realizing that others would not understand it.

By around age 4 or so, another fundamental shift in cognitive development takes place. This stage of the preoperational period is often referred to as the *period of decentration*, when the child begins to increasingly see the world from the point of view of other people. This shift reflects increased cognitive and communicative capabilities and the increasing degree of social engagement with other children as well as with adults. The child discovers that their thoughts/feelings/reactions may not be the same as that of others. Although children continue, in some respects, to be constrained in their thinking, there is an increased accommodation to reality. Concepts of justice and moral development remain somewhat simplistic (immanent justice, an eye-for-an eye approach is favored) and the child cannot yet make allowances for special situations or instances where important rules can, and should, be violated. Perception continues to have major importance in the child's construction of reality. Often, the child can attend only to one aspect/dimension of a situation at a time. Similarly, although children are aware of familiar routines and sequences, temporal understanding remains limited. There can also be difficulties in differentiating fantasy/reality and the advent of more truly imaginative play contributes to a refinement of the child's thinking.

In the **Concrete Operational Phase** (roughly ages 7–11 or 12), thought becomes increasingly sophisticated but remains, in important ways, constrained by concrete reality (i.e., actual problems/issues rather than more hypothetical problems). During this time, children acquire several important abilities. They have a more detailed understanding of transitivity (e.g., if Jim is bigger than Sally and Sally is bigger than Pete, then Jim is bigger than Pete). Children at this age also become more able to understand important aspects of classification of objects, for example, sorting objects by and along any number of characteristic features. They also understand the reversibility, for example, of mathematical operations and can start to take into account multiple issues in solving a problem. They also have a firm knowledge of conservation—for example, changing the length of a piece of clay does not actually change its size. Socially, the increased ability to "decenter" gives the child strong social-cognitive capacities to anticipate based on other people's knowledge and to make predictions.

The period of **Formal Operations** (roughly ages 11–12 and up) is the final period of cognitive development in Piaget's view. The major difference from the previous phase is the ability to increasingly grasp abstract problems. Conclusions can be drawn logically without a need for actual demonstration. The child becomes capable of highly abstract thought and can see the world not only as it is but also how it might be (presumably accounting for much of the youthful ardor for change). The adolescent has an ability to solve hypothetical problems and no longer needs to rely on trial and error but can use deduction and hypothetical reasoning. The adolescent also has a more sophisticated approach to issues of judgment, issues of long-term planning, and increasingly sophisticated social skills. The adolescents' increased self-awareness can also result in increased self-consciousness, an awareness of their personal uniqueness, and self-awareness.

Piaget's account of development has been highly influential. Initial interest in his theory lagged, particularly in the United States, because his approach was so foreign to American developmental psychology. His work has had important implications for understanding many areas of development in addition to cognition. It has inspired several lines of work, for example, on moral development in children, that have become major areas of study in their own right and his work underscores, for health professionals dealing with children, the importance of considering the level of the child's understanding in dealing with clinical problems. This can be reflected in phenomena as diverse as the toddler's difficulties with toileting, children's understanding of death as an irreversible phenomenon, of seeing illness as a punishment for the child's transgressions, and even in adolescents for difficulties in dealing with chronic health problems.

Some important objections to aspects of Piaget's theory have also been raised. As he himself noted, the issue of how change/transition occurs from one stage to another remains an issue. His focus is very much on cognitive development with lesser emphasis on other areas and very little concern for emotional or sexual development, or, for that matter, for the role of family and culture. Other psychologists have advocated different approaches to children's understanding of domain-specific knowledge and for understanding language in development.

Learning Theory

This body of work has developed in a more collaborative way over the past century and is grounded in a large body of work on how children (and others) learn and remember. Starting with Pavlov's description of classical conditioning and then extended into many other types of learning, this approach became much more concerned with overt behavior rather than underlying, imputed psychological constructs. Although lacking in some ways the grand theoretical vision of Freud's or Piaget's body of work learning theory has great applicability, for example, in teaching children with learning problems like autism (Chapter 7) and, increasingly, in clinical psychology where cognitive behavior therapy (Chapter 28) relies heavily on learning-based approaches in treatment.

Learning theory focuses on overt behavior and its antecedents and consequences. This functional perspective helps us understand how behaviors are maintained over time and what factors in the environment contribute to behavior maintenance, and change.

Pavlov's study of classical conditioning represented the earliest approach to the scientific study of learning. In his model, a stimulus like food (unconditioned stimulus) that elicited a reflexive response like salivation in his dog (unconditioned response) was paired with a stimulus like the sound of a bell (conditioned stimulus) that otherwise would not elicit a response. But with repeated learning, the bell comes to elicit the response without a need for the unconditioned stimulus. It should be noted that, in this case, the association is new but the response itself, salivation, is not a new one. Pavlov's work was extended to clinical work (and children) by Jones and Watson (see Jones, 1924), who showed that this phenomenon could be used to account for phobia. They, and others subsequently, have noted that the avoidance behavior induced by a phobia prevents extinction from occurring, thus helping the maintenance of the phobia.

Classical conditioning has also been used in models of other conditions like depression and mood problems, addictive phenomena, and psychosomatic problems. Therapy methods based on aspects of classical conditioning include desensitization, exposure training, and counter conditioning among others (see Chapter 28). Operant conditioning focuses on acquisition of new behaviors and relies heavily on the work of B. F. Skinner, whose work elegantly demonstrated how new behaviors could be acquired and shaped through the use of systematic reinforcement. The fundamental notion is straightforward in that responses are shaped by consequences. Positive reinforcement is any consequence that is rewarding whereas negative reinforcement involves the removal of a negative experience, although punishment is some consequence that decreases the probability of a behavior. Skinner's work (e.g., Skinner, 1953) and that of many others have also shown the importance of the timing or "schedule" of reinforcement. It can, for example be continuous (every time a button is pressed, a reward is dispensed) or intermittent (e.g., every third time the button is pressed, the happy event happens). Variable reinforcement is particularly effective (the reason students check their mailbox so much!). The timing of the reinforcement can also be systematically varied. Often in initially producing or "shaping" a behavior, more frequent reinforcement is used but, over time, is shifted to a variable model—the latter being particularly effective in maintaining behavior.

Similar principles apply to the elimination of a behavior (extinction). For extinction to occur, a previous reinforcement is withheld or decreased (often, this is initially associated with an early increase in the behavior, a phenomenon called "extinction burst"). Elimination of a problem behavior also may be facilitated by simultaneous work on the acquisition (and systematic reinforcement of) a new behavior—sometimes one incompatible with the problem behavior. Other work conducted within the learning theory perspective has focused on observational learning (e.g., the ability of children to learn simply through observation) as well as on aversive conditioning. In actual work with patients, therapy using behavioral principles focuses on a careful analysis of the entire behavior and its antecedents and consequences. A number of treatment approaches are available including applied behavior analysis and parent management training (see Kazdin, 2000).

METHODS OF RESEARCH

As a field, developmental psychopathology has drawn on multiple sources of information and the perspectives of many different disciplines in its attempt to understand children's development and psychopathology (see Chapter 2). Although integrating these diverse perspectives sometimes presents practical challenges, it also has stimulated considerable interdisciplinary and cross-disciplinary work that adds to the intellectual excitement of work in this field. Over the past several decades, research accomplishments in a number of different areas have translated into innovations in treatments and advanced our knowledge base. In the concluding section of this chapter, we highlight some of this work; the reading list at the end of the chapter provides resources for readers seeking additional information.

Advances in statistical methods and epidemiologic research have been made on several fronts. Solid normative data continues to help frame the broad (and sometimes narrow) range of normative development and contribute to better measure of maladaptive behaviors and psychiatric disorders. This work has helped clarify the role of risk factors and their significance in child psychopathology. At the global level, such surveys have also drawn attention to the focus on global aspects of child mental health problems. These data are important in terms of service planning and, sadly, often underscore the unavailability of appropriate supports and the need for new models of care. Epidemiologic data also have underscored the frequent onset of adult disorders in childhood or adolescence. Epidemiologic work is also strongly related to advances in measurement, assessment, and statistics, for example, with development of more reliable and valid screeners and assessment instruments (Fombonne, 2018).

Statistical approaches have also become much more sophisticated with advances that allow for more rigorous experimental control and examination of new models of statistical analysis. The increased sophistication of epidemiologic and statistical methods has also been reflected in the growing body of work on evidence-based treatments (Hamilton, 2007). For child psychiatry, this is a particular challenge because research data may be sparse, different informants (child, parent, and teacher) may have different views, and results from the many different research traditions may not always fit easily in the more traditional model of evidence-based medicine. Despite these concerns, this is a clearly growing body of expertise (see Chapter 2) and will have increasing importance in the coming decade.

Neurobiologic work has also drawn on multiple disciplines and research traditions including genetics, neuroimaging, neurochemistry, and other branches of neuroscience. Within genetics, it has become increasingly clear that multiple genes interact with environmental factors and, possibly, epigenetic influences in the expression of clinical disorder (Stevens et al., 2018). This makes the identification of disease-related genes somewhat difficult. Accordingly, a number of strategies have been utilized including linkage, association, and molecular cytogenetic approaches. These have used both common and rare variation approaches. Particularly over the last several years, significant progress in the identification of risk alleles has been made, for example, for Tourette's disorder (Chapter 16) and autism (Chapter 7). Advances in genetic technology and the increased availability of large, well-characterized samples likely will only accelerate the productivity of this work. The potential for exploring ways in which genes can be expressed in the brains and behavior (e.g., in animal models) is also very helpful in fostering our understanding of specific mechanisms of gene-brain-behavior interactions (Stevens et al., 2018). Although the possibility of gene therapy remains in the future, advances in our genetic understanding, particularly for the single-gene disorders, make this no longer seem impossible.

Advances in neurobiology and psychopharmacology have helped expand our understanding of brain mechanisms and now hold the promise of better and more effective targeted treatments. These advances have been, in part, based on the knowledge gained in genetics, particularly (at least so far) for the single-gene disorders like Rett's and Fragile x syndrome. But now, and certainly in the future, this understanding may be extended to the more complex disorders like autism, mood and anxiety, and attention deficit disorders. Work in this area has moved in several directions. One line has focused on neuronal circuitry, neural transmission, and intracellular signaling. Both the short- and long-term effects of pharmacologic intervention on brain function and structures remind us of the complex ways in which various factors interact relative to pathogenesis of disorders.

Although it has faced some significant challenges, pediatric neuroimaging work has also blossomed over the past decade. The practical challenges include, particularly for functional imaging methods, the difficulties that even normal children have in remaining still—difficulties that become much more formidable when the child's neurodevelopmental problems entail difficulties in attention, engagement, and activity level. A body of work on approaches to coping with these problems through teaching, desensitization, and advance preparation has yielded impressive results in terms of our ability to engage children in a range of scanning procedures. For very young children, scanning during sleep is another possibility. Other challenges come with the understandable limitations that research design and ethics raise, for example, for PET scanning in children given that radiation is involved in contrast to MRI or fMRI. Still others come from the potential methodologic and conceptual issues that complicate the interpretation of imaging data that typically tell us more about macroscopic brain structure and activity rather than finer structures.

In neuroimaging, one major challenge arises with regard to distinguishing cause from aftereffect, that is, presumably chronic illness itself leads to brain adaptation and change. This is a particular issue when cross-sectional designs are employed and such studies are among the most common. Thus, larger volume of a specific brain region might represent compensation effects. To some extent, this issue can be dealt with by including analyses of other measures, for example, symptom severity. Developmental issues are also important, making longitudinal studies particularly relevant. Finally, the frequent comorbidity of disorders (see Chapter 4) also presents specific challenges for neuroimaging and other studies

References

*Indicates Particularly Recommended

*Boswell, J. (1989). *Kindness of strangers*. University of Chicago Press.
*Candland, D. K. (1993). *Feral children and clever animals: Reflections on human nature*. Oxford University Press.
Darwin, C. (1859). *On the origin of species by means of natural selection*. John Murray.
Darwin, C. (1871). *The expression of the emotions in man and animals*. John Murray.
Darwin, C. (1877). A biographical sketch of an infant. *Mind*, 2(7), 285–294. https://doi.org/10.1093/mind/os-2.7.285
Erikson, E. (1997). *The life cycle completed*. W. W. Norton & Co.
Fombonne, E. (2018). Epidemiology. In A. Martin, M. Bloch, & F. R. Volkmar (Eds.), *Lewis's child and adolescent psychiatry: A comprehensive textbook* (5th ed., pp. 205–225). Wolters Kluwer.
Freud, A. (1936). *The ego and the mechanisms of defense* (Vol. II). International Universities Press, Inc.
Freud, A. (1946). *The psycho-analytic treatment of children*. Imago Publishing.
Freud, S. (1955). Analysis of a phobia in a five-year-old boy. In J. E. Strachey (Ed.), *The standard edition of the complete psychological works of Sigmund Freud* (Vol. X, pp. 3–149). Hogarth Press.

Freud, S. (1962). *Three essays on the theory of sexuality.* Basic Books. Strachey, J. (Trans.). (1996). *Drei abhandlungen zur sexualtheorie.* Fischer. [Reprint of the 1905 edition.]

Gesell, A., Thompson, H., & Amatruda, C. S. (1938). *The psychology of early growth.* The Macmillan Company.

Gould, S. J. (1996). *The mismeasure of man.* W. W. Norton & Co.

Hamilton, J. (2007). Evidence-based practice as a conceptual framework. In A. Martin & F. R. Volkmar (Eds.), *Lewis's child and adolescent psychiatry: A comprehensive textbook* (4th ed., pp. 124–139). Lippincott Williams & Wilkins.

Hunt, J. M. (1961). *Intelligence and experience.* The Ronald Press.

Jones, M. C. (1924). A laboratory study of fear: The case of Peter. *Pedagogical Seminary, 31,* 308–315. https://doi.org/10.1080/08856559.1924.9944851

Kanner, L. (1935). *Child psychiatry.* Charles C. Thomas.

Klein, M. (1932). *The psychoanalysis of children.* Hogarth Press.

Piaget, J. (1932). *The moral judgment of the child.* Kegan Paul, Trench.

Piaget, J. (1952). *The origins of intelligence in children.* International University Press. (Original work published 1936.)

Piaget, J. (1955). *The child's construction of reality.* Routledge and Kegan Paul.

Piaget, J. (1962). *Play, dreams and imitation in childhood.* W. W. Norton & Co.

Skinner, B. F. (1953). *Science and human behavior.* Simon and Shuster.

Stevens, H., Leckman, J., Lombrosso, P., & Vaccarino, F. M. (2018). From genes to brain: Developmental neurobiology. In A. Martin, M. Bloch, & F. R. Volkmar (Eds.), *Lewis's child and adolescent psychiatry: A comprehensive textbook* (5th ed., p. 247). Wolters Kluwer.

Volk, A. A., & Atkinson, J. A. (2013). Infant and child death in the human environment of evolutionary adaptation. *Evolution and Human Behavior, 34*(3), 182–192. https://doi.org/10.1016/j.evolhumbehav.2012.11.007

Suggested Readings

Doroshow, D. B. (2018). A history of child psychiatry. In A. Martin, M. Bloch, & F. R. Volkmar (Eds.), *Lewis's child and adolescent psychiatry: A comprehensive textbook* (5th ed., pp. 21–25). Wolters Kluwer.

Fernandez, T., & State, M. W. (2007). Assessing risk: Gene discovery. In A. Martin, M. Bloch, & F. R. Volkmar (Eds.), *Lewis's child and adolescent psychiatry: A comprehensive textbook* (5th ed., pp. 189–199). Lippincott Williams & Wilkins.

Fombonne, E. (2018). Epidemiology. In A. Martin, M. Bloch, & F. R. Volkmar (Eds.), *Lewis's child and adolescent psychiatry: A comprehensive textbook* (5th ed., pp. 205–225). Wolters Kluwer.

Hale, N. G. (1971). *Freud and the Americans: The beginning of psychoanalysis in the United States, 1876–1917.* Oxford University Press.

Hamilton, J. (2007). Evidence-based practice as a conceptual framework. In A. Martin & F. R. Volkmar (Eds.), *Lewis's child and adolescent psychiatry: A comprehensive textbook* (4th ed., pp. 124–139). Lippincott Williams & Wilkins.

Hogan, J. D. (2000). Developmental psychology: History of the field. *Encyclopedia of Psychology, 3,* 9–13. https://doi.org/10.1037/10518-003

Kazdin, A. E. (2000). Developing a research agenda for child and adolescent psychotherapy. *Archive of General Psychiatry, 57,* 829–835. https://doi.org/10.1001/archpsyc.57.9.829

Lombroso, P. J., & Leckman, J. F. (2007). Molecular basis of select childhood psychiatric disorders. In A. Martin & F. R. Volkmar (Eds.), *Lewis's child and adolescent psychiatry: A comprehensive textbook* (4th ed., pp. 200–213). Lippincott Williams & Wilkins.

Musto, D. F. (2007). Prevailing and shifting paradigms: A historical perspective. In A. Martin & F. R. Volkmar (Eds.), *Lewis's child and adolescent psychiatry: A comprehensive textbook* (4th ed., pp. 11–16). Lippincott Williams & Wilkins.

Robbins, S. J., Schwartz, B., & Wasserman, E. A. (2001). *Psychology of learning and behavior* (5th ed.). W. W. Norton & Co.

Sears, R. R. (1975). *Your ancients revisited: A history of child development.* University of Chicago Press.

Singer, D. G., & Revenson, T. A. (1996). *A Piaget primer: How a child thinks* (rev ed.). Plume (Penguin Books).

Strachey, J. (1965/1933). *Introductory lectures on psycho-analysis.* W. W. Norton & Co.

The MRI Unit at Columbia University and New York State Psychiatric Institute. (2007). *Neuroimaging methods in the study of childhood psychiatric disorders.* Author.

Volkmar, F. R. (2005). Charles Darwin (1809–1882). *American Journal of Psychiatry, 162,* 249.

CHAPTER 2 ■ PERSPECTIVES FROM TYPICAL CHILD DEVELOPMENT

■ INTRODUCTION

Development occurs throughout the life cycle, and although we frequently focus on some particular aspect of development (cognitive, motor, and so on), in reality developmental processes are fundamentally interrelated. The term *maturation* is often used to describe the sequential pattern of growth but both experience (nurture) and endowment (nature) interact in complex ways. As described in Chapter 1, various approaches, methods, and theories have been used to understand development. For many investigators, the development of the embryo and fetus has served as a model for subsequent development with the various processes interacting reciprocally. One of the observations consistent with this view is the awareness that early development of motor skills move in top-down (cephalocaudal or head to toe) and center-out (proximodistal) fashion so that, for example, head control is achieved before trunk control before leg control and arm control is achieved before hand control.

Clearly, while the human genome gives considerable developmental potential, it also sets certain limits. Depending on the particular skill being studied, the relative dominance of genetic or experiential factors may shift so that even if a baby has good genetic potential its placement in a severely depriving environment will result in developmental delays; conversely, a child born having suffered the effects of some insult in utero such as fetal alcohol exposure may not be able to achieve normative levels of functioning no matter what environment is provided, although even here, high optimal development would be more likely in a supportive environment. It is appropriate to begin any consideration of development with a discussion of development prior to birth.

■ PRENATAL DEVELOPMENT

Development starts at conception as the zygote begins to develop actively once the egg is fertilized. Within a few days, it will have reached the uterus and implanted and may be 0.1 inches in length. Within 2 weeks, the menstrual period may be missed and may alert the mother to the pregnancy. Over the next 6 weeks, major organs and structures develop primarily following the cephalocaudal and proximodistal pattern. By about 8 weeks, the embryo is recognizably human. After this time, the fetus grows rapidly with increased differentiation. The head initially grows more actively than other parts of the body and gradually slows during fetal life, so that at birth the head is about one fourth the length of the entire body but in adulthood only about one sixth. Conversely, at birth the legs are about one third of body length, but this increases to half by adulthood.

By about the third month in utero, the fetus can swallow, make a fist, and wiggle its toes; by the fourth month, it can respond to light; and by the fifth month, loud sounds may elicit movement. Similarly, more organized behaviors, like the sucking reflex develop before birth; this is also a time when the processes like breathing, body temperature regulation, and swallowing are sufficiently organized to make life possible outside the uterus. By around 8 months, fetal fat stores accumulate rapidly. Antibodies from the mother help prevent infection postpartum.

Even before the child is born, parents begin to experience the child and are impacted by it. This happens in various ways. For the mother, the experience of fetal movement ("quickening") provokes a series of responses as the mother observes that the child may be soothed by her speech or movement. Similarly, the mother's impact on the child begins as soon as fertilization has occurred. Although intrauterine life is relatively homeostatic, it can be influenced by the mother's health (both physical and psychological) as well as by other factors. Mothers typically gain 25–30 pounds and this weight gain is important for fetal growth; mothers who do not gain appropriate weight or who are undernourished may increase the likelihood that their baby will be small. Other factors that may adversely impact the development of the child in utero include exposure to radiation, maternal infection, or exposure to drugs.

The effects of teratogens depend on several factors. These include the timing of the exposure (e.g., in some cases, these may even antedate the pregnancy). Timing of exposure and the dose also are important depending on the agent. The route of the teratogen may also be important. The effects of teratogens can be more generalized or more specific; for example, thalidomide exposure is associated with limb defects whereas alcohol exposure in utero produces a range of problems.

The adverse effects of alcohol on the developing fetus have been recognized since ancient times. Although reports on potential adverse effects on the fetus began to appear in medical literature in the 1700s, Jones and Smith in 1973 brought new attention to the significant teratogenic effects of alcohol exposure in utero. Fetal alcohol syndrome (FAS) is associated with growth deficiency, usually mild intellectual deficiency, a characteristic "flattened" face, motor problems, and other morphologic features. A number of learning difficulties are noted as are language difficulties and continued growth problems. In the United States, alcohol continues to be the most frequently used teratogen and is one of the more common causes of intellectual deficiency. Chronic alcohol abuse is associated with greater risk, and, unfortunately, mothers who drink are also likely to smoke and the latter is also a risk factor. Stopping smoking at any point in the pregnancy is beneficial but is particularly so in the first trimester. Similarly, the potentially adverse role of prescription and street drugs has been recognized. The effects of these agents vary. Phenytoin is associated with increased risk for heart defects whereas tetracycline can cause staining of teeth and interfere with bone growth. Use of drugs like cocaine is associated with increased newborn irritability and sometimes with growth retardation. Agents like heroin and methadone can result in a withdrawal syndrome in the infant.

Maternal infections can be associated with various adverse effects. Congenital rubella can lead to severe mental retardation, visual and sensory problems, as well as cardiac difficulties. AIDS is associated with a number of congenital malformations, although, fortunately, work on prevention has advanced dramatically in the more developed countries. Similarly cytomegalovirus (CMV) and toxoplasmosis may be associated with significant learning difficulties, intellectual deficiency, and a range of other problems.

Heavy metals and other environmental toxins can have teratogenic effects as can exposure to radiation. Other risks arise with both very young (teenage) or comparatively older (>35) maternal age. For older mothers, the risk for Down syndrome begins to increase substantially. Similarly, malnutrition in the mother can be associated with growth retardation and behavioral difficulties in the newborn. Other maternal health issues, for example, diabetes, can be associated with risk to the developing child.

Perinatal Variables

Prematurity is an important risk factor for subsequent developmental problems. Premature infants also present challenges for parenting and are more likely to be abused or neglected. Both preterm babies (born before the 37th week of pregnancy) and low birth weight babies (born at or near term but who are small for gestational age) have increased risk. Although babies born as early as 24 weeks now survive, lack of development of important organ systems, particularly the respiratory system, presents major challenges. Although strides have been made in supporting preterm infants, prevention continues to be a significant public health challenge.

Premature preterm infants are at increased risk for various problems including neurologic problems, retinopathy, and developmental disabilities. Cardiovascular and respiratory problems are also common. Risks increase with the degree of prematurity. Even when babies are born on time, as many as 3% of all infants exhibit significant malformations or birth defects whereas another 7% or so may exhibit less serious problems. Babies born with severe developmental difficulties often have difficulties that started even before the labor and delivery, although sometimes a traumatic birth can result in major neurologic damage.

Parents of a premature baby or one with a birth defect face a challenge. All parents worry about their baby prior to birth but the experience of having a baby with a problem can bring up a host of unpleasant feelings—anger, anxiety, even guilt. The sense of loss of the anticipated, perfect, baby can be a shock and a source of depression. The child's continued presence serves as a constant reminder of this. Reactions of the parents are a function of their own histories and personality as well as the visibility and location of the birth defect.

Responses of Parents and Family of the Newborn

Various factors shape the parents' attitudes toward the fetus and neonate. The first is their relationships with their own parents. There are several views of the ways pregnancy is experienced; these range from the idea that pregnancy is inherently a crisis to the other extreme that views pregnancy as a normal part of development. With advances in technology, mothers (and often fathers) are aware of the pregnancy at a very early stage. Often, the first picture of the fetus during ultrasound concretizes this knowledge for both parents. Fathers sometimes experience some of the symptoms of pregnancy along with their partners (in some cultures fathers may experience feelings at the time of childbirth—couvade syndrome). Some fathers will sense, and resent, the preoccupation of the mother with the pregnancy. As with mothers, the fathers' experience of being parented can play a major role, although even fathers who have had difficult parental experiences can be loving and affectionate fathers. Sometimes, prospective fathers become more anxious, for example, owing to a sense of greater responsibility or unresolved issues with their parents. Sometimes, the couple's expectations of each other are changed by the pregnancy.

In addition to the parents, other members of the family also play important roles. Around the world, probably the bulk of child rearing (apart from breastfeeding) is done by other children—usually siblings. In developed countries, grandparents, aunts, and uncles often play a major role. Parents may find this helpful or intrusive. Preparation of the sibling for the arrival of a new brother or sister varies depending on the child's age. Significant sibling conflict/rivalry is more likely in the context of a problematic parent–child relationship particularly because the mother's attention to the older child decreases.

■ INFANCY AND TODDLERHOOD

In the first weeks after birth, infants quickly become active in learning about the world. They begin to explore the environment through multiple modalities, can track moving objects, screen out irrelevant stimuli, and become active players in the "social game." For the typically developing infant, the face/voice of the parent is the most engaging thing in the environment and this early social interest sets the stage for many subsequent skills in multiple areas. Tables 2.1 and 2.2 summarize some of the landmarks of development in the first year of life.

After about 1 month of age, the infant's ability to engage in voluntary motor movement begins to increase. The infant also begins to produce more sounds and becomes increasingly differentiated in their affective responses. Between 2 and 7 months, there is increased social interaction along with an increased awareness of the nonsocial world and greater coordination of sensation and motor action. By about 4 months, imitation becomes more striking (and further consolidates social interest and attachment). Shortly thereafter, the earliest aspects of object permanence are seen so that things exist to the baby even when not visible; at around this time, the infant's awareness of cause–effect relationships also increases (see Chapter 1 for a discussion of Piaget's model of cognitive development in infancy). Both discoveries are important building blocks in social–cognitive development, that is, as the infant appreciates its own ability to impact the world and the stability of people in that world. Object permanence

TABLE 2.1

Selected Social, Communicative, and Cognitive Milestones: Birth to 1 Year of Age

Age (weeks)	Social-Affective	Communicative	Cognitive-Adaptive
0–4	Looks at face of caregiver	Makes small, throaty noises	Responds to sounds
4–8	Social smile	Babbles spontaneously	Facial response to sounds
8–12	Recognizes mother visually	Single vowels	Glances at rattle in hand
12–16	Smiles at mirror image	Coos or chuckles	Anticipatory excitement
16–20	Aware of novel situations	Laughs, vocalizes excitement	Takes rattle to mouth
20–24	Shows displeasure over loss of toy	Spontaneous social vocalization	Visual pursuit of dropped object
24–28	Plays simple interaction games	Attends to music or singing	Bangs objects on tabletop
28–32	Shows anxiety to strangers	Makes polysyllabic vowel sounds	Shakes rattle
32–36	Imitates simple adult movements	Says single syllables ("da," "ba," "ka")	Plays with two toys at the same time
36–40	Waves bye-bye	Says "dada," "mama" (nonspecific)	Uncovers toy hidden by cloth
40–44	Inhibits activity on command	Says "dada," "mama" (specific)	Combines toys in play
44–48	"Gives" toy to mirror image	Says one word besides "mama" and "dada"	Preference for certain toys over others
48–52	Initiates games with adult	Says two words beside "mama" and "dada"	Uses crayon to "dot" imitatively

Adapted with permission from Volkmar, F. R. (1995). Normal development. In H. Kaplan & B. Sadock (Eds.), *Comprehensive textbook of psychiatry* (6th ed., Vol. 2, pp. 2154–2160). Williams & Wilkins.

TABLE 2.2

Selected Motor and Self-Care Milestones: Birth to 1 Year of Age

Age (weeks)	Motor	Personal and Self-Care
0–4	Asymmetric posture	Quiets when picked up
4–8	Sometimes holds head erect	Reacts to feeding position
8–12	Rolls partway to side	Anticipates lifting
12–16	Actively holds rattle	Regards own hand
16–20	Hands engage in midline	Anticipates feeding on sight
20–24	Holds head erect and steady	Pats or fingers bottle or breast
24–28	Rolls to prone position	Drinks from cup with assistance
28–32	Transfers objects between hands	Holds objects voluntarily
32–36	Pivots while in prone position	Feeds self cracker or cookie
36–40	Sits alone with no support	Responds to "pick up" gesture
40–44	Uses index finger to secure object	Cooperates in social games
44–48	Rolls ball while sitting	Gives toy to others without release
48–52	Takes two steps independently	Releases toys to others

Adapted with permission from Volkmar, F. R. (1995). Normal development. In H. Kaplan & B. Sadock (Eds.), *Comprehensive textbook of psychiatry* (6th ed., Vol. 2, pp. 2154–2160). Williams & Wilkins.

is an important foundation for symbolic thinking and language development and the appreciation of cause–effect helps the infant gain a new appreciation of intentionality. Socially, these skills are reflected in games like peek-a-boo.

Between 7 and 9 months, the infant develops an awareness that they can be understood by others, that is, that the mother or father can understand their feelings, wishes, and desires (a phenomenon termed *intersubjectivity*). The infant's behavior also becomes more goal directed. Around this time, the infant develops more sophisticated strategies for obtaining desired ends by grouping behaviors together in a sequence. These phenomena also serve as a basis for communicative gesturing, for example, pointing at or reaching for an object while looking at the mother/father to request help in getting it. Advances in object permanence and in social skills development also help infants develop a strong sense of attachment to their caregiver (Box 2.1). This is expressed in various ways including phenomena like separation anxiety (often starting between 6 and 8 months and peaking sometime after the first birthday) and in the related phenomenon of stranger anxiety (often beginning around 8 months and peaking around age 12–18 months). Both phenomena speak to the infant's strong awareness of essential caregivers and the ability to differentiate them from strangers.

Several new milestones are usually achieved by, or shortly after, the first birthday and mark major changes in the life of the infant and family. Motor and motor coordination skills advance (see Table 2.1) such that typically by about 12 months the infant begins to be able to walk independently. Similarly, with the onset of language (usually also around this time) and greater symbolic capacities, the infant is able to hold multiple bits of information in mind and is able to appreciate new ways to solve problems by trial and error. Important foundations for language are well established by 1 year of age and include the ability to engage in reciprocal interaction, differentiated babbling, and use of sounds and intonation (prosody) typical of their native tongue. Once language acquisition starts, knowledge of words usually dramatically increases (Figures 2.1 and 2.2). Usually by age 2, the toddler's expressive vocabulary is between 50 and 75 words and increases over the next several months so that

BOX 2.1   Attachment

Although the importance of emotional connections between infants and caregivers has been known (and discussed) for centuries, only starting in the 20th century was much attention paid to the centrality of these connections for normal child development. The idea of attachment (in the sense of psychological connectedness) has come to encompass many aspects of this process. Psychological attachment is the emotional connection one person has to another (over space and time). Attachments are very specific and can be of varying degrees of strength and typically are strongly positive.

From the first moments of life, the adult and infant embark on an emotionally intense social interaction that has strong biologic and psychological aspects. In some animals (birds and mammals), particularly those that can move and walk shortly after birth, the phenomenon of "imprinting" is observed (i.e., the young animal begins to follow around the apparent parental object, whether it is a mother goose or an ethologist such as Konrad Lorenz). For other species (including humans) in which a long period of care is required before the young can move away independently, a complex series of processes occurs and is referred to by the concept of attachment.

The awareness of this phenomenon in infants came through many individuals, but particularly the British psychiatrist and psychoanalyst John Bowlby, who noted the major difficulties children had when separated from their parents because of the child's illness. He was aware of the many emerging studies on the negative effects of inappropriate early care (e.g., as in orphanages) and was not satisfied with earlier psychoanalytic views of parent–child relationships. In a very influential monograph for the World Health Organization, Bowlby suggested the critical importance of a supportive mother–child relationship, and his work and that of his student and colleague, Mary Ainsworth, stimulated considerable research on the topic over the next decades. Bowlby's work extended into many areas, including ethology, developmental psychology, and evolutionary biology (among others). Workers such as Harry Harlow demonstrated the importance of a soft, cloth mother substitute for developing rhesus monkeys, and Ainsworth developed a specific psychological paradigm (the "strange situation") that involved brief separations of young children and their mothers and observations of reunion behavior to estimate the quality of the attachment present. Bowlby's work and that of others led to closing congregate care settings for young children in the developed world.

Attachment processes are strongly developmental but are also lifelong. Various patterns of attachments in infants and toddlers have been identified along with many of the behavioral and developmental correlates of this process. Attachment can be disrupted by various factors, including a lack of an appropriate parent or parent substitute or unavailability of the parent (e.g., because of severe maternal depression). Children who have been abused may still form attachments, although the quality of the attachment may be unusual.

Reprinted with permission from Volkmar, F. R., & Martin, A. (2011). *Essentials of Lewis's child and adolescent psychiatry* (1st ed., p. 18). Lippincott Williams & Wilkins/Wolters Kluwer.

by age 3, it is between 500 and 1000 words. By this age, the typical toddler will also be using sentences of three to four words. Increased ability to use language and think symbolically give the potential for advance planning rather than trial and error.

The increased ability to use symbols also makes for a major reorganization of cognitive development after 18 months as Piaget realized. Increased cognitive abilities are also reflected

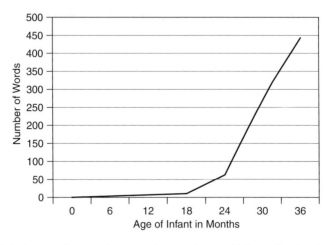

FIGURE 2.1. Typical rate of increase in expressive vocabulary of infants. Reprinted with permission from Mayes, L., Gilliam, W., & Sosinsky, L. (2007). The infant and toddler. In A. Martin & F. R. Volkmar (Eds.), *Lewis's child and adolescent psychiatry: A comprehensive textbook* (4th ed., p. 258). Lippincott Williams & Wilkins.

in phenomena like deferred (i.e., remembered) imitation. The young child begins to use symbols in play, and play begins to shift from simple functional use of materials to more abstract levels.

Various problems can negatively impact normative development. These are summarized in Table 2.3 and include problems in self-regulation (eating, sleeping, impulse control, aggression, and mood/anxiety difficulties). Given the centrality of social factors in early development, disturbances in relatedness are particularly important; these can arise as a result of environmental stress, deprivation, or with disorders like autism. Maternal/parental deprivation can arise because of problems in the parent or life circumstances. Risks arise owing to repeated changes in the primary caregiver as well as owing to abuse and neglect (see Chapter 24). The intersection of mental health and physical problems can be seen most dramatically at this age and disentangling cause–effect and relationship–individual issues can be difficult.

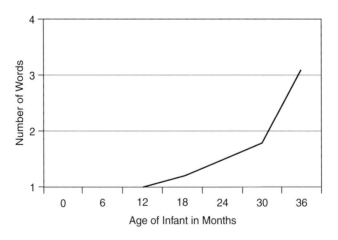

FIGURE 2.2. Typical rate of increase in number of words per sentence in infants. Reprinted with permission from Mayes, L., Gilliam, W., & Sosinsky, L. (2007). The infant and toddler. In A. Martin & F. R. Volkmar (Eds.), *Lewis's child and adolescent psychiatry: A comprehensive textbook* (4th ed., p. 258). Lippincott Williams & Wilkins.

TABLE 2.3

Forces That May Compromise Normative Developmental Processes

1. Regulatory Disturbances
   A. Sleep disturbances (frequent waking)
   B. Excessive crying or irritability
   C. Eating difficulties (finicky eating or food refusal)
   D. Low frustration tolerance
   E. Self-stimulatory/unusual movements (rocking, head banging, excessive finger sucking)
2. Social/Environmental Disturbances
   A. Failure to discriminate caregiver
   B. Apathetic, withdrawn, no expression of affect or interest in social interaction
   C. Excessive negativism
   D. No interest in objects or play
   E. Abuse, neglect, or multiple placements or caregivers
   F. Repeated or prolonged separations from caregivers
3. Psychophysiologic Disturbances
   A. Nonorganic failure to thrive
   B. Recurrent vomiting or chronic diarrhea
   C. Recurrent dermatitis
   D. Recurrent wheezing
4. Developmental Delays
   A. Specific delays (gross motor, language)
   B. General delays or arrested development
5. Genetic and Metabolic Disorders with Known Neurodevelopmental Sequelae
   A. Down syndrome
   B. Fragile X syndrome
   C. Inborn errors of metabolism
6. Exposure to Toxins
   A. Fetal alcohol syndrome
   B. Lead poisoning
7. Central Nervous System Damage
   A. Traumatic brain injuries
   B. Intraventricular hemorrhages
8. Prematurity and Serious Illnesses Early in Life

Reprinted with permission from Mayes, L., Gilliam, W., & Stout, L. (2018). The infant and toddler. In A. Martin, M. Block, & F. R. Volkmar (Eds.), *Lewis's child and adolescent psychiatry: A comprehensive textbook* (5th ed., p. 76). Wolters Kluwer.

Developmental delays can occur in isolation or across multiple areas. Problems in some areas, for example, language, may be reflected in other areas as well. Risk is increased by factors like prematurity and parental substance abuse or nonavailability. Various models of early intervention have been developed and can be helpful. Typically, mild cognitive delays are not noted until later, but more severe delays, often associated with specific genetic and metabolic disorders, can be seen. These include conditions like Down syndrome, fragile X syndrome, Prader–Willi syndrome, and so on.

THE PRESCHOOL PERIOD

As emphasized by Piaget (see Chapter 1), major changes in cognitive, communicative, and social-affective development occur between 2 and 5 years of age. The nature of language and thinking changes dramatically. These capacities are intrinsically and fundamentally interrelated so that greater cognitive capacities are reflected in new and more complex language as well as in increasingly sophisticated and nuanced social relationships. Children become more capable of understanding, and reflecting on, their own feelings and responses and can be highly verbal in indicating their wants and desires. They become much more active participants in dialogue with parents and caregivers making their thoughts, wishes, feelings, and opinions clear.

The preschool period is also a time when exposure to children other than siblings often occurs, for example, in childcare or early preschool programs. This is also a time when siblings are commonly born. Frequent behavioral–developmental difficulties in this age group can include problems with peers (particularly if the child is aggressive), anxiety problems (often around separation), and developmental delays of all types (but particularly speech–language delays). An increased awareness of the earliest manifestations of problems that come to later be diagnosed as disorders (e.g., anxiety and mood problems) has stimulated interest in the diagnosis and epidemiology of developmental and mental health problems in this age group (Egger, 2009). At the same time, there is also awareness of the potential for short- (or longer) term stresses to be reflected in behavioral and developmental change (Sosinsky et al., 2018).

During the time of explosion of words, the young child may learn about nine words each day. By the end of this time, children will have extensive vocabulary and a good sense of many aspects of correct language use including morphology, grammar, and syntax. Children at this age also have a marked capacity for learning other languages (an ability that begins to diminish, at least in terms of its ease, after about age 6). Some of the relevant milestones in development in the preschool period are summarized in Tables 2.4 and 2.5.

TABLE 2.4

Selected Social, Communicative, and Cognitive Milestones: 1–6 Years of Age

Age (years)	Social-Affective	Communicative	Cognitive-Adaptive
1.25	Shows desire to please parents	Combines words and gesture	Builds tower of two blocks
1.5	Hugs or feeds doll	Speaks in sentences	Draws imitative stroke
1.75	Shares toys or possessions	Says 50 or more words	Uses tool to attain object out of reach
2	Simple make-believe play	Jargon discarded, speech mostly intelligible	Makes simple generalizations
2.5	Identifies own mirror image	States first and last names	Matches simple shapes
3	Labels affects in self	Uses past tense, knows some songs or nursery rhymes	Designates action in pictures, copies circle
3.5	Cooperative play, games with rules	Uses adjectives and adverbs	Copies square, compares sizes
4	Assumes specific role in play	Participates in conversations appropriately	Draws person with two parts, counts three objects
4.5	Elaborate, dramatic play	Uses compound sentences	Names missing parts, counts four objects
5	Understands rules of games	Defines words, names coins	Knows days of week, counts 10 objects
6	Has "best friend"	Prints words from memory, reads simple stories	Draws person with head, neck, hands

Adapted with permission from Volkmar, F. R. (1995). Normal development. In H. Kaplan & B. Sadock (Eds.), *Comprehensive textbook of psychiatry* (6th ed., Vol. 2, pp. 2154–2160). Williams & Wilkins.

TABLE 2.5

Selected Motor and Self-Care Milestones: Age 1–6 Years

Age (years)	Motor	Personal and Self-Care
1.25	Runs well with little falling	Points to one body part
1.5	Turns knobs	Understands the meaning of "hot"
1.75	Kicks ball	Uses spoon well
2	Turns pages of book, walks up and down stairs	Pulls on simple clothing
2.5	Holds crayon with fingers	Toilet trained during the day
3	Rides tricycle	Helps put things away
3.5	Does complex block constructions	Does simple chores
4	Hops	Apologizes for unintentional mistakes
4.5	Bounces ball	Orders food in restaurant
5	Throws ball, skips well	Dresses and undresses mostly independently
6	Rides bicycle	Chooses activities independently

Adapted with permission from Volkmar, F. R. (1995). Normal development. In H. Kaplan & B. Sadock (Eds.), *Comprehensive textbook of psychiatry* (6th ed., Vol. 2, pp. 2154–2160). Williams & Wilkins.

The ability to think more abstractly and symbolically is expressed in many ways. Children begin to use drawings to represent the world (Figure 2.3 and Box 2.2). During this period, the young child also has a growing ability to organize and engage in forward planning (executive functions) that becomes important later for school success. There is a strong desire to learn, and often children take great pride in their learning and have a desire to "show off" as well as a sense of invulnerability (the latter can contribute to poor judgment and accidents). A major focus of early educational programs is the support of the child's interest in learning and exploration. Sensitive programs (and parents) are careful to arrange opportunities for learning that are mildly challenging as well as stimulating, thus helping the child to be involved in a continuous process of learning. Self-care and other "adaptive" skills also increase. Games provide important insights into the idea of rules as well as some basic abilities in recognition and manipulation of symbols that will become relevant to later school performance.

By ages 4–5, children will, for the most part, have achieved an awareness of the thoughts/feelings/beliefs of others. This accomplishment, often termed *the acquisition of a "theory of mind*," helps the child advance dramatically in the social world and opens a range of new possibilities for the child including an increased sense of self. It also is reflected in new capacities for even more sophisticated play. Play and play activities are important sources of growth for the preschool child. Rough and tumble play is common in toddlers (and indeed in many animal species), but as children become a bit older play becomes increasingly dominated by capacities for symbolic thought, language, and social issues. Children can play with language and also integrate language into their play. Because they develop the capacity for symbolic thinking, pretend play activities are no longer constrained by the actual object, that is, the object can be used as a "stand in" for anything real or imagined. Pretend play becomes increasingly complex and flexible. As play becomes more social and less "parallel" in nature (i.e., when children play independently but near each other), toys and activities are shared and become more elaborate. By around age 4, play tends to take on more complex themes and often takes the form of a story with a goal, plot, characters, and so forth.

Having solid and secure attachments to adults facilitates play and social competence. Temperament can also be important in this regard in that excessively shy and inhibited

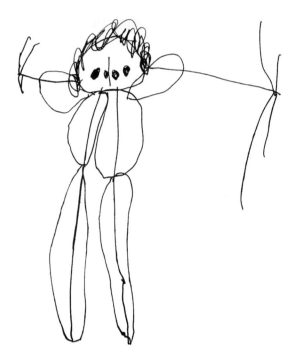

FIGURE 2.3. A 4-year-old child's drawing of her father. Note the presence of a body, head, arms, legs, and a few facial features. Children's ability to draw the human form reflects their cognitive, social, and visual-motor development and is strongly related to developmental level. Courtesy of Emily Volkmar.

BOX 2.2   Drawing Abilities

Children's ability to draw has a strong developmental component as does their ability to draw one of their favorite subjects—other people. Children who are 18–24 months old start to scribble and, over the next several months, begin to use circular strokes so that by or shortly after age 2, the child is able to copy a circle in reasonable fashion. The circle becomes the prototype for most drawing. Children who are 2 and 3 years old begin to label their drawings, and by 3–4 years of age, they start to produce rudimentary people, often with the circle as the body and stick arms and legs added on along with a smaller circle for the head. By age 3, children can typically copy a cross. Visual motor coordination continues to advance so that by age 5, children can make a reasonable copy of a square (this is also an age when hand dominance is firmly established). By 5–6 years of age, children progressively add more detail, including to the background of the image. Subsequent changes reflect increased cognitive ability as well as improved graphomotor skills so that by 9 or 10 years, children typically desire highly realistic and detailed drawings. Children may accurately depict physical disabilities or areas of somatic concern in their drawing (e.g., a child whose mother exhibits an atrophied limb might consistently portray this in their drawings). The strong developmental correlates of drawing ability are reflected in the use of activities that involve person drawing as simple proxies for overall cognitive ability.

Reprinted with permission from Volkmar, F. R., & Martin, A. (2011). *Essentials of Lewis's child and adolescent psychiatry* (1st ed., p. 23). Lippincott Williams & Wilkins/Wolters Kluwer.

children (and those who are overly active and disinhibited) can have problems with play and peer relationships (Box 2.3). Increased abilities to play also provide the potential for great insight into the child's worries, concerns, and inner experiences—a phenomenon that can be used in play interviews with younger children. For some children, play can also be used as a therapeutic tool.

It is fairly common for preschool children to have imaginary friends and companions. The child may firmly insist on the reality of these individuals. This occasionally presents some challenges for parents (and mental health professionals) but usually is harmless. It is important to keep in mind that distinctions about reality/fantasy are not well appreciated until later. Issues of independence and separation can become prominent in this age group.

Transitions can present special challenges for the toddler and preschooler and some may use transitional objects to help them deal with these transitions (Box 2.4). These difficulties are sometimes exacerbated by stresses common in this age group (parental relocation, birth of a sibling). It is important for parents (and caregivers) to appreciate the difficulties separations can cause given the limited coping skills of this age group. The preschool child may repeatedly question the parents/caregivers about separation (e.g., why the parents are leaving, where are they going); this reflects the lack of fully developed capacities for internalization and memory. Transitional objects may help in this regard and so can use of a picture or some other "token" left by the parent to remind the child that the parent will return. These difficulties can also be reflected (to some degree) around issues of transitions to new teachers, day care workers, babysitters, and so forth. Issues of separation loom large particularly when divorce or parental separation becomes a fact of the child's life. As much as possible, the principle of continuity of care should be paramount.

BOX 2.3   Temperament

As parents (particularly parents of more than one child) are aware, noteworthy individual differences are apparent in children from birth. The term *temperament* has been used to denote these relatively stable individual differences in affective "tone," responsivity, and motivation. The term has some relation to the idea of personality type as used later in life.

The work of Thomas and Chess in their longitudinal study of infants in the 1950s noted the importance of infant temperament as an enduring characteristic impacting child behavior and parent–child interaction from early in life but having some persistence throughout childhood. In thinking about temperament, they looked at features such as levels of activity, intensity of affective reactions, attention, sensitivity to the environment, and so forth. They also developed the notion of "goodness of fit" to summarize the degree to which child characteristics met parental expectations. A difficult child might, then, be one who, for one set of parents, would not be challenging but, for another, would be very challenging.

Subsequently, others have modified the concept. For example, Jerome Kagan and colleagues have focused on issues of reactivity and inhibition. Differences have been noted in long-term outcome, particularly for children who are more inhibited.

The concept can be very helpful for parents in understanding the sometimes surprising aspects of their children's individuality and responding to it appropriately. Recognition of their own temperaments and their impact on their children and their responses to their children is also helpful.

Reprinted with permission from Volkmar, F. R., & Martin, A. (2011). *Essentials of Lewis's child and adolescent psychiatry* (1st ed., p. 24). Lippincott Williams & Wilkins/Wolters Kluwer.

BOX 2.4	**Transitional Objects**

Often, by the end of the first year, typically developing children have developed a strong attachment for a "transitional object." This phenomenon was described by the British pediatrician and psychoanalyst Donald Winnicott, who noted several key features: the object is usually soft (a blanket, pillow, or stuffed animal), the child is very attached to the object and wants it with them, and the object helps with transitions (e.g., at bedtime). The presence of the actual object (not a substitute) is critically important. In his view, the object helped in the development of a sense of self (apart from the mother) and was a unique "me/not me" possession that he also saw as one aspect of a range of transitional phenomena. The child uses the object to help with separations, and the smell and feel of the object are often important. The child invariably leaves the object in various places, resulting in parental panic that it has been lost. Interestingly, children with autism often have hard rather than soft objects, and it is the class of object (e.g., any magazine, bundle of twigs) that is important for them.

Reprinted with permission from Volkmar, F. R., & Martin, A. (2011). *Essentials of Lewis's child and adolescent psychiatry* (1st ed., p. 25). Lippincott Williams & Wilkins/Wolters Kluwer.

A range of anxieties, not just around separation, often become more striking between ages 2 and 4 years. This increase in fearfulness is normative (and to some extent adaptive) and tends to happen just as stranger anxiety and separation anxiety start to diminish. Children who are well attached to their parents will look to them for support and reassurance and may be more cautious than children who are abused or neglected. Common sources of fear include issues of bedtime and are often associated with changes in routine. In some ways, the child's greater capacity for symbolic thinking also contributes, that is, children can now imagine a range of adverse outcomes. Other issues arise given children's difficulties in sorting out differences between dreams/nightmares and reality. Children in this age group often manage to feel quite powerful but also rather helpless. Even though their language skills have increased, preschoolers may have difficulty giving voice to their fears and concerns. Some children may exhibit anxiety by withdrawal, avoidance, or by being clingy whereas others become disorganized and overly active.

The mastery of aggressive impulses is a major accomplishment for most children during the preschool years. Difficulties with the modulation of aggression is a frequent cause of mental health referral in this age group. Such behavior can complicate the child's placement in day care or an educational setting. Many factors contribute to difficulties with aggression including past experience, endowment, and cognitive and language abilities. Having an ability to "use your words" gives the child much more socially acceptable alternatives to aggressive behavior; not surprisingly, children whose language development is delayed have more difficulty. The presence of important models of aggressive behavior (violent television and games, older siblings, and adults) can also exacerbate this problem. On the other hand, some degree of independence is desirable and normative. The toddler makes frequent use of words/phrases like "Mine!" and "Me do!"; temper tantrums may erupt when the child is frustrated. For some children, aggressive thoughts/feelings may be expressed more in fantasy and play than in behavior.

Preschoolers who are overly aggressive are at increased risk for a range of problems—both short and longer term. A thoughtful evaluation will include an assessment of the antecedents, behavior, and consequences of the behavior, that is, what situations elicit it and what happens as a result. This assessment should also address the potential for anxiety to contribute to the behavioral difficulties. Usually, physical aggression diminishes after age 3 while verbal aggression begins to increase. The focus of aggression also shifts with younger children being more concerned with needs whereas aggression in children in school often has a more social context. Fortunately, most aggressive 3-year-olds do not become aggressive 6-year-olds. Helping the child learn better approaches to dealing with angry (and anxious) feelings, modeling appropriate, nonaggressive behavior, and encouraging verbal expression are important.

It is increasingly common for preschoolers to be enrolled in childcare and early education programs. Given this, it is common for younger children to be referred for developmental and behavioral difficulties. Efforts have been made to bring services more directly into programs, and the availability of supports and consultants also has some advantages for mental health professionals who can see the child in more natural settings. Other models of consultation focus primarily on the classroom or behaviors that are problematic on a more general basis. Unfortunately, poor reimbursement and limited training for childcare and teaching staff is a continuing problem. Problems in the care provider, like depression, may impact their experience of (and reactions to) the child with difficulties.

▎ THE SCHOOL AGE CHILD

In the developed world, this period of development is defined by the experience of school. Peers come to be a major influence rivaling, or surpassing, parents and siblings. Although Freud referred to this as the *latency period* (presuming that sexual drives are relatively dormant until adolescence), this is an oversimplification. In some ways Erikson (1963, 1964), with his characterization of "Industry versus Inferiority" as the central developmental task, more accurately captured the challenge for this age group. School success and progress are essential for self-esteem, peer relations, and subsequent academic development. In addition to the important role of peers, effects of culture (including from media and social media) as well as societal and economic factors have more impact. Table 2.6 summarizes the considerable growth that occurs over this time.

By age 5, the brain has reached about 90% of its adult volume. The rate of growth then slows until puberty. Modification of structures continues and myelinization is almost complete by age 7 when the brain reaches about adult size. Other ongoing changes include synaptic pruning in the prefrontal cortex. Some gender differences are observed with boys having, on average, brains that are about 10% larger; other differences are observed in structures like the basal ganglia. Growth in the frontal lobe helps children be able to engage in inhibition and thus focus and process information more successfully. At the psychological level, these advances are reflected in greater coordination of motor skills, increased capacities for self-regulation, speed of information processing, and increased ability to attend. These gains are also manifest in a growing ability to read (a process typically well in place by the second grade). As noted in Chapter 1, Piaget's view of cognitive development emphasizes the move from what he termed *preoperational thinking* to more complex *operational* thought. This is reflected in greater conceptual ability and recognizing notions like conservation of number or mass (i.e., changing the shape does not change the mass of materials). The child can think of alternatives, understand hierarchies and categories, series, and master new concepts like reversibility, sequencing, and so forth. The child also can now see the world from points of view other than their own (*decentration*) and can engage in more sophisticated cognitive and social operations including advanced games and group activities. These new cognitive abilities also help children gain new understanding of biologic processes, including death that is now understood to be irreversible.

The gains are also seen in the increased sophistication of conversation. Often, there is a desire for order and ritual and many school-age children develop a need for symmetry and order as well as some ritualistic behaviors. This is a time when collecting things (insects, stamps, rocks, coins) is prominent and the collection and its ordering and reordering becomes a focus of interest.

TABLE 2.6

Characteristics of the School-Aged Child

	Child Entering First Grade (5–6 years old)	Child Completing Fifth Grade (10–11 years old)
Motor	Hop, skip, jump, throw, catch, kick a ball Reasonable balance, able to stand still and hold arms steady; stands on one foot, left and right General sense of left and right, not always consistent Able to do rapid alternating movements Mild synkinesis on fine finger movements	Hop, skip, jump, throw, catch, and kick a ball with ease Elaborates: e.g., dance steps; throw behind back or trick the receiver Balance is good; tandem walking with ease Accurate distinction of left and right No synkinesis
Writing and drawing	Able to name and copy circle, square, triangle, and cross easily Some copy diamond and asterisk. Five-pointed star is possible, if child has been exposed to this in kindergarten. Draws person with body, arms, and legs; can put detailed features, but often leaves them out Can draw house and tree, as well	Can draw circle, square, triangle, diamond, asterisk, five-pointed star Cube can be accomplished, but often only after shown how to draw it. Draws more detailed person with hands and feet, and action figures: girls with more decorative detail, boys with more action detail
Stories	About drawings, persons are largely self-referential. Even if a figure has a different name, the life circumstances are usually identical to the child's.	May draw someone who is not self and can have a story about another, even made-up family Creates complex plots, using well-developed descriptive language
Fund of knowledge (depends on exposure)	Recites alphabet; counts beyond 20; writes name, first and last Recognizes printed letters and numbers (not cursive); writes most letters and numbers; may have some reversals	Reads aloud and to self with comprehension; performs double-digit addition and subtraction in head; multiplies, divides, and does fractions on paper; knows details about historical figures, geography, natural phenomena, and body systems
Cognitive	Egocentric; idiosyncratic definitions of "scientific" observations, centration, defining by only one dimension; beginning concrete operations: conservation and classification	Conservation of number, weight, and volume; flexibility of operational skills, including reversibility
Moral	Defines right and wrong in terms of punishment and pain, or other personal and idiosyncratic rationales Interested in how the world works, including life and death, religion; uses magical thinking	Defines right and wrong through internal principles Has empathy and can weigh issues from another's position

TABLE 2.6

Characteristics of the School-Aged Child (*continued*)

	Child Entering First Grade (5–6 years old)	Child Completing Fifth Grade (10–11 years old)
Social	Enjoys the company of other children; names several friends Interactional play with rules, often externally determined Creative play is imitative Peers judged by whether they are nice to child Games of individual prowess May play on team, but cooperates based on rules rather than complex strategizing	Likely to have a best friend and a close circle of friends Activities with peers are increasingly independent of parental supervision. Able to create games and make up rules; consideration for others, particularly with girls Increasing self-reliance and responsibility Peers judged by their qualities Teamwork
Self-view	Dependent on others' descriptions	Dependent on view of success, competence, and evaluation by internal standards, as well as comparison with peers and social pressures Selects from multiple available models to define standard for "cool" for self and select friends
Sex	Interested in sexual differences; pleasure from touching oneself; generally, play with same-sex friends but comfortable with organized co-ed activities	Secondary sexual changes from Tanner stages II–V, girls usually 2 years ahead of boys Prefers same-sex friends Some awkwardness about growth (slouching, embarrassment about breast development and foot size) Wide range of pubertal onset in peer group may create challenges to individual self-esteem. Some admiration of individual members of the opposite sex versus thinking others are "yucky." Interest expressed through teasing, messages sent through others
Family	Identification with parents or siblings, primarily same sex Participates in family rituals and routines around meals and bedtimes	Compares parents with other adults, including teachers and other children's parents More independent of family rituals and routines More responsibility for household tasks, own self-care, and homework

Reprinted with permission from Combrinck-Graham, L., & Fox, G. (2018). Development of school-age children. In A. Martin, M. Block, & F. R. Volkmar (Eds.), *Lewis's child and adolescent psychiatry: A comprehensive textbook* (5th ed., p. 87). Wolters Kluwer.

Attention and "executive function" skills also increase during school age. The child is able to develop plans for action and can use private speech as well as a series of strategies to memorize, order, rehearse, and plan. The capacity for increased self-regulation is important in setting the stage for adolescence.

The topic of moral development in school-age children has been the focus of much attention starting with Piaget (see Chapter 1), who emphasized that morality at this age focused very much on "the rules" and their interpretation. Other subsequent investigators like Kohlberg (1969) talked about this as a time of "conventional morality"; this concept includes an aspect of a desire to please authority figures (parents and teachers) and the importance of rules in guiding behavior. Gender differences in moral judgment at this age are noted and may reflect some of the differences in play (with more emphasis on social interaction and empathy in girls).

For the school-age child, emotional development at this age centers on competence and the social–community environment. Competence is expected in many areas, for example, in self-care, academic, social, and physical aspects. In the view of Erikson (see Chapter 1), the major risk for the child at this age has to do with feelings of inferiority, although, at least to some extent, failures in one area can be compensated for by success in another. By the middle school years, the individual child will often have a strong sense of areas of strength and weakness and these perceptions are often quite persistent. The nature of anxiety and fear changes somewhat as children enter school age. Given their greater exposure to the world and events, they often become more worried about catastrophic events, death, and so forth. Children who struggle with issues of competence may be particularly likely to be at risk for emotional difficulties.

The role of the media, broadly defined, has been exploding in recent years. There has been considerable debate about the effects (or ill effects) of television and more recently of video games, social networking, and the internet. These activities can isolate children from interaction with family members and peers, may model inappropriate behaviors, and may provide a highly unrealistic view of the world. In addition, they are usually rather sedentary and may contribute to growing rates of obesity and lack of physical fitness in children. On the other hand, such media may be a source of comfort to some children and help consolidate connections to peers.

The peer culture has an increasingly important role in fostering socialization experiences and children's striving for acceptance and competency within their peer group. These issues are also very relevant to children's sense of self and self-concept.

Peer relationships have their own characteristic pattern of development beginning in preschool and developing, during the primary school years, into more cooperative and truly dyadic partnerships and then on to more intimate peer relationships (best friends) just before adolescence. Same-sex peers become increasingly important. Gender differences are noted with girls preferring patterns that involve greater intimacy than boys. With increasing age, the games of school-age children develop more group process features, more rules, and greater complexities. The modulation of angry and aggressive impulses becomes an important issue in dealing with peers. Children who are, or remain, more overtly aggressive are more likely to be isolated and rejected; they may form their own peer groups, but social isolation and aggression are important risk factors for subsequent development problems.

Enrollment in school for the vast majority of school-age children is a relatively new historic phenomenon. Children arrive at school with many different experiences and perspectives. Important sociocultural differences are observed as discussed at the end of this chapter. Many middle and upper class families will have children who have attended preschool, have witnessed the value of more "academic" skills in the lives of their parents, and have a strong interest in books and reading. These opportunities are often much less available to children from poor, minority, and inner-city families. Children who live in poverty also may have had very different experiences because they often must assume more responsibilities in the household. Parental background is highly related to school achievement. Children with secure attachments to their parents, who have grown up in a supportive environment, and where parents emphasize academic expectations and values are less likely to have difficulty adjusting to the demands of school. For some children, the availability of model preschool programs or Head Start may provide an important facilitation for school entry.

One of the central tasks of the early school years is gaining the ability to read. This is a complex process with both content and relational/interactional aspects (see Chapter 9). Skills needed in preparation for reading include both content and structure of books and other written materials. Children who lack a foundation of basic skills are more likely to have difficulties in learning to read. Academic material is ideally constructed in such a way as to be just at the point of "proximal development" for the child, that is, a bit (but only a bit) further than they presently are in terms of their skill sets. Both the ability of the child and the knowledge of the teacher are important in insuring successful learning. Peer learning is also important with specific methods like "cooperative learning" used to help children learn together and work as a group. Sensitive teachers will also be aware of each child's strengths, weaknesses, and learning style as well as their readiness and motivation to learn. Even when curricula are appropriate to grade level, some children will be advanced or behind. Parental involvement is also essential and for schools to be effective, they must also function as communities, which means, at least for large schools, that ways must be found to foster engagement in smaller groups. Other problems arise for children and families who must cope with chronic medical illness. In these cases, a focus on helping the child learn as effectively as possible and helping the child establish a positive view of themselves is a major goal. Children who experience repeated failure are at risk for a variety of difficulties including depression, social isolation, and further academic difficulties. Externalizing behavior disorders can also develop and may severely impact the child.

It is important to note that although schooling is the norm within the United States and more developed countries, most (90%) children in Africa and Asia are involved in work, live in extreme poverty, and have limited opportunities for education.

ADOLESCENCE

Adolescence is a time of transition defined by the intersection of several factors. The child transitions from a person with some but minimal responsibility to an adult with the entire set of responsibilities typical of adulthood. This is a time of recurrent paradox. Some adolescents will be just entering puberty, others will be well advanced. Youngsters vary significantly in their development but typically acquire physical maturity well before they have reached their adult levels of social, emotional, and intellectual maturity. Over the past century, adolescence has begun earlier. The increasing societal demands for education have resulted in an opposing trend that lengthens the process of education. In contrast to the situation a century ago, employment before age 16 is typically prohibited and school attendance required. Financial independence is usually only achieved well after high school and can continue through college and beyond. Legal issues also impact independence. Legal status represents a complicated mix of laws and regulation—younger adolescents may drive farm equipment (or even an airplane) but not a car. Similarly, a 17-year-old might be in the army when they cannot yet vote. Regulations vary from state to state and may impact things like rights to independent medical care.

Even though they are not yet financially independent, the youth market represents a substantial economic force. Adolescents are specifically targeted in television and other programming, online, and in ads—often dominated by sex and/or aggression. As King and Rutherford (2018) point out, although theories of development have tended to focus on the task of achieving independence, it is actually more accurate to discuss *interdependence*, that is, an ability to develop supportive relationships outside the immediate family. Adolescence must also be viewed in the context of culture, family, school, and community. All these factors interact so that the adolescent is influenced by the family while also influencing it.

Over the last century, different factors have impacted adolescence with a move of families from farms to cities, better health care and longer life spans, smaller families and longer periods of financial dependence on parents, and the increasing importance of social media and other information resources. As discussed near the end of this chapter, cultural factors are important as are issues of gender identification.

Puberty refers to the physical and physiologic changes that note the transition from childhood to adulthood. Physical changes include development of primary and secondary sexual characteristics along with the characteristic growth spurt. Puberty typically takes about 4–5 years in total. Girls, at least in the more developed countries, often start this process about 2 years before boys do (typically ages 9–11 for girls and 11–13 for boys). Tanner has classified the various changes in the development of secondary sex characteristics into five stages (Table 2.7). Pubertal staging can be accomplished by physical examination or self-report (although the former is more accurate). Typically, the first sign that puberty is beginning is accelerated height—this can be as much as 10 cm in a given year. The "gangling" appearance of early adolescents precedes the development of increased muscle mass and strength that is associated with later stages of puberty.

For girls, menarche is the major marker of puberty. Initially, periods may be irregular and fertility may take up to 2 years to develop. For menarche to occur, a critical body weight and fat/muscle ratio must be met. For some girls who train intensively (or have anorexia, see Chapter 17), menarche can be delayed. The average age of menarche is progressively decreasing with some racial differences noted; in developing countries, the age is later than in developed countries.

For boys, the growth of the genitalia and spermatogenesis in early and middle adolescence are associated with ejaculation (either spontaneously at night or because of masturbation). Unlike menarche, which is a frequent topic of conversation among early adolescent girls, boys typically are rather private in discussing this issue, at least in western cultures.

A large body of research has focused on the impact of early versus late maturation in boys and girls. Briefly summarized, the result of this work is that for boys, early maturation leads to greater popularity, feelings of self-esteem, and greater academic and intellectual success although possibly also incurring some risk for conduct and behavior problems possibly related to older peer group influences. For girls, the issues are more complicated. In general, it appears that girls maturing early may have more problems with self-image and are at greater risk for mood and anxiety problems. They may also be at risk for eating problems and risk taking (including sexual risk taking). Other issues impact this including culture, social class, peers, and so forth. Although popular culture frequently refers to the "raging hormones" of adolescence, evidence for an association between gonadal hormonal levels and behavioral or mental health problems is rather weak. On the other hand, often there is an increased appetite and changes in sleep patterns. Chronic sleep deprivation is not uncommon.

In Piaget's view, the period of formal operations in adolescence marks the ability to consider issues of propositional logic, deductive reasoning, hypothesis testing, etc. In other words, the adolescent is no longer constrained simply by their observation of the world, rather an appreciation of what "might be" is now possibly leading, in part to adolescent enthusiasms and idealism. Although the specifics of many aspects of Piaget's theory have been debated, there is agreement that cognitive abilities significantly increase in complexity in adolescence

TABLE 2.7

Tanner's Stages of Puberty

Stage	Boys	Girls
1	Preadolescent	Preadolescent
2	Slight amount of pubic hair, slight enlargement of penis and scrotum	Sparse pubic hair, breasts begin to develop
3	Increased pubic hair, penis longer, testes bigger	Increased pubic hair, breasts enlarged
4	Pubic hair pattern resembles adult pattern but still sparser than in adults	Abundant pubic hair (less than in adults), nipples become more prominent
5	Adult male distribution of pubic hair, adult-size testes and penis	Adult female pattern of pubic hair, breasts of mature adult

Adapted from Tanner, J. M. (1962). *Growth at adolescence* (2nd ed.). Oxford, England: Blackwell; Daniel, W. A. (1977). *Adolescents in health and disease.* St. Louis: Mosby.

because the teenager is able to consider multiple problem solutions and outcomes and process information more effectively and quickly. These cognitive changes also contributed to more sophisticated social-cognitive and moral development. Adolescents can appreciate the subtlety of moral reasoning. Despite these gains, adolescents do not, however, always make wise decisions and their judgment can be clouded by strong emotions, peer pressure, and substance use/abuse.

The physical, neurobiologic, and cognitive changes experienced herald dramatic shifts in the adolescent's relationship to their own body, to parents, peers, and self-image. Adolescence brings a number of psychological challenges. These are summarized in Table 2.8.

One of the greatest challenges comes from the major physical changes that come with adolescence. Sexual development presents opportunities for gratification and embarrassment. The adolescent will typically be very aware of similar changes in peers and evaluate themselves carefully in reference to them. The wide variation of development can pose significant issues in this regard. Girls are often particularly preoccupied with the ideal (and unrealistic) body image presented in the media. Obesity can be a problem for both sexes, although significant racial and ethnic differences are noted. Eating disorders in girls are particularly common and girls are more likely than boys to engage in measures designed to help them lose weight, for example, laxatives or vomiting. Changes in the body also pose issues for self-representation. Teenagers of both sexes spend considerable amounts of their discretionary income on products designed to improve their appearance or reach some ideal body/appearance. This can include use of supplements, exercise problems, and even anabolic steroids in boys and endless "makeovers" in girls. Other options include tattoos and piercing. In other cases, the preoccupation with a changed body and dissatisfaction can result in other behaviors, for example, cutting.

Other challenges come from major changes in relationships with parents and siblings. During adolescence, children spend less time with their parents and much more with peers. Increases in cognitive capacities and concerns about the future also typically result in some deidealization of the parents. Desire for continued closeness with parents competes with other desires for autonomy. These competing interests result in considerable ambivalence (as conveyed in books for parents of teens like *Get Out of My Life, but First Could You Drive Me and Cheryl to the Mall?*). Despite these issues, for most adolescents parents remain the primary sources of support and assistance. Even though this is true, the subjective changes in the relationship have major importance. Conflicts with parents become more frequent with disputes about rules and chores and then continue over time with new topics such as curfews, dating, and so forth. These disputes often seem to peak in mid adolescence and then decrease. Mother–daughter pairs are at particular risk in terms of frequency although father–son pairs often have more intense disputes. Mental health issues (e.g., depression) or other problems (e.g., substance abuse) can exacerbate these tensions, which take a toll on the parents as well as on the child. The apparent focus of disputes often is trivial

TABLE 2.8

Growth Tasks by Developmental Phase

The normative psychological tasks of adolescence are as follows:
- Developing a satisfactory and realistic body image
- Developing increased independence from parents and adequate capacities for self-care and regulation
- Developing satisfying relationships outside the family
- Developing appropriate control and expression of increased sexual and aggressive drives
- Identity consolidation, including a personal moral code and at least provisional plans for a vocation and economic self-sufficiency

Reprinted with permission from King, R. (2005). Adolescence. In A. Martin & F. R. Volkmar (Eds.), *Lewis's child and adolescent psychiatry: A comprehensive textbook* (4th ed., p. 282). Lippincott Williams & Wilkins.

(over hairstyle, clothes, chores, etc.); the disputes are symbolic of other issues and have considerable additional psychological meaning. For most parents, a combination of warmth and engagement coupled with a firm, expectation-based approach works best (what is often referred to as *an authoritative parenting style*). Fortunately by the time the adolescent is finishing high school and entering college, they can be more autonomous and engage in a new and more mature way with parents and family members.

Although most adolescents are healthy, their lifestyle can contribute to lifelong habits that impact health through diet, exercise, driving, sexual behaviors, and so forth. On the other hand, for some teenagers an awareness of chronic illness may significantly impact the adolescent experience and have important implications for health care. The sense of invulnerability in adolescence, coupled with a desire to fit in, may lead to noncompliance with medical treatments (see Chapter 27). For example, many teenagers with diabetes may be noncompliant with treatment. Children with other illnesses may stop or "forget" medications. The attempt to avoid or deny the reality of medical needs can further compound this problem.

Adolescence brings the new experiences of sexual desire and attraction. These can take infinite forms and are the focus of considerable research and debate in the extensive literature on this topic. Although obvious sexual behaviors are minimal prior to adolescence, they typically increase around age 10 and may initially focus on same-sex peers. In some cultures, various ceremonies and rites of passage begin as early as age 10 or 11. The ability to combine feelings of sexual interest with emotional intimacy is a major challenge for the adolescent. Over the course of adolescence, masturbation and heterosexual activities rise dramatically. Homosexual experiences are more frequent in early adolescence (slightly over a quarter of 13-year-old boys report such experience). Sexual fantasies (often initially during masturbation) are highly personal and can play an important part in the development of each adolescent's unique sexuality. As adolescence progresses, a major challenge is the introduction of erotic longings into relationships. Social and ethnic factors can have a major impact on this process. Gender differences are noteworthy. For girls, the relationship element of the encounter is critical, whereas for boys sexual gratification may be more important (but this is only a generalization and many variations on this theme are noted). The ability to fall in love is an important aspect of sexuality for the adolescent, and as they mature it may often conflict with parents over issues that involve some aspect of the child's growing sexuality, for example, appearance, dating, curfews, and so on.

Beginning with the work of Erik Erikson, there has been more attention to the centrality of the adolescent's awareness of self. More recently, the emphasis has been on self-concept and "identity" as reflected in any number of areas including social, academic, physical/athletic, and so forth. The increased cognitive abilities of the adolescent give them the capacity to view all these issues from new perspectives—including a moral perspective—and, over time, result in each individual achieving a unique view of self. Special issues arise for children coming from minority communities or where ethnic issues/concerns are strong. Other issues arise around differences in sexual orientations. In all these cases, the adolescent must develop a sense of themselves relative both to general culture and to their specific group.

Mental Health Issues in Adolescents

About one in five adolescents has a specific clinical disorder. However, a much larger number experience mood issues, problems with parents, or engage in significant risk-taking behaviors. Depression and mood problems increase during adolescence, particularly in girls. It remains unclear to what extent the emotional lability and negative emotions frequent in adolescence contribute to this problem but over one third of adolescents report issues related to depressed mood. This is more common in girls than boys possibly reflecting endocrinologic factors. Various issues including increased academic, social, and cognitive demands may contribute as can the high rates of adolescent mood variability.

Accidents and injuries associated with risk taking present another challenge for adolescents. Even though cognitive capacities increase in adolescents, this process is a long and complex one and brain mechanisms that involve forward planning and inhibition are often not yet fully established. About three fourths of deaths in individuals ages 10–24 can be attributed to activities with a significant element of risk taking (car accidents, homicide, and suicide). High rates of risk tasking are reported in national samples including drinking while driving, not wearing seat belts, carrying a weapon, and unprotected sexual encounters.

Becoming an Adult

Although the onset of adolescence is relatively clearly marked, its close is not. In earlier times, some specific event, like getting married, getting a job, or entering the army, served to close adolescence. Today, many factors blur this transition as many students move from high school to college remaining highly dependent on their parents for financial support. Marriage and employment can be postponed until after college or grad school. Arnett (1999) has proposed the term *emerging adulthood* to describe this new phenomenon. Adolescence today often is followed by a relatively long period of semi-autonomy with full independence from parents being achieved only in the late 20s and early 30s.

■ CULTURAL ISSUES

In our increasingly diverse society, cultural issues have assumed a greater role in the provision of mental health services to children (Sholevar & Joshi, 2018). Cultural psychiatry defines the impact of culture on psychiatric evaluation, diagnosis, and treatment; it also provides guidelines for culturally competent care (Mezzich et al., 1996). Early work in this area began with appreciation of cultural factors that initially applied to developing counties but today includes the awareness of the experience of children who are black, Hispanic, native American, or members of other groups within the United States (Sholevar & Joshi, 2018). Aspects of cultural psychiatry are impacted by anthropology and sociology and make us aware of differences across cultures in the conceptualization of things like time, action, the relationships of people to each other, their culture, and to the planet, as well as to interpersonal relationships. The mainstream U.S. culture does, for example, emphasize the importance of being active, autonomous, working toward some important long term-goals, and has an emphasis on nuclear as opposed to the broader extended family. There is great awareness of time and much of life revolves around a schedule and the future. In other cultures, living in the present and having a broad awareness of the extended family may be much more important. We are impacted both by the dominant mainstream culture and identification with ethnic/minority groups to varying degrees.

Our ethnic identity gives us a sense of belonging to a community but may also be the source of conflict with mainstream culture (McGoldrick et al., 1996). In the past, particularly in the United States, it was assumed that children would rapidly be incorporated into mainstream culture and this was assumed to be desirable and prevent problems related to the conflict of ethnicity and cultural values. However, subsequent work has shown that people, including children, experience psychological stress because of the partial loss of ethnic identity (Escobar, 1998; Schwoeri et al., 2003).

Clinicians must always remain culturally aware and sensitive if they wish to understand the particular experience of the individual and family in their culture of origin. In particular, increases in the degree to which the child incorporates mainstream cultures as their own may be a source of conflict with their family and culture of origin. Even as the children of immigrants rapidly become assimilated in the United States, their parents may maintain very close connections to their culture of origin. Clinicians should be aware of where the child and family stand in this process. For example, do the child and family speak English fluently and engage in activities that are typical of others, and the society at large?

Sometimes the development of a more autonomous identity leads to separation from the culture of origin and to complex and ambivalent family issues related to cultural exceptions and values. These issues can be the source of distress and guilt (Pumariega & Joshi, 2010) when parents and children adhere, to varying degrees, to their culture of origin and have a strong identification with it (Hwang, 2006).

There has been a growing appreciation of the importance of both awareness and support for cultural values while also recognizing the potential for stress and conflict in the individual child and their family. This is also increasingly appreciated at the global level because mental health services become more common in developing countries where previous resources were greatly lacking (Sholevar & Joshi, 2018) and where differences in cultural expectations are important (Stevenson et al., 1986).

Adolescence marks the transition from childhood to adult roles in different ways in all cultures and has been studied by multiple investigators since the initial observations of Margaret Mead in Samoa in the 1920s, who noted that the transition to adulthood in Samoa was gradual and nonstressful compared to that in the United States. In some cultures, there is a rapid and abrupt transition from adolescence into adulthood, sometimes with a special ceremony to mark the occasion. In the United States, the transition to adulthood is typically quite prolonged with long-term support from parents as a young person moves to college or vocational training and sometimes beyond.

As a practical matter, it is important for the clinician to be aware of any ethnic or cultural issues that may impact the child and family's understanding of mental illness or developmental difference and their willingness to accept treatments offered (Joshi et al., 2014). Tseng and Streltzer (2004) observe that in any clinical encounter, there is an interaction between the cultural background of the clinician, that of the child and family, and of the organization within which the encounter takes place. Thus the clinician should be aware of the interplay of these three cultures as it impacts their clinical work.

Training programs in all fields must emphasize the need to respect and understand the role of cultural values. Thus, in the clinical interview, the clinician should be aware of expectations, for example, for development of rapport with older family members and members of the extended family and cultural values. Indeed conducting oneself in an empathic, respectful way with an openness to understanding the perspective of others may serve as a good beginning. Language differences can present a major issue. Sometimes, the use of a translator who is quite skilled can be helpful. Other times, a less sensitive translator may hear a long response to a clinician's question and then simply respond with a yes or no, thus losing most of what was being said! Given the confidential nature of what is sometimes being discussed, be careful about the use of a family member as a translator. This can be a particularly sensitive issue when problems of abuse or sexual activity are suspected.

The clinician's formulation of the case should include their appreciation of the cultural factors that are relevant both to clinical expression and for treatment (Aggarwal, 2015). When families have recently immigrated, the family history both prior to and subsequent to the move is highly relevant. Some guidelines are available (Sholevar & Joshi, 2018). The many obstacles already in place to seeking and obtaining treatment for mental health disorders in the United States are increased in children and youth from other cultures. This contributes to underutilization of resources by ethnic minority groups (U.S. Public Health Service, 2000). Fears of stigmatization and concerns about confidentiality may further impact this problem as does ready access to services. In this regard, the attempt to provide better access to care and providers who are culturally aware and linguistically competent is highly desired (Sholevar & Joshi, 2018). An awareness of cultural issues should be particularly emphasized with consideration of psychopharmacology (Sholevar & Joshi, 2018).

■ SEXUAL MINORITY YOUTH

In considering typical development, it is also important to note the growing awareness of the presence of LGBTQ children and youth. We discuss issues of gender identity in more detail in

Chapter 20, but it is important to realize that there have been major societal shifts in thinking about this group (Telingator et al., 2018). It has now been about 50 years since homosexuality is no longer considered a disorder in the *DSM*. Over this time, there has been a growing awareness of the rights of LBGTQ individuals and their important role in society. As a new phenomenon, public and professional discourse has changed over time. Increasingly youth are rejecting simple dichotomous labels that have identified sexual orientation in the past. National population data (Liu et al., 2015) find about 10% of females and 3.5% of males (ages 14–19) have had at least one same-sex sexual experience. For sexual minority youth, the developmental challenges of adolescence are both similar to and different from that of their peers. The degree to which families and community are accepting or not can be the source of considerable distress or comfort to the person.

For communities where acceptance is limited, the youth may choose to hide their identity and sexual feelings. They may engage in heterosexual relationships in an effort to fit into the population. In one study, about half of adolescent sexual minority males and three fourths of females had heterosexual relationships antedating a same-sex experience (Telingator et al., 2018). Males were more likely than females to be aware of same-sex feelings before their heterosexual experience (Omoto & Kurtzman, 2006). As we discuss in Chapter 20, issues of sexual identity, orientation, and behavior can evolve during childhood and adolescence and the mental health clinicians should be alert to this and not simply equate a history of one form of sexual activity with a necessarily finalized identification (Telingator et al., 2018).

As Telingator et al. (2018) note, issues of sexuality, gender, and gender identification are complex and clinicians should be careful to ask their patients about their experience in sensitive and thoughtful ways. Youth who are part of sexual minority groups have increasingly formed relations through connections both locally and nationally using social media and the internet. A range of new terms is being used to self-describe sexual identity (Russell & Consolacion, 2003) and youth can have same-sex attractions, relationships, or behaviors, regardless of their specific self-identification. Parents and family members can be important sources of support and in many schools gay-straight alliances (GSA) have peers who also are important to a range of students. More positive media coverage as well as supportive friendships have been a great help as well.

SUMMARY

Development is a dynamic process in which experience and endowment interact to varying degrees and in complex ways, and major transitions and shifts that encourage or inhibit functioning occur over time. Tasks of infancy include establishment of essential social-affective bonds and acquisition of cognitive abilities like object permanence. For the toddler, issues of autonomy, language development, and behavior modulation become more prominent. As children enter the preschool and school ages, issues of peer relationship become more central as children gain increasing abilities. For the adolescent, there is a fundamental, and enduring, tension in the various forces that both encourage and inhibit development and independence. Considerable cognitive capacities give the adolescent greater awareness of the world—both as it is and should be. In Western cultures, this period has become increasingly prolonged even as sexual maturity often comes earlier.

In thinking about the individual child, it is important to keep in mind that the "normal" child exists only in an abstract way. Rather, it is the "normative" child that is typically described in chapters like this one and the astute clinician will be aware of both what is within and outside the broad range of normal. The importance of cultural factors in the experience of children and youth within the United States has been the increasingly recognized and associated with LGBTQ youth. Although no one ever meets the absolutely normal child, an awareness of what is typical is important in understanding when development seems to move outside the normal range. Clinicians should be sensitive to cultural and sexual orientation issues in dealing with children and adolescents.

References

Aggarwal, N. K. (2015). Cultural formulations in child and adolescent psychiatry. *Journal of the American Academy of Child & Adolescent Psychiatry, 49*(4), 306–309. https://doi.org/10.1016/j.jaac.2010.01.001

Arnett, J. (1999). Adolescent storm and stress, reconsidered. *The American Psychologist, 54*(5), 317–326. https://doi.org/10.1037/0003-066X.54.5.317

Egger, H. L. (2009). Psychiatric assessment of young children. *Child and Adolescent Psychiatric Clinics of North America, 18*(3), 559–580. https://doi.org/10.1016/j.chc.2009.02.004

Erikson, E. H. (1963). *Childhood and society* (2nd revised ed.). W. W. Norton & Co.

Erikson, E. H. (1994). *Identity and the life cycle.* W. W. Norton & Co.

Escobar, J. I. (1998). Immigration and mental health: Why are immigrants better off. *Archives of General Psychiatry, 55*(9), 781–782. https://doi.org/10.1001/archpsyc.55.9.781

Hwang, W.-C. (2006). Acculturative family distancing: Theory, research, and clinical practice. *Psychotherapy: Theory, Research, Practice, Training, 43*(4), 397–409. https://doi.org/10.1037/0033-3204.43.4.397

Jones, K. L., & Smith, D. W. (1973). Recognition of the fetal alcohol syndrome in early infancy. *Lancet (London, England), 302*(7836), 999–1001. https://doi.org/10.1016/s0140-6736(73)91092-1

Joshi, S. V., Pumariega, A., Reicherter, D., & Roberts, L. W. (2014). Cultural issues in ethics and professionalism. In L. Roberts & D. Reicherter (Eds.), *Professionalism and ethics: Q & A self-study guide for mental health professionals* (pp. 39–56). American Psychiatric Press, Inc.

Kohlberg, L. (1969). Stage and sequence: The cognitive-development approach to socialization. In D. A. Goslin (Ed.), *Handbook of socialization theory and research* (pp. 347–480). Rand-McNally.

Liu, G., Hariri, S., Bradley, H., Gottlieb, S. L., Leichliter, J. S., & Markowitz, L. E. (2015). Trends and patterns of sexual behaviors among adolescents and adults aged 14 to 59 years, United States. *Sexually Transmitted Diseases, 42*(1), 20–26. https://doi.org/10.1097/OLQ.0000000000000231

McGoldrick, M., Giordano, J., & Pearce, J. K. (Eds.). (1996). *Ethnicity and family therapy* (2nd ed.). Guilford Press.

Mead, M. (1928). *Coming of age in Samoa.* William Morrow Paperbacks.

Mezzich, J. E., Kleinman, A., Fabrega, H., & Parron, D. L. (Eds.). (1996). *Culture and psychiatric diagnosis: A DSM-IV perspective.* American Psychiatric Press.

Omoto, A. M., & Kurtzman, H. S. (2006). *Contemporary perspectives on lesbian, gay, and bisexual psychology. Sexual orientation and mental health: Examining identity and development in lesbian, gay, and bisexual people* (p. 323). American Psychological Association. https://doi.org/10.1037/11261-000

Pumariega, A., & Joshi, S. V. (2010). Culture and development in children and youth. *Child and Adolescent Psychiatric Clinics of North America, 19,* 661–680. https://doi.org/10.1016/j.chc.2010.08.002

Russell, S. T., & Consolacion, T. B. (2003). Adolescent romance and emotional health in the United States: Beyond binaries. *Journal of Clinical Child & Adolescent Psychology, 32*(4), 499–508. https://doi.org/10.1207/S15374424JCCP3204_2

Schwoeri, L., Sholevar, P., & Combs, M. (2003). Impact of culture and ethnicity on family interventions. In G. P. Sholevar & L. A. Schwoeri (Eds.), *Textbook of family & couples therapy: Clinical applications* (pp. 725–745). American Psychiatric Press, Inc.

Sholevar, G. P., & Joshi, S. V. (2018). Cultural child and adolescent psychiatry. In A. Martin, M. Bloch, & F. R. Volkmar (Eds.), *Lewis's child and adolescent psychiatry* (pp. 111–122). Wolters Kluwer.

Sosinsky, L. S., Gilliam, W. S., & Mayer, L. C. (2018). The preschool child. In A. Martin, M. Bloch, & F. R. Volkmar (Eds.), *Lewis's child and adolescent psychiatry* (pp. 79–85). Wolters Kluwer.

Stevenson, H. W., Azuma, H., & Hakuta, K. (1986). *Child development and education in Japan.* Freeman.

Telingator, C. J., Boyum, E. N., & Daniolos, P. T. (2018). Sexual minority youth: Identity, roles, and orientation. In A. Mart, M. Bloch, & F. R. Volkmar (Eds.), *Lewis's essentials of child and adolescent psychiatry* (pp. 138–148). Wolters Kluwer.

Tseng, W. S., & Streltzer, J. (Eds.). (2004). *Cultural competence in clinical psychiatry* (pp. 2–6). American Psychiatric Publishing.

U.S. Public Health Service. (2000). *Report of the Surgeon General's Conference on Children's Mental Health: A National Action Agenda.* Department of Health and Human Services.

Suggested Readings

Aber, J. L., Jones, S. M., & Cohen, J. (2000). The impact of poverty on the mental health and development of very young children. In C. H. Zeanah (Ed.), *Handbook of infant mental health* (pp. 113–128). The Guilford Press.

Baumrind, D. (1996). The discipline controversy revisited. *Family Relations, 45*(4), 405–414. https://doi .org/10.2307/585170

Briggs-Gowan, M. J., Carter, A. S., Bosson-Heenan, J., Guyer, A. E., & Horwitz, S. M. (2006). Are infant-toddler social-emotional and behavioral problems transient? *Journal of the American Academy of Child & Adolescent Psychiatry, 45*(7), 849–858. https://doi.org/10.1097/01.chi.0000220849.48650.59

Bronfenbrenner, U. (1986). Ecology of the family as a context for human development: Research perspectives. *Developmental Psychology, 22*(6), 723–742. https://doi.org/10.1037/0012-1649.22.6.723

Brooks-Gunn, J., & Duncan, G. J. (1997). The effects of poverty on children. *Future of Children, 7*(2), 55–71. https://doi.org/10.2307/1602387

Cameron, J. L. (2004). Interrelationships between hormones, behavior, and affect during adolescence: Understanding hormonal, physical, and brain changes occurring in association with pubertal activation of the reproductive axis. *Annals of the New York Academy of Sciences, 1021*(1), 110–123. https:// doi.org/10.1196/annals.1308.012

Carter, A. S., Briggs-Gowan, M. J., & Davis, N. O. (2004). Assessment of young children's social-emotional development and psychopathology: Recent advances and recommendations for practice. *Journal of Child Psychology & Psychiatry & Allied Disciplines, 45*(1), 109–134. https:// doi.org/10.1046/j.0021-9630.2003.00316.x

Cauce, A. M., Hiraga, Y., Mason C., Aguilar, T., Ordonez, N., & Gonzales, N. (1992). Between a rock and a hard place: Social adjustment of biracial youth. In M. P. Root (Ed.), *Racially mixed people in America* (pp. 207–222). Sage Publishing.

Chess, S., & Thomas, A. (1986). *Temperament in clinical practice*. Guilford Press.

Cicchetti, D., Rogosch, F. A., & Toth, S. L. (1998). Maternal depressive disorder and contextual risk: Contributions to the development of attachment insecurity and behavior problems in toddlerhood. *Development and Psychopathology, 10*(2), 283–300. https://doi.org/10.1017/S0954579498001618

Collins, W. A., & Steinberg, L. (2006). Adolescent development in interpersonal context. In W. Damon & R. M. Lerner (Eds.), *Handbook of child psychology* (6th ed., Vol. 3, pp. 1003–1067). John Wiley & Sons, Inc.

Combrinck-Graham, L., Fox, G. S., & Mayes, L. C. (2005). Development of school-age children. In A. Martin & F. R. Volkmar (Eds.), *Lewis's child and adolescent psychiatry: A comprehensive textbook* (pp. 267–278). Lippincott Williams & Wilkins.

Eaton, D. K., Kann, L., Kinchen, S., Ross, J., Hawkins, J., Harris, W. A., Lowry, R., McManus, T., Chyen, D., Shanklin, S., Lim, C., Grunbaum, J. A., & Wechsler, H. (2006). Youth risk behavior surveillance— United States, 2005. *Morbidity and Mortality Weekly Report. Surveillance Summaries (Washington, D.C. : 2002), 55*(5), 1–108. https://www.cdc.gov/mmwr/preview/mmwrhtml/ss5505a1.html

Eaton, D. K., Kann, L., Kinchen, S., Shanklin, S., Ross, J., Hawkins, J., Harris, W. A., Lowry, R., McManus, T., Chyen, D., Lim, C., Whittle, L., Brener, N. D., & Wechsler, H. (2010). Youth risk behavior surveillance— United States, 2009. *Morbidity and Mortality Weekly Report. Surveillance Summaries (Washington, D.C. : 2002), 59*(5), 1–142. https://www.cdc.gov/mmwr/preview/mmwrhtml/ss5905a1.html

Gilligan, C. (1982). *In a different voice: Psychological theory and women's development*. Harvard University Press.

Graham, L. C., & Fox, G. S. (2018). Development of school age children. In A. Martin, M. Bloch, & F. R. Volkmar (Eds.), *Lewis's child and adolescent psychiatry* (pp. 85–99). Wolters Kluwer.

Hart, B., & Risley, T. R. (1995). *Meaningful differences in the everyday experience of young American children*. Paul H. Brookes Publishing.

King, R. A., & Rutherford, H. J. W. (2018). Adolescence. In A. Martin, M. Bloch, & F. R. Volkmar (Eds.), *Lewis's child and adolescent psychiatry* (pp. 95–110). Wolters Kluwer.

Lerner, R., & Steinberg, L. (2004). *Handbook of adolescent psychology* (2nd ed., pp. 45–84). John Wiley & Sons, Inc.

Lewis-Fernández, R., Aggarwal, N. K., Hinton, L., Hinton, D. E., & Kirmayer, L. J. (2016). *DSM-5® handbook on the cultural formulation interview*. American Psychiatric Press, Inc.

Mayes, L. C. (1995). The assessment and treatment of the psychiatric needs of medically compromised infants: Consultation with preterm infants and their families. *Child and Adolescent Psychiatric Clinics of North America, 4*(3), 555–569. https://doi.org/10.1016/S1056-4993(18)30419-X

Mayes, L. C., Gilliam, W. S., & Stout Sosinsky, L. (2007a). The infant and toddler. In A. Martin & F. R. Volkmar (Eds.), *Lewis's child and adolescent psychiatry* (4th ed., pp. 252–260). Lippincott Williams & Wilkins.

Mayes, L. C., Gilliam, W. S., & Stout Sosinsky, L. (2007b). The preschool child. In A. Martin & F. R. Volkmar (Eds.), *Lewis's child and adolescent psychiatry* (4th ed., pp. 261–266). Lippincott Williams & Wilkins.

Mayes, L. C., Gilliam, W. S., & Stout Sosinsky, L. (2018). The infant and toddler. In A. Martin, M. Bloch, & F. R. Volkmar (Eds.), *Lewis's child and adolescent psychiatry* (pp. 70–78). Wolters Kluwer.

Petrill, S. A., Plomin, R., Defries, J. C., & Hewitt, J. K. (2003). *Nature, nurture and the transition to early adolescence.* Oxford University Press and Lippincott Williams & Wilkins.

Reiss, D., Plomin, R., Neiderhiser, J. M., & Hetherington, E. M. (2003). *The relationship code: Deciphering genetic and social influences on adolescent development (adolescent lives).* Harvard University Press.

Rutter, M. (1982). *Fifteen thousand hours: Secondary schools and their effects on children.* Harvard University Press.

Sameroff, A. J. (1987). The social context of development. In N. Eisenberg (Ed.), *Contemporary topics in development* (pp. 167–189). John Wiley & Sons, Inc.

Shaskank, A. P., & Joshi, S. V. (2018). Cultural child and adolescent psychiatry. In A. Martin, M. Bloch, & F. R. Volkmar (Eds.), *Lewis's child and adolescent psychiatry* (pp. 111–122). Wolters Kluwer.

Shaw, P., Greenstein, D., Lerch, J., Clasen, L., Lenroot, R., Gogtay, N., Evans, A., Rapoport J., & Giedd, J. (2006). Intellectual ability and cortical development in children and adolescents. *Nature, 440*(7084), 676–679. https://doi.org/10.1038/nature04513

Shonkoff, J. P., & Phillips, D. A. (2000). *From neurons to neighborhoods: The science of early childhood development.* National Academy Press.

Sosinsky, L. S., & Gilliam, W. S. (2014). Child care: How pediatricians can support children and families. In R. M. Kliegman, R. E. Behrman, H. B. Jenson, & B. F. Stanton (Eds.), *Nelson textbook of pediatrics* (20th ed., pp. 101–106.). Elsevier.

Sosinsky, L. S., Gilliam, W. S., & Mayes, L. C. (2005). The preschool child. In A. Martin & F. R. Volkmar (Eds.), *Lewis's child and adolescence psychiatry: A comprehensive textbook* (pp. 261–266). Lippincott Williams & Wilkins.

Sroufe, L., & Rutter, M. (1984). The domain of developmental psychopathology. *Child Development, 55*(1), 17–29. https://doi.org/10.2307/1129832

Steinberg, L. (2004). Risk taking in adolescence: What changes, and why? *Annals of the New York Academy of Sciences, 1021,* 51–58. https://doi.org/10.1196/annals.1308.005

Super, C. M. (1976). Environmental effects on motor development: The case of "African infant precocity." *Developmental Medicine & Child Neurology, 18*(5), 561–567. https://doi.org/10.1111/j.1469-8749.1976.tb04202.x

Super, C. M. (1980). Behavioral development in infancy. In R. L. Munroe, R. H. Munroe, & B. B. Whiting (Eds.), *Handbook of cross-cultural human development* (pp. 177–189). Garland Press.

Vygotsky, L. (1978). Tool and symbol in child development and internalization of higher psychological functions. In M. Cole, V. John-Steiner, S. Scribner, & E. Souberman (Eds.), *Mind in society* (p. 20). Harvard University Press.

Wolf, A. E. (1991). *Get out of my life, but first could you drive me and Cheryl to the mall?: A parent's guide to the new teenager.* Noonday Press.

CHAPTER 3 ■ SCIENTIFIC FOUNDATIONS OF THE FIELD

■ INTRODUCTION

As we discussed in Chapter 1, the field of developmental psychopathology has diverse roots and origins. In this chapter, we discuss some aspects of the scientific basis of the field with an emphasis on research design, the role of evidence, and epidemiology.

Morgan et al. (2018) provide an excellent review of the scientific method and research approaches. As they note, research has the goals of increasing both knowledge and clinical competence. As a general rule, for research to be regarded of the highest quality it must be peer-reviewed in a scientific journal. This means that scientifically informed peers (other researchers and clinicians) have reviewed (typically in a double-blind fashion to preserve author and reviewer anonymity) a paper for a journal and the editor then accepts, rejects, or asks for revision of the paper. This process can be tedious and has its problems but is, at present, the best and most widely used approach to vetting new scientific information. The growing reliance on serious peer-reviewed research is a major advance since the first publication by Leo Kanner of a text book in the field (Kanner, 1935). We talk more about the role of research evidence subsequently, but it is important to understand that the scientific process does not end with one paper. To be regarded as evidence based, we require multiple papers (from different places and groups) that replicate and often extend a finding. In this way, science gradually and incrementally builds knowledge.

The field of child mental health faces several complications in doing research. In some ways, the most complex and challenging work is the more basic science in areas like genetics and neurobiology, but in other ways the most complicated is the actual work with children, their parents, and teachers. This underscores the problems of having at least three potential informants for any child during a study—that is, the child, the parents, and the teacher. Some measures, like blood pressure or galvanic skin response are less subject to the problem of differences in observations and data collected, but other measures, such as questionnaires filled out by different responders, can result in highly different views depending on the nature of the study. A similar issue relates to whether we ought to rely on observed behavior or on self-reports. For some purposes, either one or both may be needed. Depending on how the study is done (e.g., with or without a control group), it may be important to think about the impact of just being in a study itself on data obtained (Shapiro & Shapiro, 2000). A whole other set of issues arise relative to qualitative compared to quantitative research.

There is a large body of work on the analysis of quantitative data (Patton, 2002). Qualitative data are more subjective in nature, for example, the child's perception of pain or of their feelings about a treatment approach (see Merriam & Tisbell, 2016). Qualitative data are typically gathered from interviews and observations, and investigators do not necessarily go on to try to apply rigorous statistical methods of analysis given the nature of the data obtained. It is important to emphasize that self-report data and ratings of behaviors or mental states by others (such as a parent rating their child's anxiety) can be quantitative or qualitative in nature. Investigators working with quantitative data are more able to apply simple and some more sophisticated statistical analyses to help understand the meaning of the data they collect. Often, they will be attempting to prove some specific idea or hypothesis.

Research usually begins with a question about a problem or issue of some kind: for example, will exercise improve adolescent depression? A host of different measures and variables might be of relevance to a study looking to address this. These might include ratings of depressed mood as well as age, gender, social status, and ethnicity of the child and family. History of depression, rating scales of depression (from the child), and reports from parents and teachers can provide many additional variables for analysis.

Data analysis for quantitative researchers usually involves well-defined statistical methods, often providing a test of the null hypothesis (i.e., no true differences are observed). Qualitative researchers are more interested in examining their data for similarities or themes that might occur among participants on a particular topic. There is always a tension between how strictly one limits the subject group and how narrowly you define the problem. If you only study boys, for example, you cannot necessarily say much about girls. There is also a tension over how little or how much information you obtain. Variables can themselves be of various types, for example, they can be continuous like age or IQ, or they can be categorical like meeting criteria for the diagnosis of depression or not.

As researchers begin to design a study, they consider both independent and dependent variables. Independent variables have to do with things like disorder status (positive or negative) whereas dependent variables have to do with the things we measure and expect to change in response to the independent variables. Thus, the independent variables are presumed to involve antecedent or possible causes of effects that we can measure in the dependent variable(s) selected (Gliner et al., 2017). Variables can also be extraneous (i.e., things not of interest to the particular study). Morgan et al. (2018) provide an excellent summary of aspects of research variables and simple methods of data description and analyses. They note that there are a number of easy ways to visually depict (plot) data that can be highly informative. Depending on the nature of the distribution of the data, statistics like measures of central tendency may be very helpful, for example, average, median, and mode as well as measures of the variation within the data like the standard deviation. For some data, for example, categorical (present/absent, yes/no) or rank order data, for example, educational attainment levels, other kinds of statistical approaches apply (see Shadish et al., 2002).

Another set of issues has to do with different types of reliability and validity in research studies. There are several kinds of reliability: interrater reliability (agreement between two observations), test–retest reliability (how stable scores are over time), and internal consistency (how well items on a test "hang together" [i.e., correlate] with each other) as well as several others (Morgan et al., 2006). In child mental health, we have the problem of differences in reporting as well as stability of scores and changes over time. A test might work well for adults but not for children. In the past there were simple approaches to assessing reliability, for example, percent agreement scores or sometimes correlations but the field has become much more sophisticated with statistics used that take chance agreement levels into account. These more robust statistics provide us with better measures to assess the instruments used in work in child mental health (Morgan et al., 2006). As the field of developmental psychopathology matures, there is also continuing refinement of research tools. For example, there is now growing recognition and appreciation of the need to collect information from multiple sources and that each informant contributes a valuable perspective (De Los Reyes et al., 2015).

The notion of validity has to do with establishing that what we are measuring truly does capture what we intend it to: for example, does a dimensional assessment of parent-reported attention-deficit hyperactivity disorder symptoms really capture how the child behaves in the classroom? Again, there are various kinds of validity and various statistical approaches to its measurement (e.g., face validity, convergent validity, divergent validity). It is possible to have a test with good reliability that is not particularly valid, for example, picking a test on which the child cannot perform the tasks at all will result in highly reliable measures (child consistently scores very low) that do not tell us much about the child's actual abilities.

Researchers try to use instruments that are well established and have high reliability and validity—and although never perfect, using these well-established measures helps ensure appropriate study design. As the measures are changed or extended in any way, for example, with a new population, different age, or different language, all these measurement issues have to be considered anew.

Quantitative research methods are of various types and can include randomized clinical trials as well as quasi-experimental descriptive and other experimental approaches (Merriam & Tisbell, 2016). The analysis of data from this kind of research tests relationships between variables and helps us answer research questions and address specific hypotheses: for example, drug X will significantly improve obsessive–compulsive disorder symptoms. For a study like this, a double-blind randomized placebo-controlled study would be the best because it provides appropriate guidance about inferring cause and effect. In a typical randomized controlled study, patients would be randomly assigned to one of two or more groups such that one group might receive the active drug (the medication of interest) while another group receives a placebo (a "sham" medication that is not expected to have any "real" effect). In this case, the independent variable is the group assignment (drug/placebo) whereas the dependent measure is the rating scale score measuring change in the severity of symptoms after treatment. Random assignment is critically important. Given ethical concerns, often at the end of a treatment trial, the "blind" will be broken, and, if effective, the drug may be offered to those who received the placebo. Other kinds of studies may be based on associations or descriptive work—these kinds of studies often precede more hypothesis-driven and rigorous randomized clinical trials. A whole set of preliminary studies would, for example, first be done in evaluating any drug before it ever reaches the stage for a rigorous placebo-controlled clinical trial (see Chapter 29). Of note, having either more than one randomized controlled clinical trial, or one large trial with multiple sites, is often very helpful in firmly establishing the evidence base of an intervention. Having a replication in a different site is a good way to ensure that the results obtained are substantive and not because of chance findings at one site.

There are several kinds of questions that can be addressed in research studies and several different approaches to study design. A hypothesis is essentially a research question about the relationship between two variables, for example, that our hypothetical drug X will improve functioning in patients with obsessive–compulsive disorder. Randomized experiments offer us the strongest evidence but quasi-experiments are also useful in giving us important information. As Morgan et al. (2018) discuss, there are many different experimental designs, some of which are much stronger than others. The choice of design raises important issues as researchers consider what their goals are and what specific questions they want to address (see Gliner et al., 2017 for discussion). Results of simple descriptive studies can inform research that adopts more rigorous controls for sources of potential bias. Depending on the nature of the design, some studies use within-subject scores or measures whereas others use between-subject measures (or sometimes both). The issues of research design are complex but very important in interpreting the results investigators obtain. Issues of sample selection and sample size are important. There are both type 1 and type 2 errors that can potentially be made. The significant values obtained in statistical analysis help protect us (partially) from making these errors. A type 1 error happens when we observe an apparent difference that really is not there, whereas a type 2 error occurs when we do not see a real difference that is there, because our study was poorly done or underpowered. The role of statistical power is an important one. For some observed effects, the strength of the effect is quite strong and even a small sample would be likely to show a statistical result; in other studies, the effect itself may be important but hard to detect and larger samples may be needed for these studies. There are ways to estimate statistical power (Cohen, 1988) as well as effect size and these are frequently used as research projects are designed. There are also good methods for assessment of the strength of an association observed beyond statistical significance. It is important to realize that what might be a statistically significant result may have little or no *clinical* significance. This can be a real problem with very large studies where chance makes for fluke findings. Of course, yet another potential source of errors, particularly for correlational approaches, is the fact that even if things are correlated that does not mean they are causally connected. For example, road temperature and lemonade consumption both go up in summer and are strongly correlated but not causally connected (both having more to do with overall temperature). A whole body of work exists focused on helping evaluate the strengths of results obtained and comparing results across studies (meta-analyses). Meta-analytic studies summarize and synthesize results of a series of studies using quantitative measures (Lipsey & Wilson, 2000). A whole body of work in medicine and other fields has used meta-analyses to help us evaluate possible treatments and whether or not they are effective. Several independent groups now routinely conduct these studies to help establish what treatments work (see evidence-based treatments later in this chapter). These offer important insights into how important findings really are. Although meta-analyses are useful, it is important to realize that they have faced some criticisms. It can be argued that combining data from different studies, even if seemingly matching in certain parameters, can sometimes yield misleading results.

Meta-analyses usually end up producing estimates of effect sizes, that is, measures of how statistically strong the results are. These can be assessed in other studies as well. Various statistics can be used to assess the strength of an effect. Particularly in behavioral studies, a strong or large effect size can provide a good indication of clinical significance. For psychotherapy research, for example, to have at least a moderate or stronger effect size is desirable. Treatments that have small effect sizes are often not regarded as really supported by evidence-based reviews (see Cohen, 1988).

■ EVIDENCE-BASED PRACTICES AND TREATMENTS

Implementation of evidence-based treatments has been an important theme in child mental health—in medicine, psychology, education, and related areas (Hamilton, 2018). Most of the actual clinical work occurs either in private practice or larger clinical settings such as community mental health clinics. The transfer of knowledge about effective mental health treatments from research settings where these treatments are developed and tested to clinical settings where these treatments are delivered to children can be a challenging process. In this section, we address issues for implementation of evidence-based treatments.

As Hamilton (2018) points out, there are several somewhat overlapping terms used in describing similar concepts: *evidence-based practice, evidence-based medicine, and evidence-based treatments/services*. Not surprisingly, *evidence-based medicine* tends to be the term used by child psychiatrists and pediatricians and is very relevant to use of medications (see Chapter 20). The term *evidence-based treatment* is more common among psychologists and is often used relative to psychotherapy or psychosocial treatments referring to better use of empirical results to improve outcomes. *Evidence-based services* and *evidence-based treatment* are the terms more commonly used in interdisciplinary treatment settings. The more general term *evidence-based practice* encompasses all these uses and thus ranges from understanding the strength of evidence supporting a treatment to its implementation in the individual case. It is worth noting that in psychology in particular, there is often an emphasis on using clearly described and rigorously implemented psychosocial or behavioral approaches as part of evidence-based treatments. This is partly because of research requirements that treatments are well defined and can be replicated by others. Given the potential for discipline-based terms to acquire highly specialized definitions within their respective disciplines, in clinical contexts, particularly interdisciplinary ones, the more general term *evidence-based practice* is usually preferred. It is very apt given the general agreement of the interdisciplinary treatment team that the care of the individual child and family, in light of all the available evidence, is the goal of the treatment plan.

One of the advantages of current digital technologies for all providers is ready access to information that evaluates treatment, and to treatment studies themselves. However, as the field of developmental psychopathology matures, new specialized treatments emerge and require use of very specific instruments or measures requiring significant training. This expertise and specialization can be more readily found in a university clinical research setting or even in a larger group practice setting but does become more challenging for the individual provider. A major increase in randomized controlled trials (RCTs) over the recent past is illustrated in Hamilton (2018). Similar increases have been seen in meta-analyses and systematic reviews that, along with RCTs, provide the fuel for making evidence-based recommendations.

There is a hierarchy of types of evidence with the strongest being RCTs and meta-analyses, to controlled studies, to case series, and finally to single cases and anecdotal clinical reports. The last category is not unimportant but clearly carries much less weight than the more scientifically informed studies. Case studies present their own complexities in that there is a tendency for only positive associations to be published (e.g., finding that syndrome X is associated with autism might be published but a paper that is titled syndrome X is *not* associated with autism is unlikely to see the light of day).

Sometimes, it is argued that rigorous research methods (Rutter et al., 1994) do not have applicability to something as individualized as psychotherapy, but, as Hamilton points out, evidence-based methods have been very effectively used to demonstrate positive effects and to help disentangle these effects (Hamilton, 2018). The importance and feasibility of conducting evidence-based practice in real-world settings have been illustrated in studies of psychotherapy with children and adolescents (Bickman et al., 1999; Weisz & Jensen, 1999). For example, data from an evidence-based system in Hawaii (the Hawaii's Child and Adolescent Mental Health Division [CAMHD]) offers a useful case in point (Daleiden & Chorpita, 2005). As Hamilton (2018) notes, there is an important backstory to the CAMHD program, starting with a federal court decision mandating an effective system of care as the stimulus for establishing a more integrated mental health and special education approach with more access for youth to a wide range of services. The initial system response to the court's decree included planning efforts and increases in service capacity, allowing more youth to access a wider variety of services, increased monitoring, and the agreement and commitment of all concerned to an awareness of evidence-based practices (Daleiden, 2004).

Two approaches are often used in understanding the overall benefits and risks of treatments and these can be used in child mental health as in other aspects of medicine. The *number needed to treat* refers to the number of individual cases you need to treat to prevent one additional bad outcome (e.g., suicide attempt, incarceration, or some other explicit indicator). This is usually expressed as a whole number and is typically done in studies with a control group. So, for example, in the treatment for adolescents with depression study, this number was 4 for the use of active medicine (fluoxetine) alone but 3 when you combined medication with cognitive behavior therapy (see Hamilton, 2018 for a detailed discussion). A different metric, the *number needed to harm* gives information on the average number of individuals who are exposed to some risk who are actually caused harm (as operationally defined over some period of time). Both numbers are usually given with a 95% confidence interval (see Hamilton, 2018 for a more extended discussion).

With the advent of evidence-based interventions and good search engines as well as free and ready access to the national library of medicine's PubMed service, most clinicians have ready access to scientific information. As Hamilton (2018) reviews extensively, it is good to have some awareness of the potential pitfalls of literature searching in evaluating available evidence. For the university-affiliated clinician, scholarly resources are readily at hand. However, a simple internet search that a patient or family is often inclined to do is several steps below a search of information like that documented in PubMed (although there are some important cautionary notes even there) and can quickly lead to misguided information, particularly in the area of mental health. For example, at the time of this writing, typing the word *autism* into Google gives about 200,000,000 hits whereas a search for autism in PubMed or some other scholarly base may show more like 40,000 peer-reviewed articles. As one can imagine, this staggering complexity is a problem for parents and youth searching for valid information. Sadly, going by the top 100 "greatest hits" is complex because a number of sites are shown that make baseless claims or ask for money to produce results (Reichow et al., 2014). As a general rule, websites that end in *.edu* or *.gov* provide potential consumers of mental health services the best information. Clinicians should be prepared these days to discuss with their patients the importance of evaluating the science behind any intervention.

There are several additional important potential sources of information. The Cochrane collaboration is named in honor of the British epidemiologist Archie Cochrane, whose 1972 book *Effectiveness and Efficiency: Random Reflections on Health Services* was a landmark in the development of clinical trials research. Cochrane was very concerned with understanding what treatments were to be regarded as well established, inefficacious or unproven, or contraindicated using the scientific evidence provided in a clinical trial. The collaboration named in his honor conducts independent research assessments on various topics with rigorous guidelines for authors who engage in these reviews and the Cochrane Database of Systematic Reviews (CDSR) has become an outstanding online resource. Some of the most useful databases and clinical resources are summarized in Table 3.1.

The issues of diagnosis are of course important ones in understanding research and these issues are addressed in this book in respective chapters on childhood psychiatric disorders and in Chapter 4 on classification and assessment. As Hamilton (2018) also notes, there is no single answer to the best approaches to diagnosis given that many different instruments are available as are the diagnostic guidelines provided by the *Diagnostic and Statistical Manual of Mental Health*. It also should be noted that implementing evidence-based treatments in complex clinical settings is not an easy task but one that does have important rewards of greater benefits for children and their families (Ferlie & Dopson, 2005).

■ PROTECTING CHILDREN IN RESEARCH

As a result of several convergent lines of research that abused human rights, a series of landmark events and reports, beginning with the Nuremberg trials after World War II, have articulated clearly some basic principles of conducting human subject research. Special issues arise for children (and others who cannot necessarily give fully informed consent like special needs populations). These issues have to do with respect for persons as autonomous individuals, balancing risks and benefits, obtaining truly informed consent for participation, ethical and scientific approval of the research proposed, assent of any minors involved, privacy and confidentiality, and any ongoing obligations the investigator may have toward the child and family—among others. As Levine summarizes (2018), there are a number of important federal laws and regulations relevant to this process, and, in research settings, an institutional review board or some other such agency is typically constituted to review and monitor research protocols. It is very important that those involved in research with children are aware of all these requirements.

■ EPIDEMIOLOGY

Epidemiologic methods have an important role in child mental health. They help in monitoring trends in developmental and psychiatric disorders in children, provide information on a host of relevant population health factors, and identify potential risk factors for conditions. Fombonne (2018) provides an excellent and more detailed review of the topic. As he notes, and as we touch on in various chapters, there are several major issues for epidemiology in dealing with child mental health problems. These include the need for multiple informants who may, and often do, disagree with each other, problems in clinical definition, the complexity of comorbidity (having more than one disorder at a time), and developmental factors (normal changes over time and the impact of development on [Rutter, 1997] clinical expression). Epidemiology is mostly observational in nature and descriptive epidemiology is centered

TABLE 3.1

Useful Databases: URLs and Availability

Site/URL	Sources/ Abstracts (A) Full Text (FT)	Classification System Used	Strengths	Weaknesses
PubMed http://www.ncbi.nlm.nih .gov/entrez/query.fcgi	Extensive medical journal base A, some FT	MeSH terms	MeSH allows specific searching	*DSM* disorders not always MeSH terms
PubMed Clinical Queries http://www.ncbi.nlm. nih.gov/entrez/query/ static/clinical.shtml	Same as PubMed	Same	Filters allow either searching for RCTs only or more sensitive search	Systematic review less well defined than in CDSR
MeSH Database http://www.ncbi.nlm .nih.gov/entrez/query .fcgi?db=mesh	MeSH "tree" of terms	Branching "tree" of terms	Allows searching with controlled vocabulary	Excludes many less medical terms (e.g., bullying)
PsycINFO, PsycARTICLES http://www.psycinfo. com/psycarticles/	Extensive psychology journal base A, fee-based FT	Index terms classification keywords	Allows very specific searching (e.g., bullying)	No RCT filter Variable quality "Publication type" filter not crisp
CRCT http://www .cochranelibrary.com/ cochrane-database-of-systematic-reviews/	All RCTs No A or FT unless UK, Australia	Keyword	Immediate discovery of RCTs on subject; uniform data presentation	Mostly via institutions in United States No charge in UK, Australia, Latin America
CDSR http://www .cochranelibrary.com/ about/central-landing-page.html	Only if SR completed A but no FT	Keyword	Uniform data presentation Updated	Limited regarding child psychiatry
JAACAP www.jaacap.com	JAACAP to 1995 A. FT also if AACAP member	Keyword	Full text option Highly specific Included in AACAP membership	Limited to one journal No filters
EBMH Online http://ebmh.bmjjournals .com/	EB Mental Health. First 150 words available; FT requires subscription	Keyword	Preappraised evidence only	Requires subscription for full access; mixed with adult literature

CDSR, Cochrane Database of Systematic Reviews; RCT, randomized controlled trial.
Reprinted with permission from Hamilton, J. (2018). Evidence-based practice as a conceptual framework. In A. Martin, M. Block, & F. R. Volkmar (Eds.), *Lewis's child and adolescent psychiatry: A comprehensive textbook* (5th ed., p. 189). Wolters Kluwer.

on rates of disease, whereas analytic epidemiology is more concerned with identification of risk and potential etiologies of disease. Clinical epidemiology studies various factors that are involved in the expression of disease and the factors that predict outcome.

The field began in the 1800s with the first appreciation of how cholera was being transmitted in London through contaminated drinking water in only certain community wells (Johnson, 2006). In psychiatry, early work focused on issues like suicide, and, in medicine, on topics like the association of smoking and lung cancer. Over the past decades, epidemiology has become much more sophisticated in its approaches to understanding health and mental health problems. Historically, the interest in child mental health disorders began with the work of Rutter and his collogues in the 1960s when they studied children on the Isle of Wight (Rutter, 1989, 1997; Rutter et al., 1976). They used a two-stage approach with a large population screen followed by a more focused assessment of a subsample of cases. This landmark series of studies became a model for subsequent work particularly in its attention to issues of reliability and validity, multiple informants, and longitudinal change.

Incidence is the rate of new cases in a population over a specific time period. Incidence rates can be complicated to interpret and thus cumulative incidence is often used. This is determined by taking the number of all new cases over a total population for a period of time. This number can be used to predict risk of a disease over some period of time. In contrast, the term *prevalence* refers to the proportion of a population who have a specific characteristic in a given time period. Prevalence thus is concerned with disease status rather than onset. It tells us what part of the population at any given time has an illness. Various forms of prevalence are identified. One might, for example, be interested in lifetime prevalence of a disorder like schizophrenia or in estimates of prevalence by intervals of 3, 6, or 9 months for mood disorders.

Different kinds of approaches to epidemiologic research exist. In cohort studies, a group of individuals is followed over some period of time, for example, studies of smokers who go on to develop lung cancer. These studies can be expensive to conduct, especially for disorders that are present at very low rates. Case control studies compare two groups of cases, for example, those with and without a specific condition relative to some feature or features. The selection of control groups is a major complication for this kind of study. Cross-sectional studies examine large and epidemiologically representative samples evaluating illnesses/disease status at various points in time so that estimates of prevalence rates can be obtained as cases are followed. These kinds of studies can also examine variables like gender, social class, urban versus rural setting, and so forth.

Complications for epidemiologic studies include things like the impact of treatment, difficulties of early diagnosis, and so forth. Ecologic studies focus on the group rather than the individual, for example, the classroom, the neighborhood, or counties to compare rates of illness or difficulties. Although comparisons of rates across locations might seem simple, a number of problems arise, for example, there may be unappreciated confounding variables. However, these comparisons are relatively easy to make. Other kinds of design are available as well.

In epidemiologic studies, issues of sampling are critical and sampling techniques are based on computational models of varying degrees of complexity (Fombonne, 2018). In some countries, like Denmark, and to a lesser extent other European Economic Community countries, case registries and electronic databases are maintained that help facilitate access, particularly to potential patient populations, and these can be particularly useful for less common disorders.

Statistical and Sample Considerations

Error of various kinds can reduce the precision of estimates obtained. A common approach to deal with this issue is to increase the size of the sample studied. This does, of course, involve a tradeoff given the costs entailed in larger samples. Missing data present another problem for research involving longitudinal studies. There may be specific factors that impact dropout rates (Fombonne, 2018). Various statistical approaches can be helpful in evaluating results obtained in epidemiologic studies, for example, the use of confidence intervals or odds ratios gives us some sense of how much confidence we can have in the results obtained. When epidemiologists observe an association, for example, of a risk factor with an illness, it is important to evaluate the strength of the effect observed—usually designated as small, medium, or large. Small effects may still be meaningful, particularly on the population level, but as we have discussed earlier, detecting small statistical effects requires large samples. And it is also possible that very large samples might yield statistically significant small effects that might not be easy to interpret in clinically meaningful ways.

Different kinds of bias can also impact results obtained in epidemiologic studies. This might include selection biases because some groups might be less likely to participate in the study than others, or differential dropout in longitudinal research where some groups of subjects might be more likely to discontinue their participation than other groups. Another kind of bias arises as a result of subject movement, for example, migration into or out of a specific area and loss of subjects to study. Issues of selection bias are a special problem for case control studies. Measurement errors, classification errors, and recall bias are some other examples of biases that epidemiologists have to grapple with. Finally, confounding variables are ones that might lead to overestimates or underestimates of association. The ultimate meaning of all these research issues is that replication of studies is always important to increase confidence in any given result.

Sensitivity/Specificity—Issues for Screening and Diagnostic Instruments

The issue of best approaches to screening for mental health disorders in epidemiologic studies is a complex one. Increasingly, there are searches for potential biomarkers of specific mental health conditions, but, in the meantime, most screening instruments are assessed relative to some standard—for example, the diagnosis by an experienced clinician. Primary screeners are usually focused on more general issues, for example, developmental delay, whereas secondary screeners focus on specific conditions like attention-deficit hyperactivity disorder or autism. As noted by Fombonne (2018), schools are often used as a location for screening studies but other approaches to recruitment are available, for example, focusing on households (Bird et al., 1988). It is typical for screening instruments to yield some score that then can be categorized into disorder present or absent. One of the major goals of data analyses for these instruments is determining what scores/thresholds work the best relative to some standard. This gives us an end result of a table that shows disorder present or absent as compared to the result of the specific test/instrument. (See Table 3.2.)

This two-by-two table presents the calculation of several important descriptive statistics: sensitivity (the number of true positives assessed as positive), specificity (the number of

TABLE 3.2

Typical Results of a Screening Exercise

	Cases D	Normal $\bar{D}$	
Test positive: T+	a	b	a + b
Test negative: T−	c	d	c + d
	a + c	b + d	a + b + c + d = N

True positives: TP = a False negatives: FN = c D = diseased
False positives: FP = b True negatives: TN = d $\bar{D}$ = nondiseased
Sensitivity (or rate of true positives: RTP): Se = a/a + c = p(T + /D)
Specificity (or rate of true negatives: RTN): Sp = d/b + d = p(T − /$\bar{D}$)
Rate of false negatives: RFN = c/a + c = p(T − /D)
Rate of false positives: RFP = b/b + d = p(T + /$\bar{D}$)
Prevalence: P = a + c/N = p(D)
Positive predictive value: PPV = a/a + b = p(D/T+)
Negative predictive value: NPV = d/c + d = p($\bar{D}$/T−)

Reprinted with permission from Fombonne, E. (2018). Epidemiology. In A. Martin, M. Block, & F. R. Volkmar (Eds.), *Lewis's child and adolescent psychiatry: A comprehensive textbook* (5th ed., p. 218). Wolters Kluwer.

true negatives relative to those assessed negative), and a number of other important test descriptors. There are always tradeoffs in developing assessment instruments and screeners, but the general goal is to have a good balance of sensitivity and specificity; in some situations, one or the other of these may be the most important although usually a reasonable balance is sought (see Fombonne, 2018). Depending on how a study is done and a sample obtained, there may be a major gap in terms of generalizing results to the greater population.

Survey Instruments and Rates of Psychopathology

The planning of epidemiologic studies requires precise methods to ascertain "cases" of the disorder being studied (Verhulst & Koot, 1995; Achenbach & Edelbrock, 1981). A definition of "caseness" must be adopted and is very much central to the study goals. For example, a survey of autism to identify representative cases for inclusion in genetic studies will require detailed phenotypic assessments, precise diagnostic subtyping, and exclusion of autistic syndromes associated with known medical disorders. If, on the other hand, the goal of the autism survey is to generate estimates of special educational needs for service planning, then a less restrictive and broader approach to caseness may be more suitable. Following the adoption of the most appropriate concept of the disorder, decisions must be made about the choice of various assessment procedures and instruments to evaluate caseness in study participants.

As we discuss in Chapter 4, both dimensional and categorical approaches are used in studies of epidemiology (as well as in clinical work). The dimensional approaches, for example, severity of anxiety, add an important metric of severity and also let investigators estimate the best approaches to establish cutoff points for categorical estimates of disorder. As Fombonne (2018) points out, it is important to realize that survey and interviews, as well as dimensional instruments, can be used for both purposes, for example, of categorical and dimensional approaches.

A number of excellent instruments are available to use in epidemiologic work with children. These include instruments focused on specific disorders, for example, Tourette's or obsessive–compulsive disorder, as well as more general ratings scales such as Achenbach's Child Behavior Checklist, one of the oldest more general ones that remains in common use both for research and clinical work (Achenbach & Rescorla, 2000). Other instruments developed for children focus more specifically on *DSM* diagnosis, for example, the diagnostic interview for children and adolescents (Reich, 2000).

Epidemiologic studies typically find high rates of behavioral problems but the relationships of specific problems to disorders can be difficult to sort out. Some problem behaviors, such as suicidal thoughts, may be important to understand and identify because these have much stronger relationships to clinical referral, even when the rest of the symptoms of possible psychiatric disorders cannot be ascertained in epidemiologic studies.

Clearly, psychopathology (as variously defined) is relatively common in children and youth (see Table 3.3), with most studies suggesting prevalence rates of 10% to 20%.

In their review of a number of studies, Verhulst and Koot (1995) found an overall rate of about 13% with a relatively even balance between emotional and behavioral problems. As Fombonne (2018) points out, many of these surveys do not include information on children and youth with neurodevelopmental problems such as intellectual disability; so, even though we know these groups do indeed have significant mental health difficulties in addition to their neurodevelopmental problems (see Chapters 6–9), the exact rates are difficult to ascertain. If the focus shifts to use of mental health services, it becomes apparent that children and youth with behavioral problems are common users of mental health services (Fombonne, 2018). This underscores that clinical samples are not necessarily representative of the larger population.

■ CONCLUSION

In this chapter, we have reviewed aspects of the scientific method as they relate to designing and conducting studies most relevant to this field of developmental psychopathology. These include how we frame the questions we ask or hypotheses, what measures we use, and how we go about doing the study as well as getting informed consent. For work on developmental

TABLE 3.3

Prevalence Findings from Recent Epidemiologic Surveys

Authors/Year	Site	Age	N	Instruments/ Diagnosis	Period	Prevalence		
						Any Emotional Disorder	Any Behavioral Disorder	Any Disorder
Anderson et al. (1987)	Dunedin, New Zealand	11	925	DISC-C/DSM-III	1 year	7.3	11.6	17.6
Offord et al. (1987)	Ontario, Canada	4–16	2679	Structured interview/ DSM-III like	6 month	—	—	18.1
Bird et al. (1988)	Puerto Rico	4–16	777	DISC/DSM-III	6 month	—	—	17.9
Esser et al. (1990)	Mannheim, Germany	8	1444	Clinical interview/ ICD-9	6 month	6	6	16.2
Morita et al. (1990)	Gunma Prefecture, Japan	12–15	1999	Isle of Wight interview/ICD-9	3 month	—	—	15.0
Jeffers and Fitzgerald (1991)	Dublin, Ireland	9–12	2029	Isle of Wight interview/ICD-9	3 month	—	—	25.4
Fergusson et al. (1993)	Christchurch, New Zealand	15	986	DISC/DSM-III-R	—	—	—	22.1[C] 13.0[P]
Lewinsohn et al. (1993)	Oregon, USA	16–18	1710	K-SADS/DSM-III-R	Current	—	1.8	9.6
Fombonne (1994)	Chartres, France	6–11	2441	Isle of Wight module/ICD-9	3 month	5.9[P]	6.5[P]	12.4[P]
Costello et al. (1996)	Great Smoky Mountains, North Carolina, USA	9, 11, 13	4500	CAPA/DSM-III-R	3 month	6.8	6.6	20.3
Verhulst et al. (1997)	Nationwide, Netherlands	13–18	780	DISC C & P/ DSM-III-R	6 month	—	7.9[C or P] 0.9[C & P]	35.5[C or P] 4.0[C & P]

(continued)

TABLE 3.3

Prevalence Findings from Recent Epidemiologic Surveys (*continued*)

Simonoff et al. (1997)	Virginia, USA	8–16	2762	CAPA/DSM-III-R	3 month	8.9	7.1	14.2
Steinhausen et al. (1998)	Zurich, Switzerland	7–16	1964	DISC-P/DSM-III-R	6 month	—	6.5	22.5
Breton et al. (1999)	Quebec, Canada	6–14	2400	Dominic-DISC2/DSM-III-R	6 month	—	—	19.9[P] 15.8[C]
Ford et al. (2003)	Nationwide, England and Wales	5–15	10,438	DAWBA/ICD-10	3 month	4.3 0.9[a] 3.8[b]	5.9	9.5
Costello et al. (2003)	Great Smoky Mountains, North Carolina, USA	9–16	6674	CAPA/DSM-IV	3 month	6.8[c, C or P]	7.0[C or P]	13.3[C or P]
Canino et al. (2004)	Puerto Rico	4–17	1897	DISC-IV/DSM-IV	12 month	3.4[b, C or P] 6.6.9[c, C or P]	11.1[C or P]	16.4[C or P]

C, based on child as informant; P, based on parent as informant.

[a] Any depressive disorder.

[b] Any anxiety disorder.

[c] Any serious emotional disturbance.

Reprinted with permission from Fombonne, E. (2018). Epidemiology. In A. Martin, M. Block, & F. R. Volkmar (Eds.), *Lewis's child and adolescent psychiatry: A comprehensive textbook* (5th ed., p. 213). Wolters Kluwer.

psychopathology, the processes of change and developmental issues are always a central concern. An additional major challenge is the nature of the data we work with (quantitative or qualitative) and the fact that usually we will have multiple sources of information or informants, for example, child, parent, and teacher.

As the field has progressed, we have met many challenges in understanding which treatments work and how well they work. Issues of evidence-based treatment and practice have become increasingly important. As we note, it is important not to confuse statistically significant with clinical significant. The latter is of major importance. It is also important to realize that the best kinds of data that support our confidence in results are those that come from multiple randomized placebo controlled studies (in different locations for purposes of replication) and in meta-analytic studies. In the not so distant past, evidence was what our teachers taught based on their experience and training, was the basis for clinical practice. We now know that there are much better approaches for individual practitioner and clinical teams in considering the increasing array of options open to them for treatment. When clinical groups "get it together," they can usually treat children well and document change using evidence-based approaches.

There are a number of important aspects of developmental psychopathology that require epidemiologic studies. These include the age at which the disorder first manifested (i.e., age of onset). This has often been a feature of diagnostic criteria, although it is usually retrospective and thus subject to some aspects of bias in parental recall. Prevalence rates will vary depending on age of onset and earlier onset may, at times, indicate greater severity. Yet other problems and issues arise relative to special populations, for example, how best to understand psychopathology in individuals with cognitive impairments. There are many challenges and opportunities offered by epidemiologic research to understand how risk factors, adversity, and mitigating and positive experiences interact in the expression of psychopathology.

References

Achenbach, T. M., & Edelbrock, C. S. (1981). Behavioral problems and competencies reported by parents of normal and disturbed children aged four through sixteen. *Monographs of the Society for Research in Child Development*, 46(1), 82. https://doi.org/10.2307/1165983

Achenbach, T. M., & Rescorla, L. A. (2000). *Manual for the ASEBA preschool forms and profiles.* University of Vermont Department of Psychiatry.

Anderson, J. C., Williams, S., McGee, R., & Silva, P. A. (1987). DSM-III disorders in preadolescent children. Prevalence in a large sample from the general population. *Archives of General Psychiatry*, 44(1), 69–76. https://doi.org/10.1001/archpsyc.1987.01800130081010

Bickman, L., Noser, K., & Summerfelt, W. (1999). Long-term effects of a system of care on children and adolescents. *Journal of Behavior Health Services and Research*, 26(2), 185–202. https://doi.org/10.1007/BF02287490

Bird, H. R., Canino, G., Rubio-Stipec, M., Gould, M. S., Ribera, J., Sesman, M., Woodbury, M., Huertas-Goldman, S., Pagan, A., Sanchez-Lacay, A., & Moscoso, M. (1988). Estimates of the prevalence of childhood maladjustment in a community survey in Puerto Rico. The use of combined measures [published erratum appears in *Archives of General Psychiatry*, 1994 May;51(5):429]. *Archives of General Psychiatry*, 45(12), 1120–1126. https://doi.org/10.1001/archpsyc.1988.01800360068010

Breton, J. J., Bergeron, L., Valla, J. P., Berthiaume, C., Gaudet, N., Lambert, J., St-Georges, M., Houde, L., & Lépine, S. (1999). Quebec child mental health survey: Prevalence of DSM-III-R mental health disorders. *Journal of Child Psychology and Psychiatry, and Allied Disciplines*, 40(3), 375–384.

Canino, G., Shrout, P. E., Rubio-Stipec, M., Bird, H. R., Bravo, M., Ramirez, R., Chavez, L., Alegria, M., Bauermeister, J. J., Hohmann, A., Ribera, J., Garcia, P., & Martinez-Taboas, A. (2004). The DSM-IV rates of child and adolescent disorders in Puerto Rico: Prevalence, correlates, service use, and the effects of impairment. *Archives of General Psychiatry*, 61(1), 85–93. https://doi.org/10.1001/archpsyc.61.1.85

Cohen, J. (1988). *Statistical power analysis for the behavioral sciences* (2nd ed.). Lawrence Erlbaum Associates.

Costello, E. J., Angold, A., Burns, B. J., Erkanli, A., Stangl, D. K., & Tweed, D. L. (1996). The great smoky mountains study of youth. Functional impairment and serious emotional disturbance. *Archives of General Psychiatry*, 53(12), 1137–1143. https://doi.org/10.1001/archpsyc.1996.01830120077013

Costello, E. J., Mustillo, S., Erkanli, A., Keeler, G., & Angold, A. (2003). Prevalence and development of psychiatric disorders in childhood and adolescence. *Archives of General Psychiatry*, 60(8), 837–844. https://doi.org/10.1001/archpsyc.60.8.837

Daleiden, E. L. (2004). *Child status measurement: System performance improvements during fiscal years 2002–2004.* State of Hawaii Department of Health, Child and Adolescent Mental Health Division.

Daleiden, E. L., & Chorpita, B. F. (2005). From data to wisdom: Quality improvement strategies supporting large-scale implementation of evidence-based services. *Child & Adolescent Psychiatric Clinics of North America, 14*(2), 329–350. https://doi.org/10.1016/j.chc.2004.11.002

De Los Reyes, A., Augenstein, T. M., Wang, M., Thomas, S. A., Drabick, D. A. G., Burgers, D. E., & Rabinowitz, J. (2015). The validity of the multi-informant approach to assessing child and adolescent mental health. *Psychological Bulletin, 141,* 858–900. https://doi.org/10.1037/a0038498

Esser, G., Schmidt, M. H., & Woerner, W. (1990). Epidemiology and course of psychiatric disorders in school-age children—results of a longitudinal study. *Journal of Child Psychology and Psychiatry, and Allied Disciplines, 31*(2), 243–263. https://doi.org/10.1111/j.1469-7610.1990.tb01565.x

Fergusson, D. M., Horwood, L. J., & Lynskey, M. T. (1993). Prevalence and comorbidity of *DSM-III-R* diagnoses in a birth cohort of 15 year olds. *Journal of the American Academy of Child and Adolescent Psychiatry, 32*(6), 1127–1134. https://doi.org/10.1097/00004583-199311000-00004

Ferlie, E., & Dopson, S. (2005). Studying complex organizations in health care. In S. Dopson & L. Fitzgerald (Eds.), *Knowledge to action? Evidence-based health care in context* (pp. 8–26). Oxford University Press.

Fombonne, E. (1994). The Chartres study: I. Prevalence of psychiatric disorders among French school-aged children. *British Journal of Psychiatry, 164,* 69–79. https://doi.org/10.1192/bjp.164.1.69

Fombonne, E. (2018). Epidemiology. In A. Martin, F. R. Volkmar, & M. H. Bloch (Eds.), *Lewis's child and adolescent psychiatry: A comprehensive textbook* (5th ed., pp. 205–225). Wolters Kluwer.

Ford, T., Goodman, R., & Meltzer, H. (2003). The British Child and Adolescent Mental Health Survey 1999: The prevalence of *DSM-IV* disorders. *Journal of the American Academy of Child and Adolescent Psychiatry, 42*(10), 1203–1211. https://doi.org/10.1097/00004583-200310000-00011

Gliner, J. A., Morgan, G. A., & Leech, N. J. (2017). *Research methods in applied settings: An integrated approach to design and analysis.* Routledge.

Hamilton, J. (2018). Evidence-based practice as a conceptual framework. In A. Martin, F. R. Volkmar, & M. H. Bloch (Eds.), *Lewis's child and adolescent psychiatry: A comprehensive textbook* (5th ed., pp. 179–194). Wolters Kluwer.

Jeffers A., & Fitzgerald M. (1991). *Irish families under stress* (Vol. 2). Dublin, Eastern Health Board.

Johnson, S. A. (2006). *The ghost map: The story of London's most terrifying epidemic and how it changed science, cities, and the modern world.* Penguin Books.

Kanner, L. (1935). *Child psychiatry.* CC Thomas.

Levine, R. J. (2018). Respect for children as research subjects. In A. Martin, F. R. Volkmar, & M. H. Bloch (Eds.), *Lewis's child and adolescent psychiatry: A comprehensive textbook* (5th ed., pp. 195–204). Wolters Kluwer.

Lewinsohn, P. M., Rohde, P., Seeley, J. R., & Fischer, S. A. (1993). Age-cohort changes in the lifetime occurrence of depression and other mental disorders. *Journal of Abnormal Psychology, 102*(1), 110–120. https://doi.org/10.1037//0021-843x.102.1.110

Lipsey, M. W., & Wilson, D. B. (2000). *Practical meta-analysis.* Sage Publishing.

Merriam, S. B., & Tisbell, E. J. (2016). *Qualitative research: A guide to design and implementation.* Jossey-Bass.

Morgan, G. A., Gliner, J. A., & Harmon, R. J. (2006). *Understanding and evaluating research in applied and clinical settings.* Lawrence Erlbaum Associates.

Morgan, G. A., Gliner, J. A., & Harmon, R. J. (2018). Understanding research methods and statistics: A primer for clinicians. In A. Martin, F. R. Volkmar, & M. H. Bloch (Eds.), *Lewis's child and adolescent psychiatry: A comprehensive textbook* (5th ed., pp. 159–178). Wolters Kluwer.

Morita, H., Suzuki, M., & Kamoshita, S. (1990). Screening measures for detecting psychiatric disorders in Japanese secondary school children. *Journal of Child Psychology and Psychiatry, and Allied Disciplines, 31*(4), 603–617. https://doi.org/10.1111/j.1469-7610.1990.tb00800.x

Offord, D. R., Boyle, M. H., Szatmari, P., Rae-Grant, N. I., Links, P. S., Cadman, D. T., Byles, J. A., Crawford, J. W., Blum, H. M., & Byrne, C. (1987). Ontario Child Health Study. II. Six-month prevalence of disorder and rates of service utilization. *Archives of General Psychiatry, 44*(9), 832–836. https://doi.org/10.1001/archpsyc.1987.01800210084013

Patton, M. Q. (2002). *Qualitative research and evaluation methods* (3rd ed.). Sage Publishing.

Pianta, R., & Caldwell, C. (1990). Stability of externalizing symptoms from kindergarten to first grade and factors related to instability. *Development and Psychopathology, 2*(3), 247–258. https://doi.org/10.1017/S0954579400000754

Reich, W. (2000). Diagnostic interview for children and adolescents (DICA). *Journal of the American Academy of Child and Adolescent Psychiatry, 39*(1), 59–66. https://doi.org/10.1097/00004583-200001000-00017

Reichow, B., Gelbar, N. W., Mouradjian, K., Shefcyk, A., & Smith, I. C. (2014). Characteristics of international websites with information on developmental disabilities. *Research in Developmental Disabilities, 35*(10), 2293–2298. https://doi.org/10.1016/j.ridd.2014.05.028

Rutter, M. (1989). Isle of Wight revisited: Twenty-five years of child psychiatric epidemiology. *Journal of the American Academy of Child and Adolescent Psychiatry, 28*(5), 633–653. https://doi.org/10.1097/00004583-198909000-00001

Rutter, M. (1997). Comorbidity: Concepts, claims and choices. *Criminal Behaviour & Mental Health, 7*(4), 265–285. https://doi.org/10.1002/cbm.190

Rutter, M., Bailey, A., Bolton, P., & Le Couteur, A. (1994). Autism and known medical conditions: Myth and substance. *Journal of Child Psychology and Psychiatry, and Allied Disciplines, 35*(2), 311–322. https://doi.org/10.1111/j.1469-7610.1994.tb01164.x

Rutter, M., Tizard, J., Yule, W., Graham, P., & Whitmore, K. (1976). Research report: Isle of Wight Studies, 1964–1974. *Psychological Medicine, 6*(2), 313–332. https://doi.org/10.1017/s003329170001388x

Shadish, W. R., Cook, T. D., & Campbell, D. T. (2002). *Experimental and quasi-experimental designs for generalized casual influence.* Houghton Mifflin.

Shapiro, A. K., & Shapiro, E. (2000). *The powerful placebo: From ancient priest to modern physician.* Johns Hopkins University Press.

Simonoff, E., Pickles, A., Meyer, J. M., Silberg, J. L., Maes, H. H., Loeber, R., Rutter, M., Hewitt, J. K., & Eaves, L. J. (1997). The Virginia twin study of adolescent behavioral development. Influences of age, sex, and impairment on rates of disorder. *Archives of General Psychiatry, 54*(9), 801–808. https://doi.org/10.1001/archpsyc.1997.01830210039004

Steinhausen, H. C., Meier, M., & Angst, J. (1998). The Zurich long-term outcome study of child and adolescent psychiatric disorders in males. *Psychological Medicine, 28*(2), 375–383. https://doi.org/10.1017/s0033291797005989

Verhulst, F. C., & Koot, H. M. (1995). *The epidemiology of child and adolescent psychopathology.* Oxford University Press.

Verhulst, F. C., van der Ende, J., Ferdinand, R. F., & Kasius, M. C. (1997). The prevalence of *DSM-III-R* diagnoses in a national sample of Dutch adolescents. *Archives of General Psychiatry, 54*(4), 329–336. https://doi.org/10.1001/archpsyc.1997.01830160049008

Weisz, J. R., & Jensen, P. S. (1999). Efficacy and effectiveness of child and adolescent psychotherapy and pharmacotherapy. *Mental Health Services Research, 1,* 125–157. https://doi.org/10.1023/a:1022321812352

Suggested Readings

Fombonne, E. (1992). Parent reports on behavior and competencies among 6–21-year-old French children. *European Child & Adolescent Psychiatry, 1*(4), 233–243. https://doi.org/10.1007/BF02094184

Gudmundsson, O. O., Magnusson, P., Saemundsen, E., Lauth, B., Baldursson, G., Skarphedinsson, G., & Fombonne, E. (2013). Psychiatric disorders in an urban sample of preschool children. *Child and Adolescent Mental Health, 18*(4), 210–217. https://doi.org/10.1111/j.1475-3588.2012.00675.x

Hawley, K., & Weisz, J. (2005). Youth versus parent working alliance in usual clinical care: Distinctive association with retention, satisfaction, and treatment out-come. *Journal of Clinical Child and Adolescent Psychology, 34*(1), 117–128. https://doi.org/10.1207/s15374424jccp3401_11

Kirk, R. E. (2001). Promoting good statistical practices: Some suggestions. *Educational and Psychological Measurement, 61,* 213–218. https://doi.org/10.1177/00131640121971185

Maziade, M., Cote, R., Boutin, P., Bernier, H., & Thivierge, J. (1987). Temperament and intellectual development: A longitudinal study from infancy to four years. *American Journal of Psychiatry, 144*(2), 144–150. https://doi.org/10.1176/ajp.144.2.144

McLeod, B. D., & Weisz, J. R. (2010). The therapy process observational coding system for child psychotherapy-strategies scale. *Journal of Clinical Child and Adolescent Psychology, 39*(3), 436–443. https://doi.org/10.1080/15374411003691750

Moffitt, T. E. (1993). Adolescence-limited and life-course-persistent antisocial behavior: A developmental taxonomy. *Psychology Review, 100*(4), 674–701. https://doi.org/10.1037/0033-295X.100.4.674

Pianta, R., & Caldwell, C. (1990). Stability of externalizing symptoms from kindergarten to first grade and factors related to instability. *Development and Psychopathology, 2*(3), 247–258. https://doi.org/10.1017/S0954579400000754

Tremblay, R. E., Nagin, D. S., Seguin, J. R., Zoccolillo, M., Zelazo, P. D., Boivin, M., Pérusse, D., & Japel, C. (2004). Physical aggression during early childhood: Trajectories and predictors. *Pediatrics, 114*(1), 43–50. https://doi.org/10.1542/peds.114.1.e43

CHAPTER 4 ■ CLASSIFICATION AND ASSESSMENT

■ PRINCIPLES OF CLASSIFICATION

Classification helps us to be better observers and to formulate hypotheses and principles. Shared approaches to classification help us communicate more effectively and develop better theories. In mental health disciplines, and indeed in medicine in general, the process of giving a label may be associated with some sense of relief on the part of the patient or the patient's parents when the patient is a child. Assigning a label, however, does not imply having an explanation. Like all human theories, classification approaches have their limitations or can be misused. There is no single "right" way to classify disorders in childhood. Systems vary, depending on the purpose of classification and what is being classified. Official diagnostic systems, such as the World Health Organization's *International Classification of Diseases (ICD-11)* (World Health Organization, 2019–2020) and the American Psychiatric Association's *Diagnostic and Statistical Manual (DSM-5)* (American Psychiatric Association, 2013) are generally categorically oriented. The dimensional approaches that are based on considerations of how behaviors or emotional traits are distributed in the population are quite useful for understanding psychopathology. To be useful, classification schemes must provide adequate descriptions of disorders (so they can be reliably differentiated from each other) and must be useful across the range of age and severity. Deviant behavior itself does not necessarily constitute a disorder unless it is a manifestation of dysfunction within the individual person that significantly impaired this person's life.

■ MODELS OF CLASSIFICATION

Various approaches to classification can be used (Table 4.1). These are not necessarily incompatible with each other. For example, a continuous variable such as IQ or blood pressure can be used to define levels of severity (e.g., of intellectual disability) or disorder (hypertension).

The issue of which model works best depends on the specific situation. For example, structured rating scales and diagnostic interviews have been developed for many disorders. In addition, a series of well-designed, psychometrically sound structured interviews "keyed" to *DSM-5* diagnostic concepts have been developed; these are particularly useful and often required in research studies (Angold et al., 2018). Another approach has focused on assessment

TABLE 4.1

Approaches to Classification

Categorical approaches	Presence or absence of disorder Examples: autism, appendicitis
Dimensional approaches	Assess dimensions of function or dysfunction Examples: intelligence, hypertension
Ideographic approaches	Focus on the individual person Examples: individualized education plan

of psychopathology with derivation of more basic "factors" such as internalizing and externalizing disorders on the Child Behavior Checklist (Achenbach, 1966). Such instruments have both research and clinical utility and may have importance for screening but do not usually translate straightforwardly into *DSM*-type diagnoses, which require integration of clinically relevant information by an expert (or at least experienced clinician). As we shall discuss later, different informants—parents, teachers, and the children themselves—can, and often do, provide different information that can inform assessment and diagnoses in important and complementary ways.

Developmental issues are also of considerable importance in classifying disorders in children and adolescents (and occasionally adults). Disorders such as autism and attention-deficit hyperactivity disorder (ADHD) originate during specific times of development, and other disorders, such as Tourette's disorder, and age of onset and developmental trajectory can provide important diagnostic context. In other cases, preexisting disorders may complicate the diagnosis of other conditions (e.g., a child with oppositional defiant disorder who goes on to develop depression in adolescence, which might be overlooked owing to a history of irritability). For some forms of developmental psychopathology, diagnostic guidelines have a strong developmental orientation, but for others, the nature of the symptoms predominates.

Theoretically based classification systems tended to be more common in the past. For example, Anna Freud had a model of classification based on her psychoanalytically informed understanding of child development (Freud, 1965). More phenomenologically based classification systems can be traced to Kraeplin's delineation of schizophrenia and bipolar disorder (Hoff, 2015). Theoretically based classification systems tend to be most useful for clinicians working with that specific theoretical framework, but they may be less useful for clinicians who do not share the same orientation. For several decades, the official classification systems, such as the one reflected in the *Diagnostic and Statistical Manual* of the American Psychiatric Association, have focused less on theories and more on research-based approaches to classification.

It is generally recognized that there is no single "right" way to classify disorders in childhood (Rutter, 1965). Classification systems vary depending on the purpose of classification and what is being classified. "Official" diagnostic systems have tended to adopt, on the whole, a categorical approach, but a dimensional approach would be equally applicable, though perhaps less useful for clinical purposes.

It is often assumed that classification systems of psychopathology are developed to approximate some ideal diagnostic system in which the cause could be directly related to clinical condition. This is not, in fact, the case, because the cause need not be included in classification systems. Different etiologic factors may result in rather similar conditions, and the same etiologic factor may be associated with a range of clinical conditions. With a few exceptions (e.g., posttraumatic stress disorders), etiologic factors are not generally included in official diagnostic systems.

Environmental or contextual factors are particularly important in understanding childhood psychopathology. Thus, variables such as family, school, or cultural setting can serve as major modifiers of clinical presentation. For example, a child who had attentional difficulties because of an inappropriate school placement should not have a diagnosis of attention-deficit disorder. Contextual variables are particularly problematic in disorders of infancy and early childhood in which child and parent variables often interact with each other. Cultural differences may also be important and may interact in complex ways with child vulnerability and family variables.

Finally, it should be emphasized that *disorders*, not children, are classified. This may seem a subtle point, but it is not. There are potential negative effects (and positive ones) related to labeling. Clearly, it is children, and not labels, who need help, and it is not appropriate to equate people with their problems. Labels can have some social stigma or other untoward effects or may be associated with more realistic expectations on the part of parents and teachers and provision of potentially more appropriate services.

■ IDEOGRAPHIC APPROACHES

Ideographic approaches to diagnosis are common in clinical practice. In the broader sense of clinical diagnosis, most clinicians target certain problems or issues for intervention that relate only in part to categorical or even dimensional diagnosis (Bostic et al., 2018). In some ways, such approaches are more practical in clinical setting or in conjunction with certain forms of psychotherapy such as family counseling. Ideographic approaches that require careful documentation of signs and history of clinical issues as well as detailed description of contexts that may affect or be affected by symptoms such as family, school, and neighborhood are also an important part of clinical case formulation (Henderson & Martin, 2018). Beyond the individual cases, the utility of ideographic approaches is limited to, for example, research purposes, where information needs to be communicated concisely and systematically.

■ RESEARCH ISSUES

As official classification systems have become more complex and sophisticated, issues of reliability and validity have assumed increasing importance. For example, both the *DSM-5* and the *ICD-10* use results of large national or international field trials in providing definitions of disorders. Categorical and dimensional approaches to classification share certain statistical concerns, including validity and reliability. *Validity* refers to the extent to which the diagnostic category captures the phenomena it purports to (e.g., does the diagnostic category have some meaning relative to course and treatment or family history or associated conditions?) *Reliability* refers to the ability of different individuals to use the diagnostic approach in the same way. This is also referred to as inter-rater reliability, a statistical index that addresses an important question about a diagnosis such as whether two doctors who examine the child within a relatively short interval (e.g., in the same week) would arrive at the same diagnosis. As with validity, various kinds of reliability are identified, and these are impacted by various factors, including who is conducting the assessment as well as variability in symptoms and time course of the disorder. Test–retest reliability refers to a question of whether or not diagnosis remains the same or changes if assessments are conducted on two occasions separated by a longer period. This issue of test–retest reliability is linked to the issues of stability and chronicity of mental health disorders. For example, conditions such as ADHD and obsessive-compulsive disorder tend to remain relatively stable over extended periods if untreated. And some disorders such as Tourette's syndrome or major depression can go through periods of remission and exacerbation. The waxing and waning course may be an important classification feature of the disorder that needs to be reflected in diagnostic assessment.

Various *statistical techniques* have been applied to data derived from assessment methods (Nunnally & Bernstein, 1994). These techniques are theoretically of considerable interest in that they can provide more rational and empirical approaches to the derivation of diagnostic schemes. The fundamental assumption of such techniques is that the variables of interest lie along some dimension of function and dysfunction that all persons exhibit to some degree. For many types of problems, this assumption is probably justified, such as relative to anxiety or depression. However, the usefulness of such techniques is limited in important ways. In the first place, these methods are highly dependent on both the sample and the type of data entered in the analysis. For example, *factor analysis* of an instrument designed to detect conduct problems would not likely produce a factor related to anxiety and vice versa (Fabrigar & Wegener, 2012). Similarly, cluster analysis of even a very large normative sample would not likely produce a cluster that corresponded to autism, given the low base rate of this disorder in the population.

In summary, classification in child and adolescent psychiatry has multiple meanings and functions. Complications in the classification of child and adolescent disorders are myriad: The child is often not the person complaining, different kinds of data may be used in making a diagnosis, developmental factors may have a major impact on the expression of disorders, and certain features (e.g., beliefs in fantasy figures) are normative at certain ages but not at others. Additional complications are posed by the unintended, but no less real, uses to which diagnostic concepts are put, such as their inclusion in legislation and their use as mandates for services in educational programs or for purposes of insurance reimbursement for services. Different kinds and levels of classification are needed for different purposes.

■ RESEARCH DOMAIN CRITERIA (RDOC) FRAMEWORK

The Research Domain Criteria (RDoC) approach is a relatively new initiative that has been launched by the National Institute of Mental Health (NIMH) in order to gather empirical data to ultimately develop a new classification of psychopathology based on the dimensions of neurobiology and behavior that cut across traditional categories of mental disorders (Insel et al., 2010; Sanislow, 2020). In contrast to the *DSM* and *ICD* classification systems, which are intended for clinical use, the RDoC approach is intended for researchers to provide a working model to stimulate research on the core dimensions (or constructs) of psychopathology. First, in 2009, an NIMH work group devised a proposal for a new system and outlined five major domains of functioning such as cognition and emotions and units of analysis ranging from genes to neural circuits to behavior. Then, five groups of experts in basic and behavioral sciences representing each of the domains were convened for a series of workshops and asked to determine and define specific dimensions to be included in each domain. In order to be included, the domains (e.g., "fear") had to reflect validated behavioral functions and show evidence for a neural circuit or system responsible for implementing this function.

The ensuing RDoC constructs are organized in a two-dimensional matrix of five domains that include constituent constructs in the rows and seven units of analysis as the columns (Cuthbert, 2015). The *units of analysis* include genes, molecules, cells, circuits, physiology, behavior, and self-report, reflecting a range of methodologic approaches from genetics to psychology. The first three levels of analysis pertain to the neurobiologic mechanism of circuitry essential to each construct. In turn, neural circuit is a central unit that can be studied with neuroimaging methods such as functional magnetic resonance imaging or indices of circuit activity such as fear-potentiated startle. Physiology refers to variables such as event-related potentials or heart rate variability that can be validated as indirect measures of neural circuits. Measures of observable behavior and performance on laboratory task are grouped under the unit of analysis termed "behavior." Lastly, self-report category is reserved for interviews, rating scales, and other psychometric instruments of various aspects of the construct of interest that represent signs and symptoms of psychopathology. This emphasis on the multifaceted characterization of constructs is part of the RDoC's aim to incorporate methods of genetics, neuroscience, and cognitive science into the future classification scheme of mental disorders.

The RDoC constructs are grouped into domains of functioning that reflect key aspects of emotion, motivation, cognition, social behavior, and regulatory systems (National Institute of Mental Health, 2020). The first domain, *negative valence systems*, includes constructs defined by responses to acute threat ("fear"), potential threat ("anxiety"), sustained threat, loss, and frustration. The second domain, *positive valence system,* contains constructs defined by reward learning and habit formation. For example, approach motivation construct encompasses goal pursuit behaviors subserved by the mesolimbic dopamine system. A dysfunction of this system can lead to abnormally low (e.g., avolition) or high (e.g., addition) goal-directed behaviors. Another construct within this domain, called "habit," is viewed as a manifestation of reinforcement learning where repetitive motor or cognitive behaviors occur and manifest without serving an adaptive goal. The *cognitive systems domain* encompasses six broad constructs: attention, perception, declarative memory, language, cognitive control, and working memory. The *social processes domain* includes constructs that bridge social behavior with neural circuits of attachment, social dominance and perception, and understanding of self and others. For example, facial communication may include receptive aspects of facial affect recognition and productive aspects of eye contact and gaze following. The neural underpinnings of these behaviors have been studied with an array of neuroimaging and electrophysiologic methods in order to establish biomarkers of psychiatric disorders such as ASD and schizophrenia. The fifth domain includes *arousal and regulatory systems* that subserve many of the other domains and are central in sleep and wakefulness.

The RDoC framework is based on three core assumptions: (1) mental illnesses are presumed to be disorders of brain circuits, (2) neuroscience tools can identify the pathophysiology, and (3) the discovery of biosignatures will supplement diagnoses based on clinical signs and symptoms and direct assessment and treatment of mental illness. Since its inception, the RDoC approach has stimulated an increasing body of research on developing and validating the proposed constructs along the lines that are outlined in the RDoC matrix. In addition, RDoC offers a new perspective to study co-occurring disorders. For example, autism commonly co-occurs with anxiety, but when using symptom-based criteria, it is hard to know whether anxiety is a true comorbidity or a feature of autism. However, measures that have been validated to test relevant functions within anxiety/fear circuitry and social brain networks can provide an alternative way to characterize anxiety in autism (Lau et al., 2020).

■ DIAGNOSTIC ASSESSMENT

Clinical and diagnostic evaluation of children and adolescents should carefully consider the context of functioning within the family, school, peer, cultural, and community settings with a goal of identifying specific forms of psychopathology and developing an appropriate treatment plan if one is needed. Depending on the reason for referral and presenting concerns, the examiner may need to prioritize areas for assessment and intervention (e.g., the presence of suicidal thoughts or high-risk behaviors). Some assessments are conducted for a very specific purpose (e.g., custody assessments or evaluation of suicidal risk of a child in the emergency department) and require very specialized expertise. More typically, the diagnostic assessment process requires the examiner to take a broad view, taking into account presenting complaints (of the child, parents, teachers, or others), the child's history and level of development, and family and cultural factors.

The assessment of a child differs from the psychiatric assessment of an adult in several important ways. Typically, parents or sometimes schools have initiated a referral, and the child may or may not be as troubled by the problem. The assessment also depends on the child's chronologic age and developmental level so that the approach to a preschool child will often involve play or games; a school-age child may prefer some combination of discussion and activities; and an interview with an adolescent may be more like that of the adult. It is important that the child understand, at whatever level they can, the purpose of the assessment and that, as appropriate, the clinician conduct interviews in a way designed to facilitate discussion. Unlike adults, children can act very differently depending on the setting. A child who is having real trouble sitting still in school may be well behaved and popular on the playground. As a result, it is important to collect information from different sources, including the child, parent(s), and school. Consequently, a major task for the clinician becomes the reconciliation of views when they diverge. Also, as a result of this process, the clinician needs to form a working relationship with multiple parties while maintaining, as appropriate, the child and family's confidentiality. In contrast to interviews with adults, developmental issues can loom large either as presenting complaints (e.g., continued temper tantrums or delayed speech) or as important considerations in the assessment itself (e.g., a child with autism who is minimally verbal). For younger children without developmental delays, it is important that the clinician have an awareness of normative cognitive processes and common childhood fears, beliefs, and fantasies. The assessment should, of course, be tailored to the circumstances of the individual case, but several key components should be considered (Table 4.2) with the aim of identifying the variables relevant to the child's presentation.

TABLE 4.2

Content Components of The Psychiatric Assessment of Children and Adolescents

Content Component	Primary Informant	Additional Resources
Reason for referral	Usually parent or guardian; sometimes school or legal agency	Letter from school or other agency seeking evaluation
History of problem(s)	Child and parent	Referral source; contact from primary care provider
Past problems	Child and parent	Structured interviews; screening scales
Comorbid symptoms	Child and parent	Structured interviews; screening scales
Substance use	Child, parent	Laboratory screening (as relevant)
Previous assessment or treatment(s)	Child, parent, clinicians	Mental health records
Child's development, including psychomotor, cognitive, interpersonal, emotional, moral, trauma, harm (to self and others)	Parents, school staff	School records, including special education evaluations; home video (as relevant)
Family history	Parent	Genogram
Medical history	Parent, health care provider(s)	Review of symptoms checklist; laboratory tests (as relevant)
Child's strengths	Parent, child, teachers, coaches, peers	Activity video (e.g., sports, music); cognitive, school, neuropsychological testing
Child's media diet	Parent, child, caregivers, siblings	Media diary; apps on phone; YouTube viewing history
Environmental supports	Parent, child, adults familiar to child	Activity schedules (scouting, teams); after-school or summer programs; mentorships such as Big Brother or Big Sister relationships
Mental status exam	Child, clinician's observations during assessment	Mini-Mental State Examination

Adapted with permission from Bostic, J. Q., Potter, M. P., & King, R. A. (2018). Clinical assessment of children and adolescents: Content and structure. In A. Martin, M. H. Bloch, & F. R. Volkmar (Eds.), *Lewis's child and adolescent psychiatry: A comprehensive textbook* (5th ed., p. 300). Wolters Kluwer.

Typically, the assessment begins with a review of the reasons for referral. This helps clarify the nature of the presenting problem(s) and expectations for what the assessment will provide. The history can be obtained from relevant persons and perspectives (e.g., child, parents, other family members, school personnel). The examiner should be alert to the context or circumstance in which problem behavior emerges. In some fundamental way, the examiner tries to assemble, and constantly revise, a narrative with attention first paid to the "facts" as they present themselves (the who, what, where, and when of the narrative) with an eventual formulation (the why). The clinician should be alert to important clues about what sets off or maintains problem behaviors. A history of previous treatment should be included if relevant. At some time, the examiner will also wish to obtain a developmental history to help clarify any potential developmental difficulties contributing to current problems and any long-standing issues that may shed light on current problems.

A review of the past history should put current problems in an historical context (e.g., is this a new problem, an exacerbation of an old one, or some new problem that arises in the context of some other difficulty?). Comorbidity or co-occurrence of multiple mental health problems and disorders is now considered a rule rather than an exception in psychopathology (Angold et al., 1999). It is often noted that children (and parents) typically have not read the *DSM*, and clinical presentations usually include a range of difficulties that might not clearly align with diagnostic criteria. Accordingly, an important part of the assessment reflects the clinician's judgment, based on history and presentation, of how the presenting symptoms can be placed in a broader context. For example, although attentional problems are a hallmark of attention-deficit disorder (Chapter 10), they can also be seen in children with anxiety, ASD, depression, or bipolar disorder. Difficulty paying attention may arise because of environmental factors and social factors such the effects of racism-related stress on the mental health of African American and other racial and ethnic minority youth (Jones & Neblett, 2017).

The medical history should include attention to the pregnancy, labor, and delivery. Sometimes, parental expectations of the child even before birth may be relevant. Complications during delivery or the neonatal period should be noted, as should any relevant medical conditions, hospitalizations, surgeries, and so forth. Response to medications and allergies to medications should be elicited. The clinician should be alert to any factors in the history that might contribute to current difficulties (e.g., a child with a history of significant prematurity who might be at risk for learning difficulties). Any sensory vulnerabilities should be noted (e.g., a child with recurrent ear infections who might present with language delay). The medical history should include a review of any significant accidents or injuries and any potential sequelae.

Family history should include a review of the parents' own histories of developmental or psychiatric problems, parenting styles, marital style, and methods for conflict resolution. Relevant cultural, ethnic, religious, or other information should be noted. Recent, or enduring, stresses and, for that matter, supports should be noted. Family moves can be disruptive of peer relationships and stressful for parents and children alike. Sometimes, the death of a familiar figure (e.g., a grandparent) significantly changes child care patterns. If parents are divorced or if there has been chronic or sporadic marital conflict, it is important that the examiner attend to parental perceptions of how these have impacted the child. If a child is adopted, the history, to the extent available, of the child before the adoption is relevant. The child's understanding of the adoption should also be obtained. The clinician should be clear about the family constellation and inquire about other individuals present. A genogram can be helpful in this process.

Depending on the child's age and level of maturity, other issues may merit review. If the child is approaching adolescence or if adolescence is already well established, it is important to inquire about pubertal development. In some situations (e.g., eating problems), measures of height and weight can be very relevant. The child's use or exposure to alcohol, cigarettes, or illegal substances should also be reviewed. With increasing media use, the issues of screen time and impact of online activity on child mental health have been receiving increasing research and clinical attention (Madigan et al., 2019). Careful evaluation of media use should now be a part of any clinical assessment of children and adolescents (Shafi et al., 2018).

It is helpful for clinicians to have both a general conceptual model of psychopathology to follow during the assessment and a specific plan for the initial clinical encounter. This helps to structure the assessment process itself and the written summary that should follow. It is important that the child and family members understand exactly what is involved in a psychiatric assessment. Unlike a visit to the pediatrician, a visit to a psychiatrist or other mental health professional is fraught with psychological "baggage" that may interfere with the assessment process. Accordingly, clarity and transparency on the part of the interviewer is extremely helpful.

Often, parents may come for an initial interview without the child. This allows for both a review of the presenting problem and the child's history and a chance for parents to convey their own concerns, expectations, and misconceptions. It can also provide an opportunity for talking with the parents about exactly what they will tell their child before the child comes to the assessment. The child may have major misconceptions about what is involved in speaking with a mental health provider. They may worry that the parents are going to hospitalize them or send them away or that the assessment is a form of punishment. The child may be burdened with some secret—or not so secret—fear. It would help if parents could openly discuss their hopes for the meeting and indicate, if it is appropriate, what they know about what will happen and who the child will see. For younger children, information from the parents (e.g., about the child's favorite activities, TV shows, or games) may serve as an "ice breaker" for the clinician. Any special needs of the child should be discussed along with confidentiality issues.

During the initial interview, parents should be helped to elaborate, in their own words, their understanding of their child's difficulties and how they have evolved over time. If there are major differences in perception (e.g., between the mother and father or between a parent and teacher), it is important that everyone have a chance to voice their own perspectives.

In addition to areas of weakness or vulnerability, it is also important to inquire about the areas of strength and potential resources for the child. The former may include interests and hobbies or any areas of information that children may volunteer about themselves. The latter may take the form of people who have special relationships with the child or cultural or social resources such as the presence of a supportive religious or ethnic community.

A host of factors can complicate the valuation process. These include problems in the parents (e.g., highly divergent expectations or perspectives on the problem). Sometimes, sadly, often in custody situations, the child can become a "target" of parental struggle. As with the child, the specific developmental and personality issues of the parents may color the assessment process.

The clinician should be very sensitive to the potential for parents to feel embarrassed or ashamed (i.e., that they have failed in some way because their child has some problem or need). The clinician should be actively listening to parental concerns and to how these concerns are colored by the parents' own history. Some important aspects of the topics for parent and child interviewing are summarized in Table 4.3.

THE MENTAL STATUS EXAMINATION

The mental status examination (MSE) is a key component of the psychiatric assessment. It provides a perspective based on direct interaction as to how the child presents themselves. The MSE should include a description of how the child presents themselves (well organized, tidy, or studiously the reverse). How easy is it to engage the child? How cooperative are they? How do they act and interact with the clinician? What is the child's speech like? Are there concerns about mood or thought process disturbance? Although usually written up as a separate section from this history, the MSE is usually highly dependent on observations made throughout the assessment. Some aspects of the MSE require specific inquiry (orientation, memory, fund of knowledge, and so forth), but others can be collected continuously throughout the assessment. Table 4.4 provides an overview of components of the MSE. Depending on the results of initial examination, other assessments (e.g., of cognition, speech-communication functioning, academic skills, or learning problems) may require specific investigation.

TABLE 4.3

Sample Clinician Questions

Component	Example Parent Questions ("Yes" responses warrant follow-up questions to clarify acts, context, intentions, and consequences.)	Example Child Questions ("Yes" responses warrant follow-up questions to clarify acts, context, intentions, consequences, and learning from these events.)
Reason for referral	Whose idea was it that [child] might need this evaluation? Who is most concerned about [child's] behavior? What do you/they hope this evaluation will accomplish?	What did your parent(s) tell you about coming here today? Who wanted you to meet with me today? What did they say to you about us meeting? How do you feel about being here?
History of problem(s)	When did you first notice [child's] problem? How did the problem develop over time? How did you understand [child's] behavior?	What do you wish would be different? What is not going well for you? What do you think is making this such a hard time?
Functional assessment of problem behaviors	Where does the problem behavior occur most often? How does the problem impact [child] at home? At school? With peers? Is the problem behavior worse in one of these places? What usually occurs right before the problem behavior? What happens after [child] does [problem behavior]? How do [parent, teacher, peers, friends] respond? Has anything changed to make the behavior worse or better?	When and where does the problem occur? What happens when you [exhibit symptoms]? What usually happens right before you [exhibit symptom]? How does your [parent, teacher, friends] respond when you [exhibit symptom]? How do you feel after you [exhibit symptom]?
Past problems	Did [child] have any problems this severe at an earlier point? What other significant difficulties has [child] had in the past?	Have you had any times before where things were difficult? Has anyone ever been worried about you?

Comorbid symptoms	Does [child] have any other symptoms that trouble you? Does [child] have any other symptoms that interfere at home, school, or with friends? Have others identified any other problems they've noticed with [child]?	Is there anything else going on that you wish were different? Do you feel bad in any other ways? Do you have any difficulty sleeping, eating, or going to the bathroom? Is there anything you worry about? How often do you feel sad? Do you wish anything were different with your peers, family members, or teachers?
Substance use history	Has your child done anything to suggest use of substances? Have you detected your child to be drunk, high, or stoned/on drugs? Have you seen or found any drug paraphernalia that might be your child's? Has your child spoken about drinking, smoking, or substance use?	Have you ever been around any substances (alcohol, tobacco, marijuana, and so on)? Have you ever tried tobacco? Alcohol? Any other drugs? Do they help in any way? Have you ever been high, stoned, or intoxicated? Has that ever led to any problems for you? Have you ever tried to stop? How did that go?
Previous treatment(s)	What all has been attempted to address this in the past? Has [child] received any treatment(s) in the past for emotional or behavioral concerns?	Has anyone tried to help you with this before? Have you talked with anyone about these difficulties before? Have you ever taken any medicines for these difficulties?
Developmental History		
Basic functions	How did [child] progress with sleep? Did [child] always sleep through the night? How has [child's] appetite been? Has [child] ever been overweight? How do you feel about [child's] size or weight? What do you tell [child] about their weight or appearance? How did toilet training progress with [child]? Has [child] had periods of wetting or soiling?	Do you have any trouble falling asleep? Staying asleep? How do you sleep through the night? Do you need or use a night-light? Do you like it better when someone sleeps with you? How is your appetite? How do you feel about the way you look? What do others (peers, parents) say about your appearance? Do you have any difficulties going to the bathroom?

(continued)

TABLE 4.3

Sample Clinician Questions (*continued*)

Component	Example Parent Questions ("Yes" responses warrant follow-up questions to clarify acts, context, intentions, and consequences.)	Example Child Questions ("Yes" responses warrant follow-up questions to clarify acts, context, intentions, consequences, and learning from these events.)
Psychomotor development	When did [child] start walking? What sports or activities has [child] participated in? Which ones have gone well? Not so well?	How do you do in sports? How do you do when you play with friends your age? Do you have any problems playing games, sports, music, or dancing?
Cognitive development	Did [child] show interest in things you pointed to? Did [child] point things out to you? When did [child] begin preschool or school? How did that go? How did [child] do with reading? With math? With writing? In which subjects did [child] do particularly well? Which subjects were more difficult? How did [child] do each year in school? Did [child] ever receive any special educational services? Has [child] ever been suspended, expelled, or asked to leave school? Did [child] ever have any periods of excessive absences? Has [child] even had any summer school or after-school tutoring? Is there anything [child] particularly enjoys or does well at in school?	Which subjects do you like best at school? Which subjects do you do best in at school? How do you like reading? Math? Writing? Is anything at school really hard for you to do? Is there anything you have trouble understanding? How do you get along with the other kids in your class? With your teacher? Has anyone ever helped you with school work? What do they do? Have you ever had to take any classes over? Have you ever done any grades over? Have you ever gone to school during the summer?

Interpersonal development	How did [child] relate to you as a child? How did [child] respond to your requests or directions? When did [child] start interacting with other children? Did [child] have any significant attachments or relationships to others that ended? What kind of friends does [child] have at this point? How does [child] get along with these children? Does [child] get invited to play dates, birthday parties, or sleep-overs?	Who are some of your good friends now (when and where met, what do you do together, how often, and so on)? How often do you and [friend] play together? How long do you stay at [friend's house]? Do you spend the night at [friend's house]? How does that go (What do you do)? Any rough spots between you and other kids? How come? Have you lost any good friends (because of moves, misunderstandings, and so on)?
Emotional development	Does [child] recognize when they are sad, really happy, etc.? How does [child] soothe themselves when unhappy or in a bad mood? What is the child's prevailing or most common mood? How does the child respond to unexpected changes? Disappointments? Frustrations? Anxieties or depressed moods?	How often do you feel sad? Mad? Worried? Does anything in particular make you sad, mad, or worried? What do you do when you are feeling that way? Can you do anything to stop yourself from getting sad, mad, or worried? How do you calm yourself down?
Moral development	Does [child] recognize right from wrong? Does [child] describe any "moral principles" that guide their actions? How does [child] contend with mistakes or when confronted about doing something wrong? Has [child] ever deliberately hurt any animals or other kids? Bullied or been bullied by other kids? Does [child] show remorse after hurting someone? Does [child] anticipate consequences of their decisions?	Do you ever do things that you wish you hadn't? Do you ever hurt others even if it's not on purpose? What do you wish will happen when you [hit other, say something really mean, break or steal someone's toy]? What does happen when you do something that hurts or upsets [someone else]? Can you keep yourself from hitting or getting back at someone if you want to?

(continued)

TABLE 4.3
Sample Clinician Questions (*continued*)

Component	Example Parent Questions ("Yes" responses warrant follow-up questions to clarify acts, context, intentions, and consequences.)	Example Child Questions ("Yes" responses warrant follow-up questions to clarify acts, context, intentions, consequences, and learning from these events.)
Trauma history	Has [child] ever been hurt or injured? Has [child] ever witnessed anything really bad or frightening? Has [child] described frightening dreams/nightmares? Has [child] ever made unusual comments about sex? Have you [parent] had any traumatic experiences that remind you of what [child] is going through?	Have you ever been hurt? Injured? Have you ever seen anything really bad? Frightening? Have you ever seen anyone get hurt badly? Do you ever have scary dreams or nightmares? Do you ever see or hear something that reminds you of something really scary? Has anyone ever tried to hurt you? Who did or would you tell if someone tried to hurt you?
Harm to self or others history	Has [child] ever talked about hurting themselves? Others? Has [child] ever done things to inflict pain on themselves? To hurt others? What happened? Has [child] ever been involved with school officials or police because of threats or harm toward others?	Have you ever thought about hurting yourself? Others? Have you ever hurt yourself on purpose? How did you feel after you did ___? Have you ever hurt anyone else on purpose? How did you feel about that? How do you feel about that now? Have you ever gotten into trouble with anyone for talking about hurting yourself or someone else?

Family history	What were the circumstances surrounding the conception and pregnancy with [child]? Do you treat them differently than you were treated by your parents? Did [parents] grow up in similar type families? Has anyone on father's [mother's] side of the family had depression, anxiety, problems with attention or learning, tics, substance abuse problems, or any other mental illness? Has anyone in the family had serious medical problems? Has anyone in the family ever been psychiatrically or medically hospitalized? Incarcerated? [If relevant] What was that like for [the child]? What do you think [child] has inherited from [all parents, biologic, and adoptive]?	Are you like anyone else in your family? Do you know if anyone in your family has ever felt like you do? How do your parents understand you?
Family constellation history	Have there been any times when [child's parents] were separated or together? Have any changes in the family [loss or addition of parent, loss or addition of sibling or other in the home] contributed to [child's] symptoms? What kind of contact does [child] have with [parents, grandparents, primary caregiving relatives]? What does [child] say about [other parent, caregivers]?	Have either of your parents ever been away very long? Do you miss anyone from your family? Whom do you get along best with in your home? Whom do you have the hardest time with? Why?
Medical history	Has [child] ever had any medical illnesses or serious injuries? Been hospitalized? Had any operations? Was [child] physically ill before these symptoms started? Has [child] had any physical symptoms that occur with or since the emotional symptoms? Has [child] ever been allergic to anything?	Have you ever been really sick? Have you ever had to go to the hospital (what happened?) Have you ever had any surgeries (what was that like?) Have you been physically sick since you have had problems with___?
Child's strengths	What is [child] good at? What does [child] do for fun? What does [child] do during the day? What does [child] want to do or wish they could do?	What do you most like to do? What are you really good at? What do your friends or other students think you are really good at? What would you like to be better at? Do you feel special in any way? What do you want to do when you grow up?

(continued)

TABLE 4.3

Sample Clinician Questions (*continued*)

Component	Example Parent Questions ("Yes" responses warrant follow-up questions to clarify acts, context, intentions, and consequences.)	Example Child Questions ("Yes" responses warrant follow-up questions to clarify acts, context, intentions, consequences, and learning from these events.)
Child's media use	What does [child] do for video games, social media, screen time? What does [child] watch, read, or listen to? How much time does [child] spend online or watching TV or YouTube? Listening to music? Reading books? How does screen time/video games influence [child]? What effects do you think [child's] musical choices have on them?	How much do you play video games or look things up on the internet every day? Watch TV? Listen to music? Read for fun? What do you like the most about [specific game, app, TV show, music]? Do you ever get into trouble after spending too much time online or on your iPhone?
Community and environmental supports	What is your neighborhood like? Is a language other than English spoken at home? If so, by whom, and does [child] also speak or understand that language? [If family is of recent immigrant origins], does [the child] still have close relatives there? Do they visit there often? What is the family's religious tradition? Does [the child] attend services regularly or have strong religious identifications? What activities does [child] participate in? Do you have any help or support managing these problems with [child]? How do your family members view [child's problems]? Does [child] benefit from interactions or participation with neighbors, scouting, hobbies, or shared interests with others?	Outside of your home, where are you most happy? Are there any other adults who are helpful to you or whom you like working with? Can you tell me about your best friends? Are there any kids that bother you? Is there a group you feel a part of? Whom do you "hang out" with? Is there a group you would rather be a part of? Is there any place you really like to go to feel better? How have your symptoms affected your family?

Adapted with permission from Bostic, J. Q., Potter, M. P., & King, R. A. (2018). Clinical assessment of children and adolescents: Content and structure. In A. Martin, M. H. Bloch, & F. R. Volkmar (Eds.), *Lewis's child and adolescent psychiatry: A comprehensive textbook* (5th ed., pp. 310–314). Wolters Kluwer.

TABLE 4.4

The Mental Status Examination in Children

Category	Components	What to Assess
Appearance	Physical appearance	Gender; ethnicity; age (actual and apparent); cleanliness and grooming, hair and clothing style, presence of physical anomalies, indicators of self-care and parental attentiveness; jewelry, cosmetics, adornments
	Manner of relating to clinician and parents	Ease of separation from each parent, guardedness or warming up to clinician, eagerness to please, defiance, flirtatiousness, reactions to meeting the clinician
	Activity level	Psychomotor retarded to hyperactive, sustained or episodic, goal oriented or erratic; coordination, unusual postures or motor patterns (e.g., tics, stereotypies, compulsions, catatonia, akathisia, dystonia, tremors)
	Speech	Fluency (including stuttering, cluttering, speech impediments), rate, volume, prosody
Mood	Current affect	Predominant emotion and range (constricted to labile) during the interview and appropriateness to content (e.g., giggles while talks about sibling's illness); intensity; lability
	Persisting mood	Predominant emotion over days or weeks; whether current affect is unusual or consistent with mood; whether mood is reactive to situations or the same across a range of situations
	Coping mechanisms and regulation of affect	How child manages conflict or distress, age appropriateness of responses to and dependency on parents; sexual interests, impulses, aggression; control or modulation of urges (finding alternative or socially appropriate means of satisfying urges); how child deals with frustration or when anxious
Sensorium	Orientation	Self (name), place (town, state), time (awareness of morning, day of week, month, year varies by age), situation (why at this appointment)
Intellect	Attention	Eye contact, need for redirection or repeating, how long sustained on activity, degree to which child shifts from activity to activity, distractibility (e.g., to outside noises)
	Memory	Immediate (repeat numbers, names back), short term (recall three objects at 2 and 5 minutes), long term (recall events of past week)
	Intelligence; fund of knowledge	Age-appropriate recognition of letters, vocabulary, reading, counting, computational skills; age-appropriate knowledge of geography, history, culture (e.g., celebrities, sports, movies); concrete to abstract thinking, ability to classify and categorize

(continued)

TABLE 4.4

The Mental Status Examination in Children (*continued*)

Category	Components	What to Assess
	Judgment	Especially concerning the current problems (best assessed after rapport established because initial responses may be minimization or denial); what child would do if found stamped envelope next to mailbox or a fire started in a theater; what the child would say if they saw a man with big feet
	Insight	Ability to see alternative explanations, others' points of view; locus of control (internal vs. external); defense mechanisms
Thought	Form: *coherence*	Logical, goal directed, circumstantial or tangential (consider age appropriateness), looseness of associations, word salad (incoherent, clanging, neologisms)
	Form: *speed*	Mutism, poverty of thought (long latency, thought blocking), poverty of content (perseveration), racing thoughts, flight of ideas
	Perceptions	Altered bodily experiences (depersonalization, derealization), misperception of stimulus (illusion), no stimulus (hallucination: auditory [psychosis > PTSD > organic causes], visual [dementia > delirium], olfactory [neurologic, seizure disorder] gustatory [from medicine side effects])
	Content	Obsessions (ego dystonic), delusions (ego syntonic), thoughts of harm to self or others (magical thinking and fears at night are often age-appropriate

Adapted with permission from Bostic, J. Q., Potter, M. P., & King, R. A. (2018). Clinical assessment of children and adolescents: Content and structure. In A. Martin, M. H. Bloch, & F. R. Volkmar (Eds.), *Lewis's child and adolescent psychiatry: A comprehensive textbook* (5th ed., p. 306). Wolters Kluwer.

■ PRACTICAL CONSIDERATIONS IN CLINICAL INTERVIEW

Interviewing the child is an important aspect of the assessment. It provides the child's view of the presenting problem or issues, provides an opportunity for additional history, and gives the clinician the child's perspective on the problem. Information derived from interviewing the child can be extremely helpful in developing an appropriate intervention program. The child may also reveal particular features or symptoms not necessarily either noted or commented on by the parents (e.g., movement problems and tics, thoughts of suicide, depressed mood, hallucinations). In some situations (e.g., sexual abuse), the child can be the major informant on an event. It is important to realize, particularly with younger children, that idiosyncratic or developmentally appropriate views may color the child's reporting.

It is essential that the interview be tailored to the child's language and cognitive level. In some instances (e.g., with adolescents), a lack of trust or profound desire to avoid discussion of a painfully recalled traumatic event may complicate the interview process. In instances of abuse or neglect, the knowledgeable child may rightly understand the risk of removal to an out-of-home placement. It is important that the clinician rightly position themselves as the child's advocate while maintaining an ongoing dialogue with the family. Typically, the child and parents are seen together before the interview with the child alone can proceed.

Once comfortable, the child can often readily have their parents leave (sometimes this is more of an issue for parents than for children). The use of games or play materials or other objects or materials may facilitate the transition. After the parents have left, it is usually appropriate to begin by asking the child what they understand about the purpose of the interview. This also provides a chance for the clinician to ask why the child believes parents or other adults want this process. Adolescents present some important challenges for interviewing. Often, an adolescent feels that the various adults have, in some way, colluded against them. Accordingly, it may be more helpful to have a short phone interview with the parents before the adolescent's first visit with the clinician, who can then truthfully say that they have not met the parents but have heard at least briefly from them about what the concerns are. Both parents and adolescents may have information to share only with the clinician (e.g., relative to marital issues; concerns about substance abuse; or, from the child's point of view, concerns they do not wish to share with the parents). It is important to maintain boundaries and appropriate confidentiality, always bearing in mind the importance of sharing certain kinds of information (e.g., relative to suicidality or dangerousness to others). Adolescents usually respond to a reasonably straightforward approach. Sometimes, clinicians can "overdo" their ability to relate at the same level to the adolescent patient; in reality, there are often important generational differences not always easily bridged even by well-meaning adults.

Child engagement can be a challenge. Helping the child feel more comfortable will facilitate the interview. This can be done both in the office itself and in the waiting room (e.g., with provision of a range of materials, including toys, magazines, and activities). The office should be "child friendly," and it is helpful to have drawing materials and activities such as building blocks, Jenga, or common board games that can provide an engaging backdrop for a clinical interaction. In such activities, the clinician must always maintain appropriate awareness of the goals of the setting (i.e., the investment should be in the child rather than in winning the game!). As much as possible, the child should be allowed to set the tone and direct the content of the play and interview. This can provide helpful information about the child's ability to self-organize, relate to others, and develop a narrative. Observation of the child during this time will reveal much about gross and fine motor skills, speech-communication abilities, cognitive level, affect, attention span, and so forth. Any child or adolescent can be asked about favorite activities, games, movies, books, and so forth. This discussion, particularly early on in the interview, can help "break the ice" and may also reveal common areas that the clinician can use to facilitate engagement. This discussion can also be continued over several interviews if, as is often the case, an evaluation extends over several sessions.

Direct questioning in interviewing children and adolescents requires good judgment on the part of the clinician (e.g., in regard to inquiries about information that the child may be sensitive about or reluctant to disclose). Except in emergency or urgent situations, it is preferable to allow the child to initially control the level of detail in response to direct questions. Questions posed to the child may, at times, have to be very specific, but often more open-ended questions provide information. Occasionally, particularly for younger children, helping the child establish a time frame may be useful (e.g., did this happen before you were out of school this summer?) With adolescents, issues of tact and timing are particularly important. As a general rule, the clinician should begin discussions with less threatening topics, addressing areas of the adolescent's strength rather than immediately moving to areas of difficulty. Some sensitive issues (e.g., substance abuse, sexuality, risk-taking behaviors) are intrinsically the focus of direct question. Giving the child a more general question to respond to is often a good way to begin a line of inquiry. It is important in discussions of sexuality that the clinician be sensitive to the possibility of both homosexual and heterosexual relationships and experiences (e.g., as far as possible, questions should be phrased in a way that maintains gender neutrality). Risk-taking can be approached by asking about things that were potentially dangerous or that might have gotten the child or adolescent into trouble with parents or teachers.

Ending the interview in a mutually satisfactory and collaborative way can help the child leave with a positive feeling and may facilitate subsequent clinical encounters. Often, it is helpful to signal the approach to the end of an interview and ask the child or adolescent if there are any things they would like to talk about that have not been touched on. It is also very reasonable to ask the child or adolescent if they have any questions for the examiner. Occasionally, the child will ask about the clinician's recommendations or thoughts. Usually, it is best not to be overly specific until there has been a chance to talk with the child's parents; in addition, there may be additional studies (e.g., laboratory or psychological tests) that the examiner wishes to obtain.

Confidentiality remains one of the most complicated issues for clinicians to address, particularly in relation to adolescents. On the one hand, it is important that the clinician not be a "parental spy," but, on the other hand, there may be some reporting requirements (e.g., in some cases relating to protection of the child or to insurance reimbursement). It is important before collecting any information that an explanation is provided to the adolescent or child of exactly what will be disclosed (e.g., recommendations for classroom modifications) and what may need to be confidential (e.g., sexuality). Both the child and the parents should understand that in some situations, the usual confidentiality rules do not apply.

■ FORMULATION AND INTEGRATION: THE TREATMENT PLAN

The formulation of the case provides a context for understanding the child's symptoms and life circumstances, providing a set of treatment goals to be adapted and changed in accordance with subsequent clinical encounters and additional information. A range of treatment options, including no treatment, is available. The formulation of the case should effectively communicate relevant information about the child, a rationale for the diagnosis and for treatment recommendations made. Core components of the formulation include the chief complaint, historical information, results of the present evaluation, and so forth (see Table 4.5). The formulation can vary in

TABLE 4.5

Core Components Toward a Formulation of a Treatment Plan

Component	Details
Source	Patient, collaterals
Chief complaint	What brought the patient in
History of present illness	Symptoms, course, severity, pertinent negatives
Past psychiatric history	Previous evaluations, therapies, hospitalizations, medications, and treatments; substance abuse history
Past medical history	Treatments, illnesses, hospitalizations, surgeries, medications (including home remedies, homeopathy, and so on)
Family history	Pertinent positives and negatives in the family's psychiatric and medical history
Social history	Family constellation, peer relations, interactions with the law and social services
Education history	Schools, grades, report cards, special or regular education
Developmental history	Mother's pregnancy and labor, delivery, milestones during infancy; stages of motor, cognitive, social, and behavioral development
Psychological testing	IQ, tests of adaptive functioning, speech and language evaluation
Mental status exam	Main findings
Assessment	Diagnoses, hypotheses of causality
Plan	Treatment goals and options, collaterals to contact

Adapted from Henderson, S. W., & Martin, A. (2018). Formulation and integration. In A. Martin, M. H. Bloch, & F. R. Volkmar (Eds.), *Lewis's child and adolescent psychiatry: A comprehensive textbook* (5th ed., p. 285). Wolters Kluwer.

length, breadth, and level of detail, depending on clinical circumstance. We have seen everything from two sentences ("child seen, diagnosis is autism") to a 30-page, single-spaced narrative. The typical formulation usually occupies a middle ground between these two extremes and should endeavor to help the child, parents, teachers, and other professionals understand the patient's difficulties and treatment options.

In addition to the details that have to be included in the evaluation report listed in Table 4.5, clinical formulation can follow the Four Ps model (Henderson & Martin, 2018). The model organizes information about the patient into *predisposing, precipitating, perpetuating,* and *protective* factors. *Predisposing* factors refer to past vulnerabilities such as family history, genetics, medical and psychiatric history, and chronic social stressors. Including these factors in clinical evaluation suggest that they are directly relevant to the child's current symptoms. *Precipitating* factors identify the current stressors, inciting events, and concurrent illness that may directly impact the chief complaint or a primary diagnosis. *Perpetuating* factors are those that make the current mental health disorder endure, such as the severity of the condition, compliance with treatment, deficits in coping, or exacerbating social circumstances. *Protective* factors describe a patient's strengths, resilience, and supports (Box 4.1).

A formulation based on the four perspectives would start with the clinical presentation and end with formulation of specific interventions. Clearly, different approaches to assessment and treatment will be required for different disorders and circumstances. For example, a biologic disease model approach might work well for patients with schizophrenia but much less well in dealing with stresses such as bereavement or dissatisfaction with one's life course.

Regardless of which approach is adopted, the formulation should give the clinician an opportunity to understand and explain the presenting concerns and outline an actionable treatment plan. Particularly for children and adolescents, the question of the "right" diagnosis may be clarified only over time, but diagnosis aside, the aim of the formulation should be to provide a thoughtful, sympathetic portrait of the child.

BOX 4.1   Sample Formulation

A 14-year-old boy presents to a community child mental health clinic from school, having been referred by his teacher first to a counselor after writing an essay in which he expressed suicidal ideation. Predisposing factors include a mother with a long history of depression treated with psychotherapy, a paternal uncle who committed suicide, and his parents' divorce with lengthy and often bitter custodial disputes. Precipitating factors include 3 weeks of poor sleep, decreased appetite, feelings of guilt and helplessness in the context of his parents' divorce, as well as several recent stressors, including a test in school, which he is scared he might fail. Perpetuating factors include lack of interest in any sort of treatment because of worries about stigma, his parents' denial that their conflicts affect their son, and a depression that has reached such depths that the patient is considering suicide. In his case, however, several protective factors can be identified, including the boy's popularity at school as a secretary of the student assembly and as catcher on the baseball team; his willingness to talk with a therapist after he comes in; his parents' care for his well-being despite their conflict; and the family's willingness to work together to help the boy through depression. After initial evaluation that included development of a safety plan that was discussed with the child and his parents, the boy agreed to participate in weekly psychotherapy focused on reducing depression and improving communication with the parents around topics that could trigger disagreements. Cognitive–behavioral interventions were also developed to improve sleep patterns and decrease worries about tests.

Adapted with permission from Henderson, S. W., & Martin, A. (2018). Formulation and integration. In A. Martin, M. H. Bloch, & F. R. Volkmar (Eds.), *Lewis's child and adolescent psychiatry: A comprehensive textbook* (5th ed., p. 288). Wolters Kluwer.

References

*Indicates Particularly Recommended

Achenbach, T. M. (1966). The classification of children's psychiatric symptoms: A factor-analytic study. *Psychological Monographs, 80*(7), 1–37. https://doi.org/10.1037/h0093906

American Psychiatric Association. (2013). *Diagnostic and statistical manual of mental disorders, fifth edition, (DSM-5)*. American Psychiatric Publishing.

*Angold, A., Costello, E. J., & Egger, H. (2018). Structured interviewing. In A. Martin, M. H. Bloch, & F. R. Volkmar (Eds.), *Lewis's child and adolescent psychiatry: A comprehensive textbook* (5th ed., pp. 342–354). Wolters Kluwer.

Angold, A., Costello, E. J., & Erkanli, A. (1999). Comorbidity. *Journal of Child Psychology and Psychiatry and Allied Disciplines, 40*(1), 57–87. https://doi.org/10.1111/1469-7610.00424

Bostic, J. Q., Potter, M. A., & King, R. A. (2018). Clinical assessment of children and adolescents: Content and structure. In A. Martin, M. H. Bloch, & F. R. Volkmar (Eds.), *Lewis's child and adolescent psychiatry: A comprehensive textbook* (5th ed., pp. 299–320). Wolters Kluwer.

*Cuthbert, B. N. (2015). Research Domain Criteria: Toward future psychiatric nosologies. *Dialogues in Clinical Neuroscience, 17*(1), 89–97. https://doi.org/10.31887/DCNS.2015.17.1/bcuthbert

Fabrigar, L. R., & Wegener, D. T. (2012). *Exploratory factor analysis*. Oxford University Press.

Freud, A. (1965). *Normality and pathology in childhood*. International Universities Press.

Henderson, S. W., & Martin, A. (2018). Formulation and integration. In A. Martin, M. H. Bloch, & F. R. Volkmar (Eds.), *Lewis's child and adolescent psychiatry: A comprehensive textbook* (5th ed., pp. 284–299). Wolters Kluwer.

*Hoff, P. (2015). The Kraepelinian tradition. *Dialogues in Clinical Neuroscience, 17*(1), 31–41. https://doi.org/10.31887/DCNS.2015.17.1/phoff

*Insel, T., Cuthbert, B., Garvey, M., Heinssen, R., Pine, D. S., Quinn, K., Sanislow, C., & Wang, P. (2010). Research Domain Criteria (RDoC): Toward a new classification framework for research on mental disorders. *American Journal of Psychiatry, 167*(7), 748–751. https://doi.org/10.1176/appi.ajp.2010.09091379

Jones, S. C. T., & Neblett, E. W. (2017). Future directions in research on racism-related stress and racial-ethnic protective factors for black youth. *Journal of Clinical Child and Adolescent Psychology, 46*(5), 754–766. https://doi.org/10.1080/15374416.2016.1146991

Lau, B. Y., Leong, R., Uljarevic, M., Lerh, J. W., Rodgers, J., Hollocks, M. J., South, M., McConachie, H., Ozsivadjian, A., Van Hecke, A., Libove, R., Hardan, A., Leekam, S., Simonoff, E., & Magiati, I. (2020). Anxiety in young people with autism spectrum disorder: Common and autism-related anxiety experiences and their associations with individual characteristics. *Autism, 24*(5), 1111–1126. https://doi.org/10.1177/1362361319886246

Madigan, S., Browne, D., Racine, N., Mori, C., & Tough, S. (2019). Association between screen time and children's performance on a developmental screening test. *JAMA Pediatrics, 173*(3), 244–250. https://doi.org/10.1001/jamapediatrics.2018.5056

*National Institute of Mental Health. (2020). *RDoC Matrix*. https://www.nimh.nih.gov/research/research-funded-by-nimh/rdoc/constructs/rdoc-matrix.shtml

Nunnally, J. C., & Bernstein, I. H. (1994). *Psychometric theory* (3rd ed.). McGraw-Hill.

Rutter, M. (1965). Classification and categorization in child psychiatry. *Journal of Child Psychology & Psychiatry, 6*, 71–83. https://doi.org/10.1111/j.1469-7610.1965.tb02229.x

Sanislow, C. A. (2020). RDoC at 10: Changing the discourse for psychopathology. *World Psychiatry, 19*(3), 311–312. https://doi.org/10.1002/wps.20800

Shafi, R. M. A., Romanowicz, M., & Croarkin, P. E. (2018). #SwitchedOn: A call for assessing social media use of adolescents. *The Lancet Psychiatry, 5*(11), e27. https://doi.org/10.1016/S2215-0366(18)30350-X

World Health Organization. (2019–2020). *International classification of diseases and related health problems (ICD)*. https://www.who.int/classifications/icd/en/

Suggested Readings

*Bresin, K. (2020). Toward a unifying theory of dysregulated behaviors. *Clinical Psychology Review, 80*, 101885. https://doi.org/10.1016/j.cpr.2020.101885

Caspi, A., & Moffitt, T. E. (2018). All for one and one for all: Mental disorders in one dimension. *American Journal of Psychiatry, 175*(9), 831–844. https://doi.org/10.1176/appi.ajp.2018.17121383

*Dalgleish, T., Black, M., Johnston, D., & Bevan, A. (2020). Transdiagnostic approaches to mental health problems: Current status and future directions. *Journal of Consulting and Clinical Psychology, 88*(3), 179–195. https://doi.org/10.1037/ccp0000482

Duncan, L., Comeau, J., Wang, L., Vitoroulis, I., Boyle, M. H., & Bennett, K. (2019). Research Review: Test–retest reliability of standardized diagnostic interviews to assess child and adolescent psychiatric disorders: A systematic review and meta-analysis. *Journal of Child Psychology and Psychiatry, 60*(1), 16–29. https://doi.org/10.1111/jcpp.12876

Egger, H. L. (2009). Psychiatric assessment of young children. *Child and Adolescent Psychiatric Clinics of North America, 18*(3), 559–580. https://doi.org/10.1016/j.chc.2009.02.004

Evans, S. C., Roberts, M. C., Keeley, J. W., Rebello, T. J., de la Peña, F., Lochman, J. E., Burke, J. D., Fite, P. J., Ezpeleta, L., Matthys, W., Youngstrom, E. A., Matsumoto, C., Andrews, H. F., Elena Medina-Mora, M., Ayuso-Mateos, J. L., Khoury, B., Kulygina, M., Robles, R., Sharan, P., ... Reed, G. M. (2020). Diagnostic classification of irritability and oppositionality in youth: A global field study comparing ICD-11 with ICD-10 and DSM-5. *Journal of Child Psychology and Psychiatry and Allied Disciplines, 62*(3), 303–312. https://doi.org/10.1111/jcpp.13244

*Fabiano, F., & Haslam, N. (2020). Diagnostic inflation in the *DSM*: A meta-analysis of changes in the stringency of psychiatric diagnosis from *DSM-III* to *DSM-5*. *Clinical Psychology Review, 80*, 101889. https://doi.org/10.1016/j.cpr.2020.101889

Masi, G., Milone, A., Brovedani, P., Pisano, S., & Muratori, P. (2018). Psychiatric evaluation of youths with Disruptive Behavior Disorders and psychopathic traits: A critical review of assessment measures. *Neuroscience and Biobehavioral Reviews, 91*, 21–33. https://doi.org/10.1016/j.neubiorev.2016.09.023

Rolon-Arroyo, B., Oosterhoff, B., Layne, C. M., Steinberg, A. M., Pynoos, R. S., & Kaplow, J. B. (2020). The UCLA PTSD reaction index for *DSM-5* brief form: A screening tool for trauma-exposed youths. *Journal of the American Academy of Child and Adolescent Psychiatry, 59*(3), 434–443. https://doi.org/10.1016/j.jaac.2019.06.015

Ronald, A. (2019). Editorial: The psychopathology p factor: Will it revolutionize the science and practice of child and adolescent psychiatry? *Journal of Child Psychology and Psychiatry, 60*(5), 497–499. https://doi.org/10.1111/jcpp.13063

Shulman, C., Rice, C. E., Morrier, M. J., & Esler, A. (2020). The role of diagnostic instruments in dual and differential diagnosis in autism spectrum disorder across the lifespan. *Child and Adolescent Psychiatric Clinics of North America, 29*(2), 275–299. https://doi.org/10.1016/j.chc.2020.01.002

Thapar, A., & Riglin, L. (2020). The importance of a developmental perspective in Psychiatry: What do recent genetic-epidemiological findings show? *Molecular Psychiatry, 25*(8), 1631–1639. https://doi.org/10.1038/s41380-020-0648-1

*Walter, H. J., Bukstein, O. G., Abright, A. R., Keable, H., Ramtekkar, U., Ripperger-Suhler, J., & Rockhill, C. (2020). Clinical practice guideline for the assessment and treatment of children and adolescents with anxiety disorders. *Journal of the American Academy of Child and Adolescent Psychiatry, 59*(10), 1107–1124. https://doi.org/10.1016/j.jaac.2020.05.005

CHAPTER 5 ■ AN OVERVIEW OF TREATMENT APPROACHES

■ INTRODUCTION

The modern history of treatment for psychological and psychiatric problems is often viewed as beginning with the work of Freud in the late 19th and early 20th centuries. After a brief stay at the Salpêtrière studying the work of the neurologist Martin Charcot, renowned for his work on the uses of hypnosis for "hysterical" conditions (Charcot & Goetz, 1987), Freud returned to Vienna where he began using hypnosis with patients. Within a few years, Freud abandoned hypnosis in favor of encouraging patients to freely share their thoughts ("free association") as a means of revealing unconscious psychological material (Freud, 1929). This led to the eventual development of *psychoanalysis* as a comprehensive theory of mental illness and a treatment approach.

The practice of psychoanalysis soon came to dominate the landscape of mental health care in much of the world but was not without its detractors. Among the criticisms levelled against psychoanalytic theory were the difficulty in empirically substantiating many of its claims, the variety of unconscious structures to which problems were being attributed, and the unobservable nature of core psychoanalytic constructs.

These criticisms, and others, contributed to the rise of behaviorism. Watson and Wolpe, early champions of the behaviorist approach, drew on animal research, such as the work of Pavlov, showing that responses to stimuli can be learned ("conditioned") through experience (Wolpe & Plaud, 1997). They emphasized focusing on processes that can be empirically studied in laboratory settings and applied learning principles to humans. In Watson's seminal case of Little Albert, a new fear was induced in a child by pairing a previously not frightening stimulus with a loud noise (Watson & Rayner, 1920). Mary Cover Jones demonstrated that fears can be removed through gradual exposure to a fear-inducing stimulus (Jones, 1924), and Wolpe applied the procedure clinically with the addition of progressive relaxation, laying the foundation for many current behavioral treatment interventions (Wolpe, 1958, 1961).

In the second half of the 20th century, a renewed focus on the not directly observable mental processes that impact psychological problems came about through the development, and eventual integration with behavioral approaches, of cognitive therapy (Beck, 1963). Underlying this focus on cognition were the assumptions that human beings respond to mental representations of events, rather than to the events themselves, that learning is mediated by mental processes of cognition, and that individuals form and maintain a cognitive style that impacts their learning and their susceptibility to psychological problems. Cognitive therapy aims to identify and modify such problematic thought patterns. The integration of cognitive and behavioral treatment strategies is generally referred to as cognitive behavioral therapy or CBT.

CBT itself has continued to evolve in recent decades. This process has included the expansion of CBT, as treatment protocols have been developed and studied for more and more mental health conditions, as well as the addition of various treatment components that draw from other areas. In particular, a group of interventions (often referred to as the *third wave* of behavioral treatment) emphasizes mindfulness, acceptance, and relationships—factors that do not feature in "classic" CBT (Hayes & Hofmann, 2017). Prominent in this group are acceptance and commitment therapy (Hayes et al., 2011), dialectical behavior therapy (DBT) (Linehan et al., 1999), and mindfulness-based therapies (Khoury et al., 2013).

Alongside the evolution of behavioral and cognitive approaches, the second half of the 20th century also saw the rise of family therapy as a theoretical and applied discipline. Ackerman is often credited with having published the first paper to explicitly describe treating an entire family unit (Ackerman & Sobel, 1950). Much of the early work in family therapy focused on the role of family and relationships in schizophrenia, which led to the now discredited concept of the "schizophrenogenic mother"—one who through aloofness, rejection, and guilt alongside a passive and ineffective father, was thought to induce schizophrenia in her children (Seeman, 2016). Though such direct cause and effect pathways are no longer thought to link parental behaviors and child mental illness, family therapy remains a prominent approach to treating mental problems.

TREATMENT APPROACHES

Psychodynamic Approaches

Psychodynamic treatment is a broad concept that describes a variety of specific treatment interventions that share certain underlying principles and assumptions (Luyten et al., 2015). Among these are an emphasis on internal and unconscious conflicts between aspects of the patient's psyche; the view that mental problems stem from experiences early in life; the view that individuals develop "defenses" or processes that emerge to reduce the distress caused by the internal conflicts; the assumption that problematic dynamics will emerge and play out in the patient–therapist interactions and relationship; and the belief that achieving insight into the previously unconscious conflicts is a key to achieving therapeutic success. Psychodynamic therapies have their root in Freud's psychoanalysis but have evolved to encompass a range of specific therapies with unique theoretical and practical characteristics. Among the schools of psychodynamic therapies are, in addition to Freudian analysis, Ego Psychology (Wallerstein, 2002), Object Relations (Klein, 1984), and Self Psychology (Kohut, 1971).

The high degree to which psychodynamic treatments are tailored to individual patients generally precludes the kind of step-by-step manualization of treatment protocols that is typical in some other forms of therapy (e.g., CBT). This necessitates a particularly high level of trust in the therapist on the part of the patient, and a particularly strong emphasis on the therapeutic alliance. Patients in psychodynamic therapy are generally encouraged to speak freely and without self-censorship as a means of revealing unconscious material, and special emphasis is placed on verbalizations relating to feelings of the patient toward the therapist.

Although much of psychodynamic therapy has focused on adults, there is also a long and rich history of psychodynamic treatment for pediatric patients, often with an emphasis on the use of play. Play therapy interprets the child's verbal and nonverbal behavior during play, similar to the open and uncensored speech in treating adults. Freud first introduced the concept of using play as a therapeutic tool with children in his seminal description of Little Hans (Young-Bruehl, 2007). Through this and other work (mostly with adults), Freud developed several theories, eventually arriving at a sexual drive theory that posits the existence of sequential psychosexual stages of development. Each of the oral, anal, phallic, and genital stages is accompanied by developmental challenges for the child. Each challenge must be successfully resolved before advancing to the next stage to avoid the development of neurotic "fixations" that cause regression to the unsuccessfully completed stage during times of stress throughout life. Further advances, expansions, and competing psychodynamic approaches for treating children have been developed over the many decades since Freud disseminated his ideas, with prominent figures in the field including Anna Freud, Melanie Klein, and Donald Winnicott. Although psychodynamic treatment tends to be more client-focused than symptom-focused, specific psychodynamic interventions have been developed for certain problems including trauma.

Cognitive Behavioral Approaches

CBT is the most widely studied psychological treatment and encompasses a large number of specific interventions for a wide range of problems, with certain shared features and underlying principles. Cognitive behavioral therapies are generally focused and pragmatic, emphasizing symptom reduction through problem solving and skill building rather than the discovery of root etiologic causes of the patient's problems. Cognitive behavioral therapies assume that problems develop at least in part through learned experience and treatment is generally informed by functional analysis of causal pathways linking thoughts, emotions, and behavior. Functional analysis involves a systematic attempt to identify the antecedents (both environmental and internal) of problematic behavior patterns (Mash & Wolfe, 2019). CBT tends to be relatively brief, with many interventions having a typical length of between 10 and 20 sessions, although both shorter and longer protocols exist and are in common use.

Most cognitive behavioral therapies include most or all the following components: (1) Psychoeducation, whereby patients (and parents) are provided with information regarding their condition and regarding the treatment and its rationale; (2) Self-monitoring, whereby patients are encouraged to systematically monitor and log a target behavior or cognitive process; (3) Behavioral rehearsal and role play of desired behaviors, to replace less adaptive behavioral patterns; (4) Identification of automatic thought patterns that bias the patient's perception and interpretation of stimuli and situations; (5) Cognitive restructuring, whereby maladaptive or biased thoughts are systematically replaced with more realistic or rational ones (often achieved through a Socratic dialog with the patient or through "thought experiments"); (6) Homework, in which the patient is encouraged to practice skills learned in therapy in their natural environment and daily life.

Additional components are typical of CBT for specific problems. For example, in CBT for anxiety problems both behavioral rehearsal and homework usually emphasize systematic exposure to feared and avoided stimuli. Somatic regulation skills such as relaxing breathing and progressive muscle relaxation are also commonly part of CBT for anxiety (and some other) problems. And CBT for depression can include a focus on behavioral activation, to increase contact with rewarding experiences and activities (Cuijpers et al., 2007).

CBT for children tends to closely resemble treatment with adults and is based on the same underlying principles. Materials are adapted for the developmental stage and cognitive maturity of the child, and parents are often involved in the treatment process to provide more information for the therapist, encourage the child to practice skills at home, and reduce unhelpful parental behaviors that may be exacerbating or maintaining the symptoms.

Group Therapy

Group therapy refers to treatment provided to a number of patients simultaneously and includes both treatments that utilize the group format and interactions among group members as the key intervention strategy as well as adaptations of individual treatment modalities to group settings.

Treatments that utilize the group dynamic as the core therapeutic mechanism emphasize the experience of universality that can be attained by communicating with others experiencing relatable problems, the correction and replacement of negative interaction patterns that were formed in previous experiences such as within the family, catharsis that can be achieved by sharing one's troubles with an empathic audience, and interpersonal learning from other group members. This kind of group therapy is more commonly applied with adults than with children, but can be provided to children and can create opportunities for the development of improved social skills.

Treatments that are usually delivered in individual format, such as CBT, can also be delivered to groups (Silverman et al., 1999). In these instances, the underlying principles of the treatment do not change, but the group can benefit from many of the benefits of a group setting such as the experience of universality, the opportunity for interpersonal learning, and the catharsis of sharing challenges with others.

A thorough review and detailed description of all psychological treatments is beyond the scope of this chapter. The treatments reviewed here in brief are some of the most widely used and prominent therapeutic approaches, but many other treatments exist. Among these are family therapy (described briefly earlier and see Chapter 30), parent management training (used for externalizing problems) (Michelson et al., 2013), parent–child interaction therapy (used for externalizing, and more recently also internalizing, problems) (Zisser-Nathenson et al., 2018), habit reversal therapy (used for tic disorders) (Piacentini et al., 2010), acceptance and commitment therapy, and many others. Each of these shares the goal of reducing problematic mental health symptoms and each is supported to one extent or another by research. But what does empirical research actually say about the efficacy of psychological therapy?

Evidence-Based Treatment

An American Psychological Association taskforce defined evidence-based practice as *the integration of the best available research with clinical expertise in the context of patient characteristics, culture, and preferences* (American Psychological Association, 2005). Each component of the definition is important but any attempt to base clinical decision making on empirical evidence relies on the availability of rigorous clinical trial research. The efficacy of any treatment can be evaluated in different ways and the gold standard of efficacy research is the randomized controlled trial (RCT).

In an RCT, patients are randomly assigned to one of two or more treatment conditions, often the treatment of interest and a comparator of known efficacy or that can be expected not to be efficacious. When comparing a treatment of interest to a comparator that is not expected to be particularly efficacious, it is important that the comparator still appear to be credible in the eyes of the participating patients. This is similar to comparing a medication to a placebo pill in a drug study. An important difference however is that in psychological treatment, it is almost impossible for the patient not to know what treatment they have been assigned to, and it is entirely not possible for the therapist not to know this. In other words, the "double blind" that is maintained in drug studies is generally not possible in psychotherapeutic research. Instead a "single blind" is often maintained, by conducting clinical assessment and evaluation through independent evaluators who are not aware of the treatment assignment. Other, less demanding methods for learning about the efficacy of treatments include case studies, open clinical trials (without a randomization process and with only one treatment arm), and single-case experimental design studies. When multiple studies have been conducted to evaluate a particular treatment, meta-analyses can be used to synthesize their results and estimate the size of the intervention's effects.

Treatments can be classified based on the level of evidence that has accumulated to support their efficacy. The highest level of evidence will include meta-analyses or systematic reviews of multiple RCTs. A lower level of evidence would include findings from at least one RCT, and yet lower levels will include data from uncontrolled trials and case studies only.

Evidence for Efficacy of Psychotherapy

Many RCTs have now been conducted, examining the efficacy of different therapies for children and adolescents across a range of target problems and disorders. Numerous meta-analyses have by now also been completed and have provided strong empirical support for psychotherapy as a means of treating children and adolescents. Some of these trials and meta-analyses have demonstrated superiority of CBT over other (nonbehavioral) forms of treatment (Weisz et al., 1995), but this remains an issue of contention. Among the criticisms levelled against those who have concluded that CBT is superior to other treatments are the fact that there are many more trials of CBT than there are of other therapies, and the fact that in some cases the non-CBT approach was implemented as the comparator condition in studies evaluating CBT (Weiss & Weisz, 1995; Westen et al., 2004). The critique is that because the non-CBT approach was being used as a comparator (rather than as the treatment of interest), it may have been delivered with less care or skill than the CBT.

Among the therapies that have garnered the strongest empirical support are exposure-based CBT for anxiety and obsessive-compulsive disorders, and behavioral parent training for oppositional child behaviors. Based on results from multiple clinical trials, most children who receive these therapies (approximately two thirds to three quarters) are likely to experience significant improvement in their symptoms and related impairment, and approximately half are likely to experience complete remission (In-Albon & Schneider, 2006). Other problems for which there exist treatments that can be considered well established include depression, posttraumatic stress disorder, attention problems, autism, and bipolar disorder, among others. Of note, for many of these conditions, efficacy may be defined in terms of a reduction in problematic symptoms and a reduction in functional impairment rather than as complete remission from the disorder.

Current and Future Questions

Despite the evidence for the efficacy of psychotherapy overall, important questions remain that have yet to be satisfactorily answered. For many conditions, the comparative efficacy of different approaches remains a matter of ongoing research and debate. The *effectiveness* of many treatments is not well established. Effectiveness is distinct from efficacy in that it focuses on how well the treatment works in the real world, rather than in a research environment such as a university setting. Another question that is not yet answered for most treatments is *for whom* treatments work best, and which treatments work best for different patients. Research aiming to answer this question focuses on *moderators*, or patient characteristics that differentially predict treatment response to different treatment interventions. Identifying such moderator variables can increase the overall efficacy of treatment by helping to correctly prescribe the right kind of therapy to each patient based on their individual characteristics, rather than relying on overall average response rates. To take an oversimplified example, two treatments might have approximately identical average efficacy in the population, but if one of those treatments is working splendidly for all the male patients and none of the females, and the other treatment is completely efficacious for females but not at all for males, then identifying the moderator variable (sex) could improve overall efficacy from 50% to 100%.

Finally, *how* treatments work is also a question that is not well answered for most therapies. Here, research focuses on *mediator* variables, or steps along the causal pathway leading from the intervention to symptom reduction. Although treatments are generally based on a theoretical model for how they work to achieve the symptom reduction, in most cases these models remain hypothetical only and have not been empirically demonstrated.

SUMMARY

Psychotherapy as a scientifically informed field of clinical work and empirical research has been around for approximately 150 years. In that time, various schools of thought have given rise to a large number of specific interventions and treatment strategies for children and adolescents. Research supports the conclusion that psychotherapy can be efficacious across a broad range of psychological and psychiatric problems. Yet, important questions remain unanswered. It is not yet clear how, why, and for whom specific treatments work; many youth continue to suffer from their mental health problems even after receiving evidence-based psychotherapy; some problems do not yet have well-established treatment options. Much work remains to be done as the field of psychotherapy continues to grow and develop in the years to come.

References

*Indicates Particularly Recommended

Ackerman, N. W., & Sobel, R. (1950). Family diagnosis: An approach to the preschool child. *American Journal of Orthopsychiatry*, 20(4), 744–753. https://doi.org/10.1111/j.1939-0025.1950.tb05473.x

American Psychological Association. (2005). *Policy statement on evidence-based practice in psychology*. Retrieved February 11, 2020, from http://www.apa.org/practice/guidelines/evidence-based-statement

Beck, A. T. (1963). Thinking and depression. I. Idiosyncratic content and cognitive distortions. *Archives of General Psychiatry*, 9, 324–333. https://doi.org/10.1001/archpsyc.1963.01720160014002

Charcot, J. M., & Goetz, C. G. (1987). *Charcot, the clinician: The Tuesday lessons: Excerpts from nine case presentations on general neurology delivered at the Salpêtrière hospital in 1887–88 by Jean–Martin Charcot*. Raven Press.

Cuijpers, P., Van Straten, A., & Warmerdam, L. (2007). Behavioral activation treatments of depression: A meta-analysis. *Clinical Psychology Review*, 27(3), 318–326. https://doi.org/10.1016/j.cpr.2006.11.001

Freud, S. (1929). *Introductory lectures on psycho-analysis: A course of twenty eight lectures delivered at the University of Vienna* (rev. ed.). Allen & Unwin.

*Hayes, S. C., & Hofmann, S. G. (2017). The third wave of cognitive behavioral therapy and the rise of process-based care. *World Psychiatry*, 16(3), 245–246. https://doi.org/10.1002/wps.20442

Hayes, S. C., Strosahl, K. D., & Wilson, K. G. (2011). *Acceptance and commitment therapy: An experiential approach to behavior change*. American Psychological Association.

*In-Albon, T., & Schneider, S. (2006). Psychotherapy of childhood anxiety disorders: A meta-analysis. *Psychotherapy and Psychosomatics*, 76(1), 15–24. https://doi.org/10.1159/000096361

Jones, M. C. (1924). A laboratory study of fear: The case of peter. *The Pedagogical Seminary and Journal of Genetic Psychology*, 31(4), 308–315. https://doi.org/10.1080/08856559.1924.9944851

Khoury, B., Lecomte, T., Fortin, G., Masse, M., Therien, P., Bouchard, V., Chapleau, M-A., Paquin, K., & Hofmann, S. G. (2013). Mindfulness-based therapy: A comprehensive meta-analysis. *Clinical Psychology Review*, 33(6), 763–771. https://doi.org/10.1016/j.cpr.2013.05.005

Klein, M. (1984). *Love, guilt, and reparation, and other works, 1921–1945* (Free Press ed.). Free Press.

Kohut, H. (1971). *The analysis of the self: A systematic approach to the psychoanalytic treatment of narcissistic personality disorders*. University of Chicago Press.

Linehan, M. M., Schmidt, H., Dimeff, L. A., Craft, J. C., Kanter, J., & Comtois, K. A. (1999). Dialectical behavior therapy for patients with borderline personality disorder and drug-dependence. *The American Journal of Addictions*, 8(4), 279–292. https://doi.org/10.1080/105504999305686

Luyten, P., Mayes, L. C., Fonagy, P., Target, M., & Blatt, S. J. (2015). *Handbook of psychodynamic approaches to psychopathology*. The Guilford Press.

Mash, E. J., & Wolfe, D. A. (2019). *Abnormal child psychology* (7th ed.). Wadsworth Publishing.

*Michelson, D., Davenport, C., Dretzke, J., Barlow, J., & Day, C. (2013). Do evidence-based interventions work when tested in the "real world?" A systematic review and meta-analysis of parent management training for the treatment of child disruptive behavior. *Clinical Child and Family Psychology Review*, 16(1), 18–34. https://doi.org/10.1007/s10567-013-0128-0

Piacentini, J., Woods, D. W., Scahill, L., Wilhelm, S., Peterson, A. L., Chang, S., Ginsburg, G. S., Deckersbach, T., Dziura, J., Levi-Pearl, S., & Walkup, J. T. (2010). Behavior therapy for children with Tourette disorder: A randomized controlled trial. *JAMA*, 303(19), 1929–1937. https://doi.org/10.1001/jama.2010.607

Seeman, M. V. (2016). Schizophrenogenic mother. In J. Lebow, A. Chambers, & D. C. Breunlin (Eds.), *Encyclopedia of couple and family therapy* (pp. 1–2). Springer International Publishing.

Silverman, W. K., Kurtines, W. M., Ginsburg, G. S., Weems, C. F., Lumpkin, P. W., & Carmichael, D. H. (1999). Treating anxiety disorders in children with group cognitive-behavioral therapy: A randomized clinical trial. *The Journal of Consulting and Clinical Psychology, 67*(6), 995–1003. https://doi.org/10.1037/0022-006X.67.6.995

Wallerstein, R. S. (2002). The growth and transformation of American ego psychology. *Journal of the American Psychoanalytic Association, 50*(1), 135–169. https://doi.org/10.1177/00030651020500011401

Watson, J. B., & Rayner, R. (1920). Conditioned emotional reactions. *Journal of Experimental Psychology, 3*(1), 1–14. https://doi.org/10.1037/h0069608

*Weiss, B., & Weisz, J. R. (1995). Relative effectiveness of behavioral versus nonbehavioral child psychotherapy. *The Journal of Consulting and Clinical Psychology, 63*(2), 317–320. https://doi.org/10.1037/0022-006X.63.2.317

Weisz, J. R., Weiss, B., Han, S. S., Granger, D. A., & Morton, T. (1995). Effects of psychotherapy with children and adolescents revisited: A meta-analysis of treatment outcome studies. *Psychological Bulletin, 117*(3), 450–468. https://doi.org/10.1037/0033-2909.117.3.450

*Westen, D., Novotny C. M., & Thompson-Brenner, H. (2004). The empirical status of empirically supported psychotherapies: Assumptions, findings, and reporting in controlled clinical trials. *Psychological Bulletin, 130*(4), 631–663. https://doi.org/10.1037/0033-2909.130.4.631

Wolpe, J. (1958). *Psychotherapy by reciprocal inhibition.* Stanford University Press.

Wolpe, J. (1961). The systematic desensitization treatment of neuroses. *Journal of Nervous and Mental Disease, 132,* 189–203. https://doi.org/10.1097/00005053-196103000-00001

*Wolpe, J., & Plaud, J. J. (1997). Pavlov's contributions to behavior therapy: The obvious and the not so obvious. *American Psychologist, 52*(9), 966–972. https://doi.org/10.1037/0003-066X.52.9.966

Young-Bruehl, E. (2007). Little Hans in the history of child analysis. *The Psychoanalytic Study of the Child, 62,* 28–43. https://doi.org/10.1080/00797308.2007.11800782

Zisser-Nathenson, A. R., Herschell, A. D., & Eyberg, S. M. (2018). Parent-child interaction therapy and the treatment of disruptive behavior disorders. In J. R. Weisz & A. E. Kazdin (Eds.), *Evidence-based psychotherapies for children and adolescents* (3rd ed., pp. 103–121). The Guilford Press.

Suggested Readings

Boakes, R. A. (1984). *From Darwin to behaviourism: Psychology and the minds of animals.* Cambridge University Press.

Geissmann-Chambon, C., & Geissmann, P. (1998). *A history of child psychoanalysis.* Routledge.

Goldenberg, I., & Goldenberg, H. (1991). *Family therapy: An overview* (3rd ed.). Thomson Brooks/Cole Publishing Co.

Homeyer, L. E., & Morrison, M. O. (2008). Play therapy: Practice, issues, and trends. *American Journal of Play, 1*(2), 210–228.

McNeil, C. B., Hembree-Kigin, T. L., Anhalt, K., & Hembree-Kigin, T. L. (2010). *Parent-child interaction therapy* (2nd ed.). Springer.

Mitchell, S. A., & Black, M. J. (1995). *Freud and beyond: A history of modern psychoanalytic thought.* Basic Books.

O'Connor, K. J., Schaefer, C. E., & Braverman, L. D. (2016). *Handbook of play therapy* (2nd ed.). John Wiley & Sons, Inc.

Samelson, F. (1988). Struggle for scientific authority: The reception of Watson's behaviorism, 1913–1920. In L. T. Benjamin (Ed.), *A history of psychology: Original sources and contemporary research* (pp. 407–424). McGraw-Hill Book Company.

VandenBos, G. R., Meidenbauer, E., & Frank-McNeil, J. (2014). *Psychotherapy theories and techniques: A reader* (1st ed.). American Psychological Association.

Wampold, B. E. (2019). *The basics of psychotherapy: An introduction to theory and practice* (2nd ed.). American Psychological Association.

CHAPTER 6 ■ INTELLECTUAL DISABILITY

▨ BACKGROUND

There has been an awareness of children with significant problems in learning and development since ancient times. Individuals with less severe impairments were more easily included in agrarian and generally nonliterate societies, but more impaired children were typically viewed as a burden (Trent, 1994). With a few exceptions, care was poor and mortality rates were high. Modern interest in what is now termed *intellectual disability* (ID) began around the Enlightenment period, when issues of nature/nurture and educational practices began to be debated, e.g., as reports of feral ("wild") children began to appear (Candland, 1993). By the early 19th century, provisions had begun to be made for more humane care, and efforts to foster development began. The first state training schools were founded in the United States and provided sheltered institutional settings, often in rural areas, where cognitive demands were minimized. The delineation of specific medical syndromes associated with specific genetic or environment risk factors also led to considerable research interest in ID (Zigler & Hodapp, 2013).

Although the initial purpose of institutional settings was to provide rehabilitation and humane care, over time such facilities frequently became places for custodial care or worse—a program that has now led to emphasis on providing services within homes and communities. Conditions in these institutions deteriorated, and a series of legal cases and greater awareness of the importance of home and institutional care led to a movement, starting mainly in the 1960s, that focused on deinstitutionalization in favor of home and community care (Rothman, 2017). The passage of the Education for All Handicapped Children Act (Public Law 94-142) (see Dunn, 2013) in 1975 also mandated schools in the United States to provide free and appropriate education to all children, thus providing for inclusion of children with all disabilities in public school settings.

The development of better measures of intelligence and of adaptive skills provided better metrics for assessment and documentation of progress. In this regard, the early work of Alfred Binet was particularly important. Binet developed the idea of the "mental age" by looking at knowledge that was normatively expectable for children at certain ages. Subsequently, the concept of intelligence quotient or IQ (originally produced by dividing mental age by chronological age and multiplying by 100 and now usually derived from standardization tables) made it much easier to compare children of different ages and levels of ability (see Gould, 1996 for an excellent review). Unfortunately, in some instances the notion of IQ,

| BOX 6.1 | Howard Skeels and the Iowa Study |

In a classic study, Skeels and Dye demonstrated the importance of good care by transferring infants and young children from an orphanage to a home for the "feebleminded" to make the children "normal." This fantastic plan had been prompted by the clinical observation that children in the home for the feebleminded received considerably more stimulation than those in the orphanage. Skeels later reported major differences in outcomes for these better-cared-for children, both in childhood and in later adult life.

Reprinted with permission from Volkmar, F. R., & Martin, A. (2011). *Essentials of Lewis's child and adolescent psychiatry* (1st ed., p. 79). Lippincott Williams & Wilkins/Wolters Kluwer; Skeels, H. M., & Dye, H. B. (1939). A study of the effects of differential stimulation on mentally retarded children. *Proceedings. American Association on Mental Deficiency, 44*(1), 114–136.

particularly when it was viewed as fixed or incorrectly and inappropriately assessed, was also misused, especially within the eugenic movement.

There was considerable faith in the IQ as a valid predictor of subsequent development, that is, as a fixed measure, and this led to a number of problems.

As children were followed longitudinally, it became clear that IQ scores did not become particularly stable, in large groups of children, until around the time the child entered school (this is not surprising because IQ tests were originally designed to predict success in school) (Hunt, 1963). Studies conducted in the 1930s and 1940s, often on children in orphanages or other institutions, began to show significant effects of experience (see Box 6.1). It also became apparent that IQ alone was not an adequate predictor of adult self-sufficiency. An awareness of the importance of appropriate self-care or "adaptive" skills in real-world settings (essentially "street smarts") led the psychologist Edgar Doll to develop the Vineland Social Maturity Scale. The current version of this scale continues to serve as an important tool in the assessment of children with ID (Sparrow et al., 2016). Importantly, in contrast to IQ, adaptive skills can be readily taught, and, as will be discussed shortly, it is clear that adaptive skills have become a major predictor of adult outcome in ID.

Another line of work centered on the association of intellectual deficiency with specific patterns of dysmorphology and developmental features and led to the specification of specific syndromes of ID that we know today. These often emerged well before an awareness of the importance of human genetics or specific mechanisms, but such conditions continue to be valid until today (Jones et al., 2013). A good example is the work of Dr. Langdon Down, who reported a syndrome (now usually referred to as trisomy 21, or earlier as Down syndrome), the result of a trisomy of chromosome 21. At the time of his report, Dr. Down, of course, had no notion of chromosomes. Although his initial theoretical concept of the condition (i.e., reversion to an earlier and inferior evolutionary type) is very fundamentally flawed, his clinical observation has been remarkably robust.

Since the 1960s, a series of court cases and legal and social initiatives began to change the care of individuals with ID significantly. There has been an increasing tendency to avoid institutional placements and segregated education settings in favor of community-based school and home care. For more severely cognitively impaired individuals, this is, of course, more challenging, and special programs within school or in more segregated settings are sometimes needed. It is important to mention noteworthy variations in practice from state to state within the United States. As will be discussed shortly, important challenges for both medical and mental health care remain to be addressed—particularly in adults with ID (Whittle et al., 2018).

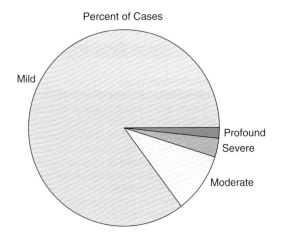

FIGURE 6.1. Levels of intellectual disability.

DIAGNOSIS, DEFINITION, CLINICAL FEATURES

Intellectual disability has had many previous diagnostic labels, mental retardation being the most recent, and earlier on terms like feebleminded, idiot, or cretin were used. The current diagnostic approaches (*DSM-5*) all define the condition essentially on the basis of the combination of subnormal intellectual functioning (see Harris, 2013), typically identified as a full-scale IQ score of 70 or below and commensurate deficits in adaptive functioning with onset before 18 years. The concept of intelligence is generally recognized to include a series of mental abilities involving problem-solving, abstract thinking, comprehension and expression of ideas, academic learning, planning, and learning from experience and so forth (Gottfredson, 1997). A number of well-developed tests of both intelligence and adaptive functioning are now available, as are guidelines for assessment and treatment (see Figure 6.1). (Siegel et al., 2020)

The current approaches in *DSM-5* (APA, 2013) attempt to de-emphasize reliance on IQ by mentioning it in text rather than criteria and to emphasize the importance of clinical assessment and the importance of various areas of functioning (conceptual, social, and practical). As in the past, various levels of ID have been specified: mild (IQ 50–70), moderate (IQ 35–49), severe (IQ 20–34), and profound (IQ < 20). Flexibility is allowed for clinical judgment. Most persons with ID in childhood are those with mild ID (about 85% of cases); the remainder of cases are comprised of those with moderate (about 10%), severe (about 4%), and profound (1%–2%) ID. In the past, the distinction was made between educable (IQ 50–70) and trainable (IQ < 50). In the past, the distinction was made between educable (IQ 50–70) and trainable (IQ < 50).

This distinction had an important function in that persons with mild ID often have psychiatric difficulties that are fundamentally similar (if generally more frequent) to those seen in the general population; this is not true for more severely impaired persons (Bouras & Holt, 2007). As noted in *DSM-5*, many individuals with mild ID can live independently as adults with minimal supports. Those with moderate ID may be independent but may also be semi-independent, needing higher levels of support. Persons with severe and profound ID need significant levels of support, the most disabled needing round-the-clock care. It is also the case that specific medical conditions associated with ID are more likely in the group with an IQ lower than 50, whereas poverty and lower socioeconomic status are more frequent in the group with mild ID (Volkmar et al., 2018). The proportion of persons with severe and profound ID is higher than would be expected given the normal curve, reflecting the impact of genetic disorders and severe medical problems on development (see Figure 6.1). Boxes 6.2 and 6.3 provide brief clinical examples of levels of ID.

BOX 6.2   **Case Report: Mild Intellectual Deficiency**

Jimmy was born at term after an uncomplicated pregnancy, labor, and delivery. His early developmental milestones were slightly delayed. Jimmy did not walk until 15 months and did not use words until he was nearly 2 years of age. His parents expressed concern to their pediatrician, and Jimmy was seen for assessment when he was 3.5 years old. At that time, developmental testing suggested borderline cognitive ability with a fairly even profile. His strengths included his social engagement and motivation to please. Various medical evaluations that were undertaken yielded uniformly negative results. There was no family history of ID, nor did Jimmy exhibit any unusual physical findings or features. Genetic consultation was noncontributory. He was enrolled in a program in which he had special supports as well as opportunities for interaction with typically developing peers. By age 8, repeat psychological testing revealed a full-scale IQ of 68, with some areas of weakness and strength becoming more pronounced. Jimmy continued to receive some special help with classes and had a modified curriculum. Starting in adolescence, he began a part-time job in a local restaurant, where he was well liked and popular. More and more of his work in school focused on vocational issues. He had some difficulties with depression and anxiety as a young adult but now lives largely independently of his parents, who see him regularly. He has an active social life and continues to enjoy his job.

Comment: Often, the diagnosis of mild ID is not made until the child is nearing entry to school or preschool. Individuals with mild ID are often able to achieve considerable independence and personal self-sufficiency, particularly when, as in this case, efforts are made to encourage community and vocational skills.

Reprinted with permission from Volkmar, F. R., & Martin, A. (2011). *Essentials of Lewis's child and adolescent psychiatry* (1st ed., p. 81). Lippincott Williams & Wilkins/Wolters Kluwer.

BOX 6.3   **Case Report: Severe Intellectual Deficiency**

Jeff was born after a term pregnancy and uncomplicated labor and delivery. He had nursing problems. His early milestones were delayed, and he had recurrent ear infections. Referral for genetics consultation was made at age 2 years because of delays and the pediatrician's concern about his unusual appearance. Jeff had a short and wide head (brachycephaly), a flattened midface, and low-set ears. He also had short but broad hands. On developmental testing, he was significantly delayed in all areas. A diagnosis of Smith–Magenis syndrome (a deletion at 17p11.2) was made by testing and was consistent with the clinical picture. Jeff enjoyed being around adults and exhibited considerable attention-seeking behavior. When frustrated, he began to engage in head banging, although this decreased as he became older. Jeff had limited communication skills, and his frustration around communication issues seemed to exacerbate his behavioral problems. Jeff also had significant sleep problems.

When he was 6 years of age, IQ testing yielded a full-scale score of 32. At that time, he had a hoarse, deep voice and still exhibited some self-injurious behaviors. He was also noted by the psychologist to exhibit an unusual "self-hug" (often seen in children with this condition). As a school-age child, his sleep problems caused the family considerable difficulties; typically, he would be up and wander the house at night but then try to sleep during the day. Fortunately, he was somewhat gregarious and outgoing, although this sometimes caused issues with strangers.

Jeff has received considerable special help in school. He had difficulties with sequencing and change but did well with structure. His family plans to help him transition to a nearby group home and sheltered workshop program when he is older.

Comment: In this deletion syndrome, there are several characteristic features, including the facial appearance, self-injury, sleep problems, and attention seeking. As adults, individuals with severe ID typically reside in group homes or other supervised care facilities.

Reprinted with permission from Volkmar, F. R., & Martin, A. (2011). *Essentials of Lewis's child and adolescent psychiatry* (1st ed., p. 82). Lippincott Williams & Wilkins/Wolters Kluwer.

EPIDEMIOLOGY AND DEMOGRAPHICS

There are important reasons for using both subnormal intellectual functioning and deficits in adaptive behavior in the definition of ID. If the IQ criterion alone is used, the expectation, based on the normal curve, would be that about 2.3% of the population should exhibit ID. In reality, this number is more reflective of children than adults. To some extent this reflects the fact that for some cognitive gains can occur and the IQ is not as fixed as was once thought and, importantly for many adults, gains in adaptive (real-world) skills mean that the person can be independent or semi-independent if the adaptive criterion is included. Figure 6.2 summarizes the differences in rates on the basis of whether or not both IQ and adaptive deficits are used to identify cases in the classic studies of Rutter and colleagues on the Isle of Wight (Rutter et al., 1976).

For severe ID, prevalence ranges from 3 to 4 cases per 1000, and for mild ID rates range from 5 to 10 children per 1000. More boys than girls are affected. Age of diagnosis varies depending on the severity of the cognitive deficits and parental awareness of normative developmental abilities. Thus, profound or severe ID is likely to be recognized early in life,

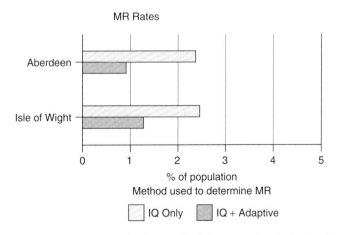

FIGURE 6.2. Isle of Wight study. From Fombonne, E., Bolton, P., Prior, J., Jordan, H., & Rutter, M. (1997). A family study of autism: cognitive patterns and levels in parents and siblings. *Journal of Child Psychology and Psychiatry, and Allied Disciplines, 38*(6), 667–683. https://doi.org/10.1111/j.1469-7610.1997.tb01694.x. Reprinted by permission of John Wiley & Sons, Inc.

whereas mild ID frequently goes unrecognized until learning difficulties are noticed in school. It should be noted that various risk factors such as prematurity, exposure to environmental toxins, as well as genetic factors can pose a risk and that there can be complex interactions between environmental and genetic factors as well (Huang et al., 2016; Simonoff et al., 1996). There are complex interactions of poverty and ID, for example, greater exposure to lead-based paint products in lower income families. For many known genetic conditions, prenatal testing can be used. At the same time, more precise methods for genetic testing have range also revealed some individuals with specific genetic syndromes who function above the ID.

ETIOLOGY AND PATHOGENESIS

The degree to which experience (nurture) or biology (nature) is involved in the pathogenies of ID has been a matter of considerable debate. A considerable body of work has focused on the presence of genetic factors or early adverse neurologic experience, for example, prematurity and obstetric risk (Huang et al., 2016). Particularly for individuals with more severe ID, medical causes are much more likely to be found—probably in about 50% of cases. The range of risk factors associated with ID is extensive, for example, from alcohol or toxin exposure in utero, to problems of early hypoxic events and genetic factors. Often, physical examination looking for the presence of specific dysmorphic features gives important clues to etiology, and an excellent clinical guide for this is available (Smith et al., 2013). For the group of individuals with mild ID, the role of experience, that is, social–cultural factors, may predominate (Zigler & Hodapp, 1986). In practice, these issues are difficult to disentangle. Clearly, some cases of mild ID undoubtedly represent the tail end of the normal, Gaussian distribution of intelligence. In many respects, work on the etiology of ID seems poised to enter a new era, with advances in genetics and neuroscience offering the potential for new models and theories (Dykens et al., 2000). Over 1000 genetic etiologies have now been identified, and this number will undoubtedly increase. Table 6.1 summarizes some of the specific forms of ID and their etiology and relevant clinical features.

Advances have also occurred in the approach to behavioral characterization, and these features may, in turn, contribute to our understanding of gene or brain function. As noted in Table 6.1, some syndromes feature unique psychiatric vulnerabilities and thus hold promise for helping to identify pathways to these psychiatric end points. There has been increased interest in relating psychiatric and behavioral difficulties to specific genetic or other etiologies. For example, the hyperphagia and compulsivity in Prader–Willi syndrome, attentional and social problems in fragile X syndrome, inappropriate laughter in Angelman's syndrome, the unusual cry in 5p-syndrome, and the self-hug in Smith–Magenis syndrome (see Dykens et al., 2000). Sometimes, aspects of syndrome expression can be related to the genetic vulnerability underlying the condition, that is, the severity of ID in fragile X syndrome and the type and severity of maladaptive behaviors in Prader–Willi syndrome. Furthermore, some of these connections between genetic disorder and behavioral outcome appear unique to a single syndrome, whereas others are "shared" between two or more syndromes. Thus, in some instances, features are relatively syndrome specific, such as the unusual hand-washing stereotypies of Rett's syndrome or the extreme hyperphasia in Prader–Willi syndrome. More often, however, features are shared in two or more conditions. Thus, attentional problems are frequent in fragile X and Williams syndrome. Understanding the nature of "dual diagnosis" is of considerable interest given its potential for shedding light on fundamental mechanisms of psychopathology (Hodapp, 1997; Mazza et al., 2020). These issues are, however, complex because the causal direction of most risk factors is unclear. Poor peer or social relations, for example, may be a precursor of psychopathology or a consequence of disruptive behavior. Other complications that increase risk include the presence of seizure disorders and impairments in sensory or motor impairments among persons with ID. For some conditions, specific genetic/biochemical or neurologic anomalies are associated with specific patterns of unusual behaviors such as severe self-injury. Demonstrable brain abnormalities, for example, as with neuroimaging, become more frequent as the degree of cognitive impairment increases.

TABLE 6.1

An Overview of Selected Conditions Associated with Intellectual Deficiency

Syndrome	Etiology	Physical/Clinical Exam	Psychological Features
Down Syndrome	Trisomy 21 (usually due to nondisjunction)	Characteristic face with wide nasal bridge, upward slanting eyebrows, simian crease, short stature, low muscle tone, cardiac and other problems	Usually relatively sociable with better verbal skills that might otherwise be expected, ↑ risk dementia in adulthood
Fetal Alcohol Syndrome	Exposure to alcohol during pregnancy	Hypoplasia of midface, microcephaly, short stature, long and smooth philtrum	Typically mild to moderate ID with increased problems in attention
Fragile X Syndrome	FMR-1 gene inactivation due to CCG repeats	Long face and large ears with high arched palate, large testes in boys	difficulties with attention and social anxiety, mild to moderate ID
Williams Syndrome	Deletion of part of long arm of chromosome 7 (about 25 genes including elastin gene)	Elfin-like face, short stature, stellate iris. Renal, cardiac, and other abnormalities	Hyperacusis, anxiety, often sociable with better verbal skills
Prader–Willi Syndrome	Deletion in 15q 11 (paternal origin in most cases)	Low tone, infants may have failure to thrive but obesity develops, small hands/feet, small testes.	compulsive eating and other behaviors (hoarding), moderate to borderline IQ range, affective lability, and agitation
Angelman's Syndrome	Deletion in 15q13 (maternal original in most cases)	Wide set mouth, thin lips, and other characteristic faces, microcephaly. Seizures frequent.	Sleep problems, stereotyped movements (hand flapping), typically profound MR
Smith–Magenis Syndrome	Deletion in chromosome 17	Broad face but midface is flattened, characteristic deep voice	Severe self-injury and hyperactivity, severe IQ range. Self-hugging
Lesch–Nyhan Syndrome	Defect in gene for hypoxanthine-guanine phosphoribosyltransferase (HGPRT), X linked	Gene defect ↑uric acid → gout, kidney problems. Movement problems.	Severe self-injury, aggression, anxiety with mild–moderate IQ delays
Phenylketonuria (PKU)	recessive defect in phenylalanine hydroxylase	High levels of phenylalanine, seizures, symptoms may not appear early in infancy	Language delay, agitation, aggression—can be prevented with diet

ID, intellectual disability; IQ, intelligence quotient.

Some conditions such as Rett's disorder are associated with gross brain atrophy, although more subtle difficulties may also be detected—particularly with the technical advances of recent years.

In addition to lack of appropriate psychosocial stimulation, other factors that can compound or exacerbate development can include low expectancies for success, learned helplessness, negative self-concept, and long-standing reinforcement of maladaptive behaviors. Problems in communication, peer difficulties, poor social judgment, isolation, and poor self-advocacy skills may also increase the risk for and complicate the treatment of associated mental health problems (Mazza et al., 2020).

Considerable research has focused on different profiles of strength or weakness in relation to specific syndromes. For example, individuals with Williams syndrome show relative strengths in specific aspects of expressive language, along with pronounced deficits in visual–spatial functioning, but, despite these problems, have remarkably good facial recognition and memory skills. Similarly, individuals with Prader–Willi syndrome show remarkable skills in solving jigsaw puzzles that may exceed those of typically developing peers. In many instances, of course, behaviors are not syndrome specific or are only partially so, for example, both fragile X and Prader–Willi syndromes appear to have relative weaknesses in certain short-term memory and sequential processing tasks whereas inattention/hyperactivity are seen in Williams and fragile X. Interestingly, significant levels of ID used to be much more commonly found in association with autism/autism spectrum disorder (see Chapter 7), but this risk appears to be decreasing with earlier detection and intervention (Bouras & Holt, 2007). Of course, persons with ID are also individuals, and within-syndrome variation studies are of considerable interest in helping us understand factors that facilitate or inhibit optimal development. Research is needed to identify the genetic, environmental, developmental, and psychosocial factors that help to explain individual behavioral differences in people with the same vulnerability.

Prevention of ID varies depending on the nature of the risk, for example, in situations of genetic origin there may be important issues of early detection of cases or of detection of risk for subsequent pregnancies or for siblings as they marry and reproduce. In other cases, the etiology may be more clearly related to environmental risk factors, for example, fetal alcohol syndrome or congenital rubella. Even when no specific etiology is identified, there is some increased risk for subsequent pregnancies, so counseling with a knowledgeable clinical geneticist is indicated (Crow & Tomie, 1998). For some disorders, such as autism, there has been a growing appreciation of genetic factors, and it now appears that for parents who have one child with autism, the risk of having a second child with autism is between 10 to 20% (see Chapter 7). Siblings of children with ID who are not themselves affected may be at increased risk of other difficulties, owing to increased family and personal stress. Support for siblings, and for their parents, is an important element of long-term treatment planning (Harris, 2010).

COURSE

The clinical presentation varies depending on many factors—particularly the level of severity. The *DSM-5* approach emphasizes functional abilities. Children with severe and profound ID have obvious delays earlier in life and thus come to diagnosis earlier; they are more likely to exhibit dysmorphic features and/or associated medical problems, and, as a group, have higher rates of behavioral and psychiatric disturbances (Buckley et al., 2020). The latter can be quite different from those seen in the general population, for example, self-injurious behaviors, unprovoked aggression, and unusual mood problems. On the other hand, those individuals with mild ID have increased rates of psychopathology of the usual types seen in normative samples. Persons with moderate levels of ID are intermediate between these two extremes. Considerable debate has revolved around how similar or different learning processes are with increasing severity of ID (Zigler & Hodapp, 2013).

Oddly, for many years there was almost a presumption that somehow ID acted to prevent the development of other problems, a phenomenon known as diagnostic overshadowing

(Reiss et al., 1982). But as researchers began to use standard interviews/rating scales with persons with mild ID (who can easily cooperate with such assessment), they realized that there was a 4- to 5-fold increase in mental health problems (White et al., 1995). Probably about 25% of persons with ID may have significant psychiatric problems; these rates are much higher if persons with salient behavior disorders are included (McKenzie et al., 2018). As can be imagined, at times issues of diagnosis are complex, but it does appear that higher rates of other mental disorders, schizophrenia, depression, and ADHD in particular, are increased relative to the general population. Various rating scales and checklists specific to psychiatric problems in this population have been developed, including for dementia in older individuals.

Outcome is related to level of severity of the ID, associated biologic or other vulnerabilities, and aspects of the individual's psychological functioning, family support, and other factors (Harris, 2010). Levels of ability to cope with the tasks of daily life are important in determining independence and self-sufficiency. Social and community supports are important. For persons with mild ID, the diagnosis is often first made on school entry but can then be "lost" as adaptive gains are made, and so the persons may be self-supporting, may marry, and may raise families but may be at increased risk for educational and behavioral problems in adult life. As adults, persons with moderate levels of ID (IQ 40–55) typically have more serious impairment. It is common for such persons to need services as adults. Moderate ID is more frequently identified in the preschool years, and medical causes are more frequently identified. Adult self-sufficiency is less likely than in mild ID, although it is possible, and many persons can live semi-independently or with partial support. In individuals with severe or profound ID case identification often occurs in infancy or early childhood. Goals for these patients include facilitating self-care and other independent living skills as far as possible. Associated medical problems and behavioral difficulties are frequent; unfortunately, problems in communication are more common and compound the problem of assessment and intervention.

■ DIFFERENTIAL DIAGNOSIS AND ASSESSMENT

The diagnosis of ID is based on the appropriate assessment of cognitive abilities and adaptive skills; clinical assessment also includes a careful developmental and family history, physical examination, and laboratory studies as appropriate (Szymaski & King, 1998). The clinician should be alert for any medical or environmental conditions that may be associated with developmental disability. For example, a strong family history of certain dysmorphic features in the child should raise the possibility of an inherited condition; a history of significant birth trauma, exposure to environmental toxins, or exposure to marked psychosocial adversity are some of the factors that should be considered (see Volkmar et al., 2018). Metabolic and genetic testing may be obtained on the basis of history and results of physical examination; for example, abnormal facial features or other physical anomalies should alert the clinician to the need for more extensive assessment. Often, the constellation of physical and developmental findings may suggest specific genetic or other condition.

Psychological assessment will usually include administration of a formal IQ test and measurement of adaptive skills as well as less formal observation. For younger children, tests of cognitive ability are often used as developmental tests; by the time a child reaches 5 years or so, the more traditional tests of intelligence can be used. Also, the emphasis in many states for very young children is on providing services for children at risk rather than, for example, assigning a precise diagnostic label. Some examples of these tests are listed in Table 6.2. Note that a distinction is made between developmental tests for younger children and intelligence tests for older children, reflecting an awareness that tests become more predictive of later intelligence as the child nears school age. Tests of intelligence usually provide an overall or "full-scale" IQ score, as well as additional scores, for example, for verbal or nonverbal abilities. Many different intelligence tests are available, and the choice of the specific test can reflect many different factors (Whittle et al., 2018). The psychologist is trained to administer the test in a standardized way, that is, to facilitate the comparison of results with normative samples.

TABLE 6.2

Tests of Intelligence and Development

Test Name	Comment
Wechsler Intelligence Scales; Wechsler Preschool and Primary Scale of Intelligence, 3rd ed. (Wechsler [WPPSI-IV], 2012); Wechsler Intelligence Scale for Children, 5th ed. (Wechsler [WISC-V], 2014), Wechsler Adult Intelligence Scale, 4th ed. (Wechsler [WAIS-IV], 2008)	Excellent series of tests covering preschool (about age 4) to adulthood; assesses a range of cognitive abilities. Some tasks are timed, which is a challenge for many children with autism and related conditions (this may actually help document need for untimed tests). Typical profiles of ability are seen in autism and Asperger's disorder.
Stanford Binet Intelligence Scale, 5th ed. (SB5) (Roid, 2003)	Excellent test; can be used with somewhat younger children. Wide age range. Nonverbal scale may underestimate abilities in some.
Kaufmann Assessment Battery for Children, 2nd ed. (KABC-II) (Kaufman & Kaufman, 2004)	Excellent test; can be used from 3 to 18 years of age. Some language is needed (but not much). Somewhat more flexible for children with ID. Many of the materials interest children with ASDs. Language demands minimized and good sensitivity to possible cultural bias.
Leiter International Performance Scale, 3rd ed. (Leiter-3) (Roid & Miller 2013)	A test originally developed for deaf children, recently revised. Provides assessment of nonverbal cognitive ability. Can be used for children with no expressive speech. Some teaching is allowed. Limitations include no verbal tasks
Mullen Scales of Early Learning (Mullen, 1995)	Can be used with very young children. Provides scores in nonverbal problem-solving, receptive and expressive language, and gross and fine motor skills. Scores from such developmental tests are usually less predictive of later abilities.
Differential Ability Scales, 2nd ed. (DAS-II) (Elliott, 2007)	Well-done test; covers wide range of ages and taps a number of different skills (not just overall IQ). Early years scales can provide an IQ for low-functioning children under 9 years old

Note: Many other tests are available, and tests are constantly being revised and reissued.
Republished with permission of John Wiley & Sons, from Volkmar, F. R., & Wiesner, L. A. (2017). *Essential clinical guide to understanding and treating autism* (1st ed., p. 320). John Wiley & Sons, Inc.; permission conveyed through Copyright Clearance Center, Inc.

Clearly, the tests chosen for assessment of intellectual functioning should be appropriate, have good reliability and validity, and be administered by appropriately trained examiners.

Measures of adaptive skills are generally based on parent or caregiver report, although, in some cases, the person may be interviewed directly. In essence, the conceptual notion is that the term *adaptive skills* refers to the performance of day-to-day activities required for personal or social self-sufficiency. The inclusion of adaptive skills in the definition of ID rests on the observation that many persons with IQ scores below 70 may, as adolescents or adults, have learned sufficient adaptive skills that enable them to function totally or largely independently. Technically, then, such individuals would not meet the criteria for ID. This situation is more typical of persons who, as children, score in the mild range. Cultural and other factors may be important considerations in terms of both selecting specific assessment instruments and making a diagnosis of ID. The presence of specific comorbid medical conditions, for example, seizures, may also complicate the diagnostic presentation. Depending on the clinical context, additional assessments, for example, from speech-communication therapists and occupational and physical therapists, may also be needed. Any comorbid psychiatric or genetic conditions should be noted.

■ TREATMENT

Treatment approaches have shifted dramatically over the past decades with more individuals living with their families, attending public schools, and staying within their communities (see Singh, 2016). For children, educational planning should be based on careful assessment and continued monitoring of progress. With appropriate support, children with ID can be included in mainstream settings, but this can be a challenge for lower cognitively functioning individuals as they become older, particularly if behavioral problems interfere. It is important that explicit attention be paid to generalization and development of skills relevant to community life and adult self-sufficiency. A variety of good evidence-based interventions are now available (Kaiser & McIntyre, 2010; Singh, 2016). These should be individualized for the specific person. Community programs are also often very helpful. Care coordination is important (Emerson et al., 2018).

Medical care should include, when possible, an awareness of any cause or associated medical condition(s) as well as knowledge of the child's strengths and weaknesses. Thus, knowing that a child has trisomy 21 has immediate and long-term implications for medical care; for example, 50% of newborns will have congenital heart problems, and there is increased risk for both leukemia and Alzheimer's disease with age. Similarly, persons with Prader–Willi syndrome also show particularly high rates of etiology-related health problems. General practice guidelines (Siegel & King, 1999) as well as specific recommendations for genetic evaluation are available (Malinowski et al., 2020).

Persons with ID are at increased risk for various psychiatric problems, and these can be a major source of distress to the individual and family and may also limit opportunities for self-sufficiency. Unmet medical and mental health needs are a major problem. Up to 75% of persons with ID who are referred for psychiatric assessment also have undiagnosed or undertreated medical conditions, and, conversely, about half receive psychotropic medications that could have behavioral side effects (Perry et al., 2018). Fortunately, both effective pharmacologic and psychological behavioral treatments are available (Cooney et al., 2018; Deutsch & Burket, 2020). Methods like cognitive behavior therapy can be used for intervention (Andrew, 2017).

The psychiatric interview of the person with ID may need to be modified, particularly for persons with more severe ID, but should still be comprehensive and multifocal. The use of specific rating scales and assessment instruments can help focus attention on these problems. Particularly in individuals with more severe and syndromic ID, the diagnostic picture can be complex because other psychiatric problems or vulnerabilities complicate the diagnostic picture. It is important that the clinician *not* overlook other difficulties that may be present and keep in mind that for individuals with ID what appears to be a small problem may, in fact, have a major impact on the person's functioning.

Transition planning should formally start in adolescence (Lima-Rodriguez et al., 2018). Most persons with ID benefit from employment or from structured programs that emphasize vocational, adaptive, or socialization skills, even after formal schooling. A goal of this planning should be to help the individual enter the workforce (Jacobs et al., 2018; Shogren & Plotner, 2012). The transition from school to work is a vulnerable stage for many persons and their families. Unlike the school years, when special education and related services (e.g., occupational, physical, and speech and language therapies) are typically provided at school under one roof, the services for adults risk being more fragmented.

Residential placements outside family homes remain an area of concern for many individuals—especially as this population of individuals with ID live longer lives, our society increasingly needs to deal with the question of who will take care of these individuals when aging parents can no longer do so. By 2030, about 1.5 million individuals with disabilities aged over 60 will be living in the United States (Shogren & Plotner, 2012).

■ SUMMARY

Considerable progress has been made in the identification and treatment of children with ID. In some ways, this field of research has become much more active over the past decade. Areas of active investigation include the study of the interplay between genetic and environmental (including psychosocial) risk factors in the origin of ID as well as the study of basic neural and genetic mechanisms in the understanding of basic processes that underlie phenotypic expression, including various forms of psychopathology. This research offers the opportunity to advance knowledge more generally about mechanisms of disorder. Although many advances have been made in the care and treatment of persons with ID, studies of treatment methods remain an important priority, as do more effective practices for care of individuals with ID.

References

American Psychiatric Association. (2013). *Diagnostic and Statistical Manual of Mental Disorders, Fifth Edition (DSM-5)*. Author.

Andrew, J. (2017). *Cognitive behaviour therapy for people with intellectual disabilities: Thinking creatively*. Palgrave Macmillan.

Bouras, N., & Holt, G. (2007). *Psychiatric behavioral disorders in intellectual and developmental disabilities* (2nd ed.). Cambridge University Press.

Buckley, N., Glasson, E. J., Chen, W., Epstein, A., Leonard, H., Skoss, R., Jacoby, P., Blackmore, A. M., Srinivasjois, R., Bourke, J., Sanders, R. J., & Downs, J. (2020). Prevalence estimates of mental health problems in children and adolescents with intellectual disability: A systematic review and meta-analysis. *Australian & New Zealand Journal of Psychiatry, 54*(10), 970–984. https://doi.org/10.1177/0004867420924101

Candland, D. K. (1993). *Feral children and clever animals: Reflections on human nature*. Oxford University Press.

Cooney, P., Tunney, C., & O'Reilly, G. (2018). A systematic review of the evidence regarding cognitive therapy skills that assist cognitive behavioural therapy in adults who have an intellectual disability. *Journal of Applied Research in Intellectual Disabilities, 31*(1), 23–42. https://doi.org/10.1111/jar.12365

Crow, Y. J., Tolmie, J. L. (1998). Recurrence risks in mental retardation. *Journal of Medical Genetics, 35*, 77–182. https://doi.org/10.1136/jmg.35.3.177

Deutsch, S. I., & Burket, J. A. (2020). Psychotropic medication use for adults and older adults with intellectual disability; selective review, recommendations and future directions. *Progress in Neuro-psychopharmacology & Biological Psychiatry, 104*, 110017. https://doi.org/10.1016/j.pnpbp.2020.110017

Dunn, D. (2013). Public Law 94-142. In F. R. Volkmar (Ed.), *Encyclopedia of autism spectrum disorders* (pp. 2468–2471). Springer.

Dykens, E. M., Hodapp, R. M., & Finucance, B. M. (2000). *Genetics and mental retardation syndromes: A new look at behavior and interventions*. Paul H. Brookes Pub. Co.

Elliott, C. D. (1990). *Differential ability scales: Introductory and technical handbook*. The Psychological Corporation.

Emerson, E., Hatton, C., Baines, S., & Robertson, J. (2018). The association between employment status and health among British adults with and without intellectual impairments: cross-sectional analyses of a Cohort study. *BMC Public Health, 18*(1), 401. https://doi.org/10.1186/s12889-018-5337-5

Fombonne, E., Bolton, P., Prior, J., Jordan, H., & Rutter, M. (1997). A family study of autism: Cognitive patterns and levels in parents and siblings. *Journal of Child Psychology & Psychiatry & Allied Disciplines, 38*(6), 667–683. https://doi.org/10.1111/j.1469-7610.1997.tb01694.x

Gottfredson, L. S. (1997). Mainstream science on intelligence: An editorial with 52 signatories, history and bibliography. *Intelligence, 24*(1), 13–23. https://doi.org/10.1016/S0160-2896(97)90011-8

Gould, S. J. (1996). *The mismeasure of man*. W. W. Norton & Co.

Harris, J. C. (2010). *Intellectual disability: A guide for families and professionals.* Oxford University Press.

Harris, J. C. (2013). New terminology for mental retardation in *DSM-5* and *ICD-11. Current Opinion in Psychiatry, 26*(3), 260–262. https://doi.org/10.1097/YCO.0b013e32835fd6fb

Hodapp, R. M. (1997). Direct and indirect behavioral effects of different genetic disorders of mental retardation. *American Journal Mental Retardation, 102,* 67–79. https://doi.org/10.1352/0895-8017(1997)102<0067:DAIBEO>2.0.CO;2

Huang, J., Zhu, T., Qu, Y., & Mu, D. (2016). Prenatal, perinatal and neonatal risk factors for intellectual disability: A systematic review and meta-analysis. *PLoS One, 11*(4), e0153655. https://doi.org/10.1371/journal.pone.0153655

Hunt, J. M. (1963). *Intelligence and experience.* Ronald Press.

Jacobs, P., MacMahon, K., & Quayle, E. (2018). Transition from school to adult services for young people with severe or profound intellectual disability: A systematic review utilizing framework synthesis. *Journal of Applied Research in Intellectual Disabilities, 31*(6), 962–982. https://doi.org/10.1111/jar.12466

Jones, K. L., Jones, M. C., and Del Campo, M. (2013). *Smith's recognizable patterns of human malformation* (7th ed.). Elsevier.

Kaiser, A. P., & McIntyre, L. L. (2010). Introduction to special section on evidence-based practices for persons with intellectual and developmental disabilities. *American Journal on Intellectual & Developmental Disabilities, 115*(5), 357–363. https://doi.org/10.1352/1944-7558-115-5.357

Kaufman, A. S., & Kaufman, N. L. (2004). *Kaufman assessment battery for children* (2nd ed.). American Guidance Service.

Lima-Rodriguez, J. S., Baena-Ariza, M. T., Dominguez-Sanchez, I., & Lima-Serrano, M. (2018). Intellectual disability in children and teenagers: Influence on family and family health. Systematic review. *Enfermeria Clinica, 28*(2), 89–102. https://doi.org/10.1016/j.enfcle.2017.10.007

Malinowski, J., Miller, D. T., Demmer, L., Gannon, J., Pereira, E. M., Schroeder, M. C., Scheuner, M. T., Tsai, A. C., Hickey, S. E., Shen, J., & ACMG Professional Practice and Guidelines Committee. (2020). Systematic evidence-based review: Outcomes from exome and genome sequencing for pediatric patients with congenital anomalies or intellectual disability. *Genetics in Medicine, 22*(6), 986–1004. https://doi.org/10.1038/s41436-020-0771-z

Mazza, M. G., Rossetti, A., Crespi, G., & Clerici, M. (2020). Prevalence of co-occurring psychiatric disorders in adults and adolescents with intellectual disability: A systematic review and meta-analysis. *Journal of Applied Research in Intellectual Disabilities, 33*(2), 126–138. https://doi.org/10.1111/jar.12654

McKenzie, K., Metcalfe, D., & Murray, G. (2018). A review of measures used in the screening, assessment and diagnosis of dementia in people with an intellectual disability. *Journal of Applied Research in Intellectual Disabilities, 31*(5), 725–742. https://doi.org/10.1111/jar.12441

Mullen, E. M. (1995). *The Mullen scales of early learning.* American Guidance Service.

Perry, B. I., Cooray, S. E., Mendis, J., Purandare, K., Wijeratne, A., Manjubhashini, S., Dasari, M., Esan, F., Gunaratna, I., Naseem, R. A., Hoare, S., Chester, V., Roy, A., Devapriam, J., Alexander, R., & Kwok, H. F. (2018). Problem behaviours and psychotropic medication use in intellectual disability: A multinational cross-sectional survey. *Journal of Intellectual Disability Research, 62*(2), 140–149. https://doi.org/10.1111/jir.12471

Reiss, S., Levitan, G. W., & Szyszko, J. (1982). Emotional disturbance and mental retardation: Diagnostic overshadowing. *American Journal of Mental Retardation, 86,* 567–574.

Roid, G. S. (2003). *Leiter international performance scale* (5th ed.). WPS.

Roid, G. M., & Miller, L. J. (2013). *Leiter international performance scale* (3rd ed.). Western Psychological Services.

Rothman, D. J. (2017). *The Willowbrook Wars: Bringing the mentally disabled into the community.* Routledge.

Rutter, M., Tizard, J., Yule, W., Graham, P., & Whitmore, K. (1976). Research report: Isle of Wight studies, 1964–1974. *Psychological Medicine, 6,* 313–332. https://doi.org/10.1017/S003329170001388X

Shogren, K. A., & Plotner, A. J. (2012). Transition planning for students with intellectual disability, autism, or other disabilities: Data from the National Longitudinal Transition Study-2. *Intellectual and Developmental Disabilities, 50*(1), 16–30. https://doi.org/10.1352/1934-9556-50.1.16

Siegel, L., & King, B. H. (1999). Practice parameters for the assessment and treatment of children, adolescents, and adults with mental retardation and comorbid mental disorders. *Journal of the American Academy of Child & Adolescent Psychiatry, 38*(12 Suppl), 5S–31S. https://doi.org/10.1016/S0890-8567(99)80002-1

Siegel, M., McGuire, K., Veenstra-VanderWeele, J., Stratigos, K., King, B., Belonci, C., Hayak, M., Keable, H., Rochill, C., & Walter, H. J. (2020). Practice parameters for the assessment and treatment of children, adolescents, and adults with mental retardation and comorbid mental disorders. *Journal of the American Academy of Child & Adolescent Psychiatry, 59*(4), 468–496. https://doi.org/10.1016/j.jaac.2019.11.018

Simonoff, E., Bolton, P., & Rutter, M. (1996). Mental retardation: Genetic findings, clinical implications, and research agenda. *Journal of Child Psychology & Psychiatry, 37,* 259–280. https://doi.org/10.1111/j.1469-7610.1996.tb01404.x

Singh, N. N. (2016). *Handbook of evidence-based practices in intellectual and developmental disabilities.* Springer.

Sparrow, S., Cicchetti, D., & Saulnier, C. A. (2016). *Vineland adaptive behavior scales* (3rd ed.). American Guidance Service.

Szymanski, L., & King, B. H. (1999). Summary of the Practice parameters for the assessment and treatment of children, adolescents, and adults with mental retardation and comorbid mental disorders. American Academy of Child and Adolescent Psychiatry. *Journal of the American Academy of Child and Adolescent Psychiatry, 38*(12), 1606–1610. https://doi.org/10.1097/00004583-199912000-00027

Trent, J. W. (1994). *Inventing the feeble mind: A history of mental retardation in the United States.* University of California Press.

Volkmar, F. R., Dykens, E., & Hodapp, R. (2018). Intellectual disability. In A. Marin, M. Bloch, & F. R. Volkmar (Eds.), *Lewis's child and adolescent psychiatry* (5th ed., pp. 434–442). Wolters Kluwer.

Wechsler, D. (2002). *Wechsler preschool and primary scale of intelligence* (3rd ed.). Pearson.

Wechsler, D. (2008). *Wechsler adults intelligence scale* (4th ed.). Pearson.

Wechsler, D. (2014). *Wechsler intelligence scale for children* (5th ed.). Pearson.

White, M. J., Nichols, C. N., Cook, R. S., Spengler, P. M., Walker, B. S., & Look, K. K. (1995). Diagnostic overshadowing and mental retardation: A meta-analysis. *American Journal of Mental Retardation, 100,* 293–298.

Whittle, E. L., Fisher, K. R., Reppermund, S., Lenroot, R., & Trollor, J. (2018). Barriers and enablers to accessing mental health services for people with intellectual disability: A scoping review. *Journal of Mental Health Research in Intellectual Disabilities, 11*(1), 69–102. https://doi.org/10.1080/19315864.2017.1408724

Zigler, E., & Hodapp, R. M. (1986). *Understanding mental retardation.* Cambridge University Press.

Zigler, E., & Hodapp, R. (2013). *Understanding mental retardation.* Cambridge University Press.

Suggested Readings

*Indicates Particularly Recommended

Baumgardner, T. L., Reiss, A. L., Freund, L. S., & Abrams, M. T. (1995). Specification of the neurobehavioral phenotype in males with fragile X syndrome. *Pediatrics, 95,* 744–752.

Binet, A., & Simon, T. (1916). *The development of intelligence in children* (E. S. Kit, Trans.). Williams & Wilkins.

Dingman, H. G., & Tarjan, G. (1960). Mental retardation and the normal distribution. *American Journal of Mental Deficiency, 64,* 991–994.

*Dykens, E. M. (1995). Measuring behavioral phenotypes: Provocations from the new genetics. *American Journal of Mental Retardation, 99*(5), 522–532.

*Dykens, E. M. (1999). Direct effects of genetic mental retardation syndromes: Maladaptive behavior and psychopathology. *International Review of Research in Mental Retardation, 22,* 1–26. https://doi.org/10.1016/S0074-7750(08)60129-9

Dykens, E. M., Cassidy, S. B., & King, B. H. (1999). Maladaptive behavior differences in Prader–Willi syndrome due to paternal deletion versus maternal uniparental disomy. *American Journal of Mental Retardation, 104,* 67–77. https://doi.org/10.1352/0895-8017(1999)104<0067:MBDIPS>2.0.CO;2

Dykens, E. M., Hodapp, R. M., & Leckman, J. F. (1994). *Behavior and development in fragile X syndrome.* Sage Publishing.

Dykens, E. M., Leckman, J. F., & Cassidy, S. B. (1996). Obsessions and compulsions in Prader–Willi syndrome. *Journal of Child Psychology & Psychiatry, 37,* 995–1002. https://doi.org/10.1111/j.1469-7610.1996.tb01496.x

Finucane, B. M., Konar, D., Haas–Givler, B., Kurtz, M. B., & Scott, C. I., Jr. (1994). The spasmodic upper body squeeze: A characteristic behavior in Smith-Magenis syndrome. *Developmental Medicine & Child Neurology, 36,* 78–83. https://doi.org/10.1111/j.1469-8749.1994.tb11770.x

Gersh, M., Goodard, S. A., Pasztor, L. M., Harris, D. J., Weiss, L., & Overhauser, J. (1995). Evidence for a distinct region causing a cat-cry in patients with 5p deletions. *American Journal of Human Genetics, 56*(5), 1404–1410.

Gottfredson, L. S. (1997). Mainstream science on intelligence: An editorial with 52 signatories, history and bibliography. *Intelligence, 24*(1), 13–23. https://doi.org/10.1016/S0160-2896(97)90011-8

*Hunt, N. (1967). *The world of Nigel Hunt.* Garrett Publications.

*Muhle, R. A., Reed, H. E., Vo, L. C., Mehta, S., McGuire, K., Veenstra-VanderWeele, J., & Pedapati, E. (2017). Clinical diagnostic genetic testing for individuals with developmental disorders. *Journal of the American Academy of Child and Adolescent Psychiatry, 56*(11), 910–913. https://doi.org/10.1016/j.jaac.2017.09.418

Polloway, E. A., Smith, J. D., Chamberlain, J., Denning, C. B., & Smith, T. E. (1999). Levels of deficits or supports in the classification of mental retardation: Implementation practices. *Education and Training in Mental Retardation and Developmental Disabilities, 34*, 200–206.

Skeels, H. M. (1966). Adult status of children with contrasting early life experiences. *Monographs of the Society for Research in Child Development, 31*(3), 1–65. https://doi.org/10.2307/1165791

Skeels, H. M., & Dye, H. B. (1939). A study of the effects of differential stimulation on mentally retarded children. *Proceedings. American Association on Mental Deficiency, 44*(1), 114–136.

Tassone, F. I., Hagerman, R. J., Ikle, D., Dyer, P. N., & Lampe, M. (1999). FMRP expression as a potential prognostic indicator in fragile X syndrome. *American Journal of Medical Genetics, 84*, 250–261. https://doi.org/10.1002/(SICI)1096-8628(19990528)84:3<250::AID-AJMG17>3.0.CO;2-4

Terman, L. M. (1911). The Binet-Simon Scale for measuring intelligence: Impressions gained by its application. *Psychological Clinic, 5*, 199–206.

VanAcker, R. (1997). Rett's syndrome. In D. J. Cohen & F. R. Volkmar (Eds.), *Handbook of autism and pervasive developmental disorders* (2nd ed., pp. 60–93). Wiley.

Verhoeven, W. M., Tuinier, S., & Curfs, L. (2003). Prader-Willi syndrome: Cycloid psychosis in a genetic subtype? *Acta Neuropsychiatrica, 15*, 32–37. https://doi.org/10.1034/j.1601-5215.2003.00006.x

Williams, C. A., Zori, R. T., Hendrickson, J., Stalker, H., Marum, T., Whidden, E., & Driscoll, D. J. (1995). Angelman syndrome. *Current Problems in Pediatrics, 25*, 216–231. https://doi.org/10.1016/S0045-9380(06)80036-8

CHAPTER 7 ■ AUTISM SPECTRUM DISORDER

■ BACKGROUND

Leo Kanner's (1943) first explicit description of the syndrome of early infantile autism remains a "classic." He described 11 children who had two common features: "autism" (living in one's own world cut off from others) and "insistence on sameness"—a term that included literal resistance to change. The latter term encompassed, to his way of thinking, some of the repetitive behaviors that he saw as the child's attempt to "maintain sameness" in the environment. His paper also mentioned many of the clinical features we see today, for example, echolalia (speech repetition), difficulties with communication including for some a total absence of spoken language. He noted that he believed the condition to be of very early onset and emphasized the lack of unusual facial features, that is, like those of children with trisomy 21. He also noted some areas of apparent strength in nonverbal tasks like puzzles.

A year after Hans Asperger (1944), a Viennese medical student also used the term *autism* to describe what he viewed as more a personality problem than a developmental disorder. His small group of cases, all boys, had difficulties in joining groups partly because of their major and intrusive circumscribed interests. The latter could include more typical interests (rocks, dinosaurs) or more esoteric ones (train schedules, American gangsters), and, in addition to complicating peer interaction, the family often found its life revolved around the interest. Asperger made the important point of noting how these interests interfered with the child's acquisition of other skills.

Effectively, these two clinical descriptions (of Kanner and Asperger), while differing in important respects, set the tension that exists today between narrow and broad views of autism, and the autism spectrum differed in many respects but did have an important point of connection: the emphasis of problems of social engagement. The debate between broad and narrow views of autism and related conditions is ongoing and is now part of a broader discussion of neurodiversity and what has been termed the *broader autism phenotype* (Ingersoll & Wainer, 2014).

In retrospect, children with something very similar to autism existed well before this description. It is quite possible that reports of so-called feral or wild children (presumed to have been reared by animals) represented the first known cases of the condition. Children who we would now likely say had autism were also noted in the 1800s as suggested by case records kept at training schools for the intellectually impaired.

Research on the conditions was slow to develop for many years. This reflected several factors. Kanner's use of the term *autism* had suggested to many a source of connection with schizophrenia, and childhood schizophrenia, although we now recognize that schizophrenia in children is vanishingly rare (see Chapter 15). Other sources of confusion arose given Kanner's early impression that children with autism did not have overall intellectual deficiency (mental retardation)—this impression reflected their often good abilities with nonverbal tasks. As time went on, it became clear that unusual IQ profiles were seen with strengths in nonverbal areas and major weaknesses in verbal ones, with older children often scoring in the intellectually deficient range. Psychoanalytic theorizing at the time autism was first described speculated that some parent–child interaction issues led to autism—a notion that led to years of unproductive psychotherapy for parents and children alike. Several key findings in the 1970s established the validity of autism and underscored the need for its official recognition: (1) autism differed from childhood schizophrenia in many; (2) autism was brain based and strongly genetic; and (3) children with autism responded better to structured teaching than unstructured psychotherapy.

■ DIAGNOSIS, DEFINITION, CLINICAL FEATURES

The growing awareness that autism was a distinctive condition led to new efforts to provide better guidelines to diagnosis. These included Rutter's (1978) synthesis of Kanner's original paper with subsequent research and the earlier efforts to provide a diagnostic checklist. The decision was made to include autism in the groundbreaking third edition of the *DSM*.

The *DSM-III* (APA, 1980) definition fostered what became an explosion of research work on autism. This definition of "infantile autism" was included in a new class of disorder—*pervasive developmental disorder* (PDD). The problem with *DSM-II* was its lack of developmental orientation; this was rectified in the *DSM-III-R* (APA, 1987) that provided a more flexible, polythetic approach to the diagnosis of "autistic disorder." Issues with this definition were addressed in the major revision of *DSM-IV* (1990), which included a field trial conducted in conjunction with the *ICD-10* revision. This field trial led to the convergence of *ICD-10* and *DSM-IV* for autism—a factor that further enhanced research and also fostered the development of new dimensional approaches to diagnosis. This approach to diagnosis also included several other conditions including Asperger's disorder, Rett syndrome, and childhood disintegrative disorder as well as a "subthreshold" category (termed PDD-NOS [not otherwise specified] in *DSM* and atypical autism in *ICD-10*) for cases not quite meeting the full criteria for autism. The definition proposed for autism included a total of 12 criteria grouped across three categories of social interaction problem, communication/play criteria, and restricted interest and repetitive behavior. Under this system, there were over 2200 ways to attain a diagnosis of autism using the provided criteria. It remained the gold standard for nearly two decades.

There were a number of differences in the overall *DSM-5* (APA, 2013) approach to diagnosis, some of which proved controversial for autism; rather than conducting a large field trial, a large set of dimensional diagnostic data derived from assessments were analyzed. The number of criteria was reduced with a combination of monothetic (for symptom areas, all criteria were needed) and polythetic (for the other symptom areas, only some were needed). As a result, the number of potential ways to achieve a diagnosis of autism was vastly reduced. Although the analysis of the large data set had many merits and of itself showed good sensitivity and specificity, criticisms quickly appeared (even before *DSM-5* was published) that suggested a major change and narrowing of the diagnostic concept. In the new *DSM-5* approach, Asperger's disorder and PDD-NOS were eliminated, and only a small number (10% or so) of these cases would now achieve a diagnosis of ASD. Even for higher cognitive functioning autism, a substantial number of cases lost their diagnosis (MC Partland et al., 2012). In the United States, in particular, this had dramatic implications for service eligibility, and as a result, a decision was made near the end of the *DSM-5* process to "grandfather in" cases with well-established previous diagnosis of autism, Asperger's, and so forth. Effectively, this created a new system while perpetuating the old one! Thus, previous diagnostic terms like *Asperger's disorder* remain in use.

A number of studies have now confirmed this problem both for the higher functioning older individuals and younger children (Smith, 2015). On the other hand, a major advance was the name change of the overall category to *autism spectrum disorder* (ASD, somewhat paradoxically termed given the more restricted diagnostic concept), but this term is more consistent with the growing awareness of the range of genetic contributions to autism and the "broader autistic phenotype." Perhaps in part concerned with just this awareness, a new *social communication disorder* (SCD) was added to the Communication Disorders section although it does not exactly converge either with the older concept of Asperger's or atypical autism/PDD-NOS (it emphasizes problems in social communication leaving out restricted interests and repetitive behaviors). Table 7.1 summarizes the history of categorical definitions of autism.

The development of a number (now over 30) of screening and diagnostic instruments has been an important advance (Lord et al., 2014). These approaches have some important advantages over categorical ones. Some are designed more as screeners, others for use in schools and educational settings, and yet others as a part of more comprehensive diagnostic assessments. It is important to realize that some of these instruments require extensive training, because some of the more widely used screening instrument studies in large populations have been disappointing and important issues of gender and possible bias have been noted.

■ EPIDEMIOLOGY AND DEMOGRAPHICS

The earliest studies of the epidemiology suggested that it was a rather rare condition on the order of 1–2 cases/1000 children, but more recent studies suggest much higher rates on the order of 1 case/145 children (Meyers et al., 2019). Several factors appear to account for this

TABLE 7.1

Evolution of the Concept of Autism/Autism Spectrum Disorder

Concept	Description
Early infantile autism (Kanner, 1943)	First described syndrome, two essential features—autism (lack of social orientation), resistance to change/insistence on sameness
Autistic personality disorder (Asperger, 1944)	Autistic personality disorder—used same word *autism* for verbal boys who had circumscribed interests that interfered with function, noted positive family history (fathers), essentially set stage for awareness of a broader autism phenotype
Infantile autism/residual infantile autism (*DSM III*, APA, 1980)	First official recognition, monothetic (all criteria had to be met), overemphasis on the "infantile" or early manifestation of autism, lacked developmental orientation; new term for overall class—*pervasive developmental disorder*
Autistic disorder (*DSM-III-R*, APA, 1987)	More and more developmental, polythetic (mix of social, communication, restricted interest) criteria, applicable across age and developmental spectrum. Probably overdiagnosed autism in the very intellectually disabled
Autistic disorder (*DSM-IV*, APA, 1990)	Retained polythetic approach, readjusted criteria based on international field trial done in conjunction with internal classification of disease 10th edition, first recognition of Asperger's as a category
Autism spectrum disorder (*DSM-5*, APA, 2013)	Moved from three categories to two (social and communication combined), mix of monothetic and polythetic, name change of category to *autism spectrum disorder*. In fact, criteria more restrictive than previously, as a result cases/children would lose label (and services). To deal with this, individuals with "well-established" diagnosis of Asperger's, etc., could retain them. But still problems persist for cases coming to diagnosis. Also, issues for diagnosis of young children and service eligibility

apparent change in rate. There are many challenges in terms of case identification, definition, sample size and methods, and so forth. Epidemiologic surveys of ASDs pose substantial challenges to researchers seeking to measure rates of ASD, particularly given the range of case definition, case identification, and case evaluation methods employed across surveys. As Fombonne and colleagues emphasize (Meyers et al., 2019), this current increase in prevalence cannot be directly attributed to actual changes in incidence of the disorder. There is fairly good evidence to suggest that a number of factors have led to changes in rates—these include changes in educational policy (i.e., inclusion of special needs children in public schools in the United States), changes in diagnostic criteria, and the marked increase in awareness of ASD in the general population as well as on the part of some parents, and the desire to have this label to increase special educational services provided. Indeed, the expansion in cases diagnosed in developed countries has risen in parallel with the growing availability of effective treatment programs. The major difficulties of undertaking good epidemiologic studies must be noted, that is, in methods of case assessment and sizes of samples. In small samples, rates are notoriously more variable. As noted earlier, the recent changes in *DSM-5* may tend to lower identified cases.

There is an apparent male predominance (at least 3–5 times more common), although this is much less pronounced in lower IQ groups and much more pronounced in high IQ cases. However, it is possible that subtle gender differences impact case identification and lead to underdiagnosis in girls. It does appear that, with usual diagnostic criteria and approaches, there is a marked male predooming in the normal range of cognitive ability—perhaps 25 or more to 1.

Cultural and ethnic issues may impact treatment and, to some extent, case detection of autism generally is remarkably similar around the world (Freeth et al., 2014). There is a growing awareness of the need for diagnosis and intervention in third world countries. The early impression that autism was more likely in children of parents with more education and higher occupational status clearly proved incorrect.

■ ETIOLOGY AND PATHOGENESIS

As noted previously, early speculation centered on psychodynamic explanations of autism. The growing body of evidence in the 1970s that autism was brain based and highly genetic changed to focus of work on the pathogenesis of the condition markedly.

A major effort has been on understanding the "autism" in autism, that is, the social brain connection (see Table 7.2). This research has centered on a number of specific brain regions that appear to be basic to understanding social information (McPartland et al., 2014).

Regions involved include the amygdala, the orbitofrontal cortex, and the ventral and lateral temporal cortexes, and supporting data have come from work in nonhuman primate electrophysiology and human neuropsychology. This work has also led to a now great volume of work on neuroimaging, particularly with fMRI and EEG processing of faces and social information (e.g., biologic movement). Well-replicated work using fMRI has shown differences in processing of the face in the fusiform facial recognition area gyrus. Similarly, work with EEG has shown differences in face processing use evoked potential and this finding may emerge as the first generally recognized biomarker of autism. Working using eye-tracking paradigms has shown marked differences in the way persons with autism view social situations—often paying less attention to the more affectively rich upper portion of the face (Figure 7.1).

The study of genetic factors in autism has similarly advanced and a number of important findings have emerged. These include the association of autism with some well-recognized genetic disorder, for example, fragile X and tuberous scleroses. Initially, it was hoped that the number of possible genes identified would be small, but this is not the case. In many ways, this finding is quite consistent with the recognition of a "broader autism phenotype." A number of candidate genes have now been identified and many of these have important functions in the brain (Yuen et al., 2019). Advances in genetic testing have also made it easier to run a broad array of genetic assays in the individual case, and perhaps 10 to 20% of cases can now be associated with some genetic finding (although sometimes of unknown etiologic significance). Family studies have also shown a strong connection of autism in the child to other conditions in family members, for example, anxiety problems and attention difficulties.

TABLE 7.2

Brain Regions Potentially Involved in Autism

Neural System	Areas	Comment/Function
Social perception system		Evolutionarily conserved and shared with other primates, refers to the initial stages in social information processing
	Superior temporal sulcus (STS)	Decoding of nonverbal social signals such as gaze direction and facial expression
	The fusiform gyrus (FFG)	Face processing
	Extrastriate body area (EBA) in lateral occipitotemporal cortex	Visual perception and recognition of the human body
	The amygdala and limbic system	Perception of emotional states and salient emotional experiences
	The orbitofrontal cortex (OFC) and ventrolateral prefrontal cortex (VLPFC)	Social reward and reinforcement
Mirror neuron system	The inferior frontal gyrus and the inferior parietal lobe (IPL)	An evolutionarily conserved system, plays an important role in action perception, understanding, and prediction
The mental state reasoning system	The medial prefrontal cortex (MPFC) and temporoparietal junction (TPJ)	Probably unique to humans Responsible for reasoning about others' thoughts

Thus, it is increasingly clear that ASDs are a collection of highly heterogeneous conditions with, perhaps, one or more final common pathways to clinical expression. With increasingly sophisticated genetic studies, it is likely that more such specific pathways will be identified. There clearly is the potential impact of some environmental factor or factors in this complex process, although to date it is the genetic factors that appear to be most robustly elucidated.

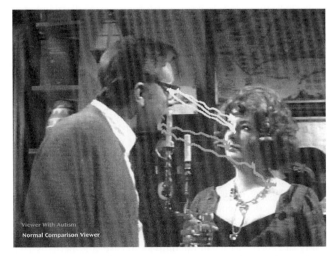

FIGURE 7.1. Differences in eye tracking in an individual with high functioning autism (*bottom line*) and a typically developing person (*top line*) watching an intensely social scene; the individual with autism focuses on the mouth losing much of the social-affective information conveyed in the top part of the face.

CLINICAL EXPRESSION

Kanner's emphasis on autism was remarkably insightful as social features remain both a hallmark of the condition and important targets for intervention and predictors of outcome. It is clear that the social difficulties are fundamental, that is, that they are not a function of intellectual disability and more likely actually contribute to it if not treated. Social problems may be an initial presenting feature as parents report difficulties engaging the child in the first year of life. Over time, the more aloof infant may become more passively accepting integration, finally developing an "active but odd" social style as seen in the most cognitively able cases.

Kanner also noted the major problem in language (or as we now appreciate in all of communication) in his first cases. Some of these children never talk or had unusual features to their language like echolalia (repetition of phrases or sentences) and pronoun reversal. The early psychodynamic speculations regarding these features came to be replaced with a better developmental understanding both of communicative and cognitive developments; for example, echolalia is now seen as a function of the child's gestalt learning style (learning things in chunks) and something to be worked with rather than a symptom to be eradicated. In the past, many individuals with ASD remained mute or largely mute throughout their lives, but with earlier detection and intervention, this number has substantially decreased. Concerns about delayed speech are another common presenting symptom at round 12–18 months. For individuals who do speak, unusual prosody (the musical aspect of speech) is common with monotonic tone, little inflection, and sometimes loud volume. Idiosyncratic language may be present, that is, a specific word or phrase, whose special meaning is known only to parents or close family members. Pragmatic language (social language) is particularly impaired, so understanding of figurative language, humor, sarcasm, and irony may be limited and become a source of great difficulties in adolescents (Paul, 2019).

The unusual difficulties with change that Kanner termed *insistence on sameness* often stand in stark contrast to sensitivity to environmental change. Unusual preoccupation or early interests—in aspects of the nonsocial world—may be seen: for example, in letters, numbers, signs, hood ornaments on cars. Sometimes, young children with autism may have an attachment object of some kind, but unlike the typically developing, this transition object is often hard rather than soft, and the specific object is less important than the category of object, for example, sticks, rocks, cars, magazines, cereal boxes. Sometimes, parents' initial clinical concern is that the child might be deaf (given language delays and failure to respond to name), but at the same time the child might respond with great anxiety to certain sounds. It is frequent for unusual sensory interests to precede more "classic" stereotyped mannerisms; the latter are almost always present by about age 3.

Early impressions of cognitive functioning were based on children's ability to do nonverbal tasks like puzzles and the notion was that children were not also intellectually disabled. Over time, it became apparent that this was not the case as nonverbal skills were often isolated areas of strengths and verbal abilities were areas of great weakness (Vivanti et al., 2019). Occasionally (maybe 10% of the time), unusual islets of ability or splinter skills like feats of memory or calendar calculation or drawing are observed (Hermelin, 2001). In the first years after autism was described, no interventions were available and many children ended up in training school or other institutions and ended up functioning in the intellectually deficient range. Now, with better and earlier interventions, progress is much more likely and a minority of cases likely end up with associated intellectual disability as adults, although (as for intellectual disability [see Chapter 6]) adaptive skills are also very major predictors of outcome.

Scatter on cognitive testing is common. Individuals with more classic autism often have the pattern of much weaker verbal and abstract abilities. Interestingly, in Asperger's syndrome, the reverse pattern may be observed (often with high degrees of knowledge about some special area of interest). In a small number of cases (perhaps 10%), some unusual or even remarkable ability may be present, for example, drawing, calculating dates, or memory. Often such "savant skills" are in contrast to overall abilities. In Asperger's disorder, areas of intense special interests are usual and the child acquires great knowledge of some topic. Often, these interests interfere with the individual's learning and impact family life, but at times these can be turned into potentially valuable vocational skills. At times, these interests lead to problems with the legal system.

TABLE 7.3

Symptoms of Autism in the First 3 Years of Life

	0–12 Months	12–36 Months
Social	Limited ability to anticipate being picked up Low frequency of looking at people Limited interest in interactional games Limited affection toward familiar people Content to be left alone Limited range of facial expression	Abnormal eye contact Limited social referencing Limited interest in other children Limited social smile Low frequency of looking at people Limited sharing of affect/enjoyment
Play	Little interest in interactive games	Limited functional play No pretend play Limited motor imitation
Communication	Poor response to name (does not respond to call) Does not frequently look at objects held by others	Low frequency of verbal or nonverbal communication Failure to share interests (e.g., through pointing, sharing, giving, showing) Poor response to name Failure to respond to communicative gestures (pointing, giving, showing) Use of others' body as a tool (pulls hand to desired object without making eye contact, as if *hand* rather than person obtains object)
Restricted interests/behaviors	Mouths objects excessively Does not like to be touched	Unusual sensory behaviors Hyper-/hyposensitivity to sounds, texture, tastes, visual stimuli Hand or finger mannerisms Inappropriate use of objects Repetitive interest/play

Republished with permission of Annual Reviews, Inc. from Volkmar, F. R., Chawarska, K., & Klin, A. (2005). Autism in infancy and early childhood. *Annual Review of Psychology, 56*, 315–336; permission conveyed through Copyright Clearance Center, Inc.

Kanner originally suggested that autism was congenital and this still seems likely to be the case, although perhaps 20% of parents will report a period of normal development followed by development of more autistic-like symptoms. Some of the early warning signs of autism are listed in Table 7.3. In a very small number of cases, there is a profound regression after some years of development. Both *DSM-IV* and *ICD-10* included the concept for childhood disintegrative disorder to this group of cases and, unfortunately, they appear to have a much worse prognosis.

■ COURSE

As noted previously, parents are typically worried about their child's development in the first year of life—typical concerns centering on language delay or possible deafness. However, the first screening instruments (at present) only begin to be useful around 18 months so that delay in diagnosis is relatively common. In addition, some children seem to develop normally for a time and then lose skills. Sometimes, children at ages 1 or 2 will exhibit the more typical social communication problems but not yet all the unusual behaviors (although sometimes exhibiting precursors to these behaviors, for example, staring at fans or fixating on some object more than on parents and family members). However, by age 3, the vast majority of children with ASD will exhibit the diagnosis and often intervention would have started even before that time because of language delay. Early diagnosis is increasingly common and schools are mandated to provide services after the age of 3.

Young children with autism may exhibit an aloof social style, although sometimes the more cognitively able are more passively accepting of social interaction or are somewhat one sided and eccentric as they mature. Behavioral difficulties often increase during childhood and may further increase in adolescence before diminishing in young adulthood. It does appear that with earlier diagnosis and more effective interventions, the overall outcome has improved (Magiati & Howlin, 2019). Although the *DSM-5* definition of ASD is somewhat restricting in the broader sense of the autistic spectrum, it is very clear that a tremendous range of features and symptoms are exhibited. See Boxes 7.1 and 7.2 for illustrative case descriptions of ASD (previously autistic disorder) and Asperger's disorder.

BOX 7.1   Case Report—Autistic Disorder

John was the second of two children born to middle-class parents after a normal pregnancy, labor, and delivery. As an infant, John appeared undemanding and relatively placid; motor development proceeded appropriately, but language development was delayed. Although his parents indicated that they were first concerned about his development when he was 18 months of age and still not speaking, in retrospect they noted that, in comparison to their previous child, he had seemed relatively uninterested in social interaction and the social games of infancy. Stranger anxiety had never really developed, and John did not exhibit differential attachment behaviors toward his parents. Their pediatrician initially reassured John's parents that he was a "late talker," but they continued to be concerned. Although John seemed to respond to some unusual sounds, the pediatrician obtained a hearing test when John was 24 months old. Levels of hearing appeared adequate for development of speech, and John was referred for developmental evaluation. At 24 months, motor skills were age appropriate and John exhibited some nonverbal problem-solving skills close to age level. His language and social development, however, were severely delayed, and he was noted to be resistant to changes in routine and unusually sensitive to aspects of the inanimate environment. His play skills were quite limited and he used play materials in unusual and idiosyncratic ways. His older sister had a history of some learning difficulties, but the family history was otherwise negative. A comprehensive medical evaluation revealed a normal EEG and CT scan; genetic screening and chromosome analysis were normal as well.

John was enrolled in a special education program, where he gradually began to speak. His speech was characterized by echolalia, extreme literalness, a monotonic voice quality, and pronoun reversal. He rarely used language in interaction and remained quite isolated. By school age, John had developed some evidence of differential attachments to family members; he also had developed a number of self-stimulatory behaviors and engaged in occasional periods of head banging. Extreme sensitivity to change continued. Intelligence testing revealed marked scatter, with a full-scale IQ in the moderately retarded range. As an adolescent, John's behavioral functioning deteriorated, and he developed a seizure disorder. Now an adult, he lives in a group home and attends a sheltered workshop. He has a rather passive interactional style but exhibits occasional outbursts of aggression and self-abuse.

Comment: With earlier intervention, more children with autism are doing better. Unfortunately in this case, although the child developed speech, his overall outcome has not been as good as might have been hoped.

Reprinted with permission from Martin, A., Volkmar, F. R., & Bloch, M. H. (2018). *Lewis's child and adolescent psychiatry* (5th ed.). Wolters Kluwer.

| **BOX 7.2** | **Case Report: Asperger Disorder** |

Tom was an only child. Birth, medical, and family histories were unremarkable. His motor development was somewhat delayed, but communicative milestones were within normal limits. His parents became concerned about him at age 4 when he was enrolled in a nursery school and was noted to have marked difficulties in peer interaction that were so pronounced that he could not continue in the program. In grade school, he was enrolled in special education classes and was noted to have some learning problems. His greatest difficulties arose in peer interaction; he was viewed as markedly eccentric and had no friends. His preferred activity, watching the weather channel on television, was pursued with great interest and intensity. On examination at age 13, he had markedly circumscribed interests and exhibited pedantic and odd patterns of communication with a monotonic voice quality. Psychological testing revealed an IQ within the normal range with marked scatter evident. Formal communication examination revealed age-appropriate skills in receptive and expressive language, but marked impairment in pragmatic language skills. Tom has now gone on to college where he has, with considerable support, done well.

Comment: Preservation of language (if not always communication) skills in Asperger's presents some important strengths for treatment.

Reprinted with permission from Volkmar, F. R., & Martin, A (2011). Autism and related disorders. In *Essentials of child and adolescent psychiatry* (1st ed., p. 71). Lippincott Williams & Wilkins/Wolters Kluwer.

■ DIFFERENTIAL DIAGNOSIS AND ASSESSMENT

The differential diagnosis of autism includes intellectual deficiency, communication disorders, severe deprivation, and sensory impairment. For the person with intellectual deficiency not associated with autism, social skills are usually on par with cognitive development. In the communication disorders (apart from the new "SCD"—see Chapter 8), social skills are generally preserved. Tests of both vision and hearing can now be conducted readily even with infants. Guidelines for genetic assessment are also available.

Although many areas of difficulty can often be identified on testing, it is also important to look for areas of strength that can be built upon in treatment planning. Often more socially based, verbal abilities are most impaired, whereas other less verbal areas may be much stronger. A number of specialists are involved and it is important that you "speak the same language" in working together as a team. A number of well-established assessment instruments can be used to assess intellectual level, communicative skills, academic achievement, motor skills, and so forth.; adaptive skills (i.e., generalization of knowledge to real-world settings) are particularly important.

Both screening and diagnostic instruments for autism have been developed (see 5.60, Table 7.4). It is important to realize that all these have important uses and limitations. Repeated screening is recommended at 18 and 24 months of age for ASD. However, recent studies in large population samples have been somewhat disappointing and some organizations no longer recommend routine screening given the limitations of these instruments. Ideally, more neurobiologically-based screeners using specific biomarkers may be developed.

The initial assessment should include a physical assessment with special attention to features of autism and signs of dysmorphology as well as a thorough history. Hearing and vision should be evaluated. It is best to observe the child both in structured and unstructured settings. Although the use of rating instruments and assessments specific to autism can be helpful, it is important to keep in mind that these are often most applicable to school-age children of mild to borderline intellectual levels and may not work as well for younger or older or for more and less cognitively impaired cases. Assessment procedures are summarized in Table 7.4.

TABLE 7.4

Evaluation Procedures: Autism and Pervasive Developmental Disorders

1. Historical information
   Early development and characteristics of development
   Age and nature of onset
   Medical and family history
2. Developmental and psychological assessment
   Intellectual level and profile of learning
   Communicative assessment (receptive and expressive language skills, use of nonverbal communication, pragmatic use of language)
   Adaptive behavior (ability to generalize skills to real-world settings)
   Occupational/physical therapy assessments as appropriate
3. Psychiatric examination
   Nature of social relatedness (eye contact, attachment behaviors, reciprocity, insight)
   Behavioral features (stereotypy/self-stimulation, resistance to change, unusual sensitivities to the environment)
   Language/communication difficulties (echolalia, presence of communicative speech, etc.)
   Play skills (nonfunctional use of play materials, symbolic play, and imagination)
4. Medical evaluations
   Search for associated medical conditions, genetic abnormalities, presence of seizures with additional tests as needed
   Hearing/vision test
   Additional consultation (neurologic/pediatric/genetic) as indicated by history and current presentation (see Yuen, et al., 2019, for current genetic testing recommendations)
   Other examinations (e.g., EEG, CT/MRI scan, chromosome analysis)

Reprinted with permission from Volkmar, F. R., Lord, C., & Bailey, A. (2017). Autism and pervasive developmental disorders. In A. Martin, F. R. Volkmar, & M. Lewis (Eds.), *Lewis's child and adolescent psychiatry: A comprehensive textbook* (4th ed., p. 391). Lippincott Williams & Wilkins.

As noted earlier, the stronger association with special genetic and medical conditions includes marked risk for epilepsy, which develops in about 20% of cases along with several strongly genetic conditions. For some toddlers, macrocephaly develops. Recommendations for genetic testing are frequently changing and the American College of Human Genetics updates these on a regular basis. As already noted, the "hit rate" for genetic testing is now much higher than in the past.

Kanner's initial report noted the absence of obvious physical dysmorphology. Subsequently, autism has been noted to be associated with several genetic conditions—notably, fragile X and tuberous sclerosis; and physical signs may be associated with the condition in these cases. As noted previously, the risk for onset of epilepsy is markedly increased with peaks of onset both in early childhood and again in adolescence.

▉ TREATMENT

Until Public Law 94-142 in the United States, public education was not a right for disabled children. Before it was passed, research had shown the importance of structured interventions, and with its passage, schools assumed the major role for psychological and other developmental interventions in autism. Before this time, parents had often organized private school programs— some of which still exist. But with the mandate for public school intervention, more and more attempts were made to develop model program interventions. Early reviews noted a handful of such programs around the country that had at least some empirical support. Over time, the number of these programs and evidence-based intervention techniques has increased markedly. With advances in research on both diagnosis and intervention, a number of practice guidelines also began to appear (McClure, 2014; Volkmar et al., 2014).

A number of educational and behavioral treatment models have been established as evidence based (Odom et al., 2019). The quality of this evidence varies and criteria for whether or not a treatment is evidence based will vary depending on the rules for study inclusion. For example, behavior approaches through applied behavior analysis have been very well studied—usually in single case pre–post designs. These methods have now come into common use and are particularly helpful for more cognitively impaired children who need "learning to learn" skills and exhibit problem behaviors. Other programs, for example, the Early STAART, are more developmentally focused and offer some advantages in working with younger children; these programs often have the strongest independent data (i.e., apart from parent- and treater-based data). Another approach combines both developmental and behavioral approaches; this pivotal response approach focuses on key behaviors that foster development and learning and has strong parent involvement. Finally, the Division TEACCH statewide model is eclectic in nature combining many different methods in a comprehensive program; parts of it have been shown to be evidence based. Table 7.5 summarizes some of the program with at least some evidence base as they exist today.

A host of specific intervention techniques have also been evaluated. These range from behavioral interventions to assistant technology, social skills training, language–communication interventions, and so on. Many treatment modalities occupy a somewhat gray area and often are referred to as emerging interventions. Given the nature of autism, social skills interventions have been a major focus of work and include peer-based interventions (often used with young children), social skills group(s), and specific instructional methods and curricula (used for school-age and older children) as well as individual instruction. For children who do not yet speak, a host of augmentative approaches, both low and high tech, can be used. For more cognitively able children, the focus is often on enhancing social language (pragmatic) skills. Organization issues (what psychologists often term *executive functions*) are another major area of intervention—the use of tablets, organizers, schedules, and special computer/software programs can be helpful.

Pharmacologic interventions also can be helpful (Mooney et al., 2019). These can be used to reduce irritability in younger children and to deal with attentional programs when these are present. As children age, other psychiatric conditions, notably anxiety and depression, emerge and can be amenable to both drug treatment and specific psychotherapeutic approaches. Of course, no drug will make up for an inadequate school program. The usual practice in

TABLE 7.5

Overview of Model Programs

Type of Program	Example	Brief Overview	Supporting Evidence
Behavioral	Lovass early intensive intervention	Uses behavioral techniques to foster desired behaviors	Many single case studies
Developmental	Early Start or Jasper	Focus on acquitting of important developmental behaviors	Well-designed studies with independent assessment
Hybrid approaches	Pivotal response	Combines both developmental and behavioral aspects	Very good evaluation including controlled trials
Eclectic	Division TEACCH Program	Pulls treatment methods from various sources	Parts of the program have been evaluated in controlled studies

schools of collecting data in an ongoing way can help inform our understanding of response to medications. Side effects such as weight gain with some of the atypical neuroleptics and agitation with stimulant medication or SSRIs are seen (see Chapter 29). At the present time, no drug treatments address the core social disability in autism, although this is an area of active research.

Parents frequently explore alternative (instead of proven treatments) or complementary (in addition to such treatment) approaches. As noted earlier, extravagant claims can be made, but it is critical that parents and providers make informed decisions with regard to use of such treatment. For many of these, the risk is that so much attention goes to exploring the alternative treatment that the child's regular intervention program suffers. On occasion, some of these are actually dangerous. One of the interesting things that has emerged with these treatments is the growing awareness of the strong impact of placebo response—that is, the nonspecific but sometimes major effects of paying more attention, expectancy effects, and so forth. This underscores the importance of thoughtfully designed well-controlled treatment studies.

■ SUMMARY

It is now over 75 years since Kanner (1943) first described the syndrome of early infantile autism. Since his initial description, much progress has been made. The pioneering studies of the 1970s showed that autism was a brain-based strongly genetic disorder that responded to structured treatment and was not related to schizophrenia. With the official recognition of autism in 1980, research began to build substantially so that now many thousands of peer-reviewed scientific papers have appeared. During this time, the prognosis of autism has begun to shift both with the discovery of structured treatment and now evidence-based approaches and the important mandates in 1975 with Public Law 94-142 for school-based services.

The understanding of the fundamental social nature of autism has remained a major focus of research. Progress has been made and autism has emerged as a singular example of a brain-based disorder of social learning. With improved detection and intervention, more children are doing increasingly well and many are now attending colleges and seeking gainful employment—a stark contract to the situation in the 1950s. Important gaps in knowledge remain—for example, there is very little work on aging in autism and treatments that address the core social vulnerability remain to be identified.

References

American Psychiatric Association. (1980). *Diagnostic and statistical manual (DSM-III)* (3rd ed.). APA Press.

American Psychiatric Association. (1987). *Diagnostic and statistical manual (DSM-III-R)* (3rd rev. ed.). APA Press.

American Psychiatric Association. (1990). *Diagnostic and statistical manual (DSM-IV)* (4th ed.). APA Press.

American Psychiatric Association. (2013). *Diagnostic and statistical manual (DSM-5)* (5th ed.). APA Press.

Asperger, H. (1944). Die "autistichen Psychopathen" im Kindersalter. *Archive fur psychiatrie und Nervenkrankheiten, 117*, 76–136.

Freeth, M., Milne, E., Sheppard, E., & Ramachandran, R. (2014). Autism across cultures: Perspectives from non-western cultures and implications for research. In F. R. Volkmar, R. Paul, S. J. Rogers, & K. A. Pelphrey (Eds.), *Handbook of autism and pervasive developmental disorders* (4th ed.). John Wiley & Sons, Inc.

Hermelin, B. (2001). *Bright splinters of the mind: A personal story of research with autistic savants.* Jessica Kingsley.

Ingersoll, B., & Wainer, A. (2014). The broader autism phenotype. In F. R. Volkmar, R. Paul, S. J. Rogers, & K. A. Pelphrey (Eds.), *Handbook of autism and pervasive developmental disorders* (4th ed.). John Wiley & Sons, Inc.

Kanner, L. (1943). Autistic disturbances of affective contact. *Nervous Child, 2*, 217–250.

Lord, C., Corsello, C., & Grzadzinski, R. (2014). Diagnostic instruments in autistic spectrum disorders. In F. R. Volkmar, R. Paul, S. J. Rogers, & K. A. Pelphrey (Eds.), *Handbook of autism and pervasive developmental disorders* (4th ed.). John Wiley & Sons, Inc.

Magiati, I., & Howlin, P. (2019). Adult life for people with autism spectrum disorders. In F. R. Volkmar (Ed.), *Autism and pervasve developmental disorders* (pp. 220–248). Cambridge University Press.

McClure, I. (2014). Developing and implementing practice guidelines. In F. R. Volkmar, R. Paul, S. J. Rogers, & K. A. Pelphrey (Eds.), *Handbook of autism and pervasive developmental disorders, volume 2: Assessment, interventions, and policy* (pp. 1014–1035). John Wiley & Sons, Inc.

McPartland, J. C., Reichow, B., & Volkmar, F. R. (2012). Sensitivity and specificity of proposed *DSM-5* diagnostic criteria for autism spectrum disorder. *Journal of the American Academy of Child & Adolescent Psychiatry, 51*(4), 368–383. https://doi.org/10.1016/j.jaac.2012.01.007

Meyers, J., Chaves, A., Hill, A. P., Zuckerman, K., & Fombonne, E. (2019). Epidemiological surveys of autism spectrum disorders. In F. R. Volkmar (Ed.), *Autism and pervasive developmental disorders* (pp. 61–88). Cambridge University Press.

Meyers, J., Chavez, A., Presmanes Hill, A., Zuckerman, K., & Fombonne, E. (2019). Epidemiological surveys of autism spectrum disorders. In F. R. Volkmar (Ed.), *Autism and pervasive developmental disorders* (3rd ed., pp. 61–88). Cambridge University Press.

Odom, S. L., Morin, K., Savage, M., & Tomaszewski, B. (2019). Behavioral and educational interventions. In F. R. Volkmar (Ed.), *Autism and the pervasive developmental disorders* (pp. 176–190). Cambridge University Press.

Paul, R. (2019). Communication and its development. In F. R. Volkmar (Ed.), *Autism spectrum disorders autism and the pervasive developmental disorders* (pp. 89–111). Cambridge University Press.

Rutter, M. (1978). Diagnosis and definition of childhood autism. *Journal of Autism & Childhood Schizophrenia, 8*(2), 139–161. https://doi.org/10.1007/BF01537863

Smith, I. C., Reichow, B., & Volkmar, F. R. (2015). The effects of *DSM-5* criteria on number of individuals diagnosed with autism spectrum disorder: a systematic review. *Journal of Autism & Developmental Disorders, 45*(8), 2541–2552. https://doi.org/https://dx.doi.org/10.1007/s10803-015-2423-8

Vivanti, G., Yerys, B. E., & Salomone, E. (2019). Psychological factors in autism spectrum disorders. In F. R. Volkmar (Ed.). *Autism and the pervasive developmental disorders* (pp. 61–89). Cambridge University Press.

Volkmar, F. R., Siegel, M., Woodbury-Smith, M., King, B., McCracken, J., State, M., & American Academy of Child and Adolescent Psychiatry (AACAP) Committee on Quality Issues (CQI). (2014). Practice parameter for the assessment and treatment of children and adolescents with autism spectrum disorder. *Journal of the American Academy of Child & Adolescent Psychiatry, 53*(2), 237–257. https://doi.org/10.1016/j.jaac.2013.10.013

Yuen, R. K. C., Szatmari, P., & Vorstman, J. A. S. (2019). The genetics of autism spectrum disorders. In F. R. Volkmar. (Ed.), *Autism and the pervasive developmental disorders* (pp. 112–128). Cambridge University Press.

Suggested Readings

Bartak, L., & Rutter, M. (1973). Special educational treatment of autistic children: A comparative study-1. Design of study and characteristics of units. *Journal of Child Psychology & Psychiatry & Allied Disciplines, 14*(3), 161–179. https://doi.org/10.1111/j.1469-7610.1973.tb01185.x

Barton, K. S., Tabor, H. K., Starks, H., Garrison, N. A., Laurino, M., & Burke, W. (2018). Pathways from autism spectrum disorder diagnosis to genetic testing. *Genetics in Medicine, 20*(7), 737–744. https://doi.org/10.1038/gim.2017.166

Brothers, L. (1990). The social brain: A project for integrating primate behavior and neurophysiology in a new domain. *Concepts in Neuroscience, 1,* 27–51.

Donvan, J., & Zuker, C. (2016). *In a different key: The story of autism.* Penguin Random House.

Folstein, S., & Rutter, M. (1977). Infantile autism: A genetic study of 21 twin pairs. *Journal of Child Psychology & Psychiatry & Allied Disciplines, 18*(4), 297–321. https://doi.org/10.1111/j.1469-7610.1977.tb00443.x

Greenberg, G. (2013). *The book of woe: The DSM and the unmaking of psychiatry.* Penguin Random House.

Ibanez, L. V., Stone, W. L., & Coonrod, E. E. (2014). Screening for autism in young children. In *Handbook of autism and pervasive developmental disorders, volume 2: Assessment, interventions, and policy* (pp. 585–608). John Wiley & Sons, Inc.

Jackson, S. L., & Volkmar, F. R. (2019). Diagnosis and definition of autism and other pervasive developmental disorders. In F. R. Volkmar (Ed.), *Autism and the pervasive developmental disorders* (pp. 1–24). Cambridge University Press.

Lord, C., Corsello, C., & Grzadzinski, R. (2014). Diagnostic instruments in autistic spectrum disorders. In F. R. Volkmar, S. J. Rogers, R. Paul, & K. A. Pelphrey (Eds.), *Handbook of autism and developmental disorders* (Vol. 2, pp. 610–650). John Wiley & Sons, Inc.

McPartland, J. C., Tillman, R. M., Yang, D. Y.-J., Bernier, R. A., & Pelphrey, K. A. (2014). The social neuroscience of autism spectrum disorder. In F. R. Volkmar, R. Paul, S. J. Rogers, & K. A. Pelphrey (Eds.), *Handbook of autism and pervasive developmental disorders* (4th ed.). John Wiley & Sons, Inc.

Muhle, R. A., Reed, H. E., Vo, L. C., Metha, S., McGuire, K., Veenstra-VanderWeele, J., & Pedapati, E. (2017). Clinical diagnostic genetic testing for individuals with developmental disorders. *Journal of the American Academy of Child and Adolescent Psychiatry, 56*(11), 910–913. https://doi.org/10.1016/j.jaac.2017.09.418

Mundy, P., & Burnette, C. (2014). Joint attention and neurodevelopmental models of autism. In F. R. Volkmar, R. Paul, S. J. Rogers, & K. A. Pelphrey (Eds.), *Handbook of autism and pervasive developmental disorders* (Vol. 1, pp. 650–681). John Wiley & Sons, Inc.

National Research Council. (2001). *Educating young children with autism*. National Academy Press.

Odom, S. L., Morin, K., Savage, M., & Tomaszewski, B. (2019). Behavioral and educational interventions. In F. R. Volkmar (Ed.), *Autism and the pervasive developmental disorders* (pp. 176–190). Cambridge University Press.

Paul, R. (2019). Communication and its development in autism spectrum disorders. In F. R. Volkmar (Ed.), *Autism and the pervasive developmental disorders* (pp. 89–111). Cambridge University Press.

Paul, R., & Fahim, D. (2015). *Let's talk*. Brooks.

Reichow, B., & Barton, E. E. (2014). Evidence-based psychosocial interventions for individuals with autism spectrum disorders. In F. R. Volkmar, R. Paul, S. J. Rogers, & K. A. Pelphrey (Eds.), *Handbook of autism and pervasive developmental disorders, volume 2: Assessment, interventions, and policy* (pp. 969–992). John Wiley & Sons, Inc.

Rutter, M. (2014). Genetic influences and autism. In F. R. Volkmar, R. Paul, S. J. Rogers, & K. A. Pelphrey (Eds.), *Handbook of autism and pervasive developmental disorders* (Vol. 1, pp. 425–452). John Wiley & Sons, Inc.

Schultz, R. T., Gauthier, I., Klin, A., Fulbright, R. K., Anderson, A. W., Volkmar, F. R., Skudlarski, P., Lacadie, C., Cohen, D. J., & Gore, J. C. (2000). Abnormal ventral temporal cortical activity during face discrimination among individuals with autism and Asperger syndrome. *Archives of General Psychiatry, 57*(4), 331–340. https://doi.org/10.1001/archpsyc.57.4.331

Silverman, A. C. (2015). *NeuroTribes: The legacy of autism and the future of neurodiversity*. Penguin Random House.

Smith, T., Oakes, L., & Selver, K. (2014). Alternative treatments. In F. R. Volkmar, R. Paul, S. J. Rogers, & K. A. Pelphrey (Eds.), *Handbook of autism and pervasive developmental disorders* (4th ed.). John Wiley & Sons, Inc.

Volkmar, F. R., Booth, L. L., McPartland, J. C., & Wiesner, L. A. (2014). Clinical evaluation in multidisciplinary settings. In F. R. Volkmar, R. Paul, S. J. Rogers, & K. A. Pelphrey (Eds.), *Handbook of autism and pervasive developmental disorders* (4th ed., pp. 661–672). John Wiley & Sons, Inc.

Volkmar, F. R., Klin, A., & McPartland, J. C. (Eds.). (2014). Asperger syndrome: An overview. In *Asperger syndrome: Assessing and treating high-functioning autism spectrum disorders* (2nd ed., pp. 1–42). Guilford Press.

Volkmar, F. R., & Nelson, D. S. (1990). Seizure disorders in autism. *Journal of the American Academy of Child & Adolescent Psychiatry, 29*(1), 127–129. https://doi.org/10.1097/00004583-199001000-00020

CHAPTER 8 ■ DISORDERS OF COMMUNICATION AND LANGUAGE

■ BACKGROUND

The ability to communicate at a very high level by a wide range of modalities—including spoken language, facial expression, tone of voice, and gesture—is a uniquely human ability. It is usually acquired early in life as a result of not only exposure but also the evolved readiness to learn to communicate. Disorders of communication can arise as disruptions in this process either in association with other problems or as more isolated and specific difficulty. Speech is one important part of the more general communication domain (see Figure 8.1 and Box 8.1). Communication also includes written communication and the use of symbols as in written language or manual sign, both of which can be used to convey information quite efficiently and durably (e.g., the hieroglyphics of the pharaohs are still readable today). Animals can communicate, for example, to signal territory, danger, attract a mate, and so forth, and some are very perceptive indeed, but they do not have the same capacities for spoken language or written communication that people do to express ideas, thoughts, and feelings.

These utterances are often totally new, that is, they are created without being previously heard. Speech is one mode of language; writing provides another form of expression. For individuals who have already learned to speak and write but then suffer impediments to speech, for example, following a stroke, written communication can be a substitute. The situation is more complicated when difficulties occur in the developmental period, that is, before these various forms of communication are established.

The investigations of Broca and Wernicke led to important discoveries about the brain localization of language functions as they studied aphasia in adults. In this approach (based largely on adults with brain damage), recognition of words came in Wernicke's area in the left temporoparietal junction and then language production occurred via Broca's area in the left inferior frontal gyrus. But with the advent of more sophisticated imaging techniques, including MRI, it is clear that this model is very much an oversimplified one (see Hagoort, 2019, for a recent and comprehensive summary).

Clinical work focused on children began in the 1900s as psychologists, speech therapists, and educators began to study similarities and differences in adults with language problems, for example, poststroke aphasia as compared to children with language problems; they also began to work on the best teaching methods. Interest in children's language as a field of study began to increase, for example, for children who were deaf or who exhibited severe language

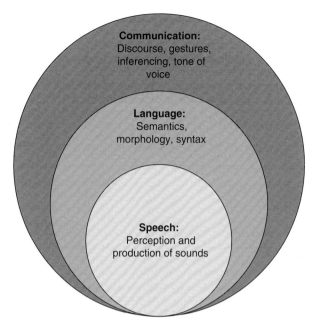

FIGURE 8.1. Relationship among speech, language, and communication and their components. Reprinted, with permission, from Simmons, E., & Paul, R. (2017). Disorders of communication. In: A. Martin, M. H. Bloch, F. R. Volkmar (Eds.), *Lewis's child and adolescent psychiatry* (5th ed., p. 451). Wolters Kluwer.

 Case Report: Language Disorder

Vinny had been noted to have delays in both his receptive and expressive language as a toddler. His family and primary care doctor adopted a *wait-and-see* attitude, in part because his father had also been language delayed and then developed normally. By the time he was 4 and entering preschool, his difficulties with language remained striking. An evaluation was obtained. Although his problem-solving abilities were at the average level and he was noted to have strengths in the area of visual learning and problem solving, auditory processing was an area of weakness, and both receptive and expressive language were significantly delayed. A diagnosis of language disorder was made and speech therapy was begun. By 6 years of age, Vinny was exhibiting attentional difficulties in first grade, and his continued language difficulties posed further obstacles for his learning. Fortunately, his reading skills turned out to be a relative area of strength for him and he used this, in part, to compensate for his language problems.

Comment: It is not unusual for children with language disorder to have other problems, commonly other learning difficulties and attentional problems. Fortunately, for this child, reading was an area of relative strength that provided some opportunities for compensatory learning.

Reprinted with permission from Volkmar, F. R., & Martin, A. (Eds.). (2011). Disorders in communication. In F. R. Volkmar (Ed.), *Essentials of Lewis's child and adolescent psychiatry* (1st ed., p. 101). Lippincott Williams & Wilkins/Wolters Kluwer.

problems. Attempts were made to start differentiating various types of child language–speech problems. Around the same period of time, interest in child language in its own right began to increase, for example, with Piaget's work on children's thinking and Chomsky's work on transformational thought (see Schoen & Paul, 2018).

■ DIAGNOSIS, DEFINITION, CLINICAL FEATURES

In the past, the term *language disorder* was used, but now it has been replaced by *communication disorder* to emphasize that problems are not limited simply to spoken language. Table 8.1 explains some key concepts/terms used in relation to language development and disorders. It should be noted that there are some important differences as well as similarities between major diagnostic systems. In the *DSM-5* approach (APA, 2013), substantial changes were made from the previous *DSM-IV* (APA, 2000) diagnoses of Expressive Language Disorder and Mixed Receptive-Expressive Language Disorder. The new *DSM-5* diagnostic categories include the following:

- **Language Disorder:** A category where problems in the acquisition and use of language occur across different communication modalities, reflecting difficulties in the understanding or production of language that are *substantially and quantifiably* below expectation based on age.
- **Social (Pragmatic) Communication Disorder (SCD):** This new concept is used when there are major problems in social pragmatic language use and it appears, in some respects, to have reflected an awareness of the increased stringency of the new *DSM-5* autism definition (see Chapter 7). There was also concern that some individuals who had previously had diagnoses of Asperger's or pervasive developmental disorder—not otherwise specified (PDD-NOS) might not be included in the new *DSM-5* autism spectrum category (children with autism spectrum disorder [ASD] are specifically excluded from the SCD diagnosis).
- **Speech Sound Disorder:** This is a category that previously would have been termed *articulation disorder*. In this category, problems in the literal production of speech sounds prevent effective communication. Other terms for this condition included phonologic disorder, articulation disorder, verbal dyspraxia, and speech apraxia. It is used when children have more than the usual delays in speech production relative to the later acquired sounds, for example, s, z, l, r, and when the articulation problems in sounds and sound combinations are more pervasive.
- **Childhood-Onset Fluency Disorder (Stuttering):** In this category, problems with fluent language production (stutter) are present and are often associated with and exacerbated by anxiety. Various patterns of dysfluencies are observed, and if the condition is more

TABLE 8.1

Key Concepts and Terms

Term	Short Definition
Pragmatics	The social use of language
Syntax	The way words are put together
Semantics	The meaning of language
Phonology	The sounds of language
Morphology	Word formation and system of word formation
Stuttering (cluttering)	Interruption of speech by repetition of sounds, words, or syllables that disrupt the easy flow of speech
Fluency	The ability to speak easily with steady flow of speech

severe, it can be associated with a range of other problems, including avoidance of certain words, unusual patterns of breathing, and articulation issues.

■ **Unspecified Communication Disorder:** This category is used in situations where the major presenting problems include aspects of communication, but the more specific criteria for the other types of communication disorder are not met.

The *DSM-5* approach builds on *DSM-IV* with some important differences. For example, with language disorder, the emphasis on whether receptive or expressive skills are more impaired is no longer made. The new social pragmatic disorder category reflects an awareness that some (if not many) individuals with problems on the autism spectrum might no longer receive an ASD diagnosis, although they still need service; the relationships and distinctions between SCD and autism remain the topic of debate (Jackson & Volkmar, 2019).

In contrast to *DSM-5*, the American Speech Hearing Association (1993) defines a language disorder as an impairment in "comprehension and/or use of a spoken, written, and/or other symbol system. The disorder may involve (1) the form of language (phonology, morphology, and syntax), (2) the content of language (semantics), and/or (3) the function of language in communication (pragmatics), in any combination" (1993, p. 40). Some clinicians have preferred to use the term *developmental language disorder* (i.e., to contrast this disorder from that of adults with onset of language problems in later life, i.e., well after language has previously been acquired). This view (more like that used in *DSM-IV*) makes a distinction between (1) mixed receptive/expressive disorders, which impair phonology, syntax, and semantics that lead to problems in expression and understanding; (2) expressive disorders, that is, when comprehension is intact but there are major problems in the production of language; and (3) higher order problems of language involving pragmatic (social language), semantic (the meaning of language), and discourse and conversation with adequate comprehension affecting spoken language (phonology; Rapin, 1996). In all these cases, some degree of functional impairment is required.

Language disorders can exist in isolation but are frequently associated with other developmental disorders. If the focus is on specific language impairments (SLIs), there is strong evidence for neurobiological factors in syndrome pathogenesis. For example, there is increased rate of concordance in monozygotic than in dizygotic twins; similarly, the risk for family members is increased. Although much speculation has centered on the role of environmental factors, the strongest associations are with lower socioeconomic status, larger family size, later birth order, and recurrent otitis media—all factors that deprive the child of language input at a critical stage in learning (Boxes 8.2 and 8.3).

BOX 8.2   **Case Report: Social Communication Disorder**

Jack is a 5-year-old boy who presented for assessment after he had difficulties with peers in nursery school. His parents reported that his early development was generally within normal limits, although his spoken language was somewhat delayed. They noted that he was often rather literal in his understanding and had problems with understanding things like jokes, sarcasm, and irony. He did well enough with adults who could accommodate his oddities, but with typical peers, he was having much more difficulty. He would tend to perseverate on his own topics of conversational interest and had trouble adjusting his communication to person and context. Ambiguous and figurative language was difficult for him. He had difficulties with understanding things like implied meanings and indirect requests. A consultation with a speech pathologist confirmed that although the form and content of his language were age appropriate, his social language was significantly delayed. He was enrolled in speech therapy for a time, with considerable work on teaching social skills. Involvement with a supportive boy scout group also helped improve his social understanding of pragmatic language.

BOX 8.3   **Speech Sound Disorder**

Larry was a pleasant but somewhat shy 4½-year-old seen for a kindergarten screening. His birth and early development were unremarkable. He had a few ear infections, but his hearing had recently been tested and was found to be within normal limits. During the screening, he had shown some articulation errors and was referred to a speech pathologist who noted difficulties with some of the later developing consonant sounds (e.g., z, sh, th, r). Sometimes, he would simply omit these sounds from words or put in other sounds in their place, for example, w for r. His difficulties became more notable when he had to string multiple words together. His speech was best articulated when he was calm and spoke in a slow, deliberate fashion. Although his parents could understand almost all of his speech, the speech pathologist suggested that likely a classroom teacher and peers might only be able to understand 80% of it. Because of this and what appeared to be his own awareness of the difficulty, speech therapy was begun with a good result. Two years later, he was having only occasional difficulties.

Comment: Often the prognosis is good, so that by age 6, many children with mild-to-moderate problems are doing well. Sometimes, problems can persist, particularly if speech becomes more complex or rapid.

Reprinted with permission from Volkmar, F. R., & Martin, A. (Eds.). (2011). Disorders in communication. In F. R. Volkmar (Ed.), *Essentials of Lewis's child and adolescent psychiatry* (1st ed., p. 101). Lippincott Williams & Wilkins/Wolters Kluwer.

If the focus is broadened beyond isolated language problems, the association with problems in overactivity and inattention is frequent. Of course, the ability to acquire language helps the child provide an inner narrative that facilitates focus, and conversely, a lack of language ability naturally may lead to difficulties with organization and attention. The nature of the role of cognitive factors has been debated, for example, some investigators suggest that the language difficulties reflect a more general deficit in symbolic representation; speed of responding also may contribute to problems in information processing. It is also the case, of course, that some individuals will simply be at the lower end of the normal range in language abilities. Other approaches have focused more specifically on difficulties in auditory information processing particularly relative to the need for rapid processing of the kind needed for speech processing and language segmentation (i.e., hearing the individual words within the stream of speech).

■ EPIDEMIOLOGY AND DEMOGRAPHICS

Perhaps 10% to 15% of children younger than 3 years of age will be delayed in language development (Schoen & Paul, 2018). Most of these (50%–80%) will eventually acquire language skills within the normal range, but some show persistent language difficulties into adulthood. As a general rule, language problems that persist after age 4 clearly warrant clinical evaluation (Tomblin et al., 1997).

Given the differences in definition and method, it is not surprising that estimates of the prevalence of specific language disorders vary widely. Expressive problems are more common than receptive ones. Boys are several (3–5) times more likely than girls to have language disorders. Data on the epidemiology of the new SCD category are quite limited, but given the likely overlap with the older PDD-NOS concept in *DSM-IV*, a rate of perhaps 1% is likely. The prevalence of speech sound disorder is greatest in toddlers and decreases to 1% to 2% as children enter school and is uncommon by the end of high school (Schoen & Paul, 2018). There is a male predominance and also familial aggregation. Stuttering also occurs more commonly in males with a general population rate of around 1%. Many younger children who stutter go on, as adults, to have fluent speech. Again, familial aggregation is noted and many

TABLE 8.2

Developmental and Mental Health Disorders Frequently Associated With Problems in Language and Communication

Other developmental disorder
Intellectual disability
Autism spectrum disorders
Other childhood-onset mental disorders
Selective mutism
Learning disorders and attention-deficit disorder
Childhood-onset psychosis
Other conditions
Deafness/hearing impairment
Child maltreatment/neglect
Fetal alcohol syndrome/drug exposure

who stutter as adults have problems with anxiety. Various methods (aggregation, pedigree, twin, adoption, and linkage studies) have provided clear evidence of genetic influences on language disorder. Complementary work also points to environmental input as a key factor that likely contributes to familial aggregation. Speech–language–communication problems often co-occur in association with a number of disorders (see Table 8.2).

Environmental and cultural factors are also important. Children reared in bilingual households will learn both languages without difficulty at a young age as long as parents are consistent (e.g., one parent speaks one language and the other parent does the other, or the native language is spoken only at home). But these children may be somewhat delayed in becoming fluent in them. Assessment by an experienced speech–language pathologist using standard measures of language communication or intelligence should take such issues into account (Paul & Lyons, 2018).

■ ETIOLOGY AND PATHOGENESIS

Neuroimaging and other neuroscience approaches have focused on differences in brain processing of language (Badcock et al., 2012). Later in life, acquired disorders, for example, aphasia after damage to Broca's area following a stroke, have clarified some aspects of localization of language process in the brain. The association of language problems with neurologic *soft signs* is further suggestive of brain involvement. Functional and structural differences have been documented in children with language disorders in those regions known to be involved in language progressing. For typically developing persons, the brain is asymmetric, with language structures tending to be larger in the left hemisphere; children with language problems typically have more symmetric hemispheres. Adults with language difficulties are more likely to have an extra sulcus in Broca's area in either brain hemisphere, although it must be emphasized that no one pattern of brain architecture has been consistently found. Onset of seizures in childhood may be associated with some language loss. Other acquired language problems can arise because of head injury or similar insults to the developing brain. Language delays can arise as a result of deafness or fluctuating hearing levels, for example, with recurrent ear infections. Exposure in utero to certain drugs or toxins may also be associated with language problems in the child. Stuttering clearly has a strong biologic component with involvement of aspects of both the central and peripheral nervous

---

BOX 8.4 | **Stuttering**

Johny, a 6-year-old boy, had started to stutter around 3 years of age. Both speech and motor milestones had been slightly delayed. As his language developed, he began to have difficulties with fluency—pausing at certain words. This problem was initially only occasional, but, over time, it became frequent and he began to repeat some sounds and was getting stuck on the initial sound in the word *h h h h help me out*. There was a strong family history of stuttering. Eventually, intervention was obtained and focused on helping Johny have better control over the rate of his speech.

Comment: It is not uncommon to observe a strong family history of stuttering. Prognostic factors, in addition to family history, include persistence of the difficulty over time, its association with other language problems, and levels of anxiety.

Reprinted with permission from Volkmar, F. R., & Martin, A. (Eds.). (2011). Disorders in communication. In F. R. Volkmar (Ed.), *Essentials of Lewis's child and adolescent psychiatry* (1st ed., p. 102). Lippincott Williams & Wilkins/Wolters Kluwer.

system, with anxiety playing a prominent role as well (see Box 8.4 for a case examples of stuttering). There is also a genetic component with increased risk in first-degree relatives.

The observation of a strong familial link in language–communication problems has led to the search for genes involved in these conditions. Several candidate genes have now been identified (Bishop et al., 1995, 2006; Reader et al., 2014; Tallal et al., 1989).

■ COURSE

Language is often delayed in children who go on to exhibit speech–language difficulties, but it is the case that some children are simply late talkers (Conti-Ramsden et al., 2012). Words may not appear until well into the second year of life, and the rate of new word acquisition is slower than usual. Language may be more like that of a younger child. A typical 2-year-old has a vocabulary of about 200 words, whereas a child with speech–language impairment may only have 20. Although vocabulary gradually increases, it frequently lags behind that of peers in school, and reading difficulties may be observed. Usually social language skills (pragmatics) are relatively preserved—social pragmatic disorder is the major exception.

Speech sound disorder (phonologic disorder) is the most common speech–communication problem—that is, difficulties with speech articulation and impaired production of developmentally expected speech sounds are present (Conti-Ramsden et al., 2012). Such a problem should not be due to cognitive disability, hearing problem, or problems with the oral-motor structures. Hearing impairments obviously can lead to language delay, and fluctuating hearing loss, for example, with recurrent ear infections, may contribute to language delay. However, in phonologic disorder, speech is marked by distortions of sounds (e.g., the *s* sound is produced but with a lisp) or omissions of sounds (e.g., *play* is pronounced *pay*) and incorrect sound substitutions (e.g., *cat* is pronounced *dat*). Young children learning language often misarticulate, but in phonologic disorder, these persist. In addition, the child may try to avoid producing some sounds or may rearrange and misorder the sounds in words or try to simplify words. More severe disorders are recognized earlier than mild ones; it is common for parents to be concerned when the child is about 4 years of age, but younger children are seen as well. Milder cases may not be picked up until the child attends school. Phonologic disorders co-occur with many conditions or may exist in isolation. About half of children with phonologic disorders will have delays in expressive language, and a smaller number will exhibit delayed language comprehension as well. Most children with phonologic disorders will *outgrow* their speech difficulties, although some continue to require services.

By school age, the child with a mild-to-moderately severe language disorder may have problems and difficulties of language organization and efficiency with problems in word retrieval, in narrative and conversation, and written language. The range of communicative functions may also be limited. The language difficulties may contribute to an impression that the child is rude or not polite, given the child's difficulty in making use of nuanced social language. Academic difficulties often center on reading and writing, although many children cope and most go on to high school or beyond and lead independent, productive lives. That being said, severe speech disorders have a much less favorable prognosis.

In stuttering, recovery, to some degree, usually occurs by adolescence so that although perhaps 1 in 30 children stutter, the rate in adolescence is 1%. Girls are more likely to recover without treatment than boys. Over time, boys are more likely to persist in stuttering. When children recover from stuttering, they typically do so in between 6 months and 3 years; in most cases, recovery occurs in 1–2 years. Boys are more likely to have stuttering associated with other communication problems, for example, problems in articulation and phonology (Conti-Ramsden et al., 2012).

Given the recency of the diagnosis, relatively little is known about SCD. To the extent that this condition shades off into what, in the past, was termed *atypical autism* or PDD-NOS, the severity of social pragmatic skills and their response to intervention are likely to be major determinants to outcome.

It should be noted that although communication disorders can exist in isolation, they are frequently associated with other developmental disorders and mental health problems. High rates of activity and attentional problems are observed. The nature of the role of cognitive factors has been debated, for example, some investigators suggest that the language difficulties reflect a more general deficit in symbolic representation; speed of responding also may contribute to problems in information processing. Leonard (1997) has argued that the difficulties may reflect abilities at the lower end of the normal range. Most investigators, however, would question this view, given the frequent association of language impairment with problems in attention and activity and with *soft* neurologic signs. Another approach to understanding etiology has focused on difficulties in auditory information processing, particularly rapid processing of the kind needed for speech processing.

■ DIFFERENTIAL DIAGNOSIS AND ASSESSMENT

As noted, language difficulties can be observed in relative isolation or in the context of other developmental problems (Schoen & Paul, 2018). For example, delays and limitations in language may be an initial sign of intellectual disability (mental retardation). In general, children with intellectual disability seem to progress through normal sequences of language acquisition, although at a slower pace. Many children with intellectual disability show language skills similar to their cognitive abilities; a fairly large group do exhibit problems in language, particularly in language production or in both reception and expression of language. Phonologic errors are more common in this group, but pragmatic (social language) skills are usually consistent with overall developmental level (in contrast to children with autism). Two of the most well-recognized syndromes of intellectual deficiency, Down syndrome and Fragile X syndrome, are associated with language problems. In other conditions, like Williams syndrome, language skills are relatively preserved—as compared to developmental level. Autism and related conditions are frequently associated with significant communication deficits (see Chapter 7). Indeed, the exclusionary rule of autism/PDD for a diagnosis of language disorder reflects the fact that communication difficulties are a core aspect of the definition of autism (see Chapter 47 for a discussion of language–communication problems in autism and related conditions). Essentially, all children with autism have some form of communication problem. In the case of autism and related conditions, the motivation to communicate is affected; although sign and other alternative forms of communication can be used, the lack of motivation presents a major problem for intervention. Diagnostic controversies surround precise delineation of syndrome groups, and borders between language disorder, learning difficulties, and ASD can become blurred.

Given their lack of access to linguistic information, children with hearing impairments are understandably at risk for language disorders. A wide variation is observed in the oral ability of children with hearing impairments. Clearly, with appropriate supports, for example, amplification through hearing aids, it may be possible to substantially improve the auditory signal. Cochlear implants and other aids can also be used to help individuals who would otherwise be deaf. Indeed, the earlier use of cochlear implants facilitates language development in children born with severe hearing loses (Tomblin et al., 1999).

For the child with a hearing impairment, language development follows the usual sequence, although typically it is greatly delayed. This delay is observed in all areas, including articulation, spoken, and written language. In contrast to the child with ASD, the child with hearing impairment usually will not have major problems in social communication. Given the language difficulties, reading and writing are often adversely affected, and the typical reading level of adolescents with uncorrected hearing impairments is usually at the third- or fourth-grade level; use of cochlear implants results in higher levels of achievement (Giddan & Milling, 1999; Paul & Quigley, 1994).

Many different tests of speech–language–communication abilities are available for individuals of different ages (see Paul & Lyons, 2018, for a review). It is important to understand the aims and intended uses of the specific instrument, for example, the results of widely used tests of vocabulary (either receptive or expressive) may not convey the severity of actual communication levels. Various kinds of assessment measures are used. These include screening measures, parent report–based tests, standardized tests of general language functioning, and tests for specific areas of combination like expressive or receptive vocabulary as well as assessments of specific areas of communication; newer tests assess even more complex aspects of language, for example, the child's social language use or understanding of higher order language features, such as figurative or ambiguous language (Paul & Lyons, 2018). Typically, the tests are administered by a speech–language pathologist or psychologist. Similarly, nonverbal intelligence can be estimated from traditional tests of intelligence or tests specifically designed to assess nonverbal abilities (Schoen & Paul, 2018; see Table 8.3).

The clinician should be aware of other conditions frequently associated with speech–language problems. As noted previously, this includes hearing loss, mental retardation, autism or a related condition, and other psychiatric problems like ADHD. Some physical difficulties can contribute to communication problems (e.g., cleft palate, apraxia, cerebral palsy). And, as noted earlier, maternal substance abuse can be a risk factor as is child maltreatment. Audiometric testing by a certified audiologist should be used to verify that hearing is intact. Chronic ear infections can be associated with speech–language problems, but it is important not to attribute this as the sole cause of difficulty because it appears that by itself recurrent otitis media does not significantly increase the risk of language disorder in otherwise typically developing children (Paul & Lyons, 2018).

The speech pathologist will conduct an assessment of factors that can impact the speech mechanism and also will typically assess the morphology, symmetry, and alignment of the facial features as well as structures involved in speech. Phonologic disorders can be diagnosed through formal testing in which the speech pathologist will assess the child's ability to produce target words by naming objects or pictures. Phonologic problems frequently coexist with other language disorders. For a diagnosis of language disorder individually administered, standardized tests should be used. In stuttering, phonologic, receptive, and expressive language skills are age appropriate. If stuttering coexists with other speech and language problems, it may be appropriate to see if the dysfluency persists after other problems are resolved. Because preschool children commonly have dysfluency, it is often sensible to follow the child before recommending speech therapy; if, however, the child appears to show signs of struggle or self-consciousness, then referral is indicated.

TABLE 8.3

Selected Frequently Used Speech–Language–Communication Assessment Instruments

Name	Comment
Peabody Picture Vocabulary Test, 4th ed. (PPVT-4; Dunn & Dunn, 2007)	Measures receptive vocabulary (what the child understands): The score may underestimate the child's actual language ability. Age range is 2½–90 years.
Expressive One-Word Picture Vocabulary Test, 4th ed. (EOW-PVT; Martin & Brownell, 2011)	Measures naming ability (what the child can label): This score may overestimate the child's actual language ability. Age range is 2–80+ years.
Reynell Developmental Language Scales, US ed. (Reynell & Gruber, 1990)	Provides measures of actual language use. Scores are often lower than when single-word vocabulary is assessed. It provides scores for verbal comprehension and expressive language. Materials are attractive to children. Age range is from 3 years to 7 years, 6 months.
Preschool Language Scale-4 (PLS-4; Zimmerman et al., 2002)	Assesses receptive and expressive language. It is frequently used in schools and is a direct assessment. It is also a good instrument for younger children. Age range is 2 weeks to <7 years.
Comprehensive Assessment of Spoken Language (CASL; Carrow-Woolfolk, 1999)	Only a verbal or nonverbal (pointing) response is required (no reading or writing ability expected). It includes tests of various language abilities, such as pragmatic ability (social language use) and figurative language. Age range is 3–21 years.
Clinical Evaluation of Language Fundamentals, 5th ed. (CELF-5; Wiig et al., 2013)	Assesses various language skills related to school requirements. It is useful for profiles of ability in children. Age range is 3–21 years.
Test of Language Competence (TLC; Wiig & Secord, 1989)	Focuses on more complex aspects of language (e.g., ambiguity, figurative language, abstract language). Age range is 5–18 years.
Goldman-Fristoe Test of Articulation-2 (Goldman & Fristoe, 2000)	Test of articulation. Age range is 2–21 years.

Note: Many other tests are available.
Republished with permission of John Wiley & Sons, from Volkmar, F. R., & Wiesner, L. A. (2017). *Essential clinical guide to understanding and treating autism* (1st ed.). John Wiley & Sons, Inc.; permission conveyed through Copyright Clearance Center, Inc.

TREATMENT

Assessment and interventions provided by speech–language therapists are frequently needed (Schoen & Paul, 2018). Several excellent recent summaries of treatment approaches are provided in the Suggested Reading list. Therapeutic work will vary depending on the nature of the presenting problem, for example, work on articulation for some children; for others, pragmatic language may be targeted through social skills training. Treatment should follow a careful assessment with the goal of clarifying the presence of any additional conditions, for example, hearing impairment, intellectual disability, autism, or anxiety disorder. Apart from selective mutism (which is now treated as an anxiety disorder; see Chapter 12), the treatment of speech–communication disorders typically involves individual or small group therapy provided by a certified speech or language pathologist. Given the frequency of comorbid conditions and difficulties, it is not uncommon for educational tutoring, social skills training, and/or psychiatric intervention to be used as well. Intervention methods include both behavioral and educational approaches. Some clinicians may be more likely to use a strictly behavioral approach, whereas others will use a more child-centered model with many opportunities for incidental learning. Most of the time, a mix of these two is used. Effectiveness has been demonstrated in several small studies, but more work is needed on treatment efficacy, particularly relative to the choice of treatment methods for the individual child. For many children with milder difficulties, for example, with immature articulation, significant improvement can occur with the passage of time. For persons who have chronic stuttering, severity fluctuates, with stuttering becoming more severe when the person is pressed to communicate, is stressed, or is anxious (Mulcahy et al., 2008).

Although general anxiety reduction techniques are not particularly effective, reducing stress while speaking may be helpful. Speech therapy can be helpful as a single treatment modality. Psychotherapy is not effective as such, although it may help with secondary effects related to the impact of a communication problem.

Manual sing language can be used, particularly in cases where a parent is deaf. This method provides an ability to communicate visually rather than with spoken language. Within the community of the hard of hearing, there is considerable debate regarding the role of manual sign language versus oral language instruction. In general, deaf children without cochlear implants who are taught sign will develop higher level language skills than those who were taught speech. Both greater speech and sign language abilities are associated with a positive outcome. Cochlear implant use has had a major impact (Colletti et al., 2011; Peng et al., 2004; Roeser, 1988).

Various complementary and alternative approaches to treatment are available and sometimes make extravagant claims of dramatic improvement; data for such interventions are generally sparse or, in some cases, convincingly negative. Clinicians should help parents make informed treatment decisions and encourage healthy skepticism.

■ SUMMARY

Because of the central nature of speech–language–communication in organizing experience and learning from the world, disorders of communication can have a significant impact on the child's development and increase risk for other disorders.

The clinician should be alert to the presence of speech–language difficulties in young children. Many are developmental in nature and resolve without intervention. However, language is typically delayed in children who go on to exhibit speech–language difficulties. Words may not appear until well into the second year of life, and the rate of new word acquisition is slower than usual. A typical 2-year-old has a vocabulary of about 200 words, whereas the child with speech–language impairment may only have 20. Although vocabulary gradually increases, it frequently lags behind that of peers in school and reading difficulties may be observed. Usually, social language skills (pragmatics) are relatively preserved.

Phonologic disorders are the most common speech–communication problems and involve difficulties with speech articulation and impaired production of developmentally expected speech sounds (Schoen & Paul, 2018). These problems are also frequent in typically developing younger children just learning speech, but in phonologic disorders, they are more frequent and persist longer than usual. The child may try to avoid producing some sounds or may rearrange and misorder the sounds in words or try to simplify words. More severe disorders are recognized earlier than mild ones; it is common for parents to be concerned when the child is about 4 years of age, but younger children are seen, although milder cases may not be picked up until school attendance.

By school age, the child with a mild-to-moderately severe language disorder may have subtle difficulties of language organization and efficiency with problems in word retrieval as well as in conversation and narrative, with a more limited range of communicative functions. Although academic problems are frequent and can persist, most children go on to high school or beyond and lead independent, productive lives. That being said, severe speech disorders have a much less favorable prognosis.

In stuttering, recovery usually occurs by adolescence. But a gender difference is observed, with girls more likely to recover without treatment than boys. Effective treatments for speech–language–communication disorders are available, and often additional attention is needed for associated emotional or behavioral problems. Research on specific genetic and neural mechanisms of these disorders is likely to yield important new insights in the years ahead (Hagoort, 2019).

References

*Indicates Particularly Recommended

American Psychiatric Association. (2000). *Diagnostic and statistical manual (DSM-IV)* (4th ed.). APA Press.

American Psychiatric Association. (2013). *Diagnostic and statistical manual (DSM-5)* (5th ed.). APA Press.

American Speech Language-Hearing Association. (1993). Definitions of communication disorders and variations. Ad Hoc Committee on Service Delivery in the Schools. *ASHA Supplement, 35*(3, Suppl 10), 40–41. https://www.asha.org/policy/RP1993-00208/

Badcock, N. A., Bishop, D. V., Hardiman, M. J., Barry, J. G., & Watkins, K. E. (2012). Co-localization of abnormal brain structure and function in specific language impairment. *Brain Language, 120*, 310–320. https://doi.org/10.1016/j.bandl.2011.10.006

Bishop, D. V., Adams, C., & Norbury, C. F. (2006). Distinct genetic influences on grammar and phonological short-term memory: Evidence from 6-year-old twins. *Genes, Brain and Behavior, 5*, 158–169. https://doi.org/10.1111/j.1601-183X.2005.00148.x

*Bishop, D. V., North, T., & Donlan, C. (1995). Genetic basis of specific language impairment: Evidence from a twin study. *Developmental Medicine and Child Neurology, 37*, 56–71. https://doi.org/10.1111/j.1469-8749.1995.tb11932.x

Carrow-Woolfolk, E. (1999). *Comprehensive assessment of spoken language (CASL)*. American Guidance Service.

Colletti, L., Mandalà, M., Zoccante, L., Shannon, R. V., & Colletti, V. (2011). Infants versus older children fitted with cochlear implants: Performance over 10 years. *International Journal of Pediatric Otorhinolaryngology, 75*, 504–509. https://doi.org/10.1016/j.ijporl.2011.01.005

Conti-Ramsden, G., St Clair, M. C., Pickles, A., & Durkin, K. (2012). Developmental trajectories of verbal and non-verbal skills in individuals with a history of SLI: From childhood to adolescence. *Journal of Speech, Language, and Hearing Research, 55*, 1716–1735. https://doi.org/10.1044/1092-4388(2012/10-0182)

Dunn, L. M., & Dunn, D. M. (2007). *The Peabody picture vocabulary test* (3rd ed.). American Guidance Service.

Giddan, J. J., & Milling, L. (1999). Comorbidity of psychiatric and communication disorders in children. *Child and Adolescent Psychiatry Clinics of North America, 8*, 19–36. https://doi.org/10.1016/S1056-4993(18)30194-9

Goldman, S., & Fristoe, M. (2000). *Goldman-Fristoe test of articulation 2*. American Guidance Service.

*Hagoort, P. (Ed.). (2019). *Human language: From gene to brain and to behavior*. MIT Press.

Jackson, S. L., & Volkmar, F. R. (2019). Diagnosis and definition of autism and other pervasive developmental disorders. In F. R. Volkmar (Ed.), *Autism and the pervasive developmental disorders* (pp. 1–24). Cambridge University Press.

Leonard, L. (1997). *Children with specific language impairment*. MIT Press.

Martin, N. A., & Brownell, R. (2011). *Expressive one-word picture vocabulary test (EOWPVT-4)*. Western Psychological Services.

Mulcahy, K., Hennessey, N., Beilby, J., & Byrnes, M. (2008). Social anxiety and the severity and typography of stuttering in adolescents. *Journal of Fluency Disorders, 33*, 306–319. https://doi.org/10.1016/j.jfludis.2008.12.002

*Paul, R., & Lyons, M. (2018). Assessing communication. In A. Martin & F. R. Volkmar (Eds.), *Lewis's child and adolescent psychiatry: A comprehensive textbook* (5th ed., pp. 451–460). Wolters Kluwer.

Paul, P., & Quigley, S. (1994). *Language and deafness*. Singular Publishing Group.

Peng, S. C., Spencer, L. J., & Tomblin, J. B. (2004). Speech intelligibility of pediatric cochlear implant recipients with 7 years of device experience. *Journal of Speech, Language, and Hearing Research, 47*, 1227–1236. https://doi.org/10.1044/1092-4388(2004/092)

Rapin, I. (1996). Practitioner review: Developmental language disorders: A clinical update. *Journal of Child Psychology & Psychiatry & Allied Disciplines, 37*(6), 643–655. https://doi.org/10.1111/j.1469-7610.1996.tb01456.x

Reader, R., Covill, L., Nudel, R., & Newbury, D. (2014). Genome-wide studies of specific language impairment. *Current Behavioral Neuroscience Reports, 1*(4), 242–250. https://doi.org/10.1007/s40473-014-0024-z

Reynell, J., & Gruber, C. (1990). *Reynell developmental language scales* (U.S. ed.). Western Psychological Services.

Roeser, R. (1988). Cochlear implants and tactile aids for the profoundly deaf student. In R. J. Roeser & M. P. Downs (Eds.), *Auditory disorders in school children* (pp. 260–280). Thieme Medical Publishers.

*Schoen, E., & Paul, R. (2018). Disorders of communication. In A. Martin, M. Block, & F. R. Volkmar (Eds.), *Lewis's child and adolescent psychiatry* (5th ed., pp. 336–341). Wolters Kluwer.

Tallal, P., Ross, R., & Curtiss, S. (1989). Familial aggregation in specific language impairment. *Journal of Speech, Language, and Hearing Disorders, 54*, 167–173. https://doi.org/10.1044/jshd.5402.167

Tomblin, J. B., Records, N. L., Buckwalter, P., Zhang, X., Smith, E., & O'Brien, M. (1997). Prevalence of specific language impairments in kindergarten children. *Journal of Speech, Language, and Hearing Research, 40*, 1245–1260. https://doi.org/10.1044/jslhr.4006.1245

Tomblin, J. B., Spencer, L., Flock, S., Tyler, R., & Gantz, B. (1999). A comparison of language achievement in children with cochlear implants and children using hearing aids. *Journal of Speech, Language, and Hearing Research, 42*, 497–509. https://doi.org/10.1044/jslhr.4202.497

Wiig, E. H., & Secord, W. (1989). *Test of language competence*. Psychological Corporation.

Wiig, E. L., Semel, E., & Secord, W. (2013). *Clinical evaluation of language fundamentals (CELF-5)* (5th ed.). Pearson.

Zimmerman, I. L., Steiner, V. G., & Pond, R. E. (2002). *Preschool language scale-4*. Psychological Corporation.

Suggested Readings

*Baker, E., & McLeod, S. (2011). Evidence-based practice for children with speech sound disorders: Part 1. Narrative review. *Language, Speech, Hearing Services in Schools, 42*(2), 102–139. https://doi.org/10.1044/0161-1461(2010/09-0075)

Beitchman, J. H., & Brownlie, E. B. (2014). Language disorders in children and adolescents. In D. Wedding (Ed.), *Advances in psychotherapy: Evidence-based practice*. Hogrefe Publishing Corp.

*Bishop, D. V. (1997). *Uncommon understanding: Development and disorders of language comprehension in children*. Psychology Press.

Bishop, D. V. (2009). Genes, cognition, and communication: Insights from neurodevelopmental disorders. *Annals of the New York Academy of Sciences, 1156*, 1–18. https://doi.org/10.1111/j.1749-6632.2009.04419.x

Bishop, D. V., & Snowling, M. J. (2004). Developmental dyslexia and specific language impairment: Same or different? *Psychological Bulletin, 130*(6), 858–886. https://doi.org/10.1037/0033-2909.130.6.858

Bowen, C. (2014). *Children's speech sound disorders* (2nd ed.). Wiley-Blackwell.

*Brownlie, E., Bao, L., & Beitchman, J. (2016). Childhood language disorder and social anxiety in early adulthood. *Journal of Abnormal Child Psychology, 44*, 1061–1070. https://doi.org/10.1007/s10802-015-0097-5

Clark, M. M., & Plante, E. (1998). Morphology of the inferior frontal gyrus in developmentally language-disordered adults. *Brain and Language, 61*, 288–303. https://doi.org/10.1006/brln.1997.1864

Cohen, N. J., Vallance, D. D., Barwick, M., Im, N., Menna, R., Horodezky, N. B., & Isaacson, L. (2000). The interface between ADHD and language impairment: An examination of language, achievement, and cognitive processing. *Journal of Child Psychology & Psychiatry, 41*, 353–362. https://doi.org/10.1111/1469-7610.00619

Colletti, L., Mandalà, M., & Colletti, V. (2012). Cochlear implants in children younger than 6 months. *Otolaryngology–Head and Neck Surgery, 147*, 139–146. https://doi.org/10.1177/0194599812441572

Dale, P. S., Price, T. S., Bishop, D. V., & Plomin, R. (2003). Outcomes of early language delay: I. Predicting persistent and transient language difficulties at 3 and 4 years. *Journal of Speech, Language, and Hearing Research, 46*(3), 544–560. https://doi.org/10.1044/1092-4388(2003/044)

Dunn, C., & Davis, B. (1983). Phonological process occurrence in phonologically disordered children. *Applied Psycholinguistics, 4*, 187–207. https://doi.org/10.1017/S0142716400004574

Evans, J. L., Viele, K., Kass, R. E., & Tang, F. (2002). Grammatical morphology and perception of synthetic and natural speech in children with specific language impairments. *Journal of Speech, Language, and Hearing Research, 45*, 494–504. https://doi.org/10.1044/1092-4388(2002/039)

Falcaro, M., Pickles, A., Newbury, D. F., Addis, L., Banfield, E., Fisher, S. E., Monaco, A. P., Simkin, Z., Conti-Ramsden, G., & SLI Consortium. (2008). Genetic and phenotypic effects of phonological short-term memory and grammatical morphology in specific language impairment. *Genes Brain Behavior, 7*(4), 393–402. https://doi.org/10.1111/j.1601-183X.2007.00364.x

*Fisher, S. E., & Scharff, C. (2009). FOXP2 as a molecular window into speech and language. *Trends in Genetics, 25*(4), 166–177. https://doi.org/10.1016/j.tig.2009.03.002

Fujiki, M., Brinton, B., & Clarke, D. (2002). Emotion regulation in children with specific language impairment. *Language, Speech, and Hearing Services in Schools, 33,* 102–111. https://doi .org/10.1044/0161-1461(2002/008)

Gillon, G. T. (2000). The efficacy of phonological awareness intervention for children with spoken language impairment. *Language, Speech, and Hearing Service in School, 31,* 126–141. https://doi .org/10.1044/0161-1461.3102.126

Guitar, B. (2013). *Stuttering: An integrated approach to its nature and treatment.* Lippincott Williams & Wilkins.

*Guitar, B., & McCauley, R. (2010). *Treatment of stuttering: Established and emerging interventions.* Lippincott Williams & Wilkins.

Kroll, R. M., De Nil, L. F., Kapur, S., & Houle, S. (1997). A positron emission tomography investigation of post-treatment brain activation in stutterers. In W. Hulstijn & H. M. F. Peters (Eds.), *Speech motor production and fluency disorders. Proceedings of the Third International Conference on Speech Motor Production and Fluency Disorders* (pp. 307–320). Elsevier.

*Law, J., Garrett, Z., & Nye, C. (2003). Speech and language therapy interventions for children with primary speech and language delay or disorder. *Cochrane Database System Review,* (3), CD004110. https://doi.org/10.1002/14651858.CD004110

Law. J., Rush, R., Schoon, I., & Parsons, S. (2009). Modeling developmental language difficulties from school entry into adulthood: Literacy, mental health, and employment outcomes. *Journal of Speech, Language, and Hearing Research, 52,* 1401–1416. https://doi.org/10.1044/1092-4388(2009/08-0142)

Liegeois, R., Mayes, A., & Morgan, A. (2014). Neural correlates of developmental speech and language disorders: Evidence from neuroimaging. *Current Developmental Disorders Reports, 1,* 215–227. https://doi.org/10.1007/s40474-014-0019-1

*Mayes, A. K., Reilly, S., & Morgan, A. T. (2015). Neural correlates of childhood language disorder: A systematic review. *Developmental Medicine & Child Neurology, 57,* 706–717. https://doi.org/10.1111/ dmcn.12714

*McCulley, E. R. J., Fey, M. E., & Gillarm, R. (Eds.). (2017). *Treatment of language disorders in children (CLI)* (2nd ed.). Paul Brooks Publishing.

McGregor, K. K., Oleson, J., Bahnsen, A., & Duff, D. (2013). Children with developmental language impairment have vocabulary deficits characterized by limited breadth and depth. *International Journal of Language & Communication Disorders, 48*(3), 307–319. https://doi.org/10.1111/1460-6984.12008

National Institute on Deafness and Other Communication Disorders. (2010). *Statistics on voice, speech, and language.* Retrieved December 7, 2015, from http://www.nidcd.nih.gov/health/statistics/pages/vsl .aspx

Norbury, C. F. (2014). Practitioner review: Social (pragmatic) communication disorder conceptualization, evidence and clinical implications. *Journal of Child Psychology and Psychiatry, 55*(3), 204–216. https:// doi.org/10.1111/jcpp.12154

*Paul, R., & Norbury, C. (2012). *Language disorders from infancy through adolescence.* Elsevier.

Prior, M., Bavin, E., Cini, E., Eadie, P., & Reilly, S. (2011). Relationships between language impairment, temperament, behavioral adjustment and maternal factors in a community sample of preschool children. *International Journal of Language & Communication Disorders, 46*(4), 489–494. https://doi .org/10.1111/j.1460-6984.2011.00003.x

*Swineford, L. B., Thurm, A., Baird, G., Wetherby, A. M., & Swedo, S. (2014). Social (pragmatic) communication disorder: A research review of this new *DSM-5* diagnostic category. *Journal of Neurodevelopment Disorder, 6*(1), 41. https://doi.org/10.1186/1866-1955-6-41

Toppelberg, C. O., & Shapiro, T. (2000). Language disorders: A 10-year research update review. *Journal of the American Academy of Child and Psychiatry, 39*(2), 143–152. https://doi.org/ 10.1097/00004583-200002000-00011

Verdon, S., McLeod, S., & Wong, S. (2015). Re-conceptualizing practice with multilingual children with speech sound disorders: People, practicalities and policy. *International Journal of Language and Communication Disorders, 50*(1), 48–62. https://doi.org/10.1111/1460-6984.12112

Yairi, E., & Ambrose, N. (2013). Epidemiology of stuttering: 21st century advances. *Journal of Fluency Disorders, 38*(2), 66–87. https://doi.org/10.1016/j.jfludis.2012.11.002

Yairi, E., Ambrose, N., & Cox, N. (1996). Genetics of stuttering: A critical review. *Journal of Speech and Hearing Research, 40,* 49–58. https://doi.org/10.1044/jshr.3904.771

Young, A. R., Beitchman, J. H., Johnson, C., Douglas, L., Atkinson, L., Escobar, M., & Wilson, B. (2002). Young adult academic outcomes in a longitudinal sample of early identified language impaired and control children. *Journal of Child Psychology and Psychiatry, 43,* 635–645. https://doi .org/10.1111/1469-7610.00052

Zebrowski, P. M. (2003). Developmental stuttering. *Pediatric Annals, 32*(7), 453–458. https://doi .org/10.3928/0090-4481-20030701-07

CHAPTER 9 ■ LEARNING DISABILITIES AND DEVELOPMENTAL COORDINATION DISORDER

LEARNING DISABILITIES

BACKGROUND

Interest in what now are termed *the learning disabilities* began in the 19th century with the increased emphasis on universal public education and with an awareness of adults with major problems in reading. This coincided with the move from a less educated to a more educated society. Early work on learning problems in the 1920s speculated that left hemisphere damage (to language centers) was involved.

Modern interest really began with Samuel Kirk who proposed the term *learning disabled* in 1963. This concept rapidly gained acceptance and the Association for Children with Learning Disabilities was formed. Awareness of children with these problems also led to an understanding that problems sometimes existed in other areas, for example, in mathematic reasoning or in writing rather than only in reading. The passage of Public Law 94-142 (the *Education for All Handicapped Children Act*) in 1975 specifically recognized learning difficulties as a disability that should be the focus of school-based intervention. Prior to that time, services in public schools were generally limited.

In terms of terminology, it is important to note that in the United Kingdom, the term *learning disability* refers to children who in the United States would be said to have *intellectual disability* or what used to be termed *mental retardation*; in the United Kingdom, the term *learning difference* is more typically used to refer to what in the United States is termed *learning disability*. Other terms like *dyslexia* (for reading problems), *dyscalculia* (for math problems), and *dysgraphia* (for writing problems) also have been used.

Children can learn in different ways, and a learning difference does not necessarily mean a child has a learning disorder. These conditions appear to be strongly brain based and have clear genetic as well as important environmental components. Individuals with learning disorders do face a number of challenges not only in school but subsequently in terms of adult occupational functioning. By their very nature, these problems usually come to attention as children enter schools, and in the United States, a multidisciplinary team often evaluates the child to establish the presence of a learning disability and develop an intervention program. Specific learning disabilities make up about 50% of all special education students (Grigorenko, 2018).

Additional difficulties arise because, in addition to legal definitions (which themselves change over time), somewhat different approaches have been taken by the many different specialties dealing with these problems. Under current law, a child who exhibits a learning disability can qualify for special help and services in school and an individualized educational program is developed once it is clear, following an assessment, that the child qualifies for such services. Changes in the legal definition of learning difficulties can have important implications for service (see Grigorenko, 2018).

■ DIAGNOSIS, DEFINITION, CLINICAL FEATURES

In 1980, *DSM-III* included a concept termed *academic skills disorder*. This concept has evolved in both *DSM* and *ICD* to encompass several different disorders. Both the *DSM-IV-TR* (APA, 2000) and *ICD-10* (WHO, 1994) used an approach based on a *discrepancy* model, that is, where the child's performance on an achievement test is significantly lower than IQ. This approach was criticized for various reasons including for being overly stringent and working less well for children with higher or lower overall intellectual ability.

The *DSM-5* approach (APA, 2013) continues to recognize three main categories of learning problems in the areas of reading, writing, or arithmetic in school-aged children. These features include the following: (1) persistence for at least 6 months even after provision of a quality evidence-based intervention; (2) achievement testing that confirms that the individual is performing significantly below age-expected levels (the level of service provided should be considered, that is, some children receiving intensive services may improve but still have learning challenges); (3) typically, these problems are observed as children enter school and academic demands increase; and (4) the problems are not due to other factors like intellectual deficiency, absenteeism or lack of schooling, sensory impairment, and so forth. The changes in *DSM-5* reflect an awareness of the response to intervention (RTI) approach in assessment and treatment of learning difficulties (Bradley et al., 2005; Denton, 2012) as well as the awareness of changes in federal mandates for schools to provide services. It should be noted that other types of learning problems, for example, nonverbal learning disability, may fall outside the *DSM-5* definition but still present challenges for learning.

■ EPIDEMIOLOGY AND DEMOGRAPHICS

Data on rates of learning disorders come from two sources—school reports of students receiving mandated services and more rigorous epidemiologic research. For school-based learning problems (see Figure 9.1), this typically ends up with estimates of 5% to 6% of school-aged children in the United States. Reading problems account for 75% to 80% of cases. It is important to recognize that rates vary markedly from school district to school district and state to state, reflecting continued differences in the approach to assessment and diagnosis of these problems (Grigorenko, 2018). Boys are twice as likely to have been recognized as having learning disability. It does appear that girls are more likely than boys to have mathematic learning problems. Rates in minority groups may be underestimated.

Research data with more rigorous and standardized case assessments show that around 1.2% of school-age children have academic difficulties; this number is reduced when schools provide high-quality teaching. Much of the available research has focused on reading difficulties and less is known about other learning problems. Changes in approach to diagnosis have influenced these estimates. Learning problems are frequently related to issues of attention, and attention deficit disorder is a common comorbid condition.

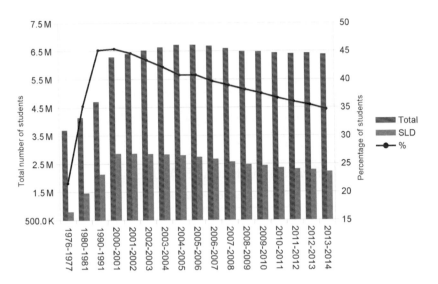

FIGURE 9.1. The absolute numbers (left axis, shown in bars) and percentage of children (right axis) diagnosed with specific learning disabilities (SLD), out of the total number of children in special education in the United States, from 1976 to 2014. Reprinted with permission from Martin, A., Volkmar, F. R., & Bloch, M. (2018). *Lewis's child and adolescent psychiatry: A comprehensive textbook* (5th ed., p. 445). Wolters Kluwer.

ETIOLOGY AND PATHOGENESIS

Genetic and neurobiological factors as well as experience play a role in the pathogenesis of learning difficulties. A large body of work has now underscored the importance of genetic factors in these conditions (Becker et al., 2017; Grigorenko, 2018; Soares et al., 2018;). Environmental factors, including prenatal ones, are important as well (Becker et al., 2017; Mascheretti et al., 2018). It appears that all these risk factors act through one or more brain mechanisms that are important in reading, writing, and mathematics skills. Extreme deprivation and lack of opportunity as well as poverty may also contribute to learning problems. Other difficulties like head trauma and treatment of childhood cancers (e.g., CNS radiation) can be implicated.

Most of the work on etiology has centered around specific reading disabilities. Various methods have been used to study the neurobiologic correlates of reading problems (Becker et al., 2017; Grigorenko, 2018). These have included MRI, EEG, genetic association studies, and so forth. As might be expected, reading skills involve a large network of brain areas predominately in the left hemisphere of the brain once they are fully established (see Figure 9.2). These involve brain regions involved in visual and auditory as well as more basic conceptual processing. The four areas that appear to be of greatest relevance to reading include the fusiform gyrus (Brodmann area (BA) 37), a portion of the middle temporal gyrus (including portions of areas 21 and 37, along with the angular gyrus (BA 39), and the posterior aspect of the superior temporal gyrus (BA 22)). Differences in brain activation have strong developmental correlates and more able readers seem to shift to frontal regions, whereas those with difficulty tend to use the most posterior ones (in the parietal and occipital regions).

There are some developmental changes in brain processing as academic skills become more well established. Over time, there is a progressive disengagement of the right hemispheric areas. In addition, there are some shifts in regional activation preferences, with frontal regions less involved over time.

Since the 19th century, there was an awareness that specific reading difficulties did, at times, strongly run in families. This has become an even more active area of investigation with the

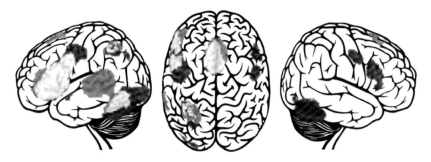

FIGURE 9.2. Surface renderings of maps of the brain circuitry for reading. *Light gray* indicates the overlapping areas of activation, *medium gray* the areas specific to children, and *dark gray* the areas specific to adults. Reprinted with permission from Martin, A., Volkmar, F. R., & Bloch, M. (2018). *Lewis's child and adolescent psychiatry: A comprehensive textbook* (5th ed.). Wolters Kluwer.

availability of more specific genetic approaches and advances in techniques of gene identification. A range of approaches have now been used including twin, sib pair, and family studies, and it now appears that multiple genes are likely involved (Grigorenko, 2018). Sites have been identified on chromosomes 15q, 6p, 2p, 6q, 3cen, 18p, 11p, 1p, and Xq; efforts are now underway to identify specific candidate genes (Riva et al., 2019; Sanchez-Moran et al., 2018). Several genes have now been identified (for more information, see Foster et al., 2015; Grigorneko, 2018).

Theoretical models for understanding specific reading disability have been elaborated within psychology and special education. Clearly, reading involves several different processes including orthography (translating the alphabetic and visual symbols), phonology (translating these symbols into speech), and semantics (translating these in turn into meaning; see Figure 9.3). Various research strategies and methods have been used to explore the various aspects of this model.

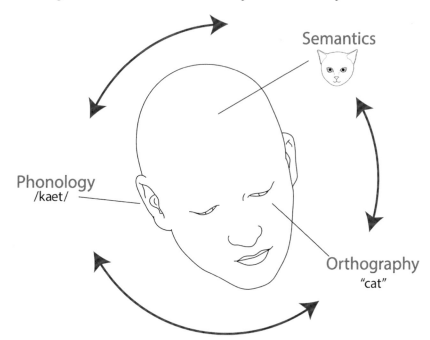

FIGURE 9.3. The componential view of reading. Reprinted with permission from Martin, A., Volkmar, F. R., & Bloch, M. (2018). *Lewis's child and adolescent psychiatry: A comprehensive textbook* (5th ed.). Wolters Kluwer.

COURSE

Given their nature, it is usual for learning problems to present in children as they enter school environments and delays or lags in specific areas are noted—usually in the ability to read. Some factors may delay recognition, for example, children who have higher cognitive abilities may present with problems later than those with lower abilities. Similarly, children whose problems are mild and whose problems are associated with other conditions might have learning difficulties that are recognized only over time.

Given the increased awareness of schools, more frequent testing, and federal mandates for service, children with significant learning challenges typically now receive special help. To some extent, this complicates our understanding of the natural history and course of the disorder. Most of the available data come from work on reading disability. Early intervention can make a difference for reading difficulties, although even with intervention, some vulnerability often persists. A large number of materials, intervention strategies, and accommodations are now available. These include special teaching methods as well as various forms of assistance ranging from very low to very high technology. For example, computers can be used for text to speech, speech to text, spell check, etc. and can provide organizational software to assist in writing as well as visual aids that help children learn to read (see Grigorenko, 2018; Shaywitz, 2020) (Box 9.1).

BOX 9.1 **Case Report Reading Disability**

Alex, a 9-year-old boy, was referred for evaluation because of persistent, and worsening, problems in school. For the past 2 years, he had been noted, by his classroom teacher, to have problems in reading and, to a lesser extent, in organization and attentional skills. He had an overall IQ in the low average range, and achievement testing had revealed somewhat lower than expected reading skills although not at the level that would have, for his school, prompted eligibility for special services.

Interview with his parents revealed a normal pregnancy and labor and delivery. Language and motor milestones had all been achieved within the normal range but slightly on the late side. As a preschool child, he seemed, at least compared to his sister, much less interested in reading and books and much more interested in rough and tumble play and various construction "projects." He particularly enjoyed helping his father around the house in carpentry and similar activities. Both his parents noted that he had some mild motor coordination problems and these were most noticeable when he was trying to play sports like softball. His father had a history of significant reading problems.

On psychological testing, his verbal IQ was in the low average range, with nonverbal skills being somewhat higher. Achievement testing revealed significant difficulties with word identification and pronunciation, and his comprehension of spoken language was poor. The psychologist also noted issues with low self-esteem and with self-organization and "executive" functions.

His school district had recently changed its approach to the diagnosis of reading disability and judged him qualified for special services. Several different interventions were put in place including procedures to help him learn to sound out words more effectively. Despite these interventions, he continued to have difficulty although he made some slow progress. A summer program was provided as was a special reading tutor and the provision of some special education services.

At the conclusion of the academic year, Alex had made important gains in his reading and his self-esteem had also improved. A specific teaching strategy had been employed to help him learn to sound out words and he was, for the first time, interested in reading on his own. He continued to need support for his reading.

DIFFERENTIAL DIAGNOSIS AND ASSESSMENT

Before 2004, the discrepancy between cognitive ability and achievement was the usual approach to diagnosis of specific learning problems. The reauthorization of the Individuals with Disabilities Education Act in 2004 gave schools the potential for alternative forms of identification. These have differed significantly in their theoretical orientation, but the most widely used approach has been the RTI model (Vaughn & Fuchs, 2003). In this approach, the students' performance is assessed relative to that of peers (the model assumes that the progress of all students is being tracked). Differences both in the absolute level of ability as well as rate of growth are assessed. Identified students are then provided individualized interventions in an attempt to maximize the student's potential. A process of reassessment and refinement then occurs over time. Supports can take place in the classroom with supplemental support, if needed, up to more focused individual support. When a child continues to fail to make expected progress with the provision of evidence-based interventions, a diagnosis of learning disorder is made.

Learning difficulties can be associated with other mental health problems including attentional difficulties as well as anxiety and depression. Association with motor coordination problems is also observed.

Given its individualized nature, there has been divergence of opinions about how the RTI is quantified. Usually, this will include norm-referenced testing at the start and end of the school year and use of explicit guidelines for when students should receive more intensive interventions. For students with identified learning disabilities, continued intervention and frequent assessment are important. One of the major difficulties for this approach has been lack of trained school teachers and staff.

TREATMENT

Although psychopharmacologic treatments may be helpful in dealing with associated comorbid conditions, for example, ADHD or depression, these do not address the underlying learning challenges. Educational interventions thus remain the mainstay of treatment. The RTI approach has some advantages in helping to clarify which approaches do and do not work for the child with a learning disorder because interventions can be continuously revised based on students' response.

A range of services can be provided in school. These can include very intensive level, for example, pullout instruction and special education classes, to less intensive support, for example, additional help in the mainstream classroom, additional help with tutoring or homework. Other treatment approaches have been concerned with addressing what are presumed to be underlying problems in information processing, attention, and so forth. Learning differences often present the child with challenges in various areas including peer interaction, and support for learning in these areas, as well as the more specifically academic challenges, can be helpful (Shaywitz, 2020).

Given the mandates for intervention, data on natural history and course of these conditions have been difficult to interpret and, as in other areas, the largest body of research work has centered on reading disability. There is some suggestion that early intervention can make a difference, although often some vulnerability persists, at least to some degree.

DEVELOPMENTAL COORDINATION DISORDER

DIAGNOSIS, DEFINITION, CLINICAL FEATURES

Children with severe, isolated motor delays have been known since antiquity. The term *cerebral palsy* has been used frequently to refer to these conditions typically associated with birth trauma or some other specific process. In the more distant past, terms like maladroitness or problems in praxis were used to refer to the broad range of motor coordination problems.

The problem can be mild or severe. More severe problems are more frequently associated with some specific medical etiology. These conditions can be associated with learning difficulties as well as other problems like attention deficit disorder. Both gross and fine motor movements are impacted and may compromise dexterity and handwriting as well as many activities of daily life.

Various terms have been used to describe children with motor coordination problems; these have included terms like dyspraxia and specific motor developmental disorder. The *DSM-IV-TR* (APA, 2000) defined developmental coordination disorder (DCD) based on the presence of motor deficits greater than expected given age or intellectual level and not due to some other condition such as an autism spectrum disorder. In the *DSM-5* approach (APA, 2013), the condition is defined on the basis of four criteria: (1) motor skills that are below age-expected levels (given reasonable opportunities for learning); (2) the difficulties are significant and interfere with learning and activities of daily life; (3) these problems must begin in the developmental period; and (4) these problems are not better explained by another medical condition. Recognition of the condition is almost always made in the first 5 years or so of life. Tests of motor functioning are well developed for school-aged children although they are lacking for both very young children and adolescents and adults.

The problems may be isolated or associated with other problems, for example, conditions—often language communication or learning disorders. The condition can be associated with attentional problems and one autism spectrum variant with a significant motor component has been described as well.

EPIDEMIOLOGY AND DEMOGRAPHICS

Estimates that 5% to 6% of school-aged children have DCD have been reported (Zwicker et al., 2012). However, one study using a more stringent approach (Lingam et al., 2009) found much lower rates. The condition is several more times common in boys than in girls (Lingam et al., 2009).

ETIOLOGY AND PATHOGENESIS

Motor skill problems can arise for many different reasons. Birth difficulties and low birth weight are risk factors (Edwards et al., 2011). Socioeconomic factors are not major risk factors. Associations with speech–language problems (particularly involving articulation and oral movements) are frequent. Associations with learning disorder are also frequent.

DIFFERENTIAL DIAGNOSIS AND ASSESSMENT

Children may present with gross and/or fine motor difficulties. The history should include discussion of pregnancy and birth problems, any relevant medications, and history of head trauma or associated medical conditions that might contribute to motor problems. Family history should include discussion of heritable motor problems (e.g., muscular dystrophy). The physical examination should note weight, height, and head circumference (micro- and macrocephaly can be associated with DCD). Other aspects of the examination should include the muscular skeletal system, a search for any neurocutaneous or retinal findings suggestive of other disorders, and neurologic assessment. Referral for neurologic evaluation may be warranted. Physical therapists can conduct standardized testing to evaluate the extent and severity of motor impairment.

TREATMENT

Occupational and physical therapy approaches can address fine and gross motor needs of individuals with motor problems. Adaptive physical education can also be used in schools.

COURSE

Children who go on to clearly have DCD may have early problems as infants in sucking and swallowing and later show delayed motor skills. They may exhibit unusual motor features like toe walking or wide-based gait. Parents may also report interference with play, and fine motor problems may become more noteworthy as children enter school. Difficulties persist into adolescence in about half of the cases. Several different factors, and their interaction, can impact outcome. Prognosis is best when motor difficulties are mild and when motor difficulties are an isolated finding, that is, when comorbid conditions are not present. Unfortunately, secondary problems, for example, peer problems and difficulties in sport, can lead to anxiety and mood difficulties.

SUMMARY

Learning difficulties and developmental coordination problems are common sources of school-based intervention services. These conditions frequently coexist, and intervention can help, although both conditions tend to persist to varying degrees. About half of all children identified as having special needs under current federal guidelines exhibit a specific learning disability—usually a reading disability. Greater awareness and increased vigilance on the part of parents and schools have led to earlier identification and potentially more effective earlier intervention. The current approaches to diagnosis no longer emphasize the older discrepancy model that has now been supplanted by changes in federal law as well as in *DSM-5* (APA, 2013). Particularly for reading disorders, progress has been made in identifying both neural pathways and potential genetic links for the condition.

References

*Indicates Particularly Recommended

American Psychiatric Association. (2000). *Diagnostic and statistical manual (DSM-IV TR)*. (4th rev. ed.). APA Press.

American Psychiatric Association. (2013). *Diagnostic and statistical manual (DSM-5)* (5th rev. ed.). APA Press.

Becker, N., Vasconcelos, M., Oliveira, V., Santos, F. C. D., Bizarro, L., Almeida, R. M. M., & Carvalho, M. R. S. (2017). Genetic and environmental risk factors for developmental dyslexia in children: Systematic review of the last decade. *Developmental Neuropsychology, 42*(7/8), 423–445. https://dx.doi.org/10.1080/87565641.2017.1374960

Bradley, R., Danielson, L., & Doolittle, J. (2005). Response to intervention. *Journal of Learning Disabilities, 38*(6), 485–486. https://doi.org/10.1177/00222194050380060201

Denton, C. A. (2012). Response to intervention for reading difficulties in the primary grades: Some answers and lingering questions. *Journal of Learning Disabilities, 45*(3), 232–243. https://doi.org/10.1177/0022219412442155

Edwards, J., Berube, M., Erlandson, K., Haug, S., Johnstone, H., Meagher, M., Sarkodee-Adoo, S., & Zwicker, J. G. (2011). Developmental coordination disorder in school-aged children born very preterm and/or at very low birth weight: A systematic review. *Journal of Developmental & Behavioral Pediatrics, 32*(9), 678–687. https://doi.org/10.1097/DBP.0b013e31822a396a

Foster, A., Titheradge, H., & Morton, M. (2015). Genetics of learning disability. *Pediatrics and Child Health, 25*(10), 450–457. https://doi.org/10.1016/j.paed.2015.06.005

Grigorenko, E. L. (2018). Learning disabilities. In A. Martin, B. Bloch, & F. R. Volkmar (Eds.), *Lewis's child and adolescent psychiatry: A comprehensive textbook* (5th ed., pp. 443–451). Wolter Kluwer.

Lingam, R., Hunt, L., Golding, J., Jongmans, M., & Emond, A. (2009). Prevalence of developmental coordination disorder using the *DSM-IV* at 7 years of age: A UK population-based study. *Pediatrics, 123*(4), e693–e700. https://doi.org/10.1542/peds.2008-1770

Mascheretti, S., Andreola, C., Scaini, S., & Sulpizio, S. (2018). Beyond genes: A systematic review of environmental risk factors in specific reading disorder. *Research in Developmental Disabilities, 82*, 147–152. https://doi.org/10.1016/j.ridd.2018.03.005

Riva, V., Mozzi, A., Forni, D., Trezzi, V., Giorda, R., Riva, S., Villa, M., Sironi, M., Cagliani, R., & Mascheretti, S. (2019). The influence of DCDC2 risk genetic variants on reading: Testing main and haplotypic effects. *Neuropsychologia, 130*, 52–58. https://doi.org/10.1016/j.neuropsychologia.2018.05.021

Sanchez-Moran, M., Hernandez, J. A., Dunabeitia, J. A., Estevez, A., Barcena, L., Gonzalez-Lahera, A., Bajo, M. T., Fuentes, L. J., Aransay, A. M., & Carreiras, M. (2018). Genetic association study of dyslexia and ADHD candidate genes in a Spanish cohort: Implications of comorbid samples. *PLoS One, 13*(10), e0206431. https://doi.org/10.1371/journal.pone.0206431

*Shaywitz, S. (2020). *Overcoming dyslexia* (2nd ed.). Knopf.

*Soares, N., Evans, T., & Patel, D. R. (2018). Specific learning disability in mathematics: A comprehensive review. *Translational Pediatrics, 7*(1), 48–62. https://doi.org/10.21037/tp.2017.08.03

Vaughn, S., & Fuchs, L. S. (2003). Redefining learning disabilities as inadequate response to instruction: The promise and potential problems. *Learning Disabilities Research & Practice, 18*(3), 137–146. https://doi.org/10.1111/1540-5826.00070

World Health Organization. (1994). Diagnostic criteria for research. In *International classification of diseases* (10th ed.). Author.

Zwicker, J. G., Missiuna, C., Harris, S. R., & Boyd, L. A. (2012). Developmental coordination disorder: A review and update. *European Journal of Paediatric Neurology, 16*(6), 573–581. https://doi.org/10.1016/j.ejpn.2012.05.005

Suggested Readings

*Deshler, D. D., Mellard, D. F., Tollefson, J. M., & Byrd, S. E. (2005). Research topics in responsiveness to intervention: Introduction to the special series. *Journal of Learning Disabilities, 38*(6), 483–484. https://doi.org/10.1177/00222194050380060101

Ehlers, S., Nyden, A., Gillberg, C., Sandberg, A. D., Dahlgren, S. O., Hjelmquist, E., & Odén, A. (1997). Asperger syndrome, autism and attention disorders: A comparative study of the cognitive profiles of 120 children. *Journal of Child Psychology, 38*(2), 207–217. https://doi.org/10.1111/j.1469-7610.1997.tb01855.x

Franklin, B. M. (1987). The first crusade for learning disabilities: The movement for the education of backward children. In T. Popkewitz (Ed.), *The foundation of the school subjects* (pp. 190–209). Falmer.

Gabrieli, J. D. E. (2009). Dyslexia: A new synergy between education and cognitive neuroscience. *Science, 325*(5938), 280–283. https://doi.org/10.1126/science.1171999

Gresham, F. M., Reschly, D. J., Tilly, W. D., Fletcher, J. M., Burns, M. K., & Christ, T. (2004). Comprehensive evaluation of learning disabilities: A response to intervention perspective. *The School Psychologist, 59*, 26–29. https://doi.org/10.1037/e537492009-006

Grigorenko, E. L. (2005). A conservative meta-analysis of linkage and linkage-association studies of developmental dyslexia. *Scientific Studies of Reading, 9*(3), 285–316. https://doi.org/10.1207/s1532799xssr0903_6

Grigorenko, E. L. (2007). Triangulating developmental dyslexia: Behavior, brain, and genes. In D. Coch, G. Dawson, & K. Fischer (Eds.), *Human behavior and the developing brain* (pp. 117–144). Guilford.

Grigorenko, E. L. (2009). Dynamic assessment and response to intervention: Two sides of one coin. *Journal of Learning Disabilities, 42*(2), 111–132. https://doi.org/10.1177/0022219408326207

Grigorenko, E. L., Wood, F. B., Meyer, M. S., Hart, L. A., Speed, W. C., Shuster, A., & Pauls, D. L. (1997). Susceptibility loci for distinct components of developmental dyslexia on chromosomes 6 and 15. *American Journal of Human Genetics, 60*(1), 27–39.

Gurney, J. G., Krull, K. R., Kadan-Lottick, N., Nicholson, H. S., Nathan, P. C., Zebrack, B., Tersak, J. M., & Ness, K. K. (2009). Social outcomes in the Childhood Cancer Survivor Study cohort. *Journal of Clinical Oncology, 27*(14), 2390–2395. https://doi.org/10.1200/JCO.2008.21.1458

Haight, S. L., Patriarca, L. A., & Burns, M. K. (2002). A statewide analysis of eligibility criteria and procedures for determining learning disabilities. *Learning Disabilities: A Multidisciplinary Journal, 11*, 39–46. https://eric.ed.gov/?id=EJ648771

Hallahan, D. P., & Mercer, C. R. (2002). Learning disabilities: Historical perspectives in identification of learning disabilities. In R. Bradley, L. Danielson, & D. P. Hallahan (Eds.), *Research to practice* (pp. 1–67). Lawrence Erlbaum.

Jordan, N. C., & Levine, S. C. (2009). Socioeconomic variation, number competence, and mathematics learning difficulties in young children. *Developmental Disabilities Research Reviews, 15*(1), 60–68. https://doi.org/10.1002/ddrr.46

Lagae, L. (2008). Learning disabilities: Definitions, epidemiology, diagnosis, and intervention strategies. *Pediatric Clinics of North America, 55*(6), 1259–1268. https://doi.org/10.1016/j.pcl.2008.08.001

Mandlawitz, M. (2006). *What every teacher should know about IDEA 2004.* Allyn & Bacon.

Mercer, C. D., Jordan, L., Allsopp, D. H., & Mercer, A. R. (1996). Learning disabilities definitions and criteria used by state education departments. *Learning Disability Quarterly, 19*(4), 217–232. https://doi.org/10.2307/1511208

Pennington, B. F. (2009). How neuropsychology informs our understanding of developmental disorders. *Journal of Child Psychology & Psychiatry & Allied Disciplines, 50*(1/2), 72–78. https://doi.org/10.1111/j.1469-7610.2008.01977.x

Price, C. J., & Mechelli, A. (2005). Reading and reading disturbance. *Current Opinion in Neurobiology, 15*(2), 231–238. https://doi.org/10.1016/j.conb.2005.03.003

Rourke, B. P., Ahmad, S. A., Collins, D. W., Hayman-Abello, B. A., Hayman-Abello, S. E., & Warriner, E. M. (2002). Child clinical/pediatric neuropsychology: Some recent advances. *Annual Review of Psychology, 53,* 309–339. https://doi.org/10.1146/annurev.psych.53.100901.135204

Semrud-Clikeman, M. (2005). Neuropsychological aspects for evaluating learning disabilities. *Journal of Learning Disabilities, 38*(6), 563–568. https://doi.org/10.1177/00222194050380061301

Shaywitz, S. E., Morris, R., & Shaywitz, B. A. (2008). The education of dyslexic children from childhood to young adulthood. *Annual Review of Psychology, 59,* 451–475. https://doi.org/10.1146/annurev.psych.59.103006.093633

Shaywitz, S. E., & Shaywitz, B. A. (2005). Dyslexia (specific reading disability). *Biological Psychiatry, 57*(11), 1301–1309. https://doi.org/10.1016/j.biopsych.2005.01.043

Shaywitz, S. E., & Shaywitz, B. A. (2008). Paying attention to reading: The neurobiology of reading and dyslexia. *Development & Psychopathology, 20*(4), 1329–1349. https://doi.org/10.1017/S0954579408000631

Sternberg, R. J., & Grigorenko, E. L. (2002). Difference scores in the identification of children with learning disabilities: It's time to use a different method. *Journal of School Psychology, 40*(1), 65–83. https://doi.org/10.1016/S0022-4405(01)00094-2

U.S. Office of Education. (1977). Assistance to states for education for handicapped children: Procedures for evaluating specific learning disabilities. *Federal Register, 42.* https://nces.ed.gov/programs/digest/d17/tables/dt17_204.30.asp

U.S. Office of Special Education and Rehabilitative Services. (2000). *History: Twenty-five years of progress in educating children with disabilities through IDEA.* US Department of Education.

CHAPTER 10 ■ ATTENTION-DEFICIT/ HYPERACTIVITY DISORDER

■ BACKGROUND

Children with difficulties in attention and impulsivity have been recognized since the mid-1800s when compulsory school attendance became the rule. The 19th-century book *Struwwelpeter*, a "morality" book for children by Heinrich Hoffmann, included the tales of Fidgety Philip, who could not sit still, and Johnny Look-in-the-Air, who could not pay attention (Struwwel, 1999). The observation of difficulties after viral encephalitis in the early 20th century led to a presumption that these problems arose as a result of some subtle or "minimal" brain damage. Bradley's observation in the 1930s that such children could improve their attention after administration of amphetamine led to one of the first pharmacologic treatments for childhood mental disorders (Bradley, 1937). This led to the use of terms like *minimal brain dysfunction* to describe the condition even though evidence of gross brain damage was not demonstrable. In 1957, Laufer used the term *hyperkinetic impulse disorder*, and, in 1970, the second edition of the *Diagnostic and Statistical Manual* (DSM) identified the syndrome as *hyperkinetic reaction* (Laufer & Denhoff, 1957). By 1980, the term *attention-deficit disorder* began to be used, as was, subsequently, the term *attention-deficit/hyperactivity disorder* (ADHD). By that time the importance of inattention symptoms had gained recognition, resulting in an appellation of *attention-deficit disorder* that can be diagnosed with or without *hyperactivity*.

■ DIAGNOSIS, DEFINITION, AND CLINICAL FEATURES

ADHD is characterized by symptoms of inattention, overactivity, and impulsivity along with deficits in the set of skills usually termed *executive functioning*. The latter are a range of abilities involved in forward planning, self-control, and delay of gratification. Although similar in some ways, there are differences in approach between the *DSM-5* (American Psychiatric Association, 2013) and the *International Classification of Diseases* (ICD-10) as well as the latest revision, *ICD-11* (World Health Organization, 2019–2020). *ICD-10* hyperkinetic disorder has been renamed ADHD and moved from the category of "behavioral and emotional disorders with childhood onset" to the category of "neurodevelopmental disorders" to recognize its developmental onset, characteristic disturbances in neurocognitive and social functions, and common co-occurrence with other neurodevelopmental disorders. Both the

DSM and *ICD* approaches provide a list of 18 symptoms that can involve both attentional problems and hyperactivity (the combined type) or only inattention *or* impulsivity. In *DSM-5*, the hyperactive type requires at least six of nine symptoms of overactivity, and the inattentive type requires at least six of nine listed symptoms of inattention. In the combined type, six of each are required. The *ICD* approach emphasizes the overactivity aspect and is more stringent in making the diagnosis when other disorders such as anxiety or depression are present. These approaches to diagnosis are summarized in Table 10.1. A notable difference in diagnostic criteria in the *DSM-5* compared to its predecessor *DSM-IV-TR* is that the age requirement for symptom onset was changed from 7 to 12 years. The distinctions between the subtypes of the disorder can be subtle, and debate continues about the best approach to conceptualizing the condition(s). For example, some children with predominately inattentive symptoms may be less active. It is the case that children whose difficulties relate to overactivity are likely to be more disruptive and thus may be more frequently referred for treatment and earlier diagnosis. For a diagnosis of ADHD to be made, the symptoms must be present in more than one setting (such as home, school, and friendships), must cause significant impairment in functioning, and cannot be exclusively attributable to another disorder or be better accounted for by it. As a practical matter, the diagnosis of ADHD should include information about symptoms and functioning from multiple sources including parents, teachers, and observations by clinicians experienced in the assessment of children with this disorder (Box 10.1).

The degree to which any one of the three major areas of difficulty—overactivity, inattention, and impulsivity—impacts the child functioning at home and in school will color the diagnostic presentation. The child's age and level of functioning are very important considerations for the diagnosis; for some children, difficulties only become apparent because of the age-expected demands placed by school for concentration and attention. Having lots of energy is not unusual for young children, and behaviors such as difficulty remaining seated, running about, and laughing and screaming loudly when having fun are expected of preschoolers. However, if older children have difficulty regulating these type of behaviors, it could be a sign of ADHD.

TABLE 10.1

Approaches to Diagnosis of Attention-Deficit/Hyperactivity Disorder in the *Diagnostic and Statistical Manual 5*

Onset and duration: Before the age of 12 years; symptoms must be present for at least 6 months.
Symptom presentation and impairment: Symptoms must be present in more than one setting and result in significant impairment; symptoms must be persistent and not attributable to developmental level and not occurring exclusively during psychosis or better explained by another disorder.
Subtypes: Three possible subtypes are identified: inattentive, hyperactive, or combined.
For the **inattentive** type, at least six symptoms of inattention (e.g., in school work, social interaction, following through on activities, troubles in organization and activities that require forward planning, readily disorganized, by extraneous environmental events)
For the **hyperactivity** type, at least six symptoms, such as inability to sit still, high activity level inappropriate to situation, trouble playing quietly, excessively verbal, trouble waiting turns, interrupts frequently, and so on
In the **combined** type, both hyperactive and inattentive symptoms are present.
Exclusionary rules: Features not attributable solely to (or occur during) schizophrenia or psychotic disorder or better viewed as part of some other condition such as anxiety or mood disorder

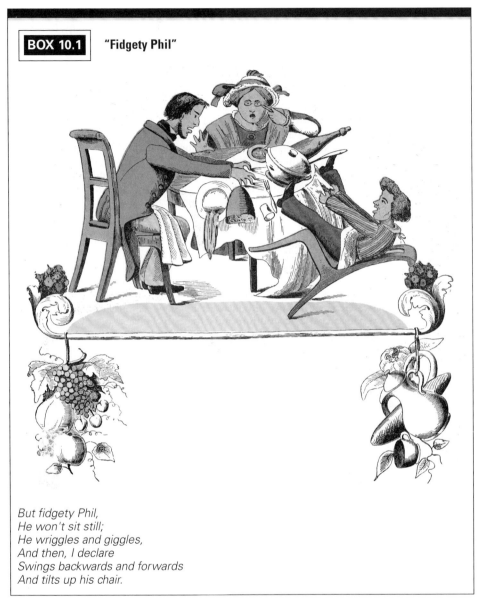

But fidgety Phil,
He won't sit still;
He wriggles and giggles,
And then, I declare
Swings backwards and forwards
And tilts up his chair.

Reproduced from Hoffmann, H. (1845). *Der Struwwelpter*. Routledge & Kegan Paul Ltd. Courtesy of the Cushing/Whitney Medical Library, Yale University School of Medicine.

As children enter kindergarten, learning to participate in structured activities and follow classroom rules can take weeks and months for most. As typically developing children show consistent progress with acquisition of new behaviors such as sitting at their desk and listening to the teachers, children with ADHD would fall behind in building such age-appropriate competencies. A lack of precision regarding how "often" a behavior or feature must be present and how "persistent" it is means that there is considerable clinical judgment involved in making the diagnosis. Also, the presence of comorbid conditions, such as learning difficulties, language problems, disruptive behavior, and so forth, frequently complicates the clinical picture. For some children, the burden of significant attentional problems and hyperactivity takes a toll on affective regulation as well as on peer relationships and social development. There has been growing awareness that, for many children, symptoms of overactivity may lessen with time, but attentional problems may persist. As a result, in adulthood, many individuals may continue to experience difficulties, although their impairment may be less immediately obvious (Nigg et al., 2020).

In the doctor's office setting, the difficulties with attention and impulsivity may not seem markedly different than those in other children, although when a child's difficulties are severe, they are often noted even in office settings. For school-age children, problems with overactivity may be most dramatic in less structured settings (e.g., gym or recess), and problems with attention are reflected in academic areas. Rating scales, checklists, and some psychological tests (discussed subsequently) may be useful in helping to clarify the diagnosis. More complex academic tasks, which require organizational skills and forward planning, are particularly impacted by problems in attention and impulsivity. This is often reflected in forgotten homework or many different projects started but never finished and can be demonstrated on psychological testing. As a practical matter, the clinician should keep in mind the core features of the condition—hyperactivity, inattention, and impulsivity—and have a reasonable sense of what is and is not within the normal range for a child of a given age (Box 10.2).

By definition, the essential feature of ADHD is a persistent pattern of inattention and/or hyperactivity-impulsivity that are developmentally inappropriate and interfere with functioning across important areas. In the *DSM-5*, the disorder must have its onset before the age of 12 years. Determination of the actual age of onset is difficult, because these data are invariably retrospective in nature. Most of the time, parents will have noted some difficulties in the preschool period, when the child may have had a "driven" quality as they rapidly explored the room. Often, parents provide detailed reports of family outings and birthday parties during which the child's difficulties have led to major disruptions. In situations in which the major difficulties relate to sustained attention and organization, it may be only when the child enters school that difficulties pose a serious obstacle for learning and lead to diagnosis. Some children have difficulty remaining seated during class. Even in situations such as recess and sports, the child's difficulties with attention and impulsivity may take a toll on social relationships. Inattention is characterized by difficulty staying focused, mind wandering off task, lacking persistence in tasks that require focused attention, and general difficulty organizing and sustaining mental effort. These symptoms are different from and should be carefully separated from lack of comprehension or noncompliance with academic assignments. In the absence of clear hyperactivity, attentional difficulties may not become obvious until middle school when academic tasks become more demanding of attentional resources. These difficulties may also continue into adulthood, and diagnosis and treatment of ADHD in adults are gaining greater recognition in the field of mental health.

EPIDEMIOLOGY AND DEMOGRAPHICS

ADHD is one of the more common psychiatric disorders, affecting approximately 5% of children and 2.5% of adults. The prevalence estimates vary across epidemiologic studies because of differences in samples, assessment methods, and diagnostic approaches. Boys are more likely to be affected than girls (2:1 or 3:1 ratio) and are more likely than girls to present with disruptive behaviors (Spetie & Arnold, 2018). Girls with ADHD are more likely to have attentional problems and more co-occurring internalizing problems, such as depression and anxiety (Rucklidge, 2010). ADHD is also found more frequently in younger children and in children from families with a lower socioeconomic status. Symptoms of hyperactivity decrease with age. As adults, many, perhaps more than 50% of individuals, continue to have symptoms. Younger individuals are more likely to show features of the hyperactive subtypes; attentional problems become more marked over time so that the combined type becomes predominant. By the junior high and high school

---

BOX 10.2   **Case Report: Attention-Deficit/Hyperactivity Disorder**

Jason, a 7-year-old boy, was referred for a clinical evaluation at the request of his teacher because of behavioral difficulties in the classroom. Jason was the third child and only boy in the family. Although not particularly worried about his behavior until he entered school, his parents did report that "his engine was running all the time." He had been enrolled in a relatively unstructured preschool program, where some concern had been expressed about his ability to "stick with" activities, although the teachers and his parents viewed him as a highly energetic and bright boy.

On entering first grade in a public-school setting, Jason had difficulty sitting still. He often did not seem to be listening to the teacher and had difficulty waiting his turn (such as when in line in the school cafeteria). His teacher was also concerned that he was behind other students in his class in emerging reading abilities. According to his parents, Jason also disliked any activities at home that required sitting and paying attention such as arts and crafts projects, and asking him to read or do his homework was a constant struggle. His parents had several discussions with the teacher and by the end of the school year asked their pediatrician if Jason's difficulties at school may require an evaluation. Following these discussions with the teacher and with Jason's pediatrician, the parents decided to seek a comprehensive clinical evaluation that included psychological testing and an evaluation by a child psychiatrist.

Psychological testing revealed an IQ in the high-average range but with lower-than-expected achievement scores. Jason had difficulty with tasks on the IQ test that required sustained attention. The psychologist also conducted a classroom observation that revealed a number of behavioral difficulties in the classroom. In addition, because of his difficulties playing sports and participating in more structured play activities, Jason also tended to be a little bit of a "loner" at recess on the playground.

As part of psychiatric evaluation, a board-certified child psychiatrist conducted a careful review of developmental milestones and medical history. Apart from several ear infections, his birth, developmental, and medical history were unremarkable. His hearing had been tested and found to be within the normal range. Regarding family history, Jason's father reported that he had attentional difficulties when he was in school and had been treated for many years with methylphenidate. On examination, Jason's behavior became more disorganized after he became more comfortable with the examiner and the setting. With support, he was able to attend the interview, but without this support, his attention was fleeting. He complained that other children in school made fun of him and said he had "ants in his pants."

Jason's behavioral and attentional difficulties persisted in the second grade and his parents decided to initiate treatment with stimulant medications along with family counseling and behavioral supports in the classroom. Because of his concern about being called out of class to the nurse's office to take medication, a long-acting stimulant was eventually prescribed and was well tolerated. Additional psychological testing was requested and resulted in several steps to improve his organization and attention in the classroom setting. By the end of the second grade, Jason's self-image and peer relationships improved.

As an adolescent, Jason's difficulties with overactivity improved, even during summers when he did not usually take medication. On the other hand, his problems with sustained attention and organization were more persistent. In college, Jason was able to obtain additional supports, including a tutor, untimed tests, and some other modifications.

Comment: Although the presenting complaint was related to classroom difficulties, the history revealed previous problems, probably dating back to the toddler years. Many features of the condition responded to stimulant medication, but even though some aspects of overactivity seemed to improve with time, other problems persisted into adolescence or adulthood. Treatment included medication, parent guidance, educational support, and other measures. A family history of the disorder is relatively common.

Adapted from Volkmar, F. R., & Martin, A. (2011). *Essentials of child and adolescent psychiatry* (p. 112). Lippincott Williams & Wilkins.

years, the inattentive type is most common. Compared with many other disorders, ADHD is often a diagnosis made by history from parents and teachers or, with adolescents and adults, by self-report. A child with ADHD can appear calm and well organized in a novel setting, so reports of parents and teachers are often used in making the diagnosis.

As noted previously, ADHD is frequently associated with other conditions including oppositional defiant or conduct disorder (~50% of cases), anxiety disorder (25%–30%), and learning disabilities (20%–25%) (Baweja & Waxmonsky, 2018; Harvey et al., 2016). The risk of developing tic disorder is also increased (Sukhodolsky et al., 2009). It is important that co-occurring disorders are carefully evaluated and documented when they are present, because they may require additional interventions apart from those for ADHD. As children with ADHD become older, they are at increased risk for mood disorders and substance abuse. Comorbidity can arise from various sources (e.g., from genetic or environmental factors that contribute to both disorders or because ADHD increases risk for other problems). Comorbid conditions can further exacerbate the negative impact of ADHD on family life, peer relationships, and academic and occupational achievements.

ETIOLOGY AND PATHOGENESIS

Both genetic and environmental factors have been implicated in the etiology of ADHD (Faraone & Larsson, 2019). Twin and adoption studies show a strong genetic component, suggesting that genetic factors account for about 60% of the heritability. Recent research has been more sophisticated in its examination of potential genetic mechanisms and neuropsychological profiles presumed to underlie syndrome expression. Various regions on the human chromosome have been implicated in available linkage studies. One line of work has focused on dopaminergic brain mechanisms. The association of ADHD with pre- and perinatal complications and with neurologic soft signs and, of course, its early history of association with the aftereffects of brain infection or trauma suggest an important role for neural mechanisms.

Table 10.2 summarizes some of the soft neurologic signs observed in ADHD.

One body of work has focused on structural and functional brain abnormalities that can be detected with various brain imaging methods. Structural brain abnormalities reported across studies have included reduced volumes in dorsolateral prefrontal cortex, caudate, pallidum, corpus callosum, and cerebellum (see Spetie & Arnold, 2018, for a detailed review). One of the most comprehensive longitudinal neuroimaging studies was conducted in a large sample of 152 children with ADHD (age range 5–18 years) and 139 age- and sex-matched controls

TABLE 10.2
Soft Neurologic Signs in Attention-Deficit/Hyperactivity Disorder

Clinical Finding	Putative Explanation
Difficulties performing repetitive motor tasks (e.g., hand flipping and foot rocking)	Impaired ability to use cognitive control to alternately inhibit and excite motor activity to maintain a regular cadence
Difficulties performing sequential timed tasks (e.g., serial thumb to finger opposition)	Impaired ability to use cognitive control to adjust motor performance flexibly in a multistep task
Difficulties maintaining gait and balance (sustained motor stance, tandem balance)	Difficulties maintaining balance, integrating proprioceptive input or body position sense, abnormal vestibular function

Adapted from Spetie, L., & Arnold, E. J. (2018). Attention-deficit/hyperactivity disorder. In A. Martin, M. H. Bloch, & F. R. Volkmar (Eds.), *Lewis's child and adolescent psychiatry: A comprehensive textbook* (5th ed., p. 371). Wolters Kluwer.

at the National Institute of Mental Health from 1991 to 2001. The patients with ADHD had significantly smaller brain volumes on the initial scan in all regions (total cerebrum; cerebellum; gray and white matter for the four major lobes: frontal–temporal, parietal, and occipital). Developmental trajectories for all structures except the caudate remained roughly parallel for patients and controls during childhood and adolescence and were unrelated to stimulant treatment (Greven et al., 2015).

Functional magnetic resonance imaging studies have identified reduced activation and connectivity in a distributed network of cortical and subcortical brain regions involved in attention, working memory, and response inhibition. For example, a recent meta-analysis of 96 task-based functional magnetic resonance imaging studies contrasting subjects with ADHD to unaffected participants revealed aberrant activity in the left pallidum/putamen and decreased activity (only in male subjects) in the left inferior frontal gyrus (Samea et al., 2019). The review also highlighted a lack of regional convergence in children/adolescents with ADHD, which might be due to heterogeneous clinical populations and various experimental designs, preprocessing, and statistical procedures in individual studies. Other neuroimaging approaches have included single-photon emission computed tomography, positron emission tomography, and proton magnetic resonance spectroscopy to focus on brain metabolism during cognitive activities. Most studies have suggested hypoperfusion of the frontal and possibly striatal areas as well as deficits in activation of inhibitory control areas. Because dopamine has had such an important apparent role in the treatment of the condition, another line of work has focused on dopamine and the dopamine transporter and has found increased binding of the transporter in the striatum of individuals with ADHD.

Changes in electroencephalograms (EEGs) and event-related potentials have also been reported. The most consistent finding has been higher levels of slow-wave activity relative to normal children with reduced alpha- and beta-wave activity. Some studies have explored the possibility of use of the EEG diagnostically to examine, for example, ratios of theta to beta activity. Related work has focused on evoked potentials, although this line of work is less advanced. There does appear to be a strong hereditary component to EEG measures. It is possible that in the future, endophenotypes might be defined using such approaches. However, it is important to underscore that EEG has been used as a research tool and it is only sensitive to detecting differences between groups of study subjects. At the time of this writing, there are no EEG procedures that can diagnose ADHD in a valid and reliable manner (Cheung et al., 2017; Loo et al., 2018).

Psychosocial adversity and other environmental factors have also been associated with ADHD. It is possible that various environmental factors interact with biologic ones to increase the risk for the disorder. Lead toxicity can, for example, lead to attentional difficulties. Similarly, maternal smoking during pregnancy increases the risk of ADHD in the child.

Neuropsychological theories of ADHD have focused on deficits in inhibitory control (a general pattern of difficulties in inhibition), working memory (ability to retain and manipulate information in short-term memory), or in delay aversion (an inability to tolerate delay). Another approach focuses on the interaction of information processing and processes such as effort, arousal, and activation (the cognitive energetic model). Another approach differentiates ADHD with and without hyperactivity and focuses on delays in information process and information retrieval (the sluggish cognitive tempo theory). Even though ADHD is often viewed as a disorder of executive functioning (planning and execution of goal-directed behavior), not all individuals with ADHD show impairment in this domain (Roberts et al., 2017). There is also increasing recognition that some neurocognitive deficits may be due to emotional processing associated with co-occurring disorders such as oppositional defiant disorder rather than with the attentional deficits conferred by ADHD.

■ DIFFERENTIAL DIAGNOSIS AND ASSESSMENT

The differential diagnosis of ADHD can be complex. Difficulties include varied symptom presentation, age-related changes, and associations with other conditions (e.g., mood problems; anxiety disorder, particularly posttraumatic stress disorder; conduct problems; and developmental difficulties of various kinds). Accordingly, careful history and examination are important.

Various parent and teacher rating instruments have been developed and standardized so that the scores for one child can be compared to the scores of children of the same age and gender (i.e., standardization sample). It is important that standardized ratings are completed by several individuals who know the child well—such as parents and two or three teachers—to obtain convergent information about ADHD symptoms across different domains of functioning. School observations conducted by trained mental health professionals are also a helpful tool in confirming ADHD diagnosis. An excellent way to collect caregiver observations is by using one of the many standardized rating scales. Probably the best ones are those that use the actual *DSM-5* symptoms rated on a standard metric, usually 0–3, from no symptom to severe. Examples include the SNAP (Swanson, Nolan, and Pelham) questionnaire (Swanson, 1992), which consists of a list of *DSM* symptoms of ADHD, and the Conners-3 long forms (Conners, 2008), which have the *DSM* symptoms embedded in a longer scale. When counting symptoms, a rating of 2 or 3 on the 0–3 scales is usually considered as the presence of the symptom. Numerous other scales are also useful and have been used in research and clinical practice.

Neuropsychological testing can also help to identify specific areas of vulnerability in individuals with ADHD (Hall et al., 2016; Nyongesa et al., 2019). These include difficulties with tasks that require response inhibition and execution, shifting of set and task, interference control, planning and organization, and working memory. A particular profile of strengths and weaknesses on tests of intelligence (IQ) such as relative weaknesses in the areas of processing speed and verbal working memory could be indicative of ADHD. Computerized assessment of sustained attention, vigilance, and response inhibition, such as the Continuous Performance Test or Test of Variables of Attention, can help to identify attentional deficits in individuals as part of clinical assessment. However, any particular score on a neurocognitive test does not automatically indicate the presence of a diagnosis. All results of paper-and-pencil and computerized neuropsychological tests should be interpreted by licensed psychologists as part of comprehensive clinical evaluation, and the diagnosis of ADHD is confirmed or disconfirmed by clinical judgment based on review of all available information.

COURSE

In more than half of the cases, symptoms persist into adulthood, although there may be changes in syndrome expression. In the adult population, the male–female discrepancy is much less marked than in childhood (Owens et al., 2017). As adults, hyperactivity symptoms often diminish substantially, persisting only as an internal experience of restlessness. However, the problems of inattention, disorganization, and distractibility are more likely to persist. An area of controversy has been the need for different diagnostic approaches or criteria in the adult population. Figure 10.1 summarizes the course of different ADHD symptoms over the life span.

Development of comorbid conditions is a risk for adults with ADHD. There is an increased risk, especially for boys and men, to develop substance abuse problems or antisocial behaviors. Difficulties with attention and impulsivity may lead to job difficulties, problems in daily living, and accidents. In women, impulsive behavior can lead to increased risk for unplanned pregnancy. Adults with ADHD may also have higher rates of mood disorders (Rasmussen & Gillberg, 2000).

TREATMENT

Given the chronic nature of the disorder, treatment must be flexible and comprehensive. The child and family should be involved in treatment planning. Both behavioral and pharmacologic treatments can be helpful. The American Academy of Pediatrics' flow chart for evaluation

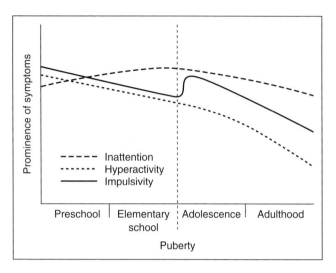

FIGURE 10.1. Course of different attention-deficit hyperactivity disorder symptoms over the life span. Hyperactivity tends to wane with maturity, being replaced by a feeling of restlessness. Impulsivity also tends to wane except for a possible blip in adolescence under the influence of "raging hormones." The most persistent cluster of symptoms is inattentiveness, with the main adult manifestations being disorganization and difficulty managing money, keeping schedules, and sticking with a relationship or job. Reproduced with permission from Arnold, L. E. (2004). *Contemporary diagnosis and management of ADHD*. Handbooks in Health Care.

and treatment is reproduced in Figure 10.2. In short- and medium-term studies, medications (stimulants and atomoxetine) typically outperform behavioral treatments. However, 75% of children with ADHD can be managed with only behavioral interventions. The combination of behavioral and pharmacologic intervention also provides some advantages. Although a number of psychoactive medications have been used to treat individuals with ADHD, only a handful have received U.S. Food and Drug Administration approval (Table 10.3). The psychostimulants and the one nonstimulant (atomoxetine) have been shown to be effective and are reasonably well tolerated (Spetie & Arnold, 2018).

For school-age children, it is common to start with a small dose of a stimulant medication and gradually increase the dose. The size of the child is only an approximate guide, and it is important to balance benefits and side effects for the individual child. For example, some children experience an "evening rebound" with stimulant medications that may be avoided by an extended-release preparation or the use of atomoxetine. These agents also have the advantage of minimizing the need for the child to take pills at school. Various side effects have been reported, including appetite suppression, troubles with sleep, irritability, and tics. Occasionally, children treated with high doses develop psychotic-like conditions, but this is uncommon. Although continuous use in nonschool settings is more frequent in recent years, the judicious use of drug holidays for stimulants (e.g., over school vacation and during the summer) provides an opportunity to provide observation in a drug-free state.

Various other agents are sometimes used in the management of individuals with ADHD. Occasionally, antipsychotic medications have been used, but they have greater risk of side effects and usually are less beneficial. Other drugs not yet Food and Drug Administration approved but with some apparent efficacy include tricyclics, monoamine oxidase inhibitors, and bupropion; these may be particularly helpful when comorbid depression or anxiety is present. In general, the danger of significant adverse effects with foods does limit the use of monoamine oxidase inhibitors in children. α-Agonists, mainly clonidine and more recently guanfacine, have been used, particularly when agitation and aggression are present; of the two, guanfacine has a longer half-life and less sedation.

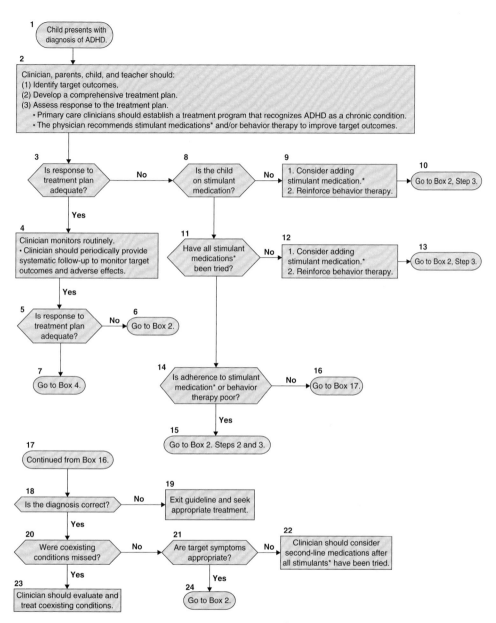

* Excluding pemoline. Another FDA-approved option is atomoxetine (Strattera©), approved since the guideline was published.
 Used with the permission of the Academy of Pediatrics. From Clinical practice guideline: treatment of the school-aged child
 with attention deficit/hyperactivity disorder. *Pediatrics* 108:1033–1044, 2001.

FIGURE 10.2. Clinical guidelines of the American Academy of Pediatrics, which were written before availability of atomoxetine, which, as a Food and Drug Administration–approved treatment for attention-deficit hyperactivity disorder, should be considered after a stimulant before resorting to off-label drugs. Reproduced with permission from American Academy of Pediatrics. (2001). Clinical practice guideline: Treatment of the school-aged child with attention-deficit/hyperactivity disorder. *Pediatrics, 108*(4), 1033–1048. Copyright © 2001 American Academy of Pediatrics.

TABLE 10.3

Drugs With Food and Drug Administration Approval for Attention-Deficit/ Hyperactivity Disorder

Generic Name	Brand Name	Usual Daily Dose, mg (mg/kg)
Stimulants		
Amphetamine (racemic), dextroamphetamine	Dexedrine Dextro Star	10–40 (0.2–0.7)
Levoamphetamine mixture	Adderall Adderall XR	5–40 (0.2–1) 5–40 (0.2–1)
Methamphetamine	Desoxyn	5–25 (0.2–0.7)
Methylphenidate, racemic	Ritalin Methylin Ritalin LA Metadate Metadate CD	10–60 (0.3–1.5) 10–60 (0.3–1.5) 20–60 (0.6–1.5) 10–60 (0.3–1.5) 20–60 (0.6–1.5)
Methylphenidate, osmotic release	Concerta	18–72 (0.4–1.8)
Dextro-threo-methylphenidate	Focalin Focalin XR	5–30 (0.2–0.7) 5–30 (0.2–0.7)
Pemoline	Cylert	37.5–112.3 (1–3)
Nonstimulant		
Atomoxetine	Strattera	18–100 (0.7–1.4)

Reproduced with permission from Arnold, L. E. (2004). *Contemporary diagnosis and management of ADHD*. Handbooks in Health Care.

Behavioral interventions include a host of interventions designed to reinforce desired behaviors, assist the child with organization, and support the child's attempts to cope adaptively. These may include visual supports, charts, organizational aids, behavioral reward systems, and so forth. These can vary from simple to much more complex systems (e.g., token economies or a daily report card from school on the child's behavior). Parenting interventions for co-occurring disruptive behaviors, such as noncompliance and irritability, can be quite helpful for preschool and school-age children with ADHD (Haack et al., 2016).

Classroom behavior management approaches and parenting interventions have been shown to be effective mostly for improving hyperactivity and impulsive behavior but have less robust effects on inattention. Over the past decade, organizational skills training (OST) has emerged as a category of behavioral interventions with a common focus on teaching children how to organize task materials (e.g., contents of the child's backpack) and time (e.g., how to pace a project that is due next week) required for academic tasks and activities of daily living. As a key component of OST programs, children are first taught what it means to be organized and to plan ahead. The organizational skills are taught using behavioral techniques including modeling, rehearsal, and contingency management. A defining feature of OST programs is the focus on concrete skills necessary to keep organized in the context of age-appropriate academic tasks. Parents are also involved in the treatment, and their role is to prompt, praise, and reward their child's learning and performance of specific skills with the intent to reinforce desirable behaviors and to promote generalization of skills to multiple contexts. Recent review of clinical trials reported that in addition to improving academic skills, OST also resulted in improved symptoms of inattention (Bikic et al., 2017).

EDUCATIONAL PLANNING AND SCHOOL SERVICES

Most children with diagnosed ADHD have some problem with academic performance; in fact, that is often what brings them to clinical attention. Although most are able to function in a regular classroom with appropriate treatment and support, some will need an individualized education plan or even a special class or resource room. This is particularly so for the 20% to 25% with comorbid learning disorders. Parents may need some coaching in obtaining appropriate educational services for the child, as is required by Public Law 94-142 (Education for All Handicapped Children Act), IDEA (Individuals with Disabilities Education Act), or Section 504 of the Civil Rights Act. Children with learning disorders are likely to be covered by the first two mandates, and those without a specific learning disorder are usually covered by Section 504, which provides for "other health impaired" (Evans et al., 2016).

DEVELOPMENT OF NOVEL TREATMENT—COGNITIVE TRAINING

Development of novel treatments for ADHD is an area of active research. Cognitive training is one such treatment that has emerged over the past 15 years based on the premise that targeted practicing of specific neurocognitive functions such as working memory or response inhibition can translate to reduction of ADHD symptoms. Despite intriguing theoretical grounding in neuroscience, most clinical trials of cognitive training failed to demonstrate meaningful clinical effects such as reduction of ADHD symptoms or change in child's adaptive functioning (Cortese et al., 2015). A notable example is a recent, large ($N = 348$) randomized controlled trial of a digital intervention delivered through a video game–like interface via at-home play for 25 min/day for 4 weeks (Kollins et al., 2020). The video game treatment resulted in a significant improvement on the Test of Variables of Attention Performance Index. There is also emerging evidence that cognitive training may alter the brain mechanisms underlying attention and cognitive control. For example, Smith et al. (2019) reported reduction in the latency of P3 evoked potential, an electrophysiologic index of response inhibition, after cognitive training in young children with ADHD. Thus, even though the current state of clinical evidence precludes recommending cognitive training as treatment for ADHD symptoms and functional impairment, there is hope that one day neuroscience-based digital treatments will have clinical utility for ADHD.

SUMMARY

ADHD is one of the most commonly encountered psychiatric disorders in children. Although significant advances in both research and treatment have been made over the past decades, in some respects, the disorder appears poorly understood. It is likely that the various factors (environmental, genetic, neurobehavioral, and developmental) contribute, in varying degrees, to the expression of the condition in each individual case. Effective treatments are available. Clinicians should be alert to the possible presence of comorbid conditions and be aware that the problems of ADHD can sometimes mask or mimic other conditions. Treatment planning should be comprehensive.

References

*Indicates Particularly Recommended

American Psychiatric Association. (2013). *Diagnostic and statistical manual of mental disorders (DSM-5)* (5th ed.). American Psychiatric Publishing.

Baweja, R., & Waxmonsky, J. G. (2018). Treatment implications for ADHD youth with mood and anxiety comorbidity. *Current Treatment Options in Psychiatry*, 5(1), 73–97. https://doi.org/10.1007/s40501-018-0135-3

*Bikic, A., Reichow, B., McCauley, S. A., Ibrahim, K., & Sukhodolsky, D. G. (2017). Meta-analysis of organizational skills interventions for children and adolescents with attention-deficit/hyperactivity disorder. *Clinical Psychology Review*, 52, 108–123. https://doi.org/10.1016/j.cpr.2016.12.004

Bradley, C. (1937). The behavior of children receiving benzedrine. *American Journal of Psychiatry, 94,* 577–585. https://doi.org/10.1176/ajp.94.3.577

Cheung, C. H. M., McLoughlin, G., Brandeis, D., Banaschewski, T., Asherson, P., & Kuntsi, J. (2017). Neurophysiological correlates of attentional fluctuation in attention-deficit/hyperactivity disorder. *Brain Topography, 30*(3), 320–332. https://doi.org/10.1007/s10548-017-0554-2

Conners, C. K. (2008). *Conners 3* (3rd ed.). Multi-Health Systems Inc.

*Cortese, S., Ferrin, M., Brandeis, D., Buitelaar, J., Daley, D., Dittmann, R. W., Holtmann, M., Santosh, P., Stevenson, J., Stringaris, A., Zuddas, A., & Sonuga-Barke, E. J. S. (2015). Cognitive training for attention-deficit/hyperactivity disorder: Meta-analysis of clinical and neuropsychological outcomes from randomized controlled trials. *Journal of the American Academy of Child and Adolescent Psychiatry, 54*(3), 164–174. https://doi.org/10.1016/j.jaac.2014.12.010

Evans, S. W., Langberg, J. M., Schultz, B. K., Vaughn, A., Altaye, M., Marshall, S. A., & Zoromski, A. K. (2016). Evaluation of a school-based treatment program for young adolescents with ADHD. *Journal of Consulting and Clinical Psychology, 84*(1), 15–30. https://doi.org/10.1037/ccp0000057

Faraone, S. V., & Larsson, H. (2019). Genetics of attention deficit hyperactivity disorder. *Molecular Psychiatry, 24*(4), 562–575. https://doi.org/10.1038/s41380-018-0070-0

*Greven, C. U., Bralten, J., Mennes, M., O'Dwyer, L., Van Hulzen, K. J. E., Rommelse, N., Schweren, L. J. S., Hoekstra, P. J., Hartman, C. A., Heslenfeld, D., Oosterlaan, J., Faraone, S. V., Franke, B., Zwiers, M. P., Arias-Vasquez, A., & Buitelaar, J. K. (2015). Developmentally stable whole-brain volume reductions and developmentally sensitive caudate and putamen volume alterations in those with attention-deficit/hyperactivity disorder and their unaffected siblings. *JAMA Psychiatry, 72*(5), 490–499. https://doi.org/10.1001/jamapsychiatry.2014.3162

Haack, L. M., Villodas, M., McBurnett, K., Hinshaw, S., & Pfiffner, L. J. (2016). Parenting as a mechanism of change in psychosocial treatment for youth with ADHD, predominantly inattentive presentation. *Journal of Abnormal Child Psychology, 45*(5), 841–855. https://doi.org/10.1007/s10802-016-0199-8

Hall, C. L., Valentine, A. Z., Groom, M. J., Walker, G. M., Sayal, K., Daley, D., & Hollis, C. (2016). The clinical utility of the continuous performance test and objective measures of activity for diagnosing and monitoring ADHD in children: A systematic review. *European Child and Adolescent Psychiatry, 25*(7), 677–699. https://doi.org/10.1007/s00787-015-0798-x

Harvey, E. A., Breaux, R. P., & Lugo-Candelas, C. I. (2016). Early development of comorbidity between symptoms of attention-deficit/hyperactivity disorder (ADHD) and oppositional defiant disorder (ODD). *Journal of Abnormal Psychology, 125*(2), 154–167. https://doi.org/10.1037/abn0000090

*Kollins, S. H., DeLoss, D. J., Cañadas, E., Lutz, J., Findling, R. L., Keefe, R. S. E., Epstein, J. N., Cutler, A. J., & Faraone, S. V. (2020). A novel digital intervention for actively reducing severity of paediatric ADHD (STARS-ADHD): A randomised controlled trial. *The Lancet Digital Health, 2*(4), e168–e178. https://doi.org/10.1016/S2589-7500(20)30017-0

Laufer, M. W., & Denhoff, E. (1957). Hyperkinetic behavior syndrome in children. *The Journal of Pediatrics, 50*(4), 463–474. https://doi.org/10.1016/S0022-3476(57)80257-1

Loo, S. K., McGough, J. J., McCracken, J. T., & Smalley, S. L. (2018). Parsing heterogeneity in attention-deficit hyperactivity disorder using EEG-based subgroups. *Journal of Child Psychology and Psychiatry and Allied Disciplines, 59*(3), 223–231. https://doi.org/10.1111/jcpp.12814

*Nigg, J. T., Karalunas, S. L., Feczko, E., & Fair, D. A. (2020). Toward a revised nosology for attention-deficit/hyperactivity disorder heterogeneity. *Biological Psychiatry: Cognitive Neuroscience and Neuroimaging, 5*(8), 726–737. https://doi.org/10.1016/j.bpsc.2020.02.005

Nyongesa, M. K., Ssewanyana, D., Mutua, A. M., Chongwo, E., Scerif, G., Newton, C. R. J. C., & Abubakar, A. (2019). Assessing executive function in adolescence: A scoping review of existing measures and their psychometric robustness. *Frontiers in Psychology, 10,* 311. https://doi.org/10.3389/fpsyg.2019.00311

Owens, E. B., Zalecki, C., Gillette, P., & Hinshaw, S. P. (2017). Girls with childhood ADHD as adults: Cross-domain outcomes by diagnostic persistence. *Journal of Consulting and Clinical Psychology, 85*(7), 723–736. https://doi.org/10.1037/ccp0000217

Rasmussen, P., & Gillberg, C. (2000). Natural outcome of ADHD with developmental coordination disorder at age 22 years: A controlled, longitudinal, community-based study. *Journal of the American Academy of Child and Adolescent Psychiatry, 39*(11), 1424–1431. https://doi.org/10.1097/00004583-200011000-00017

Roberts, B. A., Martel, M. M., & Nigg, J. T. (2017). Are there executive dysfunction subtypes within ADHD? *Journal of Attention Disorders, 21*(4), 284–293. https://doi.org/10.1177/1087054713510349

Rucklidge, J. J. (2010). Gender differences in attention-deficit/hyperactivity disorder. *Psychiatric Clinics of North America, 33*(2), 357–373. https://doi.org/10.1016/j.psc.2010.01.006

Samea, F., Soluki, S., Nejati, V., Zarei, M., Cortese, S., Eickhoff, S. B., Tahmasian, M., & Eickhoff, C. R. (2019). Brain alterations in children/adolescents with ADHD revisited: A neuroimaging meta-analysis of 96 structural and functional studies. *Neuroscience and Biobehavioral Reviews, 100,* 1–8. https://doi.org/10.1016/j.neubiorev.2019.02.011

*Smith, S. D., Crowley, M. J., Ferrey, A., Ramsey, K., Wexler, B. E., Leckman, J. F., & Sukhodolsky, D. G. (2019). Effects of Integrated Brain, Body, and Social (IBBS) intervention on ERP measures of attentional control in children with ADHD. *Psychiatry Research, 278,* 248–257. https://doi.org/10.1016/j.psychres.2019.06.021

Spetie, L., & Arnold, E. L. (2018). Attention-deficit hyperactivity disorder. In A. Martin, M. H. Bloch, & F. R. Volkmar (Eds.), *Lewis's child and adolescent psychiatriy: A comprehensive textbook* (5th ed., pp. 364–387). Wolters Kluwer.

Struwwel, P. (1999). *Fearful stories and vile pictures to instruct good little folks/stories by Heinrich Hoffman.* Feral House.

Sukhodolsky, D. G., Scahill, L., & Leckman, J. F. (2009). ADHD with Tourette syndrome. In T. E. Brown (Ed.), *ADHD comorbidities: Handbook for ADHD complications in children and adults* (pp. 293–303). American Psychiatric Press.

Swanson, J. M. (1992). *School-based assessments and interventions for ADD students.* K. C. Publishing.

World Health Organization. (2019–2020). *International statistical classification of diseases and related health problems (ICD)* (11th rev. ed.). Retrieved August 15, 2020, from https://www.who.int/classifications/icd/en/

Suggested Readings

Barkley, R. A. (2018). *Attention-deficit hyperactivity disorder: A handbook for diagnosis and treatment* (4th ed.). Guilford Press.

Bikic, A., Reichow, B., McCauley, S. A., Ibrahim, K., & Sukhodolsky, D. G. (2017). Meta-analysis of organizational skills interventions for children and adolescents with attention-deficit/hyperactivity disorder. *Clinical Psychology Review, 52,* 108–123. https://doi.org/10.1016/j.cpr.2016.12.004

Cortese, S., Ferrin, M., Brandeis, D., Buitelaar, J., Daley, D., Dittmann, R. W., Holtmann, M., Santosh, P., Stevenson, J., Stringaris, A., Zuddas, A., & Sonuga-Barke, E. J. S. (2015). Cognitive training for attention-deficit/hyperactivity disorder: Meta-analysis of clinical and neuropsychological outcomes from randomized controlled trials. *Journal of the American Academy of Child and Adolescent Psychiatry, 54*(3), 164–174. https://doi.org/10.1016/j.jaac.2014.12.010

*Faraone, S. V., Asherson, P., Banaschewski, T., Biederman, J., Buitelaar, J. K., Ramos-Quiroga, J. A., Rohde, L. A., Sonuga-Barke, E. J. S., Tannock, R., & Franke, B. (2015). Attention-deficit/hyperactivity disorder. *Nature Reviews Disease Primers, 1,* 15020. https://doi.org/10.1038/nrdp.2015.20

Greven, C. U., Bralten, J., Mennes, M., O'Dwyer, L., Van Hulzen, K. J. E., Rommelse, N., Schweren, L. J. S., Hoekstra, P. J., Hartman, C. A., Heslenfeld, D., Oosterlaan, J., Faraone, S. V., Franke, B., Zwiers, M. P., Arias-Vasquez, A., & Buitelaar, J. K. (2015). Developmentally stable whole-brain volume reductions and developmentally sensitive caudate and putamen volume alterations in those with attention-deficit/hyperactivity disorder and their unaffected siblings. *JAMA Psychiatry, 72*(5), 490–499. https://doi.org/10.1001/jamapsychiatry.2014.3162

Hall, C. L., Valentine, A. Z., Groom, M. J., Walker, G. M., Sayal, K., Daley, D., & Hollis, C. (2016). The clinical utility of the continuous performance test and objective measures of activity for diagnosing and monitoring ADHD in children: A systematic review. *European Child and Adolescent Psychiatry, 25*(7), 677–699. https://doi.org/10.1007/s00787-015-0798-x

Hoza, B., Shoulberg, E. K., Tompkins, C. L., Martin, C. P., Krasner, A., Dennis, M., Meyer, L. E., & Cook, H. (2020). Moderate-to-vigorous physical activity and processing speed: Predicting adaptive change in ADHD levels and related impairments in preschoolers. *Journal of Child Psychology and Psychiatry and Allied Disciplines, 61*(12), 1380–1387. https://doi.org/10.1111/jcpp.13227

Kollins, S. H., DeLoss, D. J., Cañadas, E., Lutz, J., Findling, R. L., Keefe, R. S. E., Epstein, J. N., Cutler, A. J., & Faraone, S. V. (2020). A novel digital intervention for actively reducing severity of paediatric ADHD (STARS-ADHD): A randomised controlled trial. *The Lancet Digital Health, 2*(4), e168–e178. https://doi.org/10.1016/S2589-7500(20)30017-0

Mattingly, G. W., Wilson, J., Ugarte, L., & Glaser, P. (2020). Individualization of attention-deficit/hyperactivity disorder treatment: Pharmacotherapy considerations by age and co-occurring conditions. *CNS Spectrums,* 1–20. https://doi.org/10.1017/S1092852919001822

*MTA Cooperative Group. (1999). A 14-month randomized clinical trial of treatment strategies for attention-deficit/hyperactivity disorder. The MTA Cooperative Group. Multimodal Treatment Study of Children with ADHD. *Archives of General Psychiatry, 56*(12), 1073–1086. https://doi.org/10.1001/archpsyc.56.12.1073

CHAPTER 11 ■ OPPOSITIONAL DEFIANT AND CONDUCT DISORDERS

For developing children, the abilities to learn self-control and to modulate aggressive impulses are important developmental tasks. This learning is fostered by the social contexts of the family, school, and peers as well as by the child's own increased capacities for symbolic thinking, appreciation of consequences, and social development. For most children, this process goes forward relatively smoothly as they learn to channel anger and frustration in appropriate ways and acquire the complex norms that govern socially approved forms of aggression such as during various contact sports. However, for some children, this process does not go so smoothly, and emotional and behavioral problems such as inappropriate anger outbursts, physical aggression, and persistent noncompliance may continue throughout childhood and into adulthood.

■ BACKGROUND

Oppositional defiant disorder (ODD) and conduct disorder (CD), sometimes termed *disruptive behavior disorders*, represent a major challenge for society, in general, and the mental health system in particular. In their historical account of CD, Jane Costello and Adrian Angold (2000) traced the questions of defining and dealing with out-of-control children to Greek philosophers and described the major changes in legal, educational, and medical views of this topic. Around the turn of the 19th century, the courts in England and the United States started to recognize that the criminal acts committed by children and adults should be treated differently, and a system of juvenile courts was established. Historically referred to as *juvenile delinquency*, the study of the criminal behavior and antisocial acts of children is more than a century old and still remains an important area for both research and clinical work. One of the earliest medical approaches was advanced from the psychodynamic perspective by August Aichhorn, the author of *Wayward Youth* (Aichhorn, 1935). The psychodynamic approach then dominated the treatment of conduct problems in the child guidance clinics in the United States for several decades. Also starting in the 1930s, developmental trajectories of anger and aggression in typically developing children were described in the work of Florence Goodenough (Goodenough, 1935) and Arnold Gesell (Gesell, 1948). Current standards for diagnosis and treatment of disruptive behavior are based on the recognition that many forms of disruptive behavior are developmentally appropriate. For example, physical aggression is normative during the first 3 years of life and can have a communicative role prior to the emergence of language. This stage is followed by a period of reduction in physical aggression between the ages of 3 and 7 years, which is paralleled by rapid acquisition of language and social–emotional skills, such as empathy and perspective taking. As the frequency of physically aggressive behavior decreases, verbally mediated disruptive behaviors such as argumentativeness and relational aggression can emerge in middle childhood. Then, as with most developmental transitions, adolescence either heralds the acquisition of social competencies that can modulate excessive aggression or sets the stage for the escalation of childhood aggression into juvenile delinquency.

In many, but not all, cases, children with disruptive behavior problems go on to have similar problems in adulthood. Early attempts to understand disruptive behavior led to speculations that such behavior represented a failure in moral development and was potentially genetic. The term *psychopathy* was used by Harvey Cleckley in 1941 to describe individuals without remorse, who had no close relationships and whose inner lives were impoverished (Cleckley, 1941). Interest in children with these difficulties increased in the early 1960s following the work of John Bowlby on early attachments of children. In an important longitudinal study, Lee Robins documented long-term stability of disruptive or "deviant" behaviors from childhood to adulthood (Robins, 1966). Early distinctions within this category had to do with the nature of the conduct problems, such as aggressive (fighting) versus nonaggressive (property destruction) and group versus individual behavior.

The term *conduct disorder* was introduced in the second edition of the *Diagnostic and Statistical Manual* (*DSM-II*) in 1968 to describe a condition in which children persistently violated the rights of others or social rules and norms. The term *oppositional defiant disorder* was introduced 12 years later in *DSM-III* and used for children whose difficulties included problems with authority figures, provocative behavior, negativity, and so forth. ODD and CD share many features, and, historically, ODD was viewed as a developmental precursor to more serious conduct problems. This view has been challenged in more recent longitudinal studies showing that angry mood in childhood can be a risk factor for mood and anxiety disorders in adulthood.

◼ DIAGNOSIS, DEFINITION, AND CLINICAL FEATURES

Current guidelines for the *DSM-5* diagnoses of ODD and CD are listed in Table 11.1. The main feature of ODD is a frequent and persistent angry or irritable mood and argumentative/defiant behavior with parents and other authority figures. The symptoms of ODD can be present in only one setting, most commonly the home. A child may show enough symptoms and be sufficiently impaired in their family functioning to meet criteria for the diagnosis. However, many symptoms of ODD can also be viewed as commonly occurring childhood behaviors so that in order to meet criteria for the disorder, the symptoms must be frequent, impairing, and present for at least 6 months. Severity of ODD can range from mild to moderate to severe, based on the number of settings (such as family, school, and peer groups) where the child's life and functioning are impaired by the ODD symptoms.

Children with CD exhibit a range of persistent behaviors that violate the basic rights of other people or major age-appropriate norms and rules. As can be seen in Table 11.1, these behaviors or symptoms of CD are grouped into four categories: aggression, property damage, deceitfulness or theft, and serious violation of rules. To meet criteria for the disorder, three or more of these symptoms must be present for at least 12 months and cause significant impairment in the child's life and functioning. Conduct problems that may develop into a full-blown disorder can appear as early as the preschool years. In contrast to the normative "terrible twos" for whom negativism and defiance is a passing phase, young children with CD repeatedly lose their tempers, are angry, are readily annoyed by others, and are typically defiant. The signs of ODD usually appear relatively early, with persistent stubbornness by age 3 and temper tantrums by age 5; the signs of CD appear somewhat later (e.g., lying may appear around age 8, bullying by age 9, and stealing by around 12 years of age). Although the

TABLE 11.1

Diagnostic Guidelines for Oppositional Defiant Disorder (ODD) and Conduct Disorder (CD) According to the *Diagnostic and Statistical Manual* (*DSM-5*)

Oppositional Defiant Disorder Symptoms
Angry/Irritable Mood
1. Often loses temper
2. Is often touchy or easily annoyed
3. Is often angry and resentful
Argumentative/Defiant Behavior
4. Argues with adults
5. Actively defies or refuses to comply with adults' requests or rules
6. Deliberately annoys people
7. Blames others for their mistakes or misbehavior
Vindictiveness
8. Spiteful or vindictive

Conduct Disorder Symptoms
Aggression Toward People and Animals
1. Often bullies, threatens, or intimidates others
2. Often initiates physical fights
3. Has used a weapon that can cause serious physical harm to others
4. Has been physically cruel to people
5. Has been physically cruel to animals
6. Has stolen while confronting a victim
7. Has forced someone into sexual activity
Destruction of Property
8. Has deliberately engaged in fire setting with the intention of causing serious damage
9. Has deliberately destroyed other's property (other than by fire setting)
Deceitfulness or Theft
10. Has broken into someone's house, building, or car
11. Often lies to obtain goods or favors or to avoid obligations (cons others)
12. Has stolen items of nontrivial value without confronting a victim
13. Often stays out at night despite parental prohibitions (beginning before age 13 years)
14. Has run away from home overnight at least twice (or once without returning)
15. Often truant from school (beginning before age 13 years)

DSM-5 ODD: Four or more of symptoms from 1 to 8, lasting at least 6 months; symptoms do not occur exclusively during a psychotic or mood disorder episode.
DSM-5 CD: Three or more symptoms in the past 12 months (at least one present in past 6 months).
Symptoms must be developmentally inappropriate in both ODD and CD.
Impairment: Symptoms must cause significant functional impairment.

Adapted with permission from Rey, J. M., Walter, G., & Soutullo, C. (2007). Oppositional defiant and conduct disorders. In A. Martin & F. R. Volkmar (Eds.), *Lewis's child and adolescent psychiatry: A comprehensive textbook* (4th ed., p. 456). Lippincott Williams & Wilkins; & Reprinted from Salmanian, M., Mohammadi, M. R., Keshavarzi, Z., & Brand, S. (2018). An update on the global prevalence of conduct disorder (2011–2017). *Journal of Forensic and Legal Medicine, 59*, 1–3. Copyright © 2018 Elsevier; with permission.

frequency of aggressive behavior tends to decrease before puberty, the risk of injury associated with aggression can increase as children grow and become physically stronger. During adolescence, physically aggressive behavior becomes particularly problematic owing to its potentially harmful impact on both the victims and the perpetrators. Antisocial behaviors such as stealing and truancy also become more prevalent in adolescence. Some children with CD exhibit decreases in problem behaviors over time, although, in general, the symptoms of CD are relatively stable.

Diagnosis of either ODD or CD should rely on information from multiple sources, including children, parents, and teachers to confirm the presence and frequency of symptoms across various contexts. Of note, although anger and irritability are the essential features of ODD, many children who meet criteria for this disorder do not endorse experiencing emotions of anger or frustration with any greater frequency than unaffected children. Instead, children with ODD may perceive others as being annoying or at fault for various problems. Similarly, children with CD may deny any wrongdoing, and clinical diagnosis of CD must rely on history and information from multiple sources. There are also minor differences in diagnoses of ODD and CD in the *DSM-5* and the *International Statistical Classification of Diseases and Related Health Problems* (*ICD-10*). The *ICD-10* and 11 (Salmanian et al., 2018) approach is explicit in suggesting that ODD is a milder form of CD. Similarities in the *DSM-5* and *ICD-10* criteria for diagnoses of disruptive behavior disorders are noteworthy, but differences arise because of requirements for symptom duration and exclusionary features. In addition to categorical approaches, dimensional methods using rating scales and checklists have been used extensively in the study of children with conduct problems. Attempts have also been made to identify specific subtypes of CD. For example, instead of the current approach (of the less severe ODD and the more severe CD), the *DSM-III* subdivided CD into three subtypes depending on the presence or absence of socialization and aggressive behavior (e.g., one subtype was unsocialized aggressive). Another approach in *DSM-III-R* was to distinguish solitary versus group types. In *DSM-IV* and *DSM-5*, there is provision for differentiating childhood versus adolescent onset (American Psychiatric Association, 2013).

The problem of comorbidity is particularly an issue for CD and ODD. Rates of several other disorders are markedly increased in association with these conditions, notably attention-deficit/hyperactivity disorder (ADHD; tenfold increase), major depression (sevenfold increase), and substance abuse (fourfold increase). It remains unclear which of the two (*DSM-5* vs. *ICD-11*) competing diagnostic approaches works best for understanding and documenting co-occurring disorders. Whereas the *DSM-5* encourages multiple diagnoses, the *ICD-11* discourages this practice. As a result, the *ICD-11* provided codes for mixed categories (World Health Organization, 2019–2020). This is not a trivial issue because boys with both ADHD and CD have early onset of problem behaviors and worse outcomes than those with CD alone.

■ EPIDEMIOLOGY AND DEMOGRAPHICS

The prevalence estimates of both ODD and CD vary depending on the study population, diagnostic criteria, assessment instruments, and informants (Moore et al., 2017; Salmanian et al., 2018). Table 11.2 summarizes recent studies using the *DSM-IV* or *DSM-5* diagnostic criteria and reveal generally consistent results, with about 5% of children and adolescents meeting criteria for either one of these conditions in the previous 3–6 months. Regarding sex differences in prevalence rates, ODD and CD rates are increased at least two- to threefold in boys relative to girls. Boys are also more likely to have an earlier age of onset of ODD/CD symptoms, with the incidence rates increasing sharply from ages 4 to 6, leveling off from ages 6 to 8, and then slowly declining from ages 8 to 14. In girls, incidence rates remain low until 11 years of age, followed by a sharp increase from age 11 to a peak at age 14. Epidemiological studies also reveal that ODD is not necessarily more prevalent in children and CD in adolescence; in fact, the prevalence estimates are rather similar in both groups.

The issue of time-related changes (cohort effects) in prevalence is of interest for these disorders given the common perception that children, particularly girls, have more recently exhibited higher rates of OCD and CD. However, the classic Isle of Wight study from the 1960s reported a rate of CD (4.2% in 10- to 11-year-old children) similar to those noted in Table 11.2. Questions about differences across countries and cultures are hard to examine in epidemiological studies, but questionnaire data on delinquent and aggressive behavior have been consistent across countries (Boxes 11.1 and 11.2).

TABLE 11.2

Point Prevalence (Percent) Oppositional Defiant Disorder (ODD) and Conduct Disorder (CD) in Recent Epidemiological Studies

Sample	Oppositional Defiant Disorder					Conduct Disorder				
	Male	Female	Children	Adolescents	Total	Male	Female	Children	Adolescents	Total
3171 Australian children ages 6 to 17 years (Sawyer et al., 2006)	3.1	2.1				4.4	1.6	4.4[a]	2.4[b]	3.0
1420 children from North Carolina ages 9 to 13 years (Costello et al., 2003)			2.0[a]	3.0[b]	2.7	4.2	1.2	2.4[a]	2.7[b]	2.7
10,438 British children ages 5 to 15 years (Ford et al., 2003)	3.2	1.4	2.6[c]	1.4[d]	2.3	2.1	0.8	0.9[c]	3.3[d]	1.5
1886 children ages 4 to 17 years in Puerto Rico (Canino et al., 2004)					2.0					5.5
1251 children ages 7 to 14 years in Brazil (Fleitlich-Bilyk et al., 2004)					3.2					2.2
6150 children, ages 7 to 9 years in Norway (Munkvold et al., 2011)	4.0	1.3	2.7		2.7					
10,148 US adolescents, ages 13 to 17 years (Kessler et al., 2012)				8.3					5.4	
1049 school students, ages 6 to 16 in Spain (Lopez-Villalobos et al., 2014)	6.8	4.3			5.6					
Average across studies	4.7	2.6	2.5	5.3	3.6	3.4	1.2	2.6	4.1	3.0

[a]9–12 years of age.
[b]13–16 years of age.
[c]5–12 years of age.
[d]13–15 years of age.

Adapted with permission from Rey, J. M., Walter, G., & Soutullo, C. (2018). Oppositional defiant and conduct disorders. In A. Martin, M. H. Bloch, & F. R. Volkmar (Eds.), *Lewis's child and adolescent psychiatry: A comprehensive textbook* (5th ed., p. 391). Wolters Kluwer.

BOX 11.1	Case Report: Oppositional Defiant Disorder

Jason, aged 7 years, was brought to the child mental health clinic by his mother with a chief complaint that he was "out of control." Jason was exhibiting frequent (usually daily) temper tantrums, which had been escalating in frequency and duration over the past year. More specifically, Jason would yell and scream when asked to do almost anything that he did not want to do. When his mother insisted in situations that she felt could not be avoided, such as brushing teeth in the morning or going to sleep at night, Jason could also throw things on the floor or stomp his feet or storm away from his mother in anger. The real precipitating event for the visit to the clinic was that, for the first time, his mother was concerned that he might hit her during their most recent argument (although he did not actually do so).

Jason lives in a single-parent household. The youngest of two sons, he has no contact with his father, who left the family when Jason was a baby. Jason has some trouble in school as academic demands have increased. He has only a few friends because he has trouble following rules during games and tolerating the demands of others. His mother works two jobs, and he is left either with various babysitters or in the after-school program because his much older brother also is working, partly to save money for vocational school. His mother reports that developmental milestones were within normal limits, although he spoke "on the late side."

On examination, Jason tends to minimize his troubles and blames his mother and "deadbeat" father for his problems. He often interrupts his mother when present with her. When seen by himself, he is personable and seems to be in a good mood. He denies feelings of depression or anxiety and appears to have adequate language and attentional skills. He and his mother confirm that it is at home where he has the most difficulty.

Comment: As in this case, children with ODD usually present clinically before about age 8 years. It is more typical for problems to be confined to one setting (often the home). Problems tend to be most noteworthy, and parents, other family members, and the child may appear well organized during the clinical interview. As symptoms become more severe, the likelihood of persistence into CD increases.

Adapted from Volkmar, F. R., & Martin, A. (2011). *Essentials of child and adolescent psychiatry* (pp. 123–124). Lippincott Williams & Wilkins.

BOX 11.2	Case Report: Conduct Disorder

Timmy, age 13 years, was brought to the emergency department by the police. He had been truant from school for several days and then ran away from home. This has happened several times during the past year. When contacted by phone, his mother's first comment was, "He is in trouble again." She relates a history of long-standing problems in behavior going back to his first year in school, when he stole some money from a teacher's purse. He has been picked up by the police several times, including once, at age 11, for shoplifting in the local mall.

Timmy is an only child. His mother reports that his early developmental milestones were normal but that he was a fussy and demanding infant "just like his father," whom she has not seen in 10 years. Timmy had special services in school, and the question of attention-deficit disorder was raised in the past, although his mother refused medications for it. His mother indicates that he is now failing school, which she says is

(continued)

not a surprise because "he never goes to class." She mentions that he hangs out with older kids on the street, and she suspects he is starting to "do drugs." His mother also notes that she was referred to child protective services when Timmy was 8 years old but that nothing came of this.

On examination, Timmy is an angry teenager who appears to be going through puberty. He minimizes his troubles and explains that life is better on the street than at home. He reports that school is a "drag" and that he does not want to have any part of it. Although angry and somewhat dismissive of the clinician, his speech is logically organized. He denies substance abuse, but toxicology screen results are positive.

Comment: Timmy exhibits a history with multiple risk factors for CD. In addition, his problems with attention and now with substance abuse are fairly frequent in children with CD. These conduct problems are, compared with many other psychiatric difficulties, some of the most difficult to treat and can be very persistent.

Adapted from Volkmar, F. R., & Martin, A. (2011). *Essentials of child and adolescent psychiatry* (pp. 123–124). Lippincott Williams & Wilkins

ETIOLOGY AND PATHOGENESIS

A host of biological and environmental factors have been implicated in the pathogenesis of ODD and CD (Table 11.3).

Approximately 50% of variability in CD is attributable to environmental factors, including prenatal, perinatal, family, and neighborhood characteristics (Fairchild et al., 2019). Maternal smoking, alcohol and drug use, and exposure to stress during pregnancy are among the most studied risk factors for childhood psychopathology, including CD and ODD. Complications during birth and exposure to early life adversity were linked to earlier onset and a more severe course of CD. Birth complications, early childhood malnutrition, and exposure to neurotoxic elements such as lead have been linked to risk of aggressive behavior, possibly mediated by neurocognitive impairments. CD and ODD are some of the few childhood psychiatric disorders with considerable evidence for family risk factors, including harsh and coercive parenting, corporal punishment, and lack of parental monitoring. Targeting and ameliorating these maladaptive family practices has become the cornerstone of some of the most effective psychosocial treatments for CD (Kazdin, 2005). Lastly, poverty, community violence, and associations with deviant peers constitute broader social risk factors for CD and delinquency. For example, in a recent epidemiological study, Moore and colleagues reported that low socioeconomic status is associated with a 3.5-fold increase in persistent versus adolescent-limited course of CD (Moore et al., 2017). It should be noted, however, that many of these environmental risk factors may not be specific for CD but rather are associated with a range of neurocognitive vulnerabilities for different forms of psychopathology. Research with large samples is needed to elucidate complex interaction among risk factors and among risk and protective factors. What might otherwise be relatively small risks in isolation may act together to multiply risk.

Regarding biological factors, twin studies suggest that approximately 50% of the variance in CD is attributable to genetic factors. A recent review by Salvatore and Dick also reports several genomic regions revealed in the genomewide linkage and association analysis and a small number of candidate genes, such as MAOA, that are associated with CD across different studies (Salvatore & Dick, 2018). Studies of gene–environment interaction also show that genetic predispositions can contribute to selection into higher risk environments and that environmental factors can alter the importance of the contribution of genetic factors to CD. Genetic factors may appear weaker in children coming from supportive environments. To complicate things further, the genetic factors may themselves act to influence the environment.

During the past 20 years, neuroimaging research with children with CD/ODD has also identified numerous brain abnormalities in a distributed network of cortical and subcortical regions (Wong et al., 2019). Compared with typically developing children without conduct problems, children with CD and ODD have been shown to have deficits in emotional processing, affective empathy, decision making, and reinforcement learning (Blair et al., 2018). Functional magnetic resonance studies (fMRI) of emotion processing demonstrate that children with CD/ODD have reduced activation in anterior cingulate, medial prefrontal cortex, as well as ventral striatum and amygdala during tasks that require viewing emotional facial expressions or empathy-eliciting situations. Poor decision making has long been considered a hallmark characteristic of CD and is thought to be based on abnormal neurocognitive processing of the positive and negative consequences of one's actions. To this end, individuals with CD were shown to have reduced activity in the key nodes of the brain reward circuitry, including striatum and ventromedial prefrontal cortex in response to positive consequences such as monetary gains. There is also reduced activity in the insula and dorsomedial prefrontal cortex in response to stimuli that should be avoided. As a result, children with CD may be particularly vulnerable to responding aggressively to frustration as well as engaging in a range of antisocial behaviors that can lead to negative consequences for both the transgressor and the recipient (Alegria et al., 2016).

There is also emerging evidence that prenatal risk factors may selectively affect brain development during childhood and contribute to the risk of disruptive behavior disorders. For example, one study (Sandman et al., 2018) reported that the level of fetal exposure to placental corticotropic-releasing hormone (pCRH), a molecule conveying maternal stress, was associated with brain development. Specifically, the concentration of pCRH at 19 weeks of gestation predicted cortical thinning in the right frontal pole at 6 to 9 years of age, which, in turn, predicted severity of conduct problems.

■ COURSE

Adult antisocial personality disorder is preceded by CD, and the relationship of the two conditions has been well recognized for many years (Pingault et al., 2013). In addition, childhood ODD and CD are associated with a range of other psychiatric difficulties in adulthood, including substance abuse, mood disorders, and psychosis. Other complications include suicide, educational problems, unemployment, and teen pregnancy. It appears that for many individuals, childhood difficulties become entrenched in a cycle of difficulties, leading to progressively less favorable outcomes. In general, the more frequent and severe the behavioral difficulties in childhood, the worse the adult outcome. Fortunately, most adolescents with CD do not go on to develop adult antisocial personality disorders. For reasons that remain unclear, these behaviors often diminish in early adult life. The relationship of childhood ODD to adult difficulties is much less clear, although recent longitudinal studies have shown that the angry/irritable mood cluster of ODD symptoms can be predictive of anxiety and mood disorders in young adults.

Given the societal and clinical significance of these conditions, considerable efforts have been made in the area of prevention (Dodge et al., 2015). It is clear that such efforts must be comprehensive and multifaceted. There are many advantages to prevention, and it is important for mental health professionals to educate policy makers about the wisdom of investing in prevention efforts. The behavioral problems associated with ODD and CD cannot be viewed in isolation. Rather, they must be addressed systematically in the context of the families, schools, and communities where they occur. Schools have a particularly important role in prevention. As noted in Table 11.3, there are many areas of potential preventive efforts. More research on prevention is needed, but the available data suggest that there is potential for improved child functioning. Many of the treatments already used can be adapted for preventive purposes.

TABLE 11.3

Summary of Factors Associated with the Development of Disruptive Behavior Disorders and Opportunities for Prevention

Risk Factor	Potential Prevention Interventions
Biological • Genetic • Low birth weight • Antenatal and perinatal complications • Brain injury, brain disease • Male sex	• Improved antenatal, prenatal, and obstetric care • Smoking cessation and drug treatment programs for parents • Programs to reduce domestic violence
Individual • Neurocognitive deficits • Difficult temperament • Emotion dysregulation • Impulsivity and hyperactivity • Attentional problems • Academic problems	• Early identification and adequate support and services for families • Quality home visiting programs that aim to facilitate attachment and enhance parenting skills • Parent management training programs • Head Start-type programs • Early speech and reading remediation programs
Family • Parental antisocial behavior or substance use • Domestic violence • Single parent, divorce • Harsh discipline, maltreatment, or neglect • Parent–child conflict • Lack of parental supervision • Excessive parental control • Maternal depression and anxiety • Early motherhood	• Quality home visitation programs • Parent management training programs • Programs to reduce domestic violence • Drug treatment programs • Child protection initiatives • Early identification and treatment of maternal depression • Prevention of teenage pregnancy • Support programs for teenage mothers
Social • Poverty • Association with deviant peers or siblings • Rejection by peers • History of victimization or of being bullied • Disorganized, disadvantaged, or high-crime neighborhoods • Dysfunctional or disorganized schools • Intense exposure to media violence	• Measures to reduce poverty and provide a social "safety net" • Enhance the quality of schools • School programs to reduce bullying and prevent behavior problems • Initiatives to reduce access to firearms and gang activities • Programs to reduce school truancy • Initiatives to enhance neighborhood cohesion • Law enforcement initiatives to reduce crime targeted at high-crime areas • Public campaigns to reduce media violence and education about how to monitor and prevent children's exposure to it

Adapted with permission from Rey, J. M., Walter, G., & Soutullo, C. (2018). Oppositional defiant and conduct disorders. In A. Martin, M. H. Bloch, & F. R. Volkmar (Eds.), *Lewis's child and adolescent psychiatry: A comprehensive textbook* (5th ed., p. 393). Wolters Kluwer.

■ DIFFERENTIAL DIAGNOSIS AND ASSESSMENT

Clinicians should be careful to use multiple sources of information and relevant questionnaires and other data in making the diagnosis of ODD or CD (Masi et al., 2018; Rey et al., 2018). Requests for assessment may come from a wide range of persons, including parents, teachers, and juvenile justice or social service agencies. It is important to clarify the purpose of the assessment and be sure that it is understood by the child or adolescent. As a group, children and adolescents with disruptive behavior disorders can be difficult to interview given their lack of compliance with authority figures and the tendency to minimize their own difficulties. Often, referral comes only after years of struggles at home or in school. It is also common to have conflicting reports from children, parents, and teachers.

Clinical evaluation of potential etiological risk factors (e.g., psychosocial adversity, parent–child problems, maternal depression, abuse) should also be conducted as part of diagnostic assessment. Information on the child's relationship with their parents and peers is important. Learning difficulties of particular profiles of neurocognitive abilities should be carefully considered because these may present special problems for diagnosis. A diagnosis of CD is not made if the difficulties are simply an understandable reaction to a problematic situation (e.g., in some situations such as high-crime areas); these behaviors may be protective and not necessarily indicative of psychopathology. It is important that the clinician keep the possibility of comorbidity in mind in assessing children and adolescents with delinquent or disruptive behaviors. As noted previously, frequent disorders also observed include ADHD, depression, substance abuse, and anxiety. Children on the autism spectrum may experience challenging behaviors, including aggression, and may run into trouble with the law often because, paradoxically, they are too rigid and rule governed or because of some isolated special interest and poor social judgment. Occasionally, a child or adolescent with an acute psychotic episode may present with a major violation of social or societal norms or a crime of violence. Similarly, individuals with bipolar disorder have high rates of behavioral difficulties. The issue of comorbid CD or ODD and bipolar disorder in prepubertal children remains very controversial. Some children with major depression or anxiety may be irritable or noncompliant. A host of norm-referenced behavioral rating scales are available for use by different informants in evaluating children with ODD or CD. Some of the best and widely used include the Achenbach System of Empirically Based Assessment (ASEBA) (Achenbach & Rescorla, 2001), the Behavioral Assessment System for Children, 3rd edition (BASC-3) (Reynolds & Kamphaus, 2004), and Strength and Difficulties Questionnaire (Goodman, 2001). The evaluation of the child or adolescent should include a careful medical history, review of educational records, and so forth. Apart from drug toxicology screens in adolescents, routine laboratory studies are not generally indicated. Occasionally, children with seizures may present with unusual behavior. Screening for sexually transmitted diseases is indicated if the child has been sexually active or sexually abused.

■ TREATMENT

Many different approaches have been used in the treatment of children with ODD or CD (Robb et al., 2020; Sukhodolsky et al., 2016). These include psychological, behavioral, and pharmacological approaches, sometimes alone but often in combination. Both the child and family may be involved in the treatment. Research on effective interventions has been increasing over the past decade, and there is more support for some treatment approaches than the other. The quality of research support of treatments for ODD/CD depends on study design, sample size, quality of outcome measure, and other clinical research characteristics that may affect the quality of research studies. As with treatments for most psychiatric disorders, fidelity to the treatment model outside the academic centers can also be problematic.

ODD and CD tend to be chronic conditions. Typically, psychosocial interventions are used initially and then continued even if medications are added. Intervening early in the disorder may be more effective (i.e., before symptom patterns are well established). Treatment should also typically involve parents and thoughtful attention to any comorbid conditions (e.g., ADHD, depression). Goals of treatment should be realistic and progressive; for example, preventing escalation or a move to another phase of difficulty, such as substance abuse, may be important as a first step in the treatment process. Attention should also be paid to school and peer groups; facilitating appropriate participation with typical peers is important.

Interestingly, children and adolescents with CD and ODD commonly present to emergency departments after a legal, parental, school, or some other crisis. Often, this has led to aggressive behavior and problems with others or destruction of property. Children who present to the emergency department with such problems are more likely to have more severe difficulties or comorbid disorders. The differentiation of ODD from CD can be difficult but usually is less relevant in the emergency situations. Crisis intervention and psychosocial interventions should be attempted before use of medications. Restraint or seclusion should be used only as a last resort.

Table 11.4 summarizes evidence for treatment efficacy in children with ODD and CD.

Parent training (PT) for disruptive behavior disorders uses positive reinforcement and aspects of social-learning theory and operant conditioning and is the most extensively researched treatment for these conditions. This method helps parents use positive reinforcement to elicit and maintain more productive child behaviors. It can produce significant improvement in both the home and school, with indirect effects in other areas such as relationships with siblings and marital satisfaction. PT has been used more in younger children, and most research on parent training for ODD has been conducted in children from ages 3 to 8 years. But parenting interventions are also essential in treatment of conduct problems in older children and adolescence, particularly in combinations with other behavioral approaches and medication in more serious forms of the disorder.

Cognitive-behavioral therapy (CBT) is another evidence-based, psychosocial treatment for childhood disruptive behavior. This treatment is conducted mostly with the child, and the goal is to teach children better strategies for regulating emotional responses to frustration as well as problem-solving skills for interpersonal conflicts. As part of treatment, children discuss situations that trigger their anger or their conflicts with parents, teachers, or peers with the therapist and then identify and role-play strategies to avoid these triggers. CBT usually consists of 12–15 sessions that are conducted in a structured yet flexible format. Adaptive therapeutic techniques and activities are directed at reducing anger outbursts and aggressive behavior. Parents are also active participants in treatment, and they learn how to reward their child's calm responses to potentially frustrating events with praise, attention, and privileges in dedicated parenting sessions. CBT has been used in a variety of settings, including schools, and as part of violence prevention interventions for children at risk for greater levels of conduct problems (Sukhodolsky & Scahill, 2012).

Multimodal interventions may augment PT and CBT in situations that require more intensive treatments or for children with specific risk factors such as academic or community problems. Sample programs include multisystemic therapy (MST) and Families and Schools Together (FAST program) (Sukhodolsky & Ruchkin, 2006). MST has been developed for adolescents with more severe conduct problems who are at risk for becoming involved with the juvenile justice system. The FAST program focuses on children with CD starting school; interventions under this program are designed to prevent worsened functioning. The MST approach is intensive with a home-based approach 7 days a week for about 4 months. This resource-intensive program appears to be cost effective. Yet another approach is to place teens in special foster care programs. These relatively short (6-month) placements may reduce subsequent criminality. Various other programs, including residential treatments and intensive wilderness or "boot camp"-type programs have not been well evaluated for treatment or prevention of conduct problems. Overall, psychosocial interventions that are focused on improving family functioning, strengthening emotion-regulation and problem-solving skills, and building positive ties within the community are most likely to benefit children with ODD/CD and their families.

TABLE 11.4

Summary of Treatments for Oppositional Defiant and Conduct Disorders

Treatment	Strength of Recommendation[a]	Quality of Evidence[b]	Comments
Psychosocial			
Parent training	***	A	Best research in young children, limited empirical data for adolescents
Cognitive-behavioral therapy	***	A	Best tested for children with moderate severity of disruptive behavior
Multisystemic therapy	**	A	Usually targets severely disordered or delinquent youth, resource intensive
FAST Track	*	B	Children starting school
Problem-solving skills training	*	B	Currently used as part of multi-component CBT interventions for anger and aggression
Therapeutic foster care	*	B	Can be used with severely conduct disordered or delinquent youth who do not respond well to other treatments
Wilderness programs, boot camps, and similar programs	#	C	Usually target severely disordered or delinquent youth. No clear research support for effectiveness
Pharmacological			
Antipsychotic drugs	**	A	Good short-term results with risperidone for children with aggressive behavior
Mood stabilizers and anticonvulsants	*	B	Heterogeneous participants (e.g., aggressive adolescents, CD with various comorbidities); inconsistent results; somewhat better data for lithium
Stimulants	#	B−	In children with comorbid ADHD
Atomoxetine	#	B−	In children with comorbid ADHD
Clonidine	#	B−	In children with comorbid ADHD
SSRIs	#	E	In children with comorbid major depression

[a]*** (good supporting evidence) through # (uncertain evidence).
[b]A (supported by meta-analysis of several, sound, randomized controlled trials) through C (systematic open studies) to E (expert opinion).
ADHD, attention-deficit/hyperactivity disorder; CD, conduct disorder; FAST, Families and Schools Together; SSRI, selective serotonin reuptake inhibitor.
Adapted from Rey, J. M., Walter, G., & Soutullo, C. (2018). Oppositional defiant and conduct disorders. In A. Martin, M. H. Bloch, & F. R. Volkmar (Eds.), *Lewis's child and adolescent psychiatry: A comprehensive textbook* (5th ed., p. 462). Wolters Kluwer.

Drug treatments are used only when other interventions fail and as part of an overall, comprehensive program (e.g., for children with other comorbid conditions such as ADHD). Pharmacotherapy should be cautious with careful monitoring. The risk of substance abuse suggests considerable care in prescribing stimulants to adolescents with CD. It is important to ensure adequate trials of medication and to avoid polypharmacy. The strength of evidence for drug treatments in summarized in Table 11.4. Frequently used medications include atypical neuroleptics such as risperidone, which may have a short-term benefit but can be associated with side effects such as weight gain and metabolic abnormalities. Mood-stabilizing medications have also been used, with less consistent results. Disruptive behavior in children with ADHD has been shown to have responded to adequate doses of stimulant medication.

■ SUMMARY

Conduct problems and oppositional behavior are important clinical and societal problems. CD, unfortunately, can be one of the most persistent childhood psychiatric diagnoses. A minority of individuals will go on to have overt antisocial personality disorder. Even for those who do not, there may be continuing difficulties both in social relationships and work settings. Although many treatments have been proposed, rigorous study of these treatments has been less common. Efforts at prevention, through many different modalities, remain important.

References

*Indicates Particularly Recommended

Achenbach, T. M., & Rescorla, L. A. (2001). *Manual for the ASEBA school-age forms & profiles.* University of Vermont, Research Center for Children, Youth, and Families.

Aichhorn, A. (1935). *Wayward youth.* Viking Press.

Alegria, A. A., Radua, J., & Rubia, K. (2016). Meta-analysis of fMRI studies of disruptive behavior disorders. *American Journal of Psychiatry, 173*(11), 1119–1130. https://doi.org/10.1176/appi .ajp.2016.15081089

American Psychiatric Association. (2013). *Diagnostic and statistical manual of mental disorders (DSM-5)* (5th ed.). American Psychiatric Publishing.

*Blair, R., Veroude, K., & Buitelaar, J. (2018). Neuro-cognitive system dysfunction and symptom sets: A review of fMRI studies in youth with conduct problems. *Neuroscience & Biobehavioral Reviews, 91,* 69–90.

Canino, G., Shrout, P. E., Rubio-Stipec, M., Bird, H. R., Bravo, M., Ramírez, R., Chavez, L., Alegría, M., Bauermeister, J. J., Hohmann, A., Ribera, J., García, P., & Martínez-Taboas, A. (2004). The *DSM-IV* rates of child and adolescent disorders in Puerto Rico: Prevalence, correlates, service use, and the effects of impairment. *Archives of general psychiatry, 61*(1), 85–93. https://doi.org/10.1001/archpsyc.61.1.85

Cleckley, H. (1941). *The masc of sanity: An attempt to clarify some issues about so-called psychopathic personality.* Mosby.

*Costello, E. J., & Angold, A. (2000). Bad behavior: An historical perspective on disorders of conduct. In J. Hill & B. Maughan (Eds.), *Conduct disorders in childhood and adolescence* (pp. 1–31). Cambridge University Press.

Costello, E. J., Mustillo, S., Erkanli, A., Keeler, G., & Angold, A. (2003). Prevalence and development of psychiatric disorders in childhood and adolescence. *Archives of General Psychiatry, 60*(8), 837–844. https://doi.org/10.1001/archpsyc.60.8.837

Dodge, K. A., Bierman, K. L., Coie, J. D., Greenberg, M. T., Lochman, J. E., McMahon, R. J., & Pinderhughes, E. E. (2015). Impact of early intervention on psychopathology, crime, and well-being at age 25. *American Journal of Psychiatry, 172*(1), 59–70. https://doi.org/10.1176/appi.ajp.2014.13060786

*Fairchild, G., Hawes, D. J., Frick, P. J., Copeland, W. E., Odgers, C. L., Franke, B., Freitag, C. M., & De Brito, S. A. (2019). Conduct disorder. *Nature Reviews Disease Primers, 5*(1), 43. https://doi .org/10.1038/s41572-019-0095-y

Fleitlich-Bilyk, B., & Goodman, R. (2004). Prevalence of child and adolescent psychiatric disorders in Southeast Brazil. *Journal of the American Academy of Child and Adolescent Psychiatry, 43*(6), 727–734. https://doi.org/10.1097/01.chi.0000120021.14101.ca

Ford, T., Goodman, R., & Meltzer, H. (2003). The British child and adolescent mental health survey 1999: The prevalence of *DSM-IV* disorders. *Journal of the American Academy of Child and Adolescent Psychiatry, 42*(10), 1203–1211. https://doi.org/10.1097/00004583-200310000-00011

Gesell, A. (1948). *Studies in child development.* Harper.

Goodenough, F. L. (1935). *Anger in young children.* The University of Minnesota Press.

Goodman, R. (2001). Psychometric properties of the strengths and difficulties questionnaire. *Journal of the American Academy of Child and Adolescent Psychiatry, 40*(11), 1337–1345. https://doi .org/10.1097/00004583-200111000-00015

Kazdin, A. E. (2005). *Parent management training: Treatment for oppositional, aggressive, and antisocial behavior in children and adolescents.* Oxford University Press.

Kessler, R. C., Avenevoli, S., McLaughlin, K. A., Green, J. G., Lakoma, M. D., Petukhova, M., Pine, D. S., Sampson, N. A., Zaslavsky, A. M., & Merikangas, K. R. (2012). Lifetime co-morbidity of *DSM-IV* disorders in the US National Comorbidity Survey Replication Adolescent Supplement (NCS-A). *Psychological Medicine, 42*(9), 1997–2010. http://www.scopus.com/inward/record .url?eid=2-s2.0-84864533614&partnerID=40&md5=a5dfd6da52a3300bc819d9bbf1a0bdb0

López-Villalobos, J. A., Andrés-De Llano, J. M., Rodríguez-Molinero, L., Garrido-Redondo, M., Sacristán-Martín, A. M., Martínez-Rivera, M. T., Alberola-López, S., & Sánchez-Azón, M. I. (2014). Prevalence of oppositional defiant disorder in Spain. *Revista de Psiquiatria Salud Mental, 7*(2), 80–87. https://doi .org/10.1016/j.rpsm.2013.07.002

Masi, G., Milone, A., Brovedani, P., Pisano, S., & Muratori, P. (2018). Psychiatric evaluation of youths with disruptive behavior disorders and psychopathic traits: A critical review of assessment measures. *Neuroscience and Biobehavioral Reviews, 91,* 21–33. https://doi.org/10.1016/j.neubiorev.2016.09.023

Moore, A. A., Silberg, J. L., Roberson-Nay, R., & Mezuk, B. (2017). Life course persistent and adolescence limited conduct disorder in a nationally representative US sample: Prevalence, predictors, and outcomes. *Social Psychiatry and Psychiatric Epidemiology, 52*(4), 435–443. https://doi.org/10.1007/ s00127-017-1337-5

Munkvold, L. H., Lundervold, A. J., & Manger, T. (2011). Oppositional defiant disorder-gender differences in co-occurring symptoms of mental health problems in a general population of children. *Journal of Abnormal Child Psychology, 39*(4), 577–587. https://doi.org/10.1007/s10802-011-9486-6

Pingault, J. B., Côté, S. M., Lacourse, E., Galéra, C., Vitaro, F., & Tremblay, R. E. (2013). Childhood hyperactivity, physical aggression and criminality: A 19-year prospective population-based study. *PLoS One, 8*(5), e62594. https://doi.org/10.1371/journal.pone.0062594

Rey, J. M., Walter, G., & Soutullo, C. (2018). Oppositional defiant and conduct disorders. In A. Martin, M. H. Bloch, & F. R. Volkmar (Eds.), *Lewis's child and adolescent psychiatry: A comprehensive textbook* (5th ed., pp. 388–398). Lippincott Williams & Wilkins.

Reynolds, C. R., & Kamphaus, R. W. (2004). *BASC-2: Behavior assessment system for children.* AGS Publishing.

*Robb, A. S., Connor, D. F., Amann, B. H., Vitiello, B., Nasser, A., O'Neal, W., Schwabe, S., Ceresoli-Borroni, G., Newcorn, J. H., Candler, S. A., Buitelaar, J. K., & Findling, R. L. (2020). Closing the gap: Unmet needs of individuals with impulsive aggressive behavior observed in children and adolescents. *CNS Spectrums,* 1–9. https://doi.org/10.1017/S1092852920001224

Robins, L. (1966). *Deviant children grown up.* Williams & Wilkins.

Salmanian, M., Mohammadi, M. R., Keshavarzi, Z., & Brand, S. (2018). An update on the global prevalence of conduct disorder (2011–2017). *Journal of Forensic and Legal Medicine, 59,* 1–3. https:// doi.org/10.1016/j.jflm.2018.07.008

Salvatore, J. E., & Dick, D. M. (2018). Genetic influences on conduct disorder. *Neuroscience and Biobehavioral Reviews, 91,* 91–101. https://doi.org/10.1016/j.neubiorev.2016.06.034

Sandman, C. A., Curran, M. M., Davis, E. P., Glynn, L. M., Head, K., & Baram, T. Z. (2018). Cortical thinning and neuropsychiatric outcomes in children exposed to prenatal adversity: A role for placental CRH? *American Journal of Psychiatry, 175*(5), 471–479. https://doi.org/10.1176/appi .ajp.2017.16121433

Sawyer, M. G., Arney, F. M., Baghurst, P. A., Clark, J. J., Graetz, B. W., Kosky, R. J., Nurcombe, B., Patton, G. C., Prior, M. R., Raphael, B., Rey, J. M., Whaites, L. C., & Zubrick, S. R. (2001). The mental health of young people in Australia: Key findings from the child and adolescent component of the national survey of mental health and well-being. *Australian and New Zealand Journal of Psychiatry, 35*(6), 806–814. https://doi.org/10.1046/j.1440-1614.2001.00964.x

Sukhodolsky, D. G., & Ruchkin, V. (2006). Evidence-based psychosocial treatments in the juvenile justice system. *Child and Adolescent Psychiatric Clinics of North America, 15*(2), 501–516. https://doi .org/10.1016/j.chc.2005.11.005

*Sukhodolsky, D. G., & Scahill, L. (2012). *Cognitive-behavioral therapy for anger and aggression in children.* Guilford Press.

Sukhodolsky, D. G., Smith, S. D., McCauley, S. A., Ibrahim, K., & Piasecka, J. B. (2016). Behavioral interventions for anger, irritability, and aggression in children and adolescents. *Journal of Child and Adolescent Psychopharmacology*, 26(1), 58–64. https://doi.org/10.1089/cap.2015.0120

Wong, T. Y., Sid, A., Wensing, T., Eickhoff, S. B., Habel, U., Gur, R. C., & Nickl-Jockschat, T. (2019). Neural networks of aggression: ALE meta-analyses on trait and elicited aggression. *Brain Structure and Function*, 224(1), 133–148. https://doi.org/10.1007/s00429-018-1765-3

World Health Organization. (2019–2020). *International classification of diseases* (11th rev. ed.). https://www.who.int/classifications/icd/en/

Suggested Readings

Blair, R. J., Leibenluft, E., & Pine, D. S. (2015). Conduct disorder and callous-unemotional traits in youth. *The New England Journal of Medicine*, 372(8), 784. https://doi.org/10.1056/NEJMc1415936

Burke, J. D., Rowe, R., & Boylan, K. (2014). Functional outcomes of child and adolescent oppositional defiant disorder symptoms in young adult men. *Journal of Child Psychology and Psychiatry*, 55(3), 264–272. https://doi.org/10.1111/jcpp.12150

Carlisi, C. O., Moffitt, T. E., Knodt, A. R., Harrington, H., Ireland, D., Melzer, T. R., Poulton, R., Ramrakha, S., Caspi, A., Hariri, A. R., & Viding, E. (2020). Associations between life-course-persistent antisocial behaviour and brain structure in a population-representative longitudinal birth cohort. *The Lancet Psychiatry*, 7(3), 245–253. https://doi.org/10.1016/S2215-0366(20)30002-X

Caspi, A., McCray, J., Moffitt, T. E., Mill, J., Martin, J., Craig, I. W., Taylor, A., & Poulton, R. (2002). Role of genotype in the cycle of violence in maltreated children. *Science*, 297(5582), 851–854. https://doi.org/10.1126/science.1072290

Connor, D. F. (2015). Pharmacological management of pediatric patients with comorbid attention-deficit hyperactivity disorder oppositional defiant disorder. *Pediatric Drugs*, 17(5), 361–371. https://doi.org/10.1007/s40272-015-0143-3

de la Osa, N., Granero, R., Domenech, J. M., Shamay-Tsoory, S., & Ezpeleta, L. (2016). Cognitive and affective components of theory of mind in preschoolers with oppositional defiance disorder. *Psychiatry Research*, 241, 128–134. https://doi.org/10.1016/j.psychres.2016.04.082

Demmer, D. H., Hooley, M., Sheen, J., McGillivray, J. A., & Lum, J. A. G. (2017). Sex differences in the prevalence of oppositional defiant disorder during middle childhood: A meta-analysis. *Journal of Abnormal Child Psychology*, 45(2), 313–325. https://doi.org/10.1007/s10802-016-0170-8

Evans, S. C., Roberts, M. C., Keeley, J. W., Rebello, T. J., de la Peña, F., Lochman, J. E., Burke, J. D., Fite, P. J., Ezpeleta, L., Matthys, W., Youngstrom, E. A., Matsumoto, C., Andrews, H. F., Elena Medina-Mora, M., Ayuso-Mateos, J. L., Khoury, B., Kulygina, M., Robles, R., Sharan, P., … Reed, G. M. (2021). Diagnostic classification of irritability and oppositionality in youth: A global field study comparing *ICD-11* with *ICD-10* and *DSM-5*. *Journal of Child Psychology and Psychiatry*, 62(3), 303–312. https://doi.org/10.1111/jcpp.13244

Ezpeleta, L., Navarro, J. B., De La Osa, N., Penelo, E., & Domènech, J. M. (2019). First incidence, age of onset outcomes and risk factors of onset of *DSM-5* oppositional defiant disorder: A cohort study of Spanish children from ages 3 to 9. *BMJ Open*, 9(3), e022493. https://doi.org/10.1136/bmjopen-2018-022493

Kim-Cohen, J., Caspi, A., Rutter, M., Tomas, M. P., & Moffitt, T. E. (2006). The caregiving environments provided to children by depressed mothers with or without an antisocial history. *American Journal of Psychiatry*, 163(6), 1009–1018. http://ajp.psychiatryonline.org/cgi/content/abstract/163/6/1009

Moffitt, T. E. (2018). Male antisocial behaviour in adolescence and beyond. *Nature Human Behavior*, 2(3), 177–186. https://doi.org/10.1038/s41562-018-0309-4

Sukhodolsky, D. G., Kassinove, H., & Gorman, B. S. (2004). Cognitive-behavioral therapy for anger in children and adolescents: A meta-analysis. *Aggression & Violent Behavior*, 9(3), 247–269. https://doi.org/10.1016/j.avb.2003.08.005

Szentiványi, D., & Balázs, J. (2018). Quality of life in children and adolescents with symptoms or diagnosis of conduct disorder or oppositional defiant disorder. *Mental Health and Prevention*, 10, 1–8. https://doi.org/10.1016/j.mhp.2018.02.001

CHAPTER 12 ■ ANXIETY DISORDERS

■ BACKGROUND

Human beings, like all other organisms, are equipped with systems for the detection of potentially harmful stimuli and for differentiating between that which is harmful and that which is necessary or rewarding. The anxiety system is a critical system that serves to promote the avoidance of risks and harm and is an important part of healthy development. When activated, anxiety impacts the various aspects of functioning, including changes to physiological functioning, cognitive functioning, emotions, and behavior. In concert, these changes can promote avoidance of risk, both imminent and more distal, and help to keep the individual safe and healthy. Risks that can trigger anxiety include not only the risk of physical harm but also psychological risks such as the risk of social humiliation and emotional distress.

Psychopathology, in the context of anxiety, occurs when the anxiety system is chronically and excessively triggered in situations that do not pose a realistic threat to the individual and when regulation of the anxiety system is impaired.

■ DIAGNOSIS, DEFINITION, AND CLINICAL FEATURES

Classification of anxiety problems into discrete diagnostic categories has evolved steadily with each successive iteration of the *Diagnostic and Statistical Manual of Mental Disorders (DSM)*, with some of the most significant changes occurring specifically in relation to the developmental psychopathology of anxiety.

DSM-III recognized three "phobic disorders" (agoraphobia [with and without panic attacks], social phobia, and "simple" phobias), panic disorder, generalized anxiety disorder, and "atypical" anxiety disorder. Also included among the anxiety disorders in *DSM-III* and *DSM-IV* was obsessive compulsive disorder. Additionally, *DSM-III* classified three anxiety disorders as commonly arising during childhood or adolescence: separation anxiety disorder, shyness disorder, and overanxious disorder.

Subsequent versions of *DSM* have refined and added to these nosological categories, leading up to the present *DSM-5* classification, which includes the following anxiety disorders: separation anxiety disorder, selective mutism, specific phobia, social anxiety disorder (social phobia), panic disorder, agoraphobia, generalized anxiety disorder, and illness anxiety disorder (which is grouped along with other somatic symptom disorders, rather than with the other anxiety disorders). *DSM-5* also recognizes substance or medication-induced anxiety disorder, anxiety disorder attributable to another medical condition, and unspecified anxiety disorder. A brief overview of the central features of the anxiety disorders follows and is summarized in Table 12.1. All the *DSM-5* anxiety disorders require that the problem be associated with significant impairment in psychosocial functioning in the domains of social relations, school and academic behavior, family functioning, or another significant area.

■ *Separation anxiety disorder*: Separation anxiety is the most frequent anxiety problem in young children but can occur at any point in development (Shear et al., 2006). It is characterized by developmentally inappropriate and impairing fear or anxiety about being separated from caregivers and other attachment figures and by excessive worry about losing them or about coming to harm during a separation (American Psychiatric Association, 2013). Children with separation anxiety disorder exhibit reluctance to separate or be separated, often insist on sleeping together with caregivers, and frequently have nightmares involving the theme of separation.

■ *Selective mutism:* Selective mutism is the consistent failure to speak in certain social situations where speech is expected, despite being able to speak in other situations (American Psychiatric Association, 2013).

■ *Specific phobia:* Specific phobias are strong fears of particular objects or situations that are excessive or exaggerated in relation to the actual risk these objects or situations pose (American Psychiatric Association, 2013). A child with a specific phobia will almost invariably seek to avoid the feared object or situation or will endure them only with significant fear and distress. In many cases, a child will meet criteria for multiple specific phobias, of different objects or situations. Common phobias include heights, dark, animals

TABLE 12.1

DSM-5 Anxiety Disorders and Key Characteristics

DSM-5 Anxiety Disorder	Key Characteristics
Separation Anxiety Disorder	• Developmentally inappropriate fear of being separated from caregivers • Nightmares with the theme of separation are common
Selective Mutism	• Consistent failure to speak in certain situations • The child is able to speak in other situations
Specific Phobia	• Strong, exaggerated fear of specific objects or situations • The child almost always seeks to avoid contact with the phobic object
Social Anxiety Disorder	• Fear of negative evaluation by others and avoidance of situations with the potential for social evaluation • Can be specific to performance situations only • Does not denote a lack of social interest, although social contact can be consistently avoided
Panic Disorder	• Recurring panic attacks lead to persistent worry about additional panic attacks • Cued panic attacks (that occur with a clearly identifiable trigger) are not symptoms of panic disorder
Agoraphobia	• Fear and avoidance of situations from which escape may be difficult in the event of developing panic-like symptoms
Generalized Anxiety Disorder	• Persistent worry that is difficult to control • The worry can impact sleep, attention, and mood
Illness Anxiety Disorder	• Preoccupation with becoming seriously ill • The worry is not aligned with actual health or risk of illness

or insects, and needles or blood, but any object can be the focus of a child's phobia. In children, in particular, the fear response may take the form of clinging to parents or having temper tantrums rather than of behaviors that more obviously denote fear.

■ *Social anxiety disorder (social phobia):* Social anxiety disorder involves persistent fear or anxiety relating to social situations that present the opportunity for real or perceived evaluation by others (American Psychiatric Association, 2013). Children with social phobia fear that they will be negatively evaluated for their performance or behavior and may fear that their anxious expression itself will contribute to this negative evaluation. For example, a child with social phobia may fear being ridiculed for blushing or stammering because of the anxiety. Social phobia leads to avoidance of social situations and interactions but does not reflect a lack of social interest in children. In most cases, children with social phobia will fear a broad range of social-evaluative situations, but in some cases the fear may be focused only on situations that involve actual performance, such as public speaking in front of an audience or classroom. Of note for developmental psychopathology, the anxiety must extend to situations that involve peers, rather than being limited to interactions with adults alone. Also of note in the context of children, shyness is a common trait in developing youth and does not necessarily indicate the presence of social phobia. Only a minority of shy children will meet the diagnostic criteria for social phobia.

■ *Panic disorder:* Panic disorder occurs when a child experiences recurring and unexpected panic attacks and becomes persistently concerned about the possibility of experiencing additional attacks in the future, usually leading to behavioral changes in the child (American Psychiatric Association, 2013). Panic attacks are brief but intense surges in fear or anxiety and are considered unexpected when they occur "out of the blue" in the absence of a clear trigger or stimulus. Panic attacks that occur in the context of a clearly identifiable trigger, for example during an encounter with a phobic object, are not symptoms of panic disorder but rather of the specific phobia. This distinction is important because all anxiety disorders can be accompanied by panic attacks, and panic disorder is diagnosed only in the context of unexpected panic attacks.

■ *Agoraphobia:* Agoraphobia is persistent anxiety and/or avoidance of situations owing to fears about not being able to easily escape the situation or to receive help in the event of developing panic-like or other incapacitating symptoms (American Psychiatric Association, 2013). Children with agoraphobia fear situations such as public transportation, open or enclosed spaces, crowds, or being alone outside of the home. In contrast to previous iterations of *DSM*, under *DSM-5* agoraphobia is diagnosed separately and irrespectively of the presence of panic disorder. Even a child who has not experienced panic attacks in the past may meet criteria for a diagnosis of agoraphobia. The avoidance of feared situations in agoraphobia can lead to highly impairing isolation and to difficulty functioning outside of the home, including school attendance.

■ *Generalized anxiety disorder:* Generalized anxiety disorder is excessive and persistent worry that is difficult to control and that adversely impacts the child's physical or psychological functioning (American Psychiatric Association, 2013). Children with generalized anxiety disorder may have difficulty sleeping at night, may become overly tired and have difficulty with attention and concentration, and may become restless and irritable. Although less common in preadolescent children than phobias and separation anxiety, generalized anxiety, and symptoms of generalized anxiety disorder, can occur even in young children.

■ *Illness anxiety disorder:* Although not grouped with the other anxiety disorders, illness anxiety disorder is an anxiety disorder in which the core diagnostic criteria center on excessive and impairing anxiety and worry (American Psychiatric Association, 2013). Illness anxiety disorder is persistent preoccupation with, and worry about, becoming seriously ill. The anxiety is not aligned with the child's actual health and risks. Somatic symptoms, such as chronic aches and pains or gastrointestinal distress, may be present but are of only mild intensity. Children with illness anxiety disorder become easily alarmed about their health and may engage in checking behaviors or may seek to avoid contact with doctors because of their fears. Children may also seek excessive reassurance from their parents about their health or help in accessing unnecessary medical examinations (Box 12.1).

| **BOX 12.1** | **Case of Separation Anxiety Disorder** |

Tommy, a 6 ½-year-old boy, was referred by his family physician because of a long-standing pattern of shyness and inhibition that had become dramatically worse on his entering school. He expressed fear that his mother would be harmed or become ill and several times had come home early from school or had tremendous difficulty separating from his mother at the start of school. His mother had a history of anxiety-related difficulties as a child and even at present described herself as rather like Tommy with many worries and concerns about the future.

When left at school, Tommy would quickly begin to complain of headaches or gastrointestinal (GI) upset. He often left the class to go to the nurse's office because he felt nausea and was afraid he would vomit in the classroom. It was a struggle for his mother to drop him off at school in the morning—he would be reluctant to bring his backpack, would lose his lunch, and would become upset on leaving the car. Tommy had never been willing to take the bus with other children on his street.

His teacher reported that when he was in school and working, his academic abilities appeared to be at age level. She was, however, concerned that his degree of difficulty with separation and his numerous physical complaints were taking a toll on his peer relationships and would eventually also impact his academic progress.

His mother noted that Tommy had a long history of anxiety-related difficulties, falling asleep only when one his parents (usually his mother) was in bed with him. He often woke during the night and would come into his parents' bed complaining of nightmares.

Although he would play with children in the neighborhood, Tommy wanted his mother to stay around, and he refused to join a soccer club because of fear of the separation it would cause. His parents also had difficulty leaving him with a babysitter.

Tommy and his parents engaged in a course of treatment focused both on his anxiety and, for his parents, on ways to help him cope more effectively and reduce their accommodation of his symptoms. Issues for the parents included a careful review of ways in which their behavior had frequently supported Tommy's anxiety and lack of independence. For Tommy, a course of CBT was helpful, combined with the work with his parents. Although he remained a somewhat anxious child, he began to be able to attend school on a regular basis and became more independent at home as well. His sleeping difficulties decreased. After Tommy had completed his treatment, his mother chose to pursue treatment for her own long-standing anxiety difficulties, which had seemed to play some role in Tommy's problems.

Reprinted with permission from Volkmar, F. R., & Martin, A. (2011). *Essentials of Lewis's child and adolescent psychiatry* (1st ed., p. 156). Lippincott Williams & Wilkins/Wolters Kluwer.

Anxiety disorders are associated with impaired functioning in children's social functioning with relatives and peers, their academic performance and achievement, their physical and mental health, their individual functioning through disrupted routines, including eating and sleep, and with high levels of personal distress (Higa-McMillan et al., 2016; Langley et al., 2013).

Impairment is not limited to the child alone. Family functioning in families of children with anxiety disorders is likewise impaired. One process that is particularly relevant to the developmental aspects of childhood anxiety is that of *family accommodation* (Jones et al., 2015; Kagan et al., 2017; Lebowitz et al., 2013; Norman et al., 2015; Reuman & Abramowitz, 2017; Thompson-Hollands et al., 2014). Family accommodation refers to the many ways in which parents modify their own behaviors to help their child avoid or alleviate anxiety. Children's natural reliance on caregivers for protection and regulation, and caregivers' powerful motivation to respond protectively to cues of childhood fear and distress contribute to the almost ubiquitous presence of family accommodation among parents of children with elevated anxiety levels. The need to maintain regular overall family functioning also contributes to high levels of family accommodation, because a child's anxiety can, when not accommodated, interfere with schedules and with the performance of everyday tasks. Thus, for example, an anxious child may have difficulty going to sleep alone, leading to parental accommodation because parents need to ensure proper sleep for the child and other family members. Likewise, parents may accommodate an anxious child by driving them to school in the morning instead of making use of the school bus, because of the need to ensure that the child arrives at school on time and that they can arrive at work on time.

Over 95% of parents of anxious children engage in regular accommodation of the child's anxiety symptoms. Despite being well intentioned and aimed at reducing the child's anxiety in the short term, family accommodation is consistently linked to higher levels of anxiety over time and to poorer overall functioning and can contribute to worse treatment outcomes (Kerns et al., 2017; Reuman & Abramowitz, 2017; Settipani, 2015; Storch et al., 2015; Zavrou et al., 2018). High levels of family accommodation also contribute to significant burden and distress for the parents and can result in high levels of intrafamilial conflict affecting all family members, including the siblings of the anxious child (Box 12.2).

BOX 12.2   Case of Generalized Anxiety

Todd, an 11-year-old boy, in the 5th grade, was referred for assessment by his primary care provider owing to symptoms she suggested might reflect an anxiety disorder. The third and final child, and only son, of professional parents, his school work began to deteriorate and had become a subject of concern to his parents. A successful participant in the martial arts and music, Todd had always been popular at school, although this year, in his private school, the level of work dramatically increased and the school shifted from what had been narrative reports to an actual report card, where he was getting B's and C's. His parents were puzzled because not only his previous narrative reports but also periodic achievement testing had suggested higher levels of academic ability. His parents initially presented their worry to the pediatrician that he had developed learning problems, but in her discussions with Todd the pediatrician noted that he complained of many worries and concerns. Although he had many physical complaints, the physical examination, including an ECG, had been unremarkable.

During the psychiatric assessment and over several sessions, Todd acknowledged being more worried about school this year, in part because he had also begun to feel pressure from his parents about college; in addition, they had suggested that he take an additional language in school. Todd had a number of somatic complaints (headaches, recurrent aches/ pains), and his parents reported that he was more irritable at home. He indicated that his worries had gradually increased but had been noteworthy over the last six months.

Review of last year's psychological testing revealed above-average intelligence and even somewhat higher achievement scores. Todd's mother, an attorney, reported a history of depression and anxiety and was currently taking an SSRI with good effect.

Todd was referred for a course of group CBT, with good results. In addition, his parents and school were encouraged to review his academic load and discontinue the additional course work. There was also an opportunity to discuss with his parents the possibility that increased expectations and premature worries about college might contribute to his anxiety. Follow-up in several months revealed that Todd was doing well in school and at home with no apparent recurrence of anxiety-related symptoms.

Reprinted with permission from Volkmar, F. R., & Martin, A. (2011). *Essentials of Lewis's child and adolescent psychiatry* (1st ed.). Lippincott Williams & Wilkins/Wolters Kluwer.

EPIDEMIOLOGY AND DEMOGRAPHICS

Taken together as a group, the anxiety disorders comprise the most common forms of developmental psychopathology (Achenbach et al., 1995; Costello et al., 2011; Merikangas et al., 2010), with onset that occurs early in life and with prevalence rates that are estimated to be as high as one third of youth by adulthood. Anxiety disorders are also commonly comorbid, both with other anxiety disorders and with nonanxiety psychopathology, in particular mood disorders (Cummings et al., 2014; Garber & Weersing, 2010; Lamers et al., 2011).

The National Comorbidity Survey Replication Adolescent Supplement (NCSA) surveyed a nationally representative sample of youth between the ages of 13 and 17, using structured interviews and confirmed the high prevalence of anxiety disorders (Kessler et al., 2009). Specific phobias were the most common anxiety disorders, followed by social anxiety disorder and separation anxiety disorder. As has been the case in some other studies, anxiety disorder prevalence in the NCSA was higher for females than for males, but this finding has not been consistent in the literature (Perou et al., 2013). Other demographic variables such as race and ethnicity have not been reliably found to predict risk of anxiety disorders (Wren et al., 2007).

Anxiety disorders in youth are more common among children of anxious parents than among those of nonanxious parents (Li et al., 2008). This is partly explained by genetic heritability, but nongenetic factors also contribute to anxiety heritability. For example, highly anxious parents may model more anxious or avoidant behavior and may exacerbate a tendency toward anxiety in children by providing high levels of family accommodation.

ETIOLOGY AND PATHOGENESIS

The precise etiology and pathogenesis of anxiety disorders in children is far from well-understood. A large number of psychological, biological, and environmental factors have been convincingly linked to the development of anxiety in children and these factors interact with each other, and very likely with other as yet unidentified factors, in complex ways (Newman et al., 2013). Even approximating a cohesive mapping of these complex relations requires additional long-term research effort. It goes almost without saying that identifying the etiology and pathogenesis of a specific child's anxiety problem is as yet not possible. Even when a particular psychological trigger for a child's anxiety is seemingly apparent, or when a deficit is identified in a particular physiological system, or when heredity is likely a significant contributor to a child's problem, it is generally a false conclusion to assume that the child's anxiety problem is actually explained by any one of these factors. The issue of heredity itself is complex, because it can include both genetic and nongenetic cross-generational transmission (Domschke & Maron, 2013; Eley, 1999; Eley et al., 2015).

Taking an historical perspective on psychological explanations for anxiety in children, some of the earliest theories were informed by psychoanalytic theory. The seminal example for this approach is that of "Little Hans," a case study in child phobia described by Freud in 1909 (Freud, 1928). Hans was a five-year-old boy with a phobia of horses. Hans' fear soon generalized, as is common in phobic disorders, to a fear of leaving the house at all because of the high prevalence of horses typical of the time. Freud posited that the fear of horses was a symbolic representation of an underlying fear of castration by the father, linked to Hans' Oedipal desire for his mother.

The emergence of behavioral learning theories of psychology during the early 20th century directed attention to the role of classical and operant conditioning as a basis for explaining the etiology of childhood anxiety disorders. The seminal experiment here was the case of "Little Albert," described by Watson in 1920 (Ollendick & Muris, 2015). Albert was a nine-month-old baby who was shown various stimuli, including a white rat, a rabbit, and a monkey, that initially did not evoke a fear response in him. After Watson paired the rat with a sudden loud noise that startled Albert, he began to show signs of fear in response to the rat, and his fear generalized to other similar stimuli. This was interpreted as evidence that childhood fears are learned responses that emerge in response to the ongoing processes of learning and conditioning.

In 1977, Rachman argued that the conditioned learning theory is insufficient to explain the etiology of childhood fears and proposed two additional pathways through which fears may be acquired: vicarious learning and the transmission of information and instruction, both of which can occur without direct contact with the feared object (Rachman, 1977). Vicarious learning occurs when a child observes the fearful response of another individual to an object or situation. Social referencing studies, such as those using the classic "visual cliff" paradigm, in which parents' facial expressions of fear caused infants to avoid crossing a raised transparent glass platform that gives the illusion of height, provide evidence for the innate tendency toward vicarious learning. Transmission of information and instruction occurs when children receive information, explicitly or implicitly, from others, in particular parents, that leads to a fearful response in the child (Box 12.3).

Alongside explicit modeling of fear and directly transmitting information, parental styles have also been linked to the development of childhood anxiety, in particular overly protective or controlling parenting and overly critical parenting styles. And parental responses to a child's actual anxiety can lead to further exacerbation of the anxiety. As noted previously, parents commonly accommodate childhood anxiety, and data suggest that high rates of accommodation can lead the child to experience increasing anxiety over time.

BOX 12.3   Case of Specific Phobia

Sheila, aged 8, was an only child. Her parents sought evaluation and treatment because of her fear of spiders, which had become increasingly severe and impactful over the past year. Sheila had always been afraid of all kinds of bugs, but for the past year her fear of spiders, in particular, had escalated considerably.

Sheila would search her room for spiders each evening before going to bed and would plead with her parents to help in the search, a process that took around half an hour each night. She also kept a light on in her room, hoping to discourage any spiders from being there. Her sleep seemed to be deteriorating, and she would wake up at night from nightmares about spiders.

When the family watched television, Sheila would make her parents promise her that they would not see anything with spiders in it, and she refused to read any book unless her parents reviewed it first to make sure there was no mention of spiders.

Sheila's family was also no longer able to go on outings or picnics because Sheila was afraid she would encounter a spider in the outdoors.

If Sheila ever did spot a spider in the house, she would panic, run from the room, and demand that her parents remove the spider, and then search the house for others.

The parents had thought the fear was a phase that would pass, but they saw it only increasing and having an ever larger impact on the whole household.

Sheila was not willing to participate in CBT because she understood from the therapist that treatment would include exposure to spider images and potentially to actual spiders.

The therapist therefore worked with Sheila's parents, encouraging them to systematically reduce their accommodations of Sheila's symptoms and to respond to her fears in a supportive manner. The parents learned to respond to Sheila by expressing both acceptance of her genuine fear and distress and confidence in her ability to cope with the fear. Sheila initially became very upset when the parents refused to accommodate by searching her room with her at night. The parents stayed firm and supportive, however, and soon she adapted to the new rules. Sheila's fear gradually decreased as the parents continued to focus on reducing accommodation and maintaining the supportive messages. After a few months of treatment, Sheila's anxiety improved significantly and treatment ended.

Biological mechanisms have also been implicated in the etiology of childhood anxiety. These mechanisms can exert their effects from the prenatal period and over the course of development (Lebowitz et al., 2016). Maternal stress during pregnancy has been linked to dysregulation in babies, measured at even a few days of age (Brouwers et al., 2001; Rieger et al., 2004; Van den Bergh et al., 2005). One hypothesis relating to the biological pathways linking stress during pregnancy to childhood anxiety centers on hormonal levels in the embryonic period (Gitau et al., 1998). Another is that maternal stress leads to restricted uterine blood flow. Some evidence exists to support each of these potential pathways (Sjostrom et al., 1997; Teixeira et al., 1999).

Although anxiety can be transmitted across generations behaviorally, through modeling, parenting style, and instruction, genetics also play a role in the etiology of child anxiety (Hettema et al., 2001). Twin studies, comparing identical and fraternal twins, have indicated that some of the variance in childhood anxiety is explained by as yet unidentified genes (Eley, 1999; Eley et al., 2015). The genetic contribution appears to be moderate but significant. Furthermore, genes and environmental factors can interact in contributing to childhood anxiety. Gene by environment interactions occur when environmental variables differentially impact different genotypes. Epigenetic effects occur when environmental variables lead to differences in the expression of particular genes. A frequently studied epigenetic mechanism is that of DNA methylation. Studies have found changes in methylation in anxiety disorders on several genes, and animal research also points to this process as a factor in the etiology of anxiety during development (Domschke & Maron, 2013; Szyf, 2015).

Neurobiological research, utilizing brain imaging procedures such as fMRI (functional magnetic resonance imaging) and EEG (electroencephalogram), is providing knowledge about the brain circuitry involved in the development and expression of childhood anxiety. Much of this research has focused on the amygdala and the prefrontal cortex and indicates that children with anxiety disorders display alterations in the functioning and regulation of these regions. Amygdala hyperactivity in response to fearful stimuli is among the most consistent findings (Guyer et al., 2008; McClure et al., 2007; Monk et al., 2008). Deficits in prefrontal control and regulation of the amygdala and weakened connectivity between the prefrontal cortex and the amygdala have also been reported repeatedly (Blackford & Pine, 2012; Kujawa et al., 2016).

Normal development involves dynamic changes in brain circuitry, with the amygdala maturing more rapidly than does the prefrontal cortex, potentially contributing to heightened risk of anxiety problems at certain development stages (Gee, 2016). Developmental changes also gradually reduce children's reliance on parents for anxiety regulation, and chronic anxiety may impede this developmental shift, leading to higher dependence on parents beyond what is normative for a given age (Gee & Casey, 2015; Gee et al., 2016).

Early adversity, including deprivation in caregiving or maltreatment, can also lead to neurobiological alterations such as increased amygdala volume and contribute to anxiety over the entire life span (Gee et al., 2013; Goff et al., 2013; Green et al., 2010; Ono et al., 2008; Tottenham et al., 2010; Zeanah et al., 2009). Such early adversity can also lead to other neurobiological changes, such as impairment in the functioning of the oxytocinergic system, which is implicated both in attachment behavior and in anxiety regulation in children.

■ COURSE

When left untreated, anxiety disorders of childhood tend to be chronic, and spontaneous remission, although possible, is relatively unlikely. It is more likely that the specific diagnostic category of anxiety disorder will change over time or that additional anxiety (and nonanxiety) diagnoses will accumulate. For example, a young child with separation anxiety may present later with social anxiety or generalized anxiety or both. Depression is also a likely sequela of untreated anxiety, and the risk of substance-related problems is significant.

Long-term outcomes of childhood anxiety are also well documented (Ramsawh et al., 2010). Anxiety in childhood predicts not only ongoing anxiety impairment well into adulthood, but also higher levels of school dropout and lower occupational achievement, higher rates of teenage pregnancy, increased need for physical and mental health care, and higher rates of suicidal behaviors (Boden et al., 2007; Kaplow et al., 2001; Kendall et al., 2010; Pine et al., 1998; Ramsawh et al., 2010; Woodward & Fergusson, 2001). These impacts lead to a societal cost for anxiety disorders estimated in billions of dollars annually.

■ DIFFERENTIAL DIAGNOSIS AND ASSESSMENT

Establishing clinical diagnoses of childhood anxiety disorders relies on clinical interview, which can be unstructured, semistructured, or structured. Best practices for deriving reliable diagnostic formulations call for the use of structured or semistructured interview schedules (Mash & Hunsley, 2005; Silverman & Ollendick, 2005). These tools make use of standardized questions that are posed to children and parents and can reduce variance related to the interviewer and to the use or interpretation of specific *DSM* criteria. The most widely used diagnostic interviews include the structured K-SADS (Schedule for Affective Disorders and Schizophrenia for School Age Children) (Kaufman et al., 1997) and DISC (Diagnostic Interview Schedule for Children) (Shaffer et al., 2000), and the semistructured ADIS C/P (Anxiety Disorders Interview Schedule, Child and Parent Versions) (Albano & Silverman, 2020).

For assessment focused on childhood anxiety, the ADIS C/P is widely considered to be the gold-standard diagnostic assessment instrument. The ADIS C/P includes modules covering the various anxiety disorders, as well as more streamlined modules for detecting other, nonanxiety, disorders. In addition to establishing the presence of symptoms matching the diagnostic criteria for each disorder, the ADIS C/P provides clinician-rated severity scales to assess the degree of severity of each disorder present on the basis of the amount of interference the disorder causes in the child's daily life. The interview is administered to children and to parents, and the information obtained is integrated in deriving the overall diagnostic and severity formulations.

Anxiety is a construct with a very broad range, from normative anxiety that every child is likely to experience from time to time to the severely impairing anxiety that can be highly debilitating for the child and family. Numerous rating scales have been developed and used for assessing the severity of anxiety in children. Among them are the RCMAS (Revised Children's Manifest Anxiety Scale) (Reynolds, 1985), the PARS (Pediatric Anxiety Rating Scale) (RUPP Anxiety Study Group, 2002), the STAIC (State-Trait Anxiety Inventory for Children), the MASC 2 (Multidimensional Anxiety Scale for Children, 2nd Version), and the SCARED (Screen for Childhood Anxiety Related Emotional Disorders) (Birmaher et al., 1997). Scales focused on specific subsets of childhood anxiety also exist. Thus, for example, the SPAIC (Social Phobia and Anxiety Inventory for Children) (Kuusikko et al., 2009) and the SASC-R (Social Anxiety Scale for Children-Revised) (La Greca & Stone, 1993) focus on the presence and severity of symptoms of social anxiety.

In addition to the presence and severity of anxiety symptoms, dimensional approaches can also be applied when considering impairment related to childhood anxiety and when considering additional constructs that make up part of the typical clinical presentation of anxiety disorders. The CAIS (Childhood Anxiety Impact Scale)(Langley et al., 2013) assesses the degree of impairment in psychosocial functioning caused by a child's anxiety problem in three major domains: school functioning, social functioning, and family functioning. Higher scores on this scale are indicative of greater impairment and can be considered separately from the severity of the anxiety symptoms themselves. For example, a child with moderately severe anxiety symptoms can sometimes be more impaired in day-to-day functioning than a child who scores higher on a scale measuring only severity of the symptoms. This can occur when a child with more severe symptoms maintains function, albeit with high levels of distress, and when a child with moderate symptoms shows more reluctance to cope with the anxiety and thus has greater avoidance and impairment.

Family accommodation, the pattern of parental entanglement in child anxiety symptoms through efforts to prevent or alleviate the symptoms, can also be dimensionally assessed. A number of rating scales have been developed for assessing family accommodation, among which the most commonly used are the FASA (Family Accommodation Scale – Anxiety) (Lebowitz et al., 2013) and its parallel child-rated version FASA-CR (Family Accommodation Scale – Anxiety Child Report)(Lebowitz et al., 2015). Both have well-established psychometric properties, including internal consistency, reliability, and convergent and divergent validity.

Another construct, separate from, but tightly linked to anxiety severity is anxiety sensitivity. Anxiety sensitivity refers to the fear of anxiety-related sensations such as rapid heart rate, because of beliefs that the sensations can have harmful physical, social, or psychological effects. Children with high levels of anxiety sensitivity perceive these sensations of anxiety as dangerous, and this in turn exacerbates the anxiety in a negative cycle. The CASI (Child Anxiety Sensitivity Index) is a rating scale that can be used to dimensionally assess the degree of anxiety sensitivity in a child (Silverman et al., 1991).

Apart from rating scales, behavioral observations and behavioral tasks are the most frequently used methods of dimensionally assessing childhood anxiety. Behavioral observations and tasks provide more objective, and in some cases naturalistic, data and can help to reduce the biases and reporting errors inherent in all self-reports. Social-evaluative tasks involve engaging the child in a socially stressful task such as reading aloud or presenting a speech, and collecting ratings, observations, and psychophysiological indicators of anxiety in response to the task (Cartwright-Hatton et al., 2003). In another approach the child is presented with a puzzle that is difficult to solve, and assessment focuses on the degree of anxiety distress in response to the challenge (Ginsburg et al., 2004).

Behavioral avoidance tasks (BAT) aim to assess the degree of actual avoidance in a child's behavior, rather than relying on self-report (Castagna et al., 2017). In a classic BAT, an individual is placed at a certain distance from a feared object, and that distance is gradually decreased up to the point at which the participant's discomfort is too great to continue, marking the level of avoidance for that person. Although informative, these BATs have limitations relating to demand characteristics inherent in a figure with some authority explicitly requesting that they approach the feared object. Classic BATs also provide limited data because only a single or very few data points are generated for each individual. Computerized BATs have been developed to address these limitations, by engaging the individual in a computerized task in which they either control an on-screen avatar or move a joystick to create approach/avoidance responses to a variety of stimuli (Klein et al., 2011). A particularly novel approach has been to use motion-tracking technology by engaging a participant in a game that requires them to move around a space physically while approaching or moving away from various stimuli and accurately tracking their location with high spatial and temporal resolution.

Another computer-based dimensional approach focuses on measuring attention bias, or the tendency of anxious individuals to attend more to fear-inducing stimuli than to neutral stimuli. To measure this bias, the "dot-probe" paradigm is used (MacLeod et al., 1986). In dot-probe, a subject is shown a computer screen, and after fixing their gaze on the center of the screen two images, one fear-inducing and the other neutral, are displayed very briefly, usually for around half a second. Then the images are removed, and in place of one of them appears a probe to which the participant responds by pressing a key or mouse button. Studies show that individuals with elevated anxiety responded more rapidly when the probe appeared in place of the fearful image than when it appeared in the location that was previously occupied by the neutral image, suggesting that their attention was already focused on the part of the screen with the fear-inducing image (Dudeney et al., 2015). This approach enables the measurement of rapid short-term processes relating to anxiety, which take place outside of conscious awareness.

Finally, another approach to dimensional assessment is to focus on underlying systems implicated in mental health conditions, which can be cross-diagnostic and implicated in multiple nosological categories. An example of this is the Research Domain Criteria (RDoC) system, developed by the National Institute of Mental Health (NIMH) to drive the next generation of research in mental health and treatment (Lebowitz et al., 2018). In RDoC, rather than focusing on particular diagnostic categories such as *DSM* diagnoses, researchers focus on a number of systems, including those for negative valence, positive valence, cognition, social processes, arousal and regulation, and sensorimotor functioning. Each of these systems includes several constructs and subconstructs and can be studied across multiple units of analysis, including genes, molecules, cells, circuitry, physiology, behavior, and self-report, using a variety of paradigms. In the context of childhood anxiety, research might focus, for example, on the constructs of fear, anxiety, or sustained threat (within the negative valence system) or on the construct of arousal (within the arousal and regulatory system). Likewise, research focused on family accommodation of childhood anxiety might focus on the construct of affiliation and attachment (within the social processes system).

TREATMENT

To date, the two treatment strategies that have garnered the strongest empirical support for their efficacy are cognitive-behavioral therapy (CBT) and pharmacological treatment (Reinblatt & Riddle, 2007; Wang et al., 2017).

CBT focuses on practicing repeated gradual exposure to feared objects or situations and on identifying maladaptive thought patterns and cognitive biases that both reflect and maintain the anxiety. For example, the tendency to focus on negative events and information rather than on the more benign, the tendency to overestimate the likelihood of negative events, and the tendency to misinterpret the behavior of others negatively. CBT teaches children to notice and monitor these "thinking traps" and to challenge and modify them through the process of cognitive restructuring.

Exposure is considered by many clinicians and researchers to be the most important element of CBT for anxiety. To practice exposure, the child and therapist construct a "fear hierarchy," which is a series of exposures including some that generate only a moderate level of anxiety and others that trigger higher levels of anxiety. The child then practices actually experiencing those situations both in session and outside of the clinical setting. Each step on the hierarchy is usually practiced several times until it no longer causes significant anxiety. Other skills often taught and practiced in CBT include physical regulation skills such as relaxing breathing and muscle relaxation.

Most psychological treatment for children also involves an element of parent guidance. Parents of children receiving CBT are provided with psychoeducation about childhood anxiety, provide the therapist with information that is useful in guiding the therapeutic process, and are encouraged to refrain from behaviors that promote avoidance in their child. Entirely parent-based treatment, without direct child involvement, can also be efficacious (Lebowitz et al., 2020). In SPACE (Supportive Parenting for Anxious Childhood Emotions), an entirely parent-based treatment, parents are taught to replace accommodating responses to child anxiety with supportive responses that convey to the child both acceptance of the distress the child is feeling and confidence in the child's ability to cope with the discomfort.

Pharmacological treatment has also proven effective at treating childhood anxiety disorders, although the consensus in the field is that in most cases psychological therapy should be attempted before introducing medication and should be provided even when a child is being medicated (Walkup et al., 2008). The frontline medications of choice are the selective serotonin reuptake inhibitors (SSRI), which are less likely to cause unwanted side effects or dependence than anxiolytics such as the benzodiazepines.

SUMMARY

Anxiety disorders are highly prevalent throughout development and most commonly have their onset in childhood. The diagnostic categorization of anxiety disorders has evolved steadily over the past decades with each version of the *DSM* introducing changes, and often new diagnostic categories. When not treated successfully, childhood anxiety disorders cause significant distress and impairment, and their long-term impact reaches well into adulthood. However, evidence-based efficacious treatments exist for childhood anxiety disorders, including cognitive-behavioral therapy (CBT), medications, and parent-based treatment approaches. The precise etiology of childhood anxiety is complex and not yet well understood. Ongoing research, including behavioral, biological, neurobiological, and genetic studies, aims to better understand the etiology and risk factors of childhood anxiety.

References

*Indicates Particularly Recommended

Achenbach, T. M., Howell, C. T., & McConaughy, S. H., & Stanger, C. (1995). Six-year predictors of problems in a national sample of children and youth: II. Signs of disturbance. *Journal of the American Academy of Child and Adolescent Psychiatry, 34*(4), 488–498. https://doi.org/10.1097/00004583-199504000-00016

Albano, A. M., & Silverman, W. K. (2020). *Anxiety disorders interview schedule (ADIS-5) child and parent interviews*. Oxford University Press.

American Psychiatric Association. (2013). *Diagnostic and statistical manual of mental disorders* (5th ed.). Author.

Birmaher, B., Khetarpal, S., Brent, D., Cully, M., Balach, L., Kaufman, J., & Neer, S. M. (1997). The screen for child anxiety related emotional disorders (scared): Scale construction and psychometric characteristics. *Journal of the American Academy of Child and Adolescent Psychiatry, 36*(4), 545–553. https://doi.org/10.1097/00004583-199704000-00018

Blackford, J. U., & Pine, D. S. (2012). Neural substrates of childhood anxiety disorders: A review of neuroimaging findings. *Child and Adolescent Psychiatric Clinics of North America, 21*(3), 501–525. https://doi.org/10.1016/j.chc.2012.05.002

Boden, J. M., Fergusson, D. M., & Horwood, L. J. (2007). Anxiety disorders and suicidal behaviours in adolescence and young adulthood: Findings from a longitudinal study. *Psychological Medicine, 37*(3), 431–440. https://doi.org/10.1017/S0033291706009147

Brouwers, E. P. M., van Baar, A. L., & Pop, V. J. M. (2001). Maternal anxiety during pregnancy and subsequent infant development. *Infant Behavior & Development, 24*(1), 95–106. https://doi.org/10.1016/s0163-6383(01)00062-5

Cartwright-Hatton, S., Hodges, L., & Porter, J. (2003). Social anxiety in childhood: The relationship with self and observer rated social skills. *Journal of Child Psychology and Psychiatry, 44*(5), 737–742. https://doi.org/10.1111/1469-7610.00159

Castagna, P. J., Davis, T. E., III, & Lilly, M. E. (2017). The behavioral avoidance task with anxious youth: A review of procedures, properties, and criticisms. *Clinical Child and Family Psychology Review, 20*(2), 162–184. https://doi.org/10.1007/s10567-016-0220-3

*Costello, E. J., Egger, H. L., Copeland, W., Erkanli, A., & Angold, A. (2011). The developmental epidemiology of anxiety disorders: Phenomenology, prevalence, and comorbidity. In W. K. Silverman & A. P. Field (Eds.), *Anxiety disorders in children and adolescents: Research, assessment and intervention* (pp. 56–75). Cambridge University Press

Cummings, C. M., Caporino, N. E., & Kendall, P. C. (2014). Comorbidity of anxiety and depression in children and adolescents: 20 years after. *Psychological Bulletin, 140*(3), 816–845. https://doi.org/10.1037/a0034733

Domschke, K., & Maron, E. (2013). Genetic factors in anxiety disorders. *Modern Trends in Pharmacopsychiatry, 29*, 24–46. https://doi.org/10.1159/000351932

Dudeney, J., Sharpe, L., & Hunt, C. (2015). Attentional bias towards threatening stimuli in children with anxiety: A meta-analysis. *Clinical Psychology Review, 40*, 66–75. https://doi.org/10.1016/j.cpr.2015.05.007

*Eley, T. C. (1999). Behavioral genetics as a tool for developmental psychology: Anxiety and depression in children and adolescents. *Clinical Child and Family Psychology Review, 2*(1), 21–36. https://doi.org/10.1023/A:1021863324202

Eley, T. C., McAdams, T. A., Rijsdijk, F. V., Lichtenstein, P., Narusyte, J., Reiss, D., Spotts, E. L., Ganiban, J. M., & Neiderhiser, J. M. (2015). The intergenerational transmission of anxiety: A children-of-twins study. *American Journal of Psychiatry, 172*(7), 630–637. https://doi.org/10.1176/appi.ajp.2015.14070818

Freud, S. (1928). Analysis of a phobia in a five-year-old boy (little hans). *Revue Française de Psychanalyse, 2*(3).

Garber, J., & Weersing, V. R. (2010). Comorbidity of anxiety and depression in youth: Implications for treatment and prevention. *Clinical Psychology: Science and Practice, 17*(4), 293–306. https://doi.org/10.1111/j.1468-2850.2010.01221.x

Gee, D. G. (2016). Sensitive periods of emotion regulation: Influences of parental care on frontoamygdala circuitry and plasticity. *New Directions for Child and Adolescent Development, 2016*(153), 87–110. https://doi.org/10.1002/cad.20166

Gee, D. G., & Casey, B. J. (2015). The impact of developmental timing for stress and recovery. *Neurobiology of Stress, 1*, 184–194. https://doi.org/10.1016/j.ynstr.2015.02.001

Gee, D. G., Fetcho, R. N., Jing, D., Li, A., Glatt, C. E., Drysdale, A. T., Cohen, A. O., Dellarco, D. V., Yang, R. R., Dale, A. M., Jernigan, T. L., Lee, F. S., Casey, B., & the PING Consortium. (2016). Individual differences in frontolimbic circuitry and anxiety emerge with adolescent changes in endocannabinoid signaling across species. *Proceedings of the National Academy of Sciences of the United States of America, 113*(16), 4500–4505. https://doi.org/10.1073/pnas.1600013113

Gee, D. G., Gabard-Durnam, L. J., Flannery, J., Goff, B., Humphreys, K. L., Telzer, E. H., Hare, T. A., Bookheimer, S. Y., & Tottenham, N. (2013). Early developmental emergence of human amygdala-prefrontal connectivity after maternal deprivation. *Proceedings of the National Academy of Sciences of the United States of America, 110*(39), 15638–15643. https://doi.org/10.1073/pnas.1307893110

*Ginsburg, G. S., Siqueland, L., Masia-Warner, C., & Hedtke, K. A. (2004). Anxiety-disorders in children: Family matters. *Cognitive and Behavioral Practice, 11*(1), 28–43. https://doi.org/10.1016/S1077-7229(04)80005-1

Gitau, R., Cameron, A., Fisk, N. M., & Glover, V. (1998). Fetal exposure to maternal cortisol. *Lancet, 352*(9129), 707–708. https://doi.org/10.1016/S0140-6736(05)60824-0

Goff, B., Gee, D. G., Telzer, E. H., Humphreys, K. L., Gabard-Durnam, L., Flannery, J., & Tottenham, N. (2013). Reduced nucleus accumbens reactivity and adolescent depression following early-life stress. *Neuroscience, 249*, 129–138. https://doi.org/10.1016/j.neuroscience.2012.12.010

Green, J. D., McLaughlin, K. A., Berglund, P. A., Gruber, M. J., Sampson, N. A., Zaslavsky, A. M., & Kessler, R. C. (2010). Childhood adversities and adult psychiatric disorders in the national comorbidity survey replication I: Associations with first onset of *DSM-IV* disorders. *Archives of General Psychiatry, 67*(2), 113–123. https://doi.org/10.1001/archgenpsychiatry.2009.186

Guyer, A. E., Lau, J. Y., McClure-Tone, E. B., Parrish, J., Shiffrin, N. D., Reynolds, R. C., Chen, G., Blair, R. J., Leibenluft, E., Fox, N. A., Ernst, M., Pine, D. S., & Nelson, E. E. (2008). Amygdala and ventrolateral prefrontal cortex function during anticipated peer evaluation in pediatric social anxiety. *Archives of General Psychiatry, 65*(11), 1303–1312. https://doi.org/10.1001/archpsyc.65.11.1303

Hettema, J. M., Neale, M. C., & Kendler, K. S. (2001). A review and meta-analysis of the genetic epidemiology of anxiety disorders. *American Journal of Psychiatry, 158*(10), 1568–1578. https://doi.org/10.1176/appi.ajp.158.10.1568

Higa-McMillan, C. K., Francis, S. E., Rith-Najarian, L., & Chorpita, B. F. (2016). Evidence base update: 50 years of research on treatment for child and adolescent anxiety. *Journal of Clinical Child and Adolescent Psychology, 45*(2), 91–113. https://doi.org/10.1080/15374416.2015.1046177

Jones, J. D., Lebowitz, E. R., Marin, C. E., & Stark, K. D. (2015). Family accommodation mediates the association between anxiety symptoms in mothers and children. *Journal of Child and Adolescent Mental Health, 27*(1), 41–51. https://doi.org/10.2989/17280583.2015.1007866

Kagan, E. R., Frank, H. E., & Kendall, P. C. (2017). Accommodation in youth with OCD and anxiety. *Clinical Psychology: Science and Practice, 24*(1), 78–98. https://doi.org/10.1111/cpsp.12186

Kaplow, J. B., Curran, P. J., Angold, A., & Costello, E. J. (2001). The prospective relation between dimensions of anxiety and the initiation of adolescent alcohol use. *Journal of Clinical Child Psychology, 30*(3), 316–326. https://doi.org/10.1207/s15374424jccp3003_4

Kaufman, J., Birmaher, B., Brent, D., Rao, U., Flynn, C., Moreci, P., Williamson, D., & Ryan, N. (1997). Schedule for affective disorders and schizophrenia for school-age children-present and lifetime version (K-SADS-PL): Initial reliability and validity data. *Journal of the American Academy of Child and Adolescent Psychiatry, 36*(7), 980–988. https://doi.org/10.1097/00004583-199707000-00021

*Kendall, P. C., Compton, S. N., Walkup, J. T., Birmaher, B., Albano, A. M., Sherrill, J., Ginsburg, G., Rynn, M., McCracken, J., Gosch, E., Keeton, C., Bergman, L., Sakolsky, D., Suveg, C., Iyengar, S., March, J., & Piacentini, J. (2010). Clinical characteristics of anxiety disordered youth. *Journal of Anxiety Disorders, 24*(3), 360–365. https://doi.org/10.1016/j.janxdis.2010.01.009

Kerns, C. E., Pincus, D. B., McLaughlin, K. A., & Comer, J. S. (2017). Maternal emotion regulation during child distress, child anxiety accommodation, and links between maternal and child anxiety. *Journal of Anxiety Disorders, 50*, 52–59. https://doi.org/10.1016/j.janxdis.2017.05.002

Kessler, R. C., Avenevoli, S., Costello, E. J., Green, J. G., Gruber, M. J., Heeringa, S., Merikangas, K. R., Pennell, B., Sampson, N. A., & Zaslavsky, A. M. (2009). Design and field procedures in the US national comorbidity survey replication adolescent supplement (NCS-A). *International Journal of Methods in Psychiatric Research, 18*(2), 69–83. https://doi.org/10.1002/mpr.279

Klein, A. M., Becker, E. S., & Rinck, M. (2011). Approach and avoidance tendencies in spider fearful children: The approach-avoidance task. *Journal of Child and Family Studies, 20*(2), 224–231. https://doi.org/10.1007/s10826-010-9402-7

Kujawa, A., Wu, M., Klumpp, H., Pine, D. S., Swain, J. E., Fitzgerald, K. D., Monk, C. S., & Phan, K. L. (2016). Altered development of amygdala-anterior cingulate cortex connectivity in anxious youth and young adults. *Biological Psychiatry: Cognitive Neuroscience and Neuroimaging, 1*(4), 345–352. https://doi.org/10.1016/j.bpsc.2016.01.006

Kuusikko, S., Pollock-Wurman, R., Ebeling, H., Hurtig, T., Joskitt, L., Mattila, M. L., Jussila, K., & Moilanen, I. (2009). Psychometric evaluation of social phobia and anxiety inventory for children (SPAI-C) and social anxiety scale for children-revised (SASC-R). *European Child and Adolescent Psychiatry, 18*(2), 116–124. https://doi.org/10.1007/s00787-008-0712-x

La Greca, A. M., & Stone, W. L. (1993). Social anxiety scale for children-revised: Factor structure and concurrent validity. *Journal of Clinical Child Psychology,* 22(1), 17–27. https://doi.org/10.1207/s15374424jccp2201_2

Lamers, F., van Oppen, P., Comijs, H. C., Smit, J. H., Spinhoven, P., van Balkom, A. J. L. M., Nolen, W. A., Zitman, F. G., Beekman, A. T. F., & Penninx, B. W. J. H. (2011). Comorbidity patterns of anxiety and depressive disorders in a large cohort study: The Netherlands study of depression and anxiety (NESDA). *The Journal of Clinical Psychiatry, 72*(3), 341–348. https://doi.org/10.4088/JCP.10m06176blu

Langley, A. K., Falk, A., Peris, T., Wiley, J. F., Kendall, P. C., Ginsburg, G., Birmaher, B., March, J., Albano, A. M., & Piacentini, J. (2014). The child anxiety impact scale: Examining parent-and child-reported impairment in child anxiety disorders. *Journal of Clinical Child and Adolescent Psychology, 43*(4), 579–591. https://doi.org/10.1080/15374416.2013.817311

*Lebowitz, E. R., Gee, D. G., Pine, D. S., & Silverman, W. K. (2018). Implications of the research domain criteria project for childhood anxiety and its disorders. *Clinical Psychology Review, 64*, 99–109. https://doi.org/10.1016/j.cpr.2018.01.005

Lebowitz, E. R., Leckman, J. F., Silverman, W. K., & Feldman, R. (2016). Cross-generational influences on childhood anxiety disorders: Pathways and mechanisms. *Journal of Neural Transmission, 123*(9), 1053–1067. https://doi.org/10.1007/s00702-016-1565-y

Lebowitz, E. R., Marin, C., Martino, A., Shimshoni, Y., & Silverman, W. K. (2020). Parent-based treatment as efficacious as cognitive-behavioral therapy for childhood anxiety: A randomized noninferiority study of supportive parenting for anxious childhood emotions. *Journal of the American Academy of Child and Adolescent Psychiatry, 59*(3), 362–372. https://doi.org/10.1016/j.jaac.2019.02.014

Lebowitz, E. R., Scharfstein, L., & Jones, J. (2015). Child-report of family accommodation in pediatric anxiety disorders: Comparison and integration with mother-report. *Child Psychiatry and Human Development, 46*(4), 501–511. https://doi.org/10.1007/s10578-014-0491-1

Lebowitz, E. R., Woolston, J., Bar-Haim, Y., Calvocoressi, L., Dauser, C., Warnick, E., Scahill, L., Chakir, A. R., Shechner, T., Hermes, H., Vitulano, L. A., King, R. A., & Leckman, J. F. (2013). Family accommodation in pediatric anxiety disorders. *Depression and Anxiety, 30*(1), 47–54. https://doi.org/10.1002/da.21998

Li, X., Sundquist, J., & Sundquist, K. (2008). Age-specific familial risks of anxiety. A nation-wide epidemiological study from Sweden. *European Archives of Psychiatry and Clinical Neuroscience, 258*(7), 441–445. https://doi.org/10.1007/s00406-008-0817-8

MacLeod, C., Mathews, A., & Tata, P. (1986). Attentional bias in emotional disorders. *Journal of Abnormal Psychology, 95*(1), 15–20. https://doi.org/10.1037/0021-843x.95.1.15

Mash, E. J., & Hunsley, J. (2005). Evidence-based assessment of child and adolescent disorders: Issues and challenges. *Journal of Clinical Child and Adolescent Psychology, 34*(3), 362–379. https://doi.org/10.1207/s15374424jccp3403_1

McClure, E. B., Monk, C. S., Nelson, E. E., Parrish, J. M., Adler, A., Blair, R. J., Fromm, S., Charney, D. S., Leibenluft, E., Ernst, M., & Pine, D. S. (2007). Abnormal attention modulation of fear circuit function in pediatric generalized anxiety disorder. *Archives of General Psychiatry, 64*(1), 97–106. https://doi.org/10.1001/archpsyc.64.1.97

Merikangas, K. R., He, J.-P., Burstein, M., Swanson, S. A., Avenevoli, S., Cui, L., Benjet, C., Georgiades, K., & Swendsen, J. (2010). Lifetime prevalence of mental disorders in U.S. adolescents: Results from the national comorbidity survey replication–adolescent supplement (NCS-A). *Journal of the American Academy of Child and Adolescent Psychiatry, 49*(10), 980–989. https://doi.org/10.1016/j.jaac.2010.05.017

Monk, C. S., Telzer, E. H., Mogg, K., Bradley, B. P., Mai, X., Louro, H. M., Chen, G., McClure-Tone, E. B., Ernst, M., & Pine, D. S. (2008). Amygdala and ventrolateral prefrontal cortex activation to masked angry faces in children and adolescents with generalized anxiety disorder. *Archives of General Psychiatry, 65*(5), 568–576. https://doi.org/10.1001/archpsyc.65.5.568

Newman, M. G., Llera, S. J., Erickson, T. M., Przeworski, A., & Castonguay, L. G. (2013). Worry and generalized anxiety disorder: A review and theoretical synthesis of evidence on nature, etiology, mechanisms, and treatment. *Annual Review of Clinical Psychology, 9*(1) 275–297. https://doi.org/10.1146/annurev-clinpsy-050212-185544

*Norman, K. R., Silverman, W. K., & Lebowitz, E. R. (2015). Family accommodation of child and adolescent anxiety: Mechanisms, assessment, and treatment. *Journal of Child and Adolescent Psychiatric Nursing, 28*(3), 131–140. https://doi.org/10.1111/jcap.12116

Ollendick, T. H., & Muris, P. (2015). The scientific legacy of Little Hans and Little Albert: Future directions for research on specific phobias in youth. *Journal of Clinical Child and Adolescent Psychology, 44*(4), 689–706. https://doi.org/10.1080/15374416.2015.1020543

Ono, M., Kikusui, T., Sasaki, N., Ichikawa, M., Mori, Y., & Murakami-Murofushi, K. (2008). Early weaning induces anxiety and precocious myelination in the anterior part of the basolateral amygdala of male balb/c mice. *Neuroscience, 156*(4), 1103–1110. https://doi.org/10.1016/j.neuroscience.2008.07.078

Perou, R., Bitsko, R. H., Blumberg, S. J., Pastor, P., Ghandour, R. M., Gfroerer, J. C., Hedden, S. L., Crosby, A. E., Visser, S. N., Schieve, L. A., Parks, S. E., Hall, J. E., Brody, D., Simile, C. M., Thompson, W. W., Baio, J., Avenevoli, S., Kogan, M. D., & Huang, L. N. (2013). Mental health surveillance among children—United States, 2005-2011. *Morbidity and Mortality Weekly Report (MMWR), 62*(02), 1–35.

Pine, D. S., Cohen, P., Gurley, D., Brook, J., & Ma, Y. (1998). The risk for early-adulthood anxiety and depressive disorders in adolescents with anxiety and depressive disorders. *Archives Of General Psychiatry, 55*(1), 56–64. https://doi.org/10.1001/archpsyc.55.1.56

*Rachman, S. (1977). The conditioning theory of fear-acquisition: A critical examination. *Behaviour Research and Therapy, 15*(5), 375–387. https://doi.org/10.1016/0005-7967(77)90041-9

Ramsawh, H. J., Chavira, D. A., & Stein, M. B. (2010). Burden of anxiety disorders in pediatric medical settings: Prevalence, phenomenology, and a research agenda. *Archives of Pediatrics and Adolescent Medicine, 164*(10), 965–972. https://doi.org/10.1001/archpediatrics.2010.170

Reinblatt, S. P., & Riddle, M. A. (2007). The pharmacological management of childhood anxiety disorders: A review. *Psychopharmacology, 191*(1), 67–86. https://doi.org/10.1007/s00213-006-0644-4

Reuman, L., & Abramowitz, J. S. (2017). Predictors of accommodation among families affected by fear-based disorders. *Child Psychiatry and Human Development, 49*(1), 53–62. https://doi.org/10.1007/s10578-017-0728-x

Reynolds, C. R. (1985). Multitrait validation of the revised children's manifest anxiety scale for children of high intelligence. *Psychological Reports, 56*(2), 402. https://doi.org/10.2466/pr0.1985.56.2.402

Rieger, M., Pirke, K. M., Buske-Kirschbaum, A., Wurmser, H., Papousek, M., & Hellhammer, D. H. (2004). Influence of stress during pregnancy on HPA activity and neonatal behavior. *Annals of the New York Academy of Sciences, 1032*(1), 228–230. https://doi.org/10.1196/annals.1314.026

RUPP Anxiety Study Group. (2002). The pediatric anxiety rating scale (PARS): Development and psychometric properties. *Journal of the American Academy of Child and Adolescent Psychiatry, 41*(9), 1061–1069. https://doi.org/10.1097/00004583-200209000-00006

Settipani, C. A., Kendall, P. C. (2017). The effect of child distress on accommodation of anxiety: Relations with maternal beliefs, empathy, and anxiety. *Journal of Clinical Child & Adolescent Psychology, 46*(6), 810–823. https://doi.org/10.1080/15374416.2015.1094741

Shaffer, D., Fisher, P., Lucas, C. P., Dulcan, M. K., & Schwab-Stone, M. E. (2000). NIMH diagnostic interview schedule for children version IV (NIMH DISC-IV): Description, differences from previous versions, and reliability of some common diagnoses. *Journal of the American Academy of Child and Adolescent Psychiatry, 39*(1), 28–38. https://doi.org/10.1097/00004583-200001000-00014

Shear, K., Jin, R., Ruscio, A. M., Walters, E. E., & Kessler, R. C. (2006). Prevalence and correlates of estimated DSM-IV child and adult separation anxiety disorder in the national comorbidity survey replication. *The American Journal of Psychiatry, 163*(6), 1074–1083. https://doi.org/10.1176/appi.ajp.163.6.1074

Silverman, W. K., Fleisig, W., Rabian, B., & Peterson, R. A. (1991). Childhood anxiety sensitivity index. *Journal of Clinical Child Psychology, 20*(2), 162–168. https://doi.org/10.1207/s15374424jccp2002_7

*Silverman, W. K., & Ollendick, T. H. (2005). Evidence-based assessment of anxiety and its disorders in children and adolescents. *Journal of Clinical Child and Adolescent Psychology, 34*(3), 380–411. https://doi.org/10.1207/s15374424jccp3403_2

Sjostrom, K., Valentin, L., Thelin, T., & Marsal, K. (1997). Maternal anxiety in late pregnancy and fetal hemodynamics. *European Journal of Obstetrics, Gynecology, and Reproductive Biology, 74*(2), 149–155. https://doi.org/10.1016/s0301-2115(97)00100-0

Storch, E. A., Salloum, A., Johnco, C., Dane, B. F., Crawford, E. A., King, M. A., McBride, N. M., & Lewin, A. B. (2015). Phenomenology and clinical correlates of family accommodation in pediatric anxiety disorders. *Journal of Anxiety Disorders, 35*, 75–81. https://doi.org/10.1016/j.janxdis.2015.09.001

Szyf, M. (2015). Nongenetic inheritance and transgenerational epigenetics. *Trends in Molecular Medicine, 21*(2), 134–144. https://doi.org/10.1016/j.molmed.2014.12.004

Teixeira, J. M., Fisk, N. M., & Glover, V. (1999). Association between maternal anxiety in pregnancy and increased uterine artery resistance index: Cohort based study. *British Medical Journal, 318*(7177), 153–157. https://doi.org/10.1136/bmj.318.7177.153

Thompson-Hollands, J., Kerns, C. E., Pincus, D. B., & Comer, J. S. (2014). Parental accommodation of child anxiety and related symptoms: Range, impact, and correlates. *Journal of Anxiety Disorders, 28*(8), 765–773. https://doi.org/10.1016/j.janxdis.2014.09.007 25261837

Tottenham, N., Hare, T. A., Quinn, B. T., McCarry, T. W., Nurse, M., Gilhooly, T., Millner, A., Galvan, A., Davidson, M. C., Eigsti, I., Thomas, K. M., Freed, P. J., Booma, E. S., Gunnar, M. R., Altemus, M., Aronson, J., & Casey, B. (2010). Prolonged institutional rearing is associated with atypically larger amygdala volume and difficulties in emotion regulation. *Developmental Science, 13*(1), 46–61. https://doi.org/10.1111/j.1467-7687.2009.00852.x

Van den Bergh, B. R., Mulder, E. J., Mennes, M., & Glover, V. (2005). Antenatal maternal anxiety and stress and the neurobehavioural development of the fetus and child: Links and possible mechanisms. A review. *Neuroscience and Biobehavioral Reviews, 29*(2), 237–258. https://doi.org/10.1016/j.neubiorev.2004.10.007

Walkup, J. T., Albano, A. M., Piacentini, J., Birmaher, B., Compton, S. N., Sherrill, J. T., Ginsburg, G. S., Rynn, M. A., McCracken, J., Waslick, B., Iyengar, S., March, J. S., & Kendall, P. C. (2008). Cognitive behavioral therapy, sertraline, or a combination in childhood anxiety. *New England Journal of Medicine, 359*(26), 2753–2766. https://doi.org/10.1056/nejmoa0804633

Wang, Z., Whiteside, S. P. H., Sim, L., Farah, W., Morrow, A. S., Alsawas, M., Barrionuevo, P., Tello, M., Asi, N., Beuschel, B., Daraz, L., Almasri, J., Zaiem, F., Larrea-Mantilla, L., Ponce, O. J., LeBlanc, A., Prokop, L. J., & Murad, M. H. (2017). Comparative effectiveness and safety of cognitive behavioral therapy and pharmacotherapy for childhood anxiety disorders: A systematic review and meta-analysis. *JAMA Pediatrics, 171*(11), 1049–1056. https://doi.org/10.1001/jamapediatrics.2017.3036

Woodward, L. J., & Fergusson, D. M. (2001). Life course outcomes of young people with anxiety disorders in adolescence. *Journal of the American Academy of Child and Adolescent Psychiatry, 40*(9), 1086–1093. https://doi.org/10.1097/00004583-200109000-00018

Wren, F. J., Berg, E. A., Heiden, L. A., Kinnamon, C. J., Ohlson, L. A., Bridge, J. A., Birmaher, B., & Bernal, M. P. (2007). Childhood anxiety in a diverse primary care population: Parent-child reports, ethnicity and scared factor structure. *Journal of the American Academy of Child and Adolescent Psychiatry, 46*(3), 332–340. https://doi.org/10.1097/chi.0b013e31802f1267

Zavrou, S., Rudy, B., Johnco, C., Storch, E. A., & Lewin, A. B. (2018). Preliminary study of family accommodation in 4-7 year-olds with anxiety: Frequency, clinical correlates, and treatment response. *Journal of Mental Health, 28*(4), 1–7. https://doi.org/10.1080/09638237.2018.1466034

Zeanah, C. H., Egger, H. L., Smyke, A. T., Nelson, C. A., Fox, N. A., Marshall, P. J., & Guthrie, D. (2009). Institutional rearing and psychiatric disorders in Romanian preschool children. *The American Journal of Psychiatry, 166*(7), 777–785. https://doi.org/10.1176/appi.ajp.2009.08091438

Suggested Readings

Chansky, T. E. (2004). *Freeing your child from anxiety: Powerful, practical strategies to overcome your child's fears, phobias, and worries.* Broadway Books.

Creswell, C., Parkinson, M., Thirlwall, K., & Willetts, L. (2017). *Parent-led CBT for child anxiety: Helping parents help their kids.* Guilford Press.

McKay, D., & Storch, E. A. (2011). *Handbook of child and adolescent anxiety disorders.* Springer Science+Business Media.

Nathan, P. E., & Gorman, J. M. (2015). *A guide to treatments that work* (4th ed.). Oxford University Press.

Steele, R. G., Elkin, T. D., & Roberts, M. C. (2008). *Handbook of evidence-based therapies for children and adolescents: Bridging science and practice. Issues in clinical child psychology.* Springer Science+Business Media.

CHAPTER 13 ■ OBSESSIVE-COMPULSIVE DISORDER

■ BACKGROUND

Metaphors used to describe the human brain, such as that of a highly efficient computer, often convey an image of impeccable organization and control. Yet the thoughts, feelings, and urges produced by the brain are actually considerably more chaotic, with little control on the part of the person experiencing them. History is replete with descriptions of individuals who struggled with or succumbed to uncontrollable thoughts that ran amok, overwhelming the capacity for organized thought or behavior. Where in the past such individuals may have been considered the victims of an evil force, such as a demon or a curse, the modern science of mental health views them as suffering from a neurologic condition stemming from the physical functioning of the brain. Attributing intrusive and uncontrollable thoughts and feelings to the actions of the central nervous system also enables the identification of a continuum in these processes— from the normative and healthy to the clinical and psychopathologic. Indeed, symptoms characteristic of obsessive-compulsive disorder (OCD) are present at some level in the general population and even somewhat elevated levels of these patterns are considered normative at some developmental stages (Garcia-Soriano et al., 2011).

Freud is often credited with providing the first cohesive description of OCD in the modern era, in his case history of a patient he nicknamed the Rat Man (Freud, 1997). The actual identity of the Rat Man, whom Freud described as a "youngish man of university education," remains in some question, but he may have been a lawyer by the name of Ernst Lanzer. The Rat Man was treated by Freud over several months, starting in 1907, because of intrusive obsessive thoughts and compulsive urges he had experienced since childhood including the eponymous obsessive thought about a form of torture involving rats. Freud provided a typically psychoanalytic explanation for the symptoms, centering around forbidden sexual and aggressive wishes and the defenses against them, and claimed at least partial success for the treatment. Despite the differences between Freud's approach and those more common today, the case of the Rat Man highlights many aspects of the disorder that are still seen as hallmark features.

▓ DIAGNOSIS, DEFINITION, CLINICAL FEATURES

OCD is the clinical term for a condition characterized by the presence of *obsessions* and/or *compulsions*. Obsessions are thoughts, urges, impulses, images, or other mental content that are intrusive in that they enter the mind unbidden and repeatedly, causing distress and impairing normal function. In children in particular, obsessions may be described as a "voice" in the mind but should be distinguished from auditory hallucinations. Children with OCD who describe their obsessions as a voice are generally able to recognize that the thoughts are emerging from their own mind and do not expect others to hear them as well (Selles et al., 2018).

Compulsions are behaviors the person feels compelled to perform, usually in rigid and repetitive fashion and often with the goal of alleviating distress stemming from the presence of an obsession. Obsessive behaviors tend to be highly ritualized and can be external behaviors performed with the body or internal behaviors performed in the mind only. Some common examples of external compulsions include saying certain words, touching or arranging objects, repeating behaviors unnecessarily (e.g., washing or cleaning), and checking that some condition is met. Examples of internal compulsions can include repeating words in the mind, counting, mentally rehearsing or reviewing, and praying. Compulsions are often, but not always, directly linked to a particular obsession. For example, a child with obsessive thoughts about harm relating to germs or contamination may feel compelled to engage in handwashing rituals whenever the obsessive thought arises. But a child without such an obsession may likewise exhibit excessive handwashing. Even when the compulsion follows a particular obsession, the content of the thought will not necessarily be directly related to the form of the obsession. For example, a child with obsessions about engaging in a forbidden, inappropriate, or harmful behavior may likewise engage in handwashing in response to the thoughts.

Obsessions and compulsions can take any form and center around any domain of content, but certain themes or "dimensions" of OCD have been identified, and most OCD symptoms will fall into these broad categories (Leckman et al., 2005). Common themes for obsessions include thoughts about harm (either befalling or perpetrated by the individual with OCD), religion, sex (less common, but not absent in young children), symmetry, numbers (e.g., magical or "good" and "bad" numbers), contamination (by germs, chemicals, or other things), and doubting (e.g., doubting whether a certain behavior such as shutting off a light was actually completed). Common themes for compulsions include checking, arranging, repeating (can include physical, verbal, or mental repetition), and cleaning.

At least a moderate level of insight, or the ability to recognize that the obsessive thoughts are unrealistic and the compulsive behaviors unnecessary, is present in the majority of individuals with OCD, including children. In a large study aggregating data from multiple sources internationally, complete lack of insight was present in only 1.4% of children with OCD, whereas approximately 90% of children had insight that was categorized as fair or better (Leckman et al., 2005).

The broad spectrum of OCD symptoms, from the normative to the highly debilitating, means that the mere presence of some such symptoms cannot be taken as indicative of psychopathology. For example, a preference for repetition, a tendency toward various forms of magical thinking, certain superstitious-like behaviors, and repeated checking behaviors are all common during childhood. Likewise, young children often manifest a preoccupation with symmetry and rules and with guilt or lying that can be similar to symptoms of OCD (Leckman et al., 2005) (Box 13.1).

Establishing a diagnosis of OCD therefore necessitates that the symptoms be developmentally unexpected and significantly impairing to some important area of functioning such as school, social interactions, or family relations or that they consume substantial time each day (American Psychiatric Association, 2013). Determining the actual amount of time consumed by OCD symptoms can be challenging however, in particular for young children or when the symptoms are primarily internal mental events.

BOX 13.1 **Obsessive-Compulsive Disorder: Overview of Diagnosis and Clinical Features in Children and Adolescents**

- Obsessions (recurrent and persistent thoughts, impulses, or images) are present, experienced as intrusive and unwanted, and usually cause marked anxiety or distress.
- Compulsions (repetitive behaviors or mental acts) are present and the individual feels compelled to perform them to reduce anxiety or prevent a feared event.
- The obsessions or compulsions are time consuming (e.g., take more than 1 hour a day) or cause significant distress or impairment to function.
- The obsessive-compulsive symptoms are not attributable to the physiologic effects of a substance or medical condition.
- Young children may not be able to articulate the aims of their compulsive acts.
- The level of insight (recognition that the obsessive beliefs are not true) is specified as "good or fair," "poor," or "absent."
- The presence of or history of a tic disorder is specified.

The impairment associated with OCD, much like the severity of symptoms, can range very broadly. In some cases, only certain aspects of functioning are meaningfully impaired and overall function is well preserved. For example, a child with OCD may be chronically late to school or other engagements because of compulsive rituals and slowness but may function at a high level once there.

Children with OCD may be high achievers in school and social interactions can also be good, though in many cases they are impacted by the symptoms. In other cases, the impairment is considerably broader and almost every aspect of function is impacted. In the most severe cases, the disorder can be completely debilitating, preventing essentially any age-appropriate function in or outside of the home. The repetition of certain rituals can also lead to physical damage such as the macerations that can occur from excessive handwashing (Box 13.2).

As with other childhood conditions, impairment is not limited to the child alone and overall family functioning is frequently significantly impaired. A child with OCD can place functional and economic burden on a family. Relations often become strained because of a child's symptoms and parents may miss work because of the need to remain with a child. Some symptoms can also lead to extra expenses as parents purchase special items or buy larger quantities of items than they otherwise would.

Parents and others in the home typically engage in family accommodation of children's OCD symptoms (Shimshoni et al., 2019). The term *accommodation* refers to any changes to the parents' behavior aimed at helping their child to avoid or lessen symptom-related distress. Common forms of accommodation in OCD include parents purchasing special items, engaging in compulsive rituals themselves, and listening to a child's "confessions." For example, parents might carry a child physically because their OCD makes them unwilling to walk in certain places or touch the floor, or they might answer repeated questions relating to the child's obsessive content. The accommodation can be extremely time consuming and children will often react negatively, including with anger or aggression, to any attempt on the parents' part to refrain from accommodating. Parents typically report high levels of distress stemming from the need to accommodate their child. Research also consistently links higher levels of accommodation to worse symptoms and indicates that accommodation is associated with worse treatment outcomes for both psychosocial and pharmacologic treatment interventions (Strauss et al., 2015).

BOX 13.2	**Case Report: Obsessive-Compulsive Disorder**

Luke is a 13-year-old boy who lives with his parents and older sister. He was referred by his primary care provider for assessment in light of long-standing difficulties. His pediatrician reported that, for as long as he had known him (since toddlerhood), Luke has been a worrier but over the last several years things had "taken a turn for the worse" and his parents were urged by the pediatrician to seek psychiatric assessment.

Luke's parents reported that he was a bright and academically successful boy who had always been "a bit of a worrier." He worried about various bad things that might happen early in life and also was very meticulous, wanting his projects and school work to be perfect. He constantly sought feedback on his performance and would repeatedly check his work—sometimes to the point that his teachers would tell him things will become worse if he fussed over them too much. With the onset of adolescence, Luke had become more worried about his appearance and cleanliness. He wanted to have a girlfriend but was worried that his body odor (not notable to his parents or physician) would turn them off to him. He would repeatedly ask his parents for reassurance that he did not smell bad and they would accommodate by providing the reassurance, often many times per day. At around this time, his entry into junior high school had also meant a somewhat more challenging academic load with more need for forward planning and less tolerance of his difficulties "getting stuck" on assignments (in contrast to the past, he now had to deal with many teachers as opposed to just one).

Even small mistakes in his work would result in his redoing his assignment. He became more meticulous about clothing and seemed to his parents more withdrawn and preoccupied. He seemed to be taking longer and longer to get things done and now seemed to lose many of his connections with peers as a result. He could spend several hours in the shower each day. Because he was unwilling to talk with his parents about his problems, they talked with his pediatrician who made the referral for psychiatric assessment.

In talking with the parents, it emerged that there was a family history of depression and a paternal uncle had Tourette's syndrome—well controlled with medication.

Reprinted with permission from Volkmar, F. R., & Martin, A. (2011). *Essentials of Lewis's child and adolescent psychiatry* (1st ed.). Lippincott Williams & Wilkins/Wolters Kluwer.

■ EPIDEMIOLOGY AND DEMOGRAPHICS

Given the heterogeneity of its presentation and the broad spectrum of symptoms across both form and severity, it is not surprising that establishing the actual prevalence rates of OCD in children and adolescents, and indeed at any age, is not straightforward and estimates have ranged quite broadly. It is likely that actual lifetime prevalence is between 1% and 2% and approximately equal for males and females, though average age of onset may be earlier for boys than for girls, leading to higher prevalence of OCD in male children (Rapoport et al., 2000). Rates of OCD in different demographic groups, including race and ethnicity, are comparable.

In general, age of onset for OCD appears to follow a bimodal distribution with two peak points. Early-onset OCD begins in the prepubertal period, usually between the ages of 6 and 10. Later-onset OCD usually begins toward the end of the teenage years or in early adulthood (Chabane et al., 2005).

Comorbidity is very common in OCD, with clinical samples showing a majority of cases having at least one comorbid psychiatric condition (Storch et al., 2008). Frequently comorbid with OCD are anxiety disorders, depression, attention and behavior problems, and other OCD-related conditions such as tic disorders and hoarding. The presence of comorbidity can increase the burden of the condition and is associated with more severe symptoms, greater impairment, and worse treatment outcomes (Geller, Biederman, Stewart, Mullin, Farrell, et al., 2003).

■ ETIOLOGY AND PATHOGENESIS

The etiology of OCD is a matter of ongoing research; its understanding is hampered by aspects of the condition and by methodologic limitations. Among these are the heterogeneity of the disorder and the possibility for multiple etiologically distinct subtypes, as well as small sample sizes in many studies and the variability in diagnostic and assessment tests used.

Genetic research supports an important role for heritability in the vulnerability to OCD. Familial studies show higher rates of OCD among first-degree relatives of individuals with OCD, compared with the general population, as well as higher rates of other OCD-related conditions such as tics, trichotillomania, and body dysmorphic disorder (Grabe et al., 2006; Pauls et al., 1995). Twin studies have also found that monozygotic (identical) twins are significantly more likely to share a diagnosis of OCD than are dizygotic (fraternal) twins (Hudziak et al., 2004). Genome-wide association studies have also supported significant heritability for OCD and are being used, along with other methodologies, to identify specific genes implicated in the etiology of the disorder (Shugart et al., 2006).

Functional and structural brain imaging studies have pointed to several neurobiological abnormalities in the brains of individuals with OCD, including in children. These findings however should be interpreted with caution until better replication using larger studies and complementary methods is available.

Much research has focused on cortico-striato-thalamo-circuitry (CSTC) (Menzies et al., 2008). These circuits, linking frontal lobe regions, the basal ganglia, and the thalamus through both excitatory and inhibitory pathways, form a loop that is critical to movement, habit formation, and decision making. Studies, in both adults and children with OCD, point to abnormalities in CSTC structure and function (Saxena & Rauch, 2000). Imbalance between the pathways that make up the CSTC may be particularly implicated in the emergence and maintenance of OCD symptoms.

The CSTC model is also well aligned with the efficacy of serotonin reuptake inhibiting (SRI) medications in reducing OCD symptoms. Augmenting serotonergic activity would reduce glutamatergic signaling and activity in system.

Much debate and no small amount of controversy has surrounded the role of infection and inflammation in the etiology of some cases of OCD. The link was first proposed in 1998 in a paper suggesting that certain acute-onset cases of pediatric OCD were associated with group A β-hemolytic streptococcal infection (Swedo et al., 1998). The paper coined the term *PANDAS* for Pediatric Autoimmune Neuropsychiatric Disorder Associated with Streptococcal infection to describe this syndrome. The issue has remained controversial because of questions surrounding the strength of the evidence for the suggested pathophysiology, the temporal relations between the highly common streptococcal infections and symptom onset or exacerbation, and the response to treatments targeting the bacteria (Leckman et al., 2011; Lougee et al., 2000). Questions relating to treatment are particularly important as the hypothesis that the immune system's response to streptococcal infection is the cause of the OCD symptoms has led to sometimes aggressive, burdensome, or expensive treatments that carry their own risks. Among these are the acute and prophylactic use of antibiotics, immunotherapy, corticosteroids, intravenous immunoglobulin and plasma exchange, and tonsillectomies (Nicolson et al., 2000). More recently, a revised classification has been proposed, termed *PANS* for Pediatric Acute-onset Neuropsychiatric Syndrome (Chang et al., 2015). A PANS diagnosis is based on the sudden onset of OCD symptoms and on the presence of certain ancillary symptoms relating to mood, behavior, sleep, urination, and sensory motor functioning, but does not require a history of streptococcal infection.

COURSE

OCD is a chronic condition that when not treated effectively will continue to cause distress and impair function for years in many, and likely most, cases. Indeed, in a study of adults with OCD, over three-quarters reported their symptoms' onset in childhood rather than adulthood (Ruscio et al., 2010). For children with comorbid mental health problems and for those that have not responded to an evidence-based treatment, likelihood of remission is even lower (Geller, Biederman, Stewart, Mullin, Martin, et al., 2003). There are however treatments for OCD that are efficacious in approximately half of the cases in clinical trials (Abramowitz et al., 2005).

DIFFERENTIAL DIAGNOSIS AND ASSESSMENT

Obsessive thoughts and rigid or compulsive behavior are typical of numerous conditions, and establishing a diagnosis of OCD relies on thorough evaluation, integrating information from multiple sources, and careful differential diagnosis. For example, patients with anorexia may experience obsessive thoughts relating to food or body weight, those with generalized anxiety disorder experience persistent worries that cause distress and are difficult to control, and those with posttraumatic stress disorder experience intrusive thoughts relating to their traumatic past. Likewise, patients with autism spectrum disorder may exhibit behavioral rigidity and compulsivity, and those with tics manifest repetitive behaviors. OCD should also be distinguished from obsessive-compulsive personality disorder, a condition that is also characterized by over-preoccupation with rules, excessive scrupulosity, and inflexibility (Table 13.1).

Assessment should include clinical interview with a clinician knowledgeable about OCD as well as the use of standardized instruments. Both the child and the parents should provide information for the evaluation. The nature of OCD symptoms causes many children, and some parents, to be reluctant to fully disclose their symptoms and it is essential to convey an

TABLE 13.1

Disorders Manifesting Obsessions and/or Compulsions

Anorexia nervosa
Body dysmorphic disorder
Delusional disorder (all types)
Depression
Hypochondriasis
Obsessive-compulsive personality disorder
Organic mental disorder[a]
Panic disorder
Pervasive developmental disorder
Phobias
Posttraumatic stress disorder
Schizophrenia
Schizotypal personality
Somatization disorder
Somatoform disorders
Trichotillomania
Tourette's syndrome

[a]Specifically arising from CNS trauma, tumors, toxins.
Reprinted with permission from Towbin, K., & Riddle, M. (2017). Obsessive compulsive disorder. In A. Martin & F. R. Volkmar (Eds.), *Lewis's child and adolescent psychiatry: A comprehensive textbook* (4th ed., p. 556). Lippincott Williams & Wilkins.

open and accepting atmosphere and to make clear that the symptoms of OCD are familiar to the clinician who will not be surprised, embarrassed, or judgmental about them (Rapoport & Inoff-Germain, 2000). For example, a child who experiences obsessive thoughts of a bizarre or sexual nature may find it very difficult to share these symptoms during the evaluation. Parents should also be reassured that irrational thoughts are an intrinsic part of the disorder. For example, parents of a child with thoughts of harming others, such as a sibling, may be reassured to learn that these are common obsessions and do not signify that the child is dangerous or will become so in the future. Indeed, providing psychoeducation to the child and family about OCD during the evaluation process can begin to have a therapeutic effect even before treatment is formally commenced.

In addition to the natural reluctance to disclose certain symptoms, children and parents may not associate some symptoms with the OCD, rather seeing them as merely habits, personality, superstitions, or "quirks." For example, a common symptom of OCD in children is the tendency to "evening out." This refers to attempts the child makes to establish a feeling of symmetry in their own body. For example, a child may "even out" their body by flexing their right hand if for some reason they flexed their left. Parents are often unaware of such symptoms and the child may omit them in their report if they do not connect them with other OCD symptoms. Relatedly, many children with OCD will attempt to achieve a feeling of "just right" in certain behaviors, for example, placing their cup down on the table *just right* with the correct amount of force. Just right symptoms are often unaccompanied by specific obsessive thoughts and are easy to miss during assessment. Reviewing a thorough list of obsessions and compulsions, rather than only asking the family what symptoms they are aware of, is an important part of the evaluation process.

The Children's Yale-Brown Obsessive Compulsive Scale (CY-BOCS) is a standardized checklist that can provide information on the nature and severity of a child's current and past OCD symptoms (Goodman, Price, Rasmussen, Mazure, Delgado, et al., 1989; Goodman, Price, Rasmussen, Mazure, Fleischmann, et al., 1989). The CY-BOCS was developed as a clinician-administered instrument but is also used as a self-report measure for children and parents. The CY-BOCS begins with checklists of common obsessions and compulsions, and patients indicate whether these symptoms are currently present or have been so in the past. Following this, several questions query the current (past week) severity of the overall symptoms, taken together as a group. The scores for these questions are summed to provide an overall severity score and cutoffs are provided for determining whether symptoms are subclinical, mild, moderate, severe, or extreme. The CY-BOCS can be readministered to gauge treatment-related changes in symptom severity.

TREATMENT

Two treatments are currently recognized as frontline evidence-based treatments for childhood OCD: cognitive-behavioral therapy (CBT) and medications. CBT for OCD is also often termed *Exposure and Response Prevention*. The key element of exposure and response prevention is practicing exposure to stimuli or situations that trigger obsessive thoughts and evoke the urge to perform a compulsive ritual while refraining from performing the compulsion (March, 1995). For example, for a child with obsessive thoughts relating to numbers who normally avoids the number 4, exposures might include saying the number 4 or doing things 4 times. Or, for a child with contamination obsessions who performs cleaning rituals after contact with things that might carry germs, exposures might include touching unclean surfaces and refraining from the cleaning compulsion. In a typical course of treatment, the patient and therapist will construct an "exposure hierarchy," which is a list of various exposures ranked in difficulty from easier to harder, and then practice each step on the hierarchy several times until it ceases to elicit significant distress.

Prior to the actual exposures, the child will receive psychoeducation, instructing them about the nature of the problem and the rationale for the treatment approach. This will usually include a discussion of how the performance of compulsive rituals, although effective in reducing the distress in the very short term, actually maintains OCD symptoms over time, trapping the child in a cycle of distress and compulsion. The child will also learn about the nature of the anxiety and the anxious response, and, in particular, that anxiety will subside independently even if the compulsion is not enacted or the situation is avoided. Many children feel or believe that avoidance and compulsive behavior are the only means of reducing their distress and will learn in treatment, through information and experience, that this is not so.

Alongside the behavioral component of exposure and response prevention, CBT also focuses on modifying maladaptive and distorted cognitions that are typical of children with OCD. Children are taught to label obsessive thoughts as such and to challenge their irrational thoughts and beliefs, and replace them with more rational thoughts, a process known as cognitive restructuring.

The frontline pharmacologic treatment for OCD, the other evidence-based treatment alongside CBT, is the use of SRIs (Geller et al., 2001; Geller, Biederman, Stewart, Mullin, Martin, et al., 2003; March et al., 1998). Selecting the specific drug of use from within the group of SRIs relies on consideration of numerous clinical factors, and a certain amount of trial and error may be required. However, it is important to ensure that a drug has been adequately trialed before introducing an alternative.

Although insufficiently efficacious on their own, it is not uncommon to augment the SRIs with atypical antipsychotic medications (Bloch & Storch, 2015). Importantly, however, these medications are associated with more serious side effects and require a high level of monitoring as well as thorough psychoeducation for the patient and family.

The efficacy of CBT for childhood OCD has been demonstrated several times in randomized clinical trials. The largest of these was the Pediatric OCD Treatment Study (POTS) (Pediatric OCD Treatment Study Team, 2004). POTS randomly assigned children to CBT, medication (sertraline), the combination of CBT and medication, or medication placebo control. Results from the study showed similar efficacy for both single therapies, with approximately 40% response. The combined treatment was somewhat more efficacious than either treatment alone, and all active treatments were more efficacious than the placebo. Other studies have demonstrated that CBT can be streamlined by focusing primarily on the behavioral exposure component of therapy, and other modalities of treatment delivery, including web-based treatment, have also been found to work (Storch et al., 2011).

■ SUMMARY

Obsessive-compulsive symptoms are common in the general population, in particular during childhood and adolescence, and should only be considered indicative of obsessive-compulsive disorder when they take up significant time, cause distress to the patient, and meaningfully impair normal functioning. Research into the etiology of OCD is ongoing and has pointed to several biological mechanisms as potentially implicated causing or maintaining this disorder. Genetic heritability contributes to the risk of OCD, but the process of identifying specific risk genes for this condition is still in early stages. Assessment is complicated by the broad heterogeneity of the condition, the possibility that multiple distinct subtypes of OCD exist, and the reluctance of some patients to openly disclose the full range of their obsessive-compulsive symptoms. Front-line evidence-based treatments for OCD in children and adolescents include cognitive-behavioral therapy, with an emphasis on exposure and response prevention (E/RP), and the use of medications, in particular serotonin reuptake inhibitors. Taken together, these treatments appear to be efficacious in approximately half of cases in clinical trials.

References

*Indicates Particularly Recommended

Abramowitz, J. S., Whiteside, S. R., & Deacon, B. J. (2005). The effectiveness of treatment for pediatric obsessive-compulsive disorder: A meta-analysis. *Behavior Therapy, 36*(1), 55–63. https://doi .org/10.1016/S0005-7894(05)80054-1

American Psychiatric Association. (2013). *Diagnostic and statistical manual of mental disorders* (5th ed.). American Psychiatric Publishing.

Bloch, M. H., & Storch, E. A. (2015). Assessment and management of treatment-refractory obsessive-compulsive disorder in children. *Journal of the American Academy of Child and Adolescent Psychiatry, 54*(4), 251–262. https://doi.org/10.1016/j.jaac.2015.01.011

Chabane, N., Delorme, R., Millet, B., Mouren, M.-C., Leboyer, M., & Pauls, D. (2005). Early-onset obsessive-compulsive disorder: A subgroup with a specific clinical and familial pattern? *Journal of Child Psychology and Psychiatry, 46*(8), 881–887. https://doi.org/10.1111/j.1469-7610.2004.00382.x

*Chang, K., Frankovich, J., Cooperstock, M., Cunningham, M. W., Latimer, M. E., Murphy, T. K., Pasternack, M., Thienemann, M., Williams, K., Walter, J., Swedo, S. E., & PANS Collaborative Consortium. (2015). Clinical evaluation of youth with pediatric acute-onset neuropsychiatric syndrome (PANS): Recommendations from the 2013 PANS Consensus Conference. *Journal of Child and Adolescent Psychopharmacology, 25*(1), 3–13. https://doi.org/10.1089/cap.2014.0084

Freud, S. (1997). Theoretical (from "notes upon a case of obsessional neurosis"). In D. J. Stein & M. H. Stone (Eds.), *Essential papers on obsessive-compulsive disorder* (pp. 45–64). New York University Press.

Garcia-Soriano, G., Belloch, A., Morillo, C., & Clark, D. A. (2011). Symptom dimensions in obsessive-compulsive disorder: From normal cognitive intrusions to clinical obsessions. *Journal of Anxiety Disorders, 25*(4), 474–482. https://doi.org/10.1016/j.janxdis.2010.11.012

Geller, D. A., Biederman, J., Stewart, S. E., Mullin, B., Farrell, C., Wagner, K. D., Emslie, G., & Carpenter, D. (2003). Impact of comorbidity on treatment response to paroxetine in pediatric obsessive-compulsive disorder: Is the use of exclusion criteria empirically supported in randomized clinical trials? *Journal of Child and Adolescent Psychopharmacology, 13*(1 Suppl), S19–S29. https://doi.org/10.1089/104454603322126313

Geller, D. A., Biederman, J., Stewart, S. E., Mullin, B., Martin, A., Spencer, T., & Faraone, S. V. (2003). Which SSRI? A meta-analysis of pharmacotherapy trials in pediatric obsessive-compulsive disorder. *American Journal of Psychiatry, 160*(11), 1919–1928. https://doi.org/10.1176/appi.ajp.160.11.1919

Geller, D. A., Hoog, S. L., Heiligenstein, J. H., Ricardi, R. K., Tamura, R., Kluszynski, S., Jacobson, J. G., & Fluoxetine Pediatric OCD Study Team. (2001). Fluoxetine treatment for obsessive-compulsive disorder in children and adolescents: A placebo-controlled clinical trial. *Journal of the American Academy of Child and Adolescent Psychiatry, 40*(7), 773–779. https://doi.org/10.1097/00004583-200107000-00011

Goodman, W. K., Price, L. H., Rasmussen, S. A., Mazure, C., Delgado, P., Heninger, G. R., & Charney, D. S. (1989). The yale-brown obsessive compulsive scale. II. Validity. *Archives of General Psychiatry, 46*(11), 1012–1016. https://doi.org/10.1001/archpsyc.1989.01810110054008

Goodman, W. K., Price, L. H., Rasmussen, S. A., Mazure, C., Fleischmann, R. L., Hill, C. L., Heninger, G. R., & Charney, D. S. (1989). The yale-brown obsessive compulsive scale. I. Development, use, and reliability. *Archives of General Psychiatry, 46*(11), 1006–1011. https://doi.org/10.1001/archpsyc.1989.01810110048007

Grabe, H. J., Ruhrmann, S., Ettelt, S., Buhtz, F., Hochrein, A., Schulze-Rauschenbach, S., Meyer, K., Kraft, S., Reck, C., Pukrop, R., Freyberger, H. J., Klosterkötter, J., Falkai, P., John, U., Maier, W., & Wagner, M. (2006). Familiality of obsessive-compulsive disorder in nonclinical and clinical subjects. *The American Journal of Psychiatry, 163*(11), 1986–1992. https://doi.org/10.1176/appi.163.11.1986

*Hudziak, J. J., van Beijsterveldt, C. E. M., Althoff, R. R., Stanger, C., Rettew, D. C., Nelson, E. C., Todd, R. D., Bartels, M., & Boomsma, D. I. (2004). Genetic and environmental contributions to the child behavior checklist obsessive-compulsive scale: A cross-cultural twin study. *Archives of General Psychiatry, 61*(6), 608–616. https://doi.org/10.1001/archpsyc.61.6.608

Leckman, J., King, R., Gilbert, D., Coffey, B., Singer, H., Dure, L., Grantz, H., Katsovich, L., Lin, H., Lombroso, P. J., Kawikova, I., Johnson, D. R., Kurlan, R. M., & Kaplan, E. (2011). Streptococcal upper respiratory tract infections and exacerbations of tic and obsessive-compulsive symptoms: A prospective longitudinal study. *Journal of the American Academy of Child and Adolescent Psychiatry, 50*(2), 108–118. https://doi.org/10.1016/j.jaac.2010.10.011

Leckman, J. F., MataixCols, D., & RosarioCampos, M. C. (2005). Symptom dimensions in OCD: Developmental and evolutionary perspectives. In J. S. Abramowitz & A. C. Houts (Eds.), *Concepts and controversies in obsessive-compulsive disorder* (pp. 3–25). Springer Science + Business Media.

Lougee, L., Perlmutter, S. J., Nicolson, R., Garvey, M. A., & Swedo, S. E. (2000). Psychiatric disorders in first-degree relatives of children with pediatric autoimmune neuropsychiatric disorders associated with streptococcal infections (pandas). *Journal of the American Academy of Child and Adolescent Psychiatry, 39*(9), 1120–1126. https://doi.org/10.1097/00004583-200009000-00011

*March, J. S. (1995). Cognitive-behavioral psychotherapy for children and adolescents with OCD: A review and recommendations for treatment. *Journal of the American Academy of Child and Adolescent Psychiatry, 34*(1), 7–18. https://doi.org/10.1097/00004583-199501000-00008

*March, J. S., Biederman, J., Wolkow, R., Safferman, A., Mardekian, J., Cook, E. H., Cutler, N. R., Domingues, R., Ferguson, J., Muller, B., Riesenberg, M., Rosenthal, M., Sallee, F. R., Wagner, K. D., & Steiner, H. (1998). Sertraline in children and adolescents with obsessive-compulsive disorder: A multicenter randomized controlled trial. *JAMA, 280*(20), 1752–1756. https://doi.org/10.1001/jama.280.20.1752

Menzies, L., Chamberlain, S. R., Laird, A. R., Thelen, S. M., Sahakian, B. J., & Bullmore, E. T. (2008). Integrating evidence from neuroimaging and neuropsychological studies of obsessive-compulsive disorder: The orbitofronto-striatal model revisited. *Neuroscience and Biobehavioral Reviews, 32*(3), 525–549. https://doi.org/10.1016/j.neubiorev.2007.09.005

Nicolson, R., Swedo, S. E., Lenane, M., Bedwell, J., Wudarsky, M., Gochman, P., Hamburger, S. D., & Rapoport, J. L. (2000). An open trial of plasma exchange in childhood-onset obsessive-compulsive disorder without poststreptococcal exacerbations. *Journal of the American Academy of Child and Adolescent Psychiatry, 39*(10), 1313–1315. https://doi.org/10.1097/00004583-200010000-00020

Pauls, D. L., Alsobrook, J. P., Goodman, W., Rasmussen, S., & Leckman, J. F. (1995). A family study of obsessive-compulsive disorder. *The American Journal of Psychiatry, 152*(1), 358–363. https://doi.org/10.1176/ajp.152.1.76 7802125

*Pediatric OCD Treatment Study Team. (2004). Cognitive-behavior therapy, sertraline, and their combination for children and adolescents with obsessive-compulsive disorder. *JAMA, 292*(16), 1969–1976. https://doi.org/10.1001/jama.292.16.1969

Rapoport, J. L., & Inoff-Germain, G. (2000). Treatment of obsessive-compulsive disorder in children and adolescents. *Journal of Child Psychology and Psychiatry and Allied Disciplines, 41*(4), 419–431. https://doi.org/10.1111/1469-7610.00627

Rapoport, J. L., Inoff-Germain, G., Weissman, M. M., Greenwald, S., Narrow, W. E., Jensen, P. S., Lahey, B. B., & Canino, G. (2000). Childhood obsessive-compulsive disorder in the NIMH MECA study: Parent versus child identification of cases. Methods for the epidemiology of child and adolescent mental disorders. *Journal of Anxiety Disorders, 14*(6), 535–548. https://doi.org/10.1016/S0887-6185(00)00048-7

Ruscio, A. M., Stein, D. J., Chiu, W. T., & Kessler, R. C. (2010). The epidemiology of obsessive-compulsive disorder in the national comorbidity survey replication. *Molecular Psychiatry, 15*(1), 53–63. https://doi.org/10.1038/mp.2008.94

Saxena, S., & Rauch, S. L. (2000). Functional neuroimaging and the neuroanatomy of obsessive-compulsive disorder. *Psychiatric Clinics of North America, 23*(3), 563–586. https://doi.org/10.1016/S0193-953X(05)70181-7

Selles, R. R., Hojgaard, D. R. M. A., Ivarsson, T., Thomsen, P. H., McBride, N., Storch, E. A., Geller, D., Wilhelm, S., Farrell, L. J., Waters, A. M., Mathieu, S., Lebowitz, E., Elgie, M., Soreni, N., & Stewart, S. E. (2018). Symptom insight in pediatric obsessive-compulsive disorder: Outcomes of an international aggregated cross-sectional sample. *Journal of the American Academy of Child and Adolescent Psychiatry, 57*(8), 615–619. https://doi.org/10.1016/j.jaac.2018.04.012

Shimshoni, Y., Shrinivasa, B., Cherian, A. V., & Lebowitz, E. R. (2019). Family accommodation in psychopathology: A synthesized review. *Indian Journal of Psychiatry, 61*(7), S93–S103. https://doi.org/10.4103/psychiatry.IndianJPsychiatry_530_18

Shugart, Y. Y., Samuels, J., Willour, V. L., Grados, M. A., Greenberg, B. D., Knowles, J. A., McCracken, J. T., Rauch, S. L., Murphy, D. L., Wang, Y., Pinto, A., Fyer, A. J., Piacentini, J., Pauls, D. L., Cullen, B., Page, J., Rasmussen, S. A., Bienvenu, O. J., Hoehn-Saric, R., ... Nestadt, G. (2006). Genomewide linkage scan for obsessive-compulsive disorder: Evidence for susceptibility loci on chromosomes 3q, 7p, 1q, 15q, and 6q. *Molecular Psychiatry, 11*(8), 763–770. https://doi.org/10.1038/sj.mp.4001847

Storch, E. A., Caporino, N. E., Morgan, J. R., Lewin, A. B., Rojas, A., Brauer, L., Larsen, M. J., & Murphy, T. K. (2011). Preliminary investigation of web-camera delivered cognitive-behavioral therapy for youth with obsessive-compulsive disorder. *Psychiatry Research, 189*(3), 407–412. https://doi.org/10.1016/j.psychres.2011.05.047

Storch, E. A., Larson, M. J., Merlo, L. J., Keeley, M. L., Jacob, M. L., Geffken, G. R., Murphy, T. K., & Goodman, W. K. (2008). Comorbidity of pediatric obsessive-compulsive disorder and anxiety disorders: Impact on symptom severity and impairment. *Journal of Psychopathology and Behavioral Assessment, 30*(2), 111–120. https://doi.org/10.1007/s10862-007-9057-x

Strauss, C., Hale, L., & Stobie, B. (2015). A meta-analytic review of the relationship between family accommodation and OCD symptom severity. *Journal of Anxiety Disorders, 33*, 95–102. https://doi.org/10.1016/j.janxdis.2015.05.006

*Swedo, S. E., Leonard, H. L., Garvey, M., Mittleman, B., Allen, A. J., Perlmutter, S., Lougee, L., Dow, S., Zamkoff, J., & Dubbert, B. K. (1998). Pediatric autoimmune neuropsychiatric disorders associated with streptococcal infections: Clinical description of the first 50 cases. *American Journal of Psychiatry, 155*(2), 264–271. https://doi.org/10.1176/ajp.155.2.264

Suggested Readings

Barrett, P. M., Farrell, L., Pina, A. A., Peris, T. S., & Piacentini, J. (2008). Evidence-based psychosocial treatments for child and adolescent obsessive-compulsive disorder. *Journal of Clinical Child and Adolescent Psychology, 37*(1), 131–155. https://doi.org/10.1080/15374410701817956

Barrett, P. M., Shortt, A., & Healy, L. (2002). Do parent and child behaviours differentiate families whose children have obsessive-compulsive disorder from other clinic and non-clinic families? *Journal of Child Psychology and Psychiatry, 43*(5), 597–607. https://doi.org/10.1111/1469-7610.00049

Barzilay, R., Patrick, A., Calkins, M. E., Moore, T. M., Wolf, D. H., Benton, T. D., Leckman, J. F., & Gur, R. C. (2019). Obsessive-compulsive symptomatology in community youth: Typical development or a red flag for psychopathology? *Journal of the American Academy of Child and Adolescent Psychiatry, 58*(2), 277–286.e4. https://doi.org/10.1016/j.jaac.2018.06.038

Blanco-Vieira, T., Santos, M., Ferrao, Y. A., Torres, A. R., Miguel, E. C., Bloch, M. H., Leckman, J. F., & do Rosario, M. C. (2019). The impact of attention deficit hyperactivity disorder in obsessive-compulsive disorder subjects. *Depression and Anxiety, 36*(6), 533–542. https://doi.org/10.1002/da.22898

Bloch, M. H. (2017). *Chapter: Managing a child with OCD who is treatment refractory The clinician's guide to cognitive-behavioral therapy for pediatric obsessive-compulsive disorder* (pp. 329–356). Elsevier Academic Press.

Franklin, M., Freeman, J. B., & March, J. S. (2019). *Treating OCD in children and adolescents: A cognitive-behavioral approach.* The Guilford Press.

Lack, C. W., Storch, E. A., Keeley, M. L., Geffken, G. R., Ricketts, E. D., Murphy, T. K., & Goodman, W. K. (2009). Quality of life in children and adolescents with obsessive-compulsive disorder: Base rates, parent-child agreement, and clinical correlates. *Social Psychiatry and Psychiatric Epidemiology, 44*(11), 935–942. https://doi.org/10.1007/s00127-009-0013-9

Lebowitz, E. R., Vitulano, L. A., Mataix-Cols, D., & Leckman, J. (2011). Editorial perspective: When OCD takes over … the family! Coercive and disruptive behaviours in paediatric obsessive compulsive disorder. *Journal of Child Psychology and Psychiatry and Allied Disciplines, 52*(12), 1249–1250. https://doi.org/10.1111/j.1469-7610.2011.02480.x

Piacentini, J. (1999). Cognitive behavioral therapy of childhood OCD. *Child and Adolescent Psychiatric Clinics of North America, 8*(3), 599–616. https://doi.org/10.1016/S1056-4993(18)30170-6

Rapoport, J. L., Inoff-Germain, G., Weissman, M. M., Greenwald, S., Narrow, W. E., Jensen, P. S., Lahey, B. B., & Canino, G. (2000). Childhood obsessive-compulsive disorder in the NIMH MECA study: Parent versus child identification of cases. Methods for the epidemiology of child and adolescent mental disorders. *Journal of Anxiety Disorders, 14*(6), 535–548. https://doi.org/10.1016/s0887-6185(00)00048-7

Storch, E. A., Geffken, G. R., & Murphy, T. K. (2007). *Handbook of child and adolescent obsessive-compulsive disorder.* Lawrence Erlbaum Associates Publishers.

Towbin, K. E., & Riddle, M. A. (2018). Obsessive-compulsive disorder. In A. Martin, M. H. Bloch, & F. R. Volkmar (Eds.), *Lewis's child and adolescent psychiatry: A comprehensive textbook* (5th ed.). Wolters Kluwer.

CHAPTER 14 ■ DEPRESSIVE AND BIPOLAR DISORDERS

■ BACKGROUND

Although described in adults since antiquity, depressive disorders were only recognized in children beginning in the 1980s. Until that time, it was assumed, largely for theoretical reasons, that children either did not develop depressive disorders or that they presented in other ways (so-called masked depression). Although childhood depression can present in ways somewhat different from that in adults, it became clear that many of the symptoms are similar and that childhood depression is a frequent and impairing disorder.

Similarly, bipolar disorder or mania was first recognized in adults in ancient Greece and described by Kraepelin in the late 19th century, but it was assumed for many years that children could not experience it. Now there is recognition that, as with depression, children can suffer from bipolar disorders. Even more so, in most adults with bipolar disorder, the origins of the disorder can be traced to childhood or adolescence.

■ DEPRESSIVE DISORDERS

Diagnosis, Definition, and Clinical Features

In the fifth edition of the *Diagnostic and Statistical Manual of Mental Disorders* (*DSM-5*) (American Psychiatric Association, 2013), depressive disorders are separated from bipolar disorder and listed in separate chapters. In children and adolescents, the hallmarks of depressive disorder include chronic, pervasive, and all-encompassing sadness, lack of pleasure in enjoyable activities, and sometimes irritability. Depressive disorders differ from transient feelings of low mood based on their degree of pervasiveness and association with impairment in daily life or important areas of functioning. *DSM-5* currently recognizes several specific depressive disorders as well as an unspecified depressive disorder and depressive disorders due to medical conditions and substance abuse. Some of the relevant clinical features of these conditions are provided in Table 14.1.

Depressive disorders exist on a continuum classified based on the number and severity of symptoms and the degree of associated functional impairment. It is also possible to use specifiers for severity (mild, moderate, severe), for the presence or absence of psychotic features, and for remission status (partial or full) for the most recent episode. For major

TABLE 14.1

Depressive Disorders in Childhood and Adolescence: An Overview of Clinical and Diagnostic Features

Major Depressive Disorder (MDD)
Five or more persistent symptoms in the areas of affect, cognition, and neurovegetative functions that occur for at least 2 weeks and represent a clear change from previous functioning. • Depressed mood may include feeling sad, empty, hopeless, and irritable. • Other affective symptoms are loss of pleasure, worthlessness, and feelings of guilt. • Cognitive symptoms include difficulty paying attention, making decisions, thoughts of death, and suicidal ideation. • Somatic symptoms may include weight loss, lack of energy, fatigue, and insomnia. To meet criteria for the diagnosis, these symptoms should cause significant distress or impairment in one or more impaired areas of functioning such as social, family, or school. Exclusionary criteria require that the symptoms are not attributable to bereavement, substance abuse, or general medical condition. • For children, irritable mood can be experienced, and failure to make appropriate weight gain (rather than weigh toss) may also be encountered. • Various specifiers are available for coding: presence of unusual features (e.g., catatonia), and severity (e.g., mild, moderate, severe).
Persistent Depressive Disorder (Dysthymia)
Major feature is chronically depressed or irritable mood (most of the day, more often than not) associated with at least two features of depression. • 1-year duration is required (for children and adolescents; 2 years for adults). • Diagnosis is not made if better accounted for by major depression episode that has been present; diagnosis is also not made if features are better accounted for by substance use or abuse or a general medical condition; and it cannot occur exclusively in association with psychotic features. • Symptoms must be a source of distress or impairment. • Onset before or after age 21 years can be specified as can atypical features.
Disruptive Mood Dysregulation Disorder (DMDD)
Severe recurrent temper outbursts manifested verbally (e.g., verbal rages) and/or behaviorally (e.g., physical aggression toward people or property) that are grossly out of proportion in intensity or duration to the situation or provocation. • The temper outbursts are inconsistent with development, and occur three or more times per week. • The mood between temper outbursts is persistently irritable or angry most of the day, nearly every day. • Temper tantrums have been present for 12 or more months, in at least two of three settings and are severe in at least one of these. • The diagnosis not made before age 6 years or after age 18 years, and age at onset of severe tantrum has to be before 10 years of age.

Reprinted with permission from Volkmar, F. R., & Martin, A. (2011). *Essentials of Lewis's child and adolescent psychiatry* (1st ed., p. 140). Lippincott Williams & Wilkins/Wolters Kluwer.

depressive disorder, a child or adolescent must exhibit one of two cardinal symptoms: (1) sad or irritable mood or (2) lack of interest and pleasure for at least 2 weeks. Youth must also have four or more other symptoms such as social withdrawal, difficulty concentrating, insomnia or hypersomnia, feelings of worthlessness, and thoughts of death or suicidal ideations.

For persistent depressive disorder, which is also called dysthymia, a depressed or irritable mood must be present for at least 1 year and be associated with at least two depressive symptoms, such as appetite (undereating or overeating) or sleep (insomnia or hypersomnia) disturbances, lack of energy, low self-esteem, difficulties with concentration or decision making, or hopeless feelings. To meet criteria for dysthymia, the child or adolescent cannot be free of these symptoms for more than 2 months at a time. Milder versions of depressive disorder and subclinical forms of depression can still lead to considerable distress and impairment (Wesselhoeft et al., 2019). Other conditions with significant depressive aspects include adjustment disorders with depressed mood (e.g., after stress) and depressive disorders associated with general medical conditions (e.g., hypothyroidism). Various other conditions associated with depression can be diagnosed but are more common in adults.

A new childhood disorder was introduced in the *DSM-5* chapter on depressive disorder: *disruptive mood dysregulation disorder* (DMDD) (Roy et al., 2014). This disorder was included in the *DSM-5* to recognize the cardinal mood feature of pediatric irritability and to address concerns about over-diagnosis of bipolar disorder based on chronic irritability. DMDD is diagnosed based on chronic and severe irritability, manifested in frequent temper outbursts with angry or depressed mood between outbursts. Temper outbursts typically occur in response to frustration or provocation and can be associated with verbal and physical aggression. DMDD is common among children seeking mental health services and the 1-year prevalence rates are estimated to be between 2% and 5%. DMDD is also highly comorbid with other childhood disorders, most notably attention deficit hyperactivity disorder (ADHD) and anxiety. Frequent temper outbursts are also a symptom in oppositional defiant disorder (ODD), and the differential diagnosis of DMDD requires the presence of persistent disruption of mood between outbursts. In addition, diagnosis of DMDD requires severe impairment in at least one setting and moderate impairment in the second setting. DMDD is considered a more severe disorder than ODD, although some diagnostic confusion between the two disorders remains as diagnosis of ODD has three specifiers—mild, moderate, and severe— based on the presence of symptoms in one, two, or three and more settings, respectively (Stringaris et al., 2018).

One of the great complications in understanding and diagnosing depression (and other mood disorders) in children and adolescents is the complex relationships among various forms of psychopathology. Anxiety disorders are very frequently observed in association with (often preceding) depression. Depression is also associated with ADHD and conduct disorder (CD) as well as with substance abuse problems and has a strong familial basis. The nature of these comorbidities remains somewhat poorly understood. It might, for example, relate to commonalities in the various conditions or might reflect the fact that our nosology is attempting overly fine-grained distinctions (Angold et al., 1999).

Epidemiology and Demographics

The yearly prevalence of depressive disorders ranges from about 1% to 2% in childhood to between 4% and 8% of adolescents. The lifetime prevalence of depression by the end of teenage years can be as high as 20%. Starting in adolescence, female predominance emerges (female: male ratio 3:1), possibly as a result of differential effects of hormones in the changes in the brain circuitry involved in emotion regulation as well as higher rates of other internalizing disorders such as anxiety disorder in girls during adolescence (Avenevoli et al., 2015).

Recent work has underscored the potential for depression in young children, although in this age group, either irritability or sadness may be prominent (Donohue et al., 2019). Before puberty, depression is strongly associated with a range of other problems, including psychosocial adversity, chronic family fighting, parental substance abuse, or criminality. In some cases, familial transmission is striking with associations to other disorders such as anxiety and bipolar disorders (Shanahan et al., 2011).

Etiology and Pathogenesis

Genetic factors are a major risk factor for depressive disorders. Studies in twins show a heritability of about 40% to 65% with higher concordance rates in identical twins. Early onset (before puberty) may be more mediated by environmental factors. Depressive disorders are also strongly related to anxiety symptoms, and there is some suggestion that anxiety symptoms might increase the risk of developing depression, perhaps via specific genetic factors (Brent, 2018).

Cognitive factors have also been implicated in the pathogenesis. In contrast to individuals without depression, those with depression tend to develop cognitive biases associated with depressive symptoms including negative view of self, future, and the world (Beck et al., 1979). These cognitive distortions and biases can exacerbate reactions to stressful life events and predict onset of exacerbation of depressive symptoms. These cognitive distortions have been identified in both children and adolescents, and they often persist even after the depressive episode has passed, posing risk for recurrence of depression. Ruminative cognitive style, which involves repetitive and passive focus on upsetting events, has been particularly strongly associated with depression in adolescence and adulthood (Nolen-Hoeksema, 1991).

Studies of twins have also shown the importance of environmental factors. Indeed, shared environmental effects appear at least as strong as genetic ones (Goodyer, 2015). For example, having a depressed mother might provide not only a genetic risk but also a model for depression. Families in which depression exists without a strong family history are more likely to have had various forms of psychosocial adversity. Similarly, child neglect and abuse increase the risk for depression as does the loss of a parent or significant other (particularly if a strong family history of mood disorder exists) (LeMoult et al., 2020). On the other hand, protective factors include good connections to family, community, and school; engagement with supportive peers; and appropriate parental expectations and supervision.

Neuroimaging studies have shown consistent differences in the structure and function of brain regions and networks in emotional processing. For example, depressed adolescents were found to have dysfunctional connectivity in the attentional networks leading to greater attention to negative emotional cues and decreased activity in prefrontal cognitive networks that inhibit subcortical regions such as the amygdala that are involved in negative emotions (Miller et al., 2015). There are also consistent findings of abnormal neural processing of reward in children and adolescents with depression, namely, reduced striatal signal during reward processing (Keren et al., 2018). These neuroimaging results were found to be associated with concurrent symptoms of sadness and low positive affect as well as with the risk of developing depressive disorder later in life (Toenders et al., 2019). Studies of the noradrenergic and serotonergic neurotransmission systems have noted some differences in children with depression. Further, there is some suggestion of differences in cortisol secretion in adolescents (Brent, 2018).

Differential Diagnosis and Assessment

Assessment of childhood and adolescent depression begins with a comprehensive evaluation of the child and often separate interviews with the parents. The focus is on both the depression and other comorbid diagnoses. As noted previously, symptoms must meet certain requirements in terms of duration and number and must be a source of impairment (e.g., on school performance or peer relationships). The focus on impairment is essential in differentiating normative mood changes from a clinical disorder. As noted previously, the *DSM-5* allows irritable mood (rather than depression *per se*) to qualify for this diagnosis in children; when irritability is the presenting symptom, the clinician should be alert to the potential for depressive disorders to present in this fashion and alert to the possibility that the child or adolescent has relatively little awareness of the impact of their irritability on others. Similarly, the parents may not initially believe the child to be depressed and may view irritability as a sign of normal adolescent "storm and stress" (although the latter is not, in fact, necessarily normative; see Chapters 3 and 11). The adolescent may have greater insight into the nuances of their emotional experiences and interpersonal situations that might be linked to the experience and expression of sadness and anger. Difficulties in school are often associated with depression in children and adolescents and may result from chronic fatigue and difficulties with concentration and memory. Similarly, weight loss or failure to gain expected weight may

BOX 14.1 **Case Study: Depressive Disorder**

Liam is a 12-year-old boy who had exhibited difficulties in school over the past year. He was seen in the emergency department and complained of chronic depression, difficulties with sleeping and attention, lack of energy, and social isolation. He was overtly depressed with a sad mood. He cried easily and talked about his difficulties in school, which seemed related to his mood problems. He recently had been refusing to go to school. The visit to the emergency department was precipitated when his mother found Liam's diary open on his computer and saw that he was writing about suicide (planning to jump in front of a train on tracks near their house). There was a strong family history of depression and anxiety problems. His mother herself had been treated for many years with a selective serotonin reuptake inhibitor, and as an adolescent, she had one episode of suicidal ideation that led to hospital admission.

After the initial assessment, Liam agreed to a no-suicide contract, and both his parents and emergency department clinician were comfortable with the arrangements the family had made to ensure his safety. Rapid follow-up was arranged with the local community mental health clinic, and he was enrolled in a partial hospital program quickly. A combination of a selective serotonin reuptake inhibitor and cognitive behavior therapy led to remission of his symptoms, and he began attending school more regularly and transitioned into a less intense outpatient treatment program. At the time of last follow-up (age 15 years), he remained on medications but was free of depression symptoms and had returned to the expected levels of social and academic achievement in school.

Reprinted with permission from Volkmar, F. R., & Martin, A. (2011). *Essentials of Lewis's child and adolescent psychiatry* (1st ed., p. 142). Lippincott Williams & Wilkins/Wolters Kluwer.

be seen (excessive weight gain is more typical in adults). Children may complain of feeling bored or worthless. Adolescents are more likely than younger children to exhibit some of the more serious features of depression including psychotic features or suicide attempts, but the latter is possible at any age (see Chapter 27). Given the complexities of how depression may present, it is common for the initial complaint to be one focused on school work, behavior change, or substance abuse; sometimes a suicide attempt or expression of suicidal thoughts is what prompts parents or teachers to seek evaluation (Box 14.1).

Comorbidity is frequent and complicates assessment. As many as half of depressed youth may have at least two comorbid conditions, and a single comorbid condition is even more frequent. For example, it is common for an anxiety disorder to precede depression and to be comorbid with it. Other frequent conditions include substance abuse, attentional disorders, and conduct problems. The presence of comorbid conditions can have important implications for treatment and thus their presence is an important aspect of the initial assessment. The clinician should also be alert to the possibility that children and adolescents with bipolar disorder may present with a depressive episode. Accordingly, careful inquiry about manic or hypomanic symptomatology should be conducted, and the clinician following the child over time should be aware of the potential for bipolar disorder to develop after an initial period of depression. In taking a history, the clinician should be alert to the importance of potential stressors (e.g., for adjustment disorder with depressed mood). Similarly, bereavement can result in depressive symptoms. Substance use and withdrawal can also be associated with irritability or feelings of depression (substance-induced mood disorder can be diagnosed, but the clinician should be alert to the possibility that the child has essentially been self-medicating depression). The role of routine laboratory tests is relatively limited with the exception of symptoms that suggest hypothyroidism, which should prompt testing. Features that suggest substance abuse or the presence of a general medical condition might prompt other laboratory studies. A host of other medical problems can include a significant component of depression (e.g., seizure disorders, infections, other endocrinologic conditions, and autoimmune disorders, among others). Children with infections such as mononucleosis may also complain of chronic fatigue, difficulties concentrating, and mood problems suggestive of depression. Finally, a variety of medications (including antibiotics, steroids, oral contraceptives, and others) can be associated with symptoms suggestive of depression. When depression can be reasonably attributed to any of these conditions, a diagnosis of mood disorder associated with a general medical condition is made.

The task of the clinician is complicated by the considerable symptom overlap between depressive disorders and a range of other conditions including eating problems associated with eating disorders (see Chapter 17); sleep problems associated with stress or other psychiatric conditions (see Chapter 21); and mood and self-esteem problems that are frequent in children with developmental, learning, or attention deficit disorders (see Chapters 7, 9, and 10).

Several rating scales and checklists are available. These include Children's Depression Rating Scale-Revised (CDRS-R) (Poznanski & Mokros, 1996), a clinician-administered assessment of various symptom areas. The CDRS-R can be used at baseline and then for monitoring treatment efficacy. The Children Depression Inventory is another popular scale that has parent-rated and child self-report forms that provide cutoff scores for severity of depression based on a large standardization sample (Kovacs, 1992).

Treatment

Current guidelines for treatment of depression in children and adolescents are informed by four large clinical trials: the Treatment of Adolescents with Depression Study (TADS [N = 439]) (March, 2004), Treatment of Resistant Depression in Adolescents (TORDIA [N = 334]) (Brent et al., 2008), Adolescent Depression Antidepressants and Psychotherapy Trial (ADAPT [N = 208]) (Goodyer et al., 2008), and Improving Mood with Psychoanalytic and Cognitive Therapies (IMPACT [N = 465]) (Goodyer et al., 2017). Recent reviews summarize well-established approaches to assessment and treatment (especially psychotherapy) of adolescent depression (Goodyer & Wilkinson, 2019) as well as approaches to treatment-resistant depression (Dwyer et al., 2020). All treatment approaches emphasize psychoeducation, family engagements, and careful assessment of high-risk behavior of harm to self or others. Children with mild forms of depression can benefit from brief evidence-based psychotherapy and supportive counseling. Moderate to severe depression can require more intensive services and combinations of psychotherapy with medication.

Cognitive behavior therapy (CBT) and interpersonal therapy (IPT) are the most extensively studied forms of treatment for depression in children and adolescents. CBT uses a range of techniques to address maladaptive cognitions and behavior patterns that contribute to depression. The emphasis is on remediation of "distortions" and use of a range of strategies to cope more effectively with negative feelings and mood states. A number of different techniques can be used, and techniques and procedures are frequently modified for children of different ages. These treatments differ in some details, such as length of treatment, which can range from weeks to months, format (individual or group), and the degree of family involvement. Numerous studies have shown CBT for depression to be superior to wait-list control groups and usual clinical care, although the effect sizes vary depending on the type of control condition, informants (e.g., child vs. parents), and setting where the study was conducted (e.g., research center, school, community clinic) (Weisz et al., 2006). However, of note, in the TADS study in which CBT was compared with fluoxetine, a combination treatment (drug plus CBT), and placebo, CBT was not better than placebo, although the combination treatment (most effective) and drug treatment alone (with fluoxetine) were. It is possible that relatively low response rate to CBT in the TADS study (35%) was due to the differential assignment of more severely affected patients to the CBT treatment group or that the particular CBT approach in this study was overly structured to accommodate unique situations of study participants. Numerous modifications to CBT procedures have been made since the early pioneering work to improve treatment elements and make CBT more compelling for a wider type of symptom profiles across various groups of children and adolescents (Hetrick et al., 2016).

IPT for adolescents (IPT-A) is the other psychotherapeutic intervention for depression with substantive empirical support (Mufson et al., 1993). This approach emphasizes the interpersonal context of depression and has some similarities with, as well differences from, CBT. The interpersonal focus of IPT-A has some unique advantages for teenagers for whom peer relationships are particularly important and peer conflicts are frequent. IPT helps teenagers resolve interpersonal problems, and increases access to social support and decreases interpersonal stress, which improves emotional processing and interpersonal skills and ultimately improves symptoms of depression. There are a number of specific techniques that can be used, such as helping the client to express emotions in specific social situations and using role play to allow the client to "test out" and improve their communication style (Lipsitz & Markowitz, 2013). Several studies have now demonstrated the benefits of this approach, and the ability to move this treatment readily into school-based mental health clinics is an important advantage.

Selective serotonin reuptake inhibitor (SSRI) antidepressants are also used in children and adolescents, with fluoxetine (Prozac) among the most intensively studied agents in this class. In the TADS, fluoxetine was more effective than either placebo or CBT. Interestingly, in that study, combined treatments were most effective overall. Although the SSRIs appear to be of greater benefit than placebo, the overall effect size was not high, reflecting a robust placebo response rate. Other SSRIs have been studied as well, although less extensively, and show benefit, although effect sizes are relatively small, possibly due to high response to placebo. Adolescents appear to respond better to medication than younger children. Side effects and adverse events are a source of concern, including higher rates of suicide-related adverse events, mostly early on in treatment (Solmi et al., 2020). Although the risk-to-benefit ratio appears to be acceptable, caution and careful monitoring, particularly early in treatment, are indicated. Other adverse effects of antidepressant medications include agitation and restlessness, sleep and gastrointestinal problems, and some risk for increased bruising.

Given the generally strongly response to placebo or supportive treatment, it appears that for mild depression, supportive counseling and education are indicated. As depressive disorders become more severe or last longer, several treatment options are available, including SSRIs, CBT, or IPT-A. Response should be assessed after a reasonable period so that a move to a different strategy can be considered if the response is not satisfactory. If the individual fails to respond to one medication, a trial of another SSRI is indicated (see Chapter 21 for more details).

Course and Prognosis

The typical duration of depression episodes ranges between 3 and 6 months and is somewhat longer in clinically referred samples. Depressive episodes are long in the presence of some comorbid conditions, including anxiety and substance abuse disorders. Other factors associated with longer durations include family history (e.g., parental depression and family discord), initial greater severity, and the presence of suicidal ideation or behavior. In about one in five cases in adolescents, depression lasts for 2 years or more (Birmaher et al., 2002).

Unfortunately, recurrence risk is high in children and particularly in adolescents (up to 70% of cases over 1–2 years). Factors that increase the risk for recurrence include parental history of early onset mood problems, lack of total remission of symptoms, social difficulties, sexual abuse history, and chronic family strife. Other risk factors for recurring depression later in life include substance abuse, CD, as well as social, occupational, and academic difficulties.

◼ BIPOLAR DISORDER

Diagnosis, Definition, and Clinical Features

There has been tremendous growth in research on pediatric bipolar disorder over the past two decades (Birmaher et al., 2018). There is clear consensus among experts that children can meet criteria for bipolar disorder, although there is continuing debate regarding the degree to which cardinal adult features (grandiosity and elated mood) present in youth (Goldstein et al., 2017). Similarly, the issues of how best to define manic episodes in terms of symptoms, duration, and cycling remain controversial.

Despite these controversies, some children and adolescents clearly meet current *DSM-5* criteria, even though these criteria were initially developed in adults. For example, many of the criteria for either a manic or hypomanic episode could be viewed as applicable to children in general, at least to some extent. For example, exuberant mood, rapid speech, and high level of activity can be developmentally appropriate for children, at least in some situations such as at birthday parties or on family vacation trips. Accordingly, in considering the diagnosis of bipolar disorder in youth, it is important that developmental factors, context, and degree of mood abnormality relative to usual mood are taken into account. Symptoms must be viewed in a developmental context as well. For example, children do not have the opportunity to make unwise business decisions or drive recklessly, and high-risk behaviors in adolescence, including sexual behaviors, may arise from a sense of invulnerability (Axelson et al., 2006).

Table 14.2 summarizes current approaches to diagnosis. More so in children than in adults, the distinction between manic and hypomanic episodes can be difficult. A consideration of developmental issues can be helpful because the threshold for minimal duration and severity may otherwise be difficult to judge. Parents, teachers, and other caregivers have important roles to play in providing information. The lack of specificity of common symptoms of mania in children is also suggested by studies comparing bipolar disorder and ADHD, with no significant differences in several symptoms including irritability, accelerated speech, distractibility, and unusual energy levels. Accordingly, a simple frequency count of symptoms does not capture the complexity of the clinical phenomenon and has some potential to mislead less experienced clinicians. Some have argued for an emphasis on the core features of elevated mood and grandiosity. Unfortunately, although these features are usually present, there is more variability in children.

Other complexities arise in relation to features such as irritability (Brotman et al., 2017). Although almost always present, it is not specific to bipolar disorder—irritability is common in children with depression, conduct problems, anxiety, and stress-related disorders. This is an area of considerable disagreement, with some advocating reliance on irritability alone (if severe) as a primary feature of bipolar disorder in youth, but others emphasizing the lack of specificity in pediatric populations. A final controversy arises regarding the degree to which features are chronic or episodic. Some investigators suggest that symptoms are long-lasting, up to several years for manic or mixed episodes. Following a series of longitudinal studies of youths with severe irritability, a new diagnosis was introduced in *DSM-5*, DMDD, to recognize the presence of severe and chronic irritability in children.

The issue of associated depressive symptoms is of great interest, particularly because most studies of adults with bipolar disorder suggest that they exhibited noteworthy depressive symptoms in their youth. Some youth with bipolar disorder have clear periods of depression sufficient to qualify for a major depressive episode, and it is sometimes the case that bipolar disorder first presents with a depressive episode. Difficulties arise relative to differentiating mixed states of depressed and elated mood from affective lability or transient dysphoria. Symptom overlap and comorbidity complicate the issue of deciding the best way to assign the diagnosis. Yet other issues arise because at times youth have some manic symptoms, but either the symptoms do not last long enough or are not sufficiently distinctive or associated with other features; therefore, the question of whether full criteria are met is unclear. Current diagnostic classification offers additional specified and unspecified categories of bipolar disorder, but further work is needed to more precisely delineate syndrome boundaries.

TABLE 14.2

Bipolar Disorders in Childhood and Adolescence: An Overview of Clinical and Diagnostic Features

Manic Episode
Elevated, expansive, or irritable mood for at least 1 week (or any duration if hospitalization is necessary).   • During the period of mood disturbance and increased energy or activity, at least three of the following symptoms must be present: inflated self-esteem or grandiosity, diminished need for sleep, pressure of speech, racing thoughts or flight of idea, decreases in attention, agitation (psychomotor or sexual, although the latter is less common in children), risk taking.   • Difficulties must cause impairment or cause hospitalization but must not be attributable to substance use or abuse or a general medical condition, and the individual cannot meet the criteria for mixed episode.
Hypomanic Episode
A distinct period of elated, expansive, or irritable mood (lasting at least 4 days) that represents a change from baseline functioning (must be a distinct change and noticed by others).   • During this period, three or more of these symptoms must be present: grandiosity, diminished need for sleep, pressure of speech, racing thoughts or flight of idea, decreases in attention, agitation or increased activities, risk taking.   • Episode is associated with unequivocal change in functioning that is uncharacteristic of the person when they are not symptomatic, but does *not* cause marked impairment or need for hospitalization.   • Symptoms are not attributable to substance use or abuse or a general medical condition.
Bipolar I Disorder
One or more manic episodes must be present. The manic episode may have been preceded and may be followed by hypomanic or major depressive episodes.   • Difficulties must cause impairment or distress.   • A number of coding modifiers can be used to specify the nature of the most recent episode, severity, features of onset, rapid cycling, and so forth.
Bipolar II Disorder
Major depressive episode(s) associated with at least one hypomanic episode but *not* a manic episode).   • Difficulties must cause impairment or distress.   • A number of coding modifiers can be used to specify the nature of the most recent episode, severity, features of onset, rapid cycling, and so forth.
Cyclothymic Disorder
Symptoms of hypomania and depression are generally present for at least 1 year (in children and adolescents).   • These must be the source of distress or impairment.   • The diagnosis is not made if symptoms are better accounted for by another disorder or if they are attributable to substance use or abuse or a general medical condition.

Reprinted with permission from Volkmar, F. R., & Martin, A. (2011). *Essentials of Lewis's child and adolescent psychiatry* (1st ed., p. 147). Lippincott Williams & Wilkins/Wolters Kluwer.

Epidemiology and Demographics

Retrospectively, more than half of adults with bipolar disorder report symptom onset before age 20 years. Epidemiologic studies suggest rates of about 1% to 2% of the general population and that these rates tend to increase with age. In clinical populations, there is considerable

---

BOX 14.2	Case Study: Bipolar Disorder

Jim is a 15-year-old boy with a history of depression and one prior suicide attempt (overdose of his mother's medication). Over the past year, he had seemed to do well in an outpatient treatment program without medication, but over the past several weeks, he had been sleeping less and had taken on unrealistic projects. In particular, he attempted to board a train without a ticket because he decided he was ready to go to college. The police became involved when he presented his father's credit card to pay for a ticket, and his degree of obvious disturbance led the police to transport him to the nearest hospital.

On meeting the clinician, Jim began to talk very rapidly about his interest in becoming a physician and a lawyer. He attempted to explain his desire to board the train to get to college, but his account was difficult to follow, and his speech was pressured. After his parents arrived, they reported that he had seemed to need less sleep over the past week and was up at night engaged in various projects. They had been somewhat concerned about his mood because of a strong family history of depression and made an appointment for him that day for follow-up but had awoken to find that Jim had left the house and left them a note saying he was going off to college.

Jim's father reported that in the past, Jim had been somewhat reserved with girls, but over the last several weeks, had been e-mailing various girls in his class nonstop asking them to go out. He had lost weight over the past several weeks as his need for food seemed to diminish.

Jim became more and more agitated in the emergency department, eventually threatening staff members. He and his parents denied substance use and a toxicology screen was negative. Jim was initially treated with an antipsychotic medication and a mood stabilizer was added later. He responded well to this regimen and was hospitalized for 10 days. Follow-up indicated that for a period of almost 2 years, he only had very mild symptoms, except for one instance when he attempted to stop his mood stabilizer and experienced a second manic episode.

Reprinted with permission from Volkmar, F. R., & Martin, A. (2011). *Essentials of Lewis's child and adolescent psychiatry* (1st ed., p. 148). Lippincott Williams & Wilkins/Wolters Kluwer.

---

variation, presumably reflecting sundry factors related to ascertainment and methodology (Van Meter et al., 2019) (Box 14.2).

Etiology and Pathogenesis

A strong role for genetic factors is suggested by the high rates of bipolar disorder in family members (8–10 times more common than in the general population). Similarly, both adoption and twin studies show strong genetic components, with children of parents who have bipolar disorder having about a sevenfold increase in risk for bipolar disorder as well as high risk of anxiety, mood, attentional, and other problems. Finally, youth with bipolar disorder have first-degree relatives with higher risk for the condition. The heritability of the condition has been estimated to be more than 80% (Birmaher et al., 2018; Estrada-Prat et al., 2019).

Structural neuroimaging studies of children with bipolar disorder reported abnormally decreased amygdala volumes and decreased gray matter volumes in the orbitofrontal and anterior cingulate cortices (Cattarinussi et al., 2019). Functional MRI studies revealed abnormally low levels of activity and connectivity in emotion processing circuitry including amygdala and ventrolateral prefrontal cortex, and "overactivity" in the self-hemispheric ventral striatum and ventrolateral prefrontal cortex and orbitofrontal cortex (vlPFC/OFC) reward processing circuitry. Neuroimaging research also aims to dissociate brain correlates of pediatric bipolar from brain signatures of other disorders. For example, a recent review of neuroimaging studies of bipolar disorder versus depression reported that the most common differences were found in the anterior cingulate cortex, insula, and dorsal striatum, brain areas that play a significant role in neural systems that support emotion processing and regulation, cognition, and reward processing (Kelberman et al., 2021).

The small literature on psychosocial risk suggests that socioeconomic stress, negative life events, and high "expressed emotion" are associated with worse outcomes.

Differential Diagnosis and Assessment

As with depressive disorder, pediatric bipolar disorder is very frequently associated with other conditions, including ADHD, disruptive behavior disorder, and anxiety disorders. In adolescents, rates of substance abuse also gradually increase. Treatment should carefully consider the implications of comorbid conditions for planning care. The variability in clinical presentation and high rates of comorbidity raise major practical problems for differential diagnosis.

Various conditions that can lead to mood variability and behavioral challenges should be considered in the differential diagnosis (and sometimes are present in addition to the bipolar disorder). In addition to the conditions noted previously, these include depressive disorders, autism and related conditions, and other psychotic conditions, particularly schizophrenia. Substance abuse and borderline personality disorder can also sometimes be confused with pediatric bipolar disorder, although the history and presentation usually help to clarify the diagnosis. Various medical conditions can present with affective and behavioral change suggestive of mania (e.g., hyperthyroidism; brain tumors and trauma; side effects of a number of medications such as antidepressants, steroids and corticosteroids, and stimulants).

ADHD can usually be differentiated based on the later onset of bipolar disorder, abrupt symptom onset, association with mood change and fluctuation in course, psychotic features, and family history. Similarly, in disruptive behavior disorder, unusual aspects of the presentation (fluctuating course), positive family history of bipolar disorder, and delusional thinking are also suggestive of bipolar disorder (See Birmaher et al., 2018 for additional discussion). The presence of more "classic" bipolar symptoms such as grandiosity and decreased need for sleep may help with differential diagnosis, as do the course of the illness and response to treatment. At the time of initial presentation, it is not always clear whether children with depressed mood and fluctuating energy levels or high-risk behaviors will go on to develop bipolar disorder. The clinician should be alert for the presence or history of symptoms suggestive of mania or hypomania. Positive family history and history of psychotic thinking or apparent manic symptoms in relation to drug treatments are further possible warning signs. In the presence of substance abuse, the clinician should be alert to the possibility that the child or adolescent is essentially self-medicating an underlying mood or other problem.

A number of approaches have been developed to systematize assessment. These include various structured and semi-structured interviews as well as checklists and rating scales. The Washington University version of the Kiddie Schedule for Affective Disorders and Schizophrenia for School Age Children (WASH-U-KSADS) has been widely used for research purposes (Geller et al., 2001). The Young Mania Rating Scale (YMRS) (Young et al., 1978) and the Child Mania Rating Scale (CMRS) (Pavuluri et al., 2006) have been used to quantify severity of bipolar disorder symptoms. Other approaches rely on diaries or "mood timelines" to chart the course of mood and its association with life events and stressors and in response to treatment.

Treatment

For some children and adolescents, hospitalization is indicated (e.g., if suicidal or homicidal symptoms, significant agitation, psychosis, substance dependence are present). In some instances (e.g., when families are unable to be supportive and stabilizing), hospitalization may be considered even if levels of symptomatology are somewhat lower than would usually prompt hospitalization.

Treatment goals and priorities vary depending on the state of the illness. In the acute situation, the primary focus is on acute symptoms; in the subsequent phases, the goal shifts to avoiding relapses and maintaining gains made. Treatment is also guided by the severity, associated conditions, age of the child or adolescent, and family and individual factors. Particularly when response is poor, it is important to be aware of other factors that may be impacting treatment (e.g., lack of compliance, associated disorders, ongoing stress). At all times, it is important to provide education and support. Preparation for potential recurrence and mood fluctuations is a part of this process for the child and parents alike. This helps improve treatment compliance and helps parents gain some perspective on the origins of frequent mood changes and steps that can be taken to help avoid recurrence. For example, parents and patients alike should be helped to understand the potential for sleep deprivation to exacerbate difficulties.

Several randomized controlled trials have evaluated pharmacologic treatments for acute manic episodes in pediatric bipolar disorder. Currently, several second-generation antipsychotics including risperidone and aripiprazole have been approved by the United States Food and Drug Administration (FDA) for the treatment of acute mania and/or mixed mania in children and adolescents in the age range of 10 to 17 years. Lithium has FDA indication for the treatment and recurrence prevention of mania in youths aged 12 and older (Findling et al., 2015). Despite the increasing number of clinical trials, pharmacologic treatment of pediatric bipolar is complicated by high rates of comorbidity. For example, in the "Treatment of Early Age Mania" study, which included 290 children aged 6 to 15 years with bipolar disorder, the rates of comorbid ADHD in this study were as high as 90% (Geller & Luby, 2019).

Expert guidelines for treatment suggest that, if possible, medications are begun at a low dose and gradually increased. The various mood stabilizers are relatively similar in the treatment of manic episodes, with up to 50% of those treated responding. The atypical antipsychotics are also effective and may provide benefit more rapidly. For an acute manic or mixed episode, the combination of mood stabilizer with atypical antipsychotic ranges from 60% to 90% response. Often, lithium or valproate is used initially with nonresponders, then switched to a different mood stabilizer, or to a combination with an atypical antipsychotic. The combination of mood stabilizers or use of mood stabilizer and antipsychotic may be indicated if symptoms are severe or there has been only a partial response to the single mood stabilizer (Birmaher et al., 2018).

There is some suggestion that, as with adults who have depression associated with bipolar disorder, mood stabilizers or atypical antipsychotics can be combined with the SSRIs, but data in children are limited. Of note, there is some suggestion that SSRIs can elicit manic or hypomanic symptoms, especially if used in isolation. At present, use of a mood stabilizer or atypical antipsychotics is frequently the initial pharmacologic intervention in depression associated with bipolar disorder (Birmaher et al., 2018).

It should be noted that many of the psychosocial interventions effective for depression also can be used in this situation. Other psychosocial interventions have been developed for children and adolescents with bipolar disorder, including special family treatment programs and CBT approaches. Psychosocial treatments can be helpful for associated conditions such as substance abuse, anxiety, and CDs.

Complex issues for treatment can arise in the presence of associated comorbid disorders, but the literature on this topic is quite limited. Attentional difficulties or other problems associated with bipolar disorder sometimes resolve or substantially diminish if the bipolar disorder is effectively treated. If this is done and attentional symptoms continue after the mood disorder is stabilized, consideration can be given to whether treatment of a comorbid condition is indicated. Both pharmacologic and nonpharmacologic treatments can be used, and it is important for clinicians to have a full sense of the entire clinical picture (e.g., sometimes clinicians use many different medications to treat symptoms that might, more parsimoniously, be thought of as manifestations of a single condition).

Psychosocial Treatments

There is also a growing number of psychosocial interventions for pediatric bipolar disorder that have been tested in randomized clinical trials including family-focused therapy (FFT); cognitive behavioral therapy (CBT), and dialectical behavior therapy (DBT). Central features of all psychosocial treatment models for pediatric bipolar disorder include psychoeducation, problem solving, and coping skills. Parents are closely engaged in their children's therapy and referred to treatment if they have clinically significant symptoms themselves. Child- and family-focused cognitive behavior therapy (CFF-CBT) is a 12-session intervention for 8- to 12-year-olds that is delivered jointly to parents and children. CFF-CBT is associated with improvement in functioning, mood symptoms, and treatment adherence (West et al., 2009). A similar but longer version of a family intervention, 21 sessions over 9 months, was shown to be effective for adolescents with bipolar disorder (Miklowitz et al., 2004). This treatment includes psychoeducation geared toward illness management, building problem-solving skills, and building communication skills to decrease stress and conflict in the family environment. DBT has also been tested in adolescents (age 12–18) with bipolar disorder and their family members. This approach includes both individual and family sessions to provide psychoeducation. DBT also focuses on building skills of mindfulness, emotion regulation, distress tolerance, interpersonal effectiveness, and parent–child problem solving (Goldstein et al., 2007). With respect to psychosocial treatment of common comorbid conditions (e.g., oppositional behaviors, substance abuse, anxiety disorder), efficacious psychosocial treatments are indicated (see Chapters 11, 12, and 22).

Course and Prognosis

Despite the various diagnostic complexities and controversies, it appears that between 70% and 100% of youth with bipolar disorder eventually recover (as defined by not having symptoms for at least 2 months). However, as many as 75% will have a recurrence in the next several years. There are frequent problems with substance abuse, legal issues, school, and family relationships. Recent research has also noted that although cycles of recovery and recurrence are noted, some youth have fluctuating courses with subsyndromal symptoms, particularly with depressive and mixed symptoms. Negative prognostic factors include early onset, comorbid conditions, the presence of familial psychopathology and low socioeconomic status, duration of symptoms, psychotic thinking, and mixed or rapid cycling (Birmaher et al., 2014).

■ SUMMARY

Depressive and bipolar disorders in children and adolescents represent a significant public health problem. These disorders often have a chronic course and can be the source of considerable morbidity and mortality. Although noteworthy progress has been made in treatment, much work remains to be done to clarify mechanisms of action and to better understand how clinical intervention can be tailored to children's individual needs. Although many children respond positively to treatment, there remains a considerable risk of relapse or of only partial treatment response. This work also has important implications for prevention, early intervention, and public health practices given the severity of the disorder and its association with suicidality. For mood disorders, high rates of comorbidity are not surprising but do present important challenges for implementation of treatment programs.

References

*Indicates Particularly Recommended

American Psychiatric Association. (2013). *Diagnostic and statistical manual of mental disorders (DSM-5)* (5th ed.). Author.

*Angold, A., Costello, E. J., & Erkanli, A. (1999). Comorbidity. *Journal of Child Psychology and Psychiatry, 40*(1), 57–87. https://doi.org/10.1111/1469-7610.00424

Avenevoli, S., Swendsen, J., He, J. P., Burstein, M., & Merikangas, K. R. (2015). Major depression in the national comorbidity survey–adolescent supplement: Prevalence, correlates, and treatment. *Journal of the American Academy of Child and Adolescent Psychiatry, 54*(1), P37–44.E32. https://doi.org/10.1016/j.jaac.2014.10.010

*Axelson, D., Birmaher, B., Strober, M., Gill, M. K., Valeri, S., Chiappetta, L., Ryan, N., Leonard, H., Hunt, J., Iyengar, S., Bridge, J., & Keller, M. (2006). Phenomenology of children and adolescents with bipolar spectrum disorders. *Archives of General Psychiatry, 63*(10), 1139–1148. https://doi.org/10.1001/archpsyc.63.10.1139

*Beck, A. T., Rush, A. J., Shaw, B. F., & Emery, G. (1979). *Cognitive therapy of depression.* Guilford Press.

Birmaher, B., Arbelaez, C., & Brent, D. (2002). Course and outcome of child and adolescent major depressive disorder. *Child and Adolescent Psychiatric Clinics of North America, 11*(3), 619–637. https://doi.org/10.1016/S1056-4993(02)00011-1

Birmaher, B., Gill, M. K., Axelson, D. A., Goldstein, B. I., Goldstein, T. R., Yu, H., Liao, F., Iyengar, S., Diler, R. S., Strober, M., Hower, H., Yen, S., Hunt, J., Merranko, J. A., Ryan, N. D., & Keller, M. B. (2014). Longitudinal trajectories and associated baseline predictors in youths with bipolar spectrum disorders. *American Journal of Psychiatry, 171*(9), 990–999. https://doi.org/10.1176/appi.ajp.2014.13121577

*Birmaher, B., Goldstein, T., Axelson, D. A., & Pavuluri, M. (2018). Bipolar spectrum disorders. In A. Martin, M. H. Bloch, & F. R. Volkmar (Eds.), *Lewis's child and adolescent psychiatry* (5th ed., pp. 483–499). Lippincott Williams & Wilkins.

Brent, D., Emslie, G., Clarke, G., Wagner, K. D., Asarnow, J. R., Keller, M., Vitiello, B., Ritz, L., Iyengar, S., Abebe, K., Birmaher, B., Ryan, N., Kennard, B., Hughes, C., DeBar, L., McCracken, J., Strober, M., Suddath, R., Spirito, A., ... Zelazny, J. (2008). Switching to another SSRI or to venlafaxine with or without cognitive behavioral therapy for adolescents with SSRI-resistant depression: The TORDIA randomized controlled trial. *JAMA, 299*(8), 901–913. https://doi.org/10.1001/jama.299.8.901

*Brent, D. A. (2018). Depressive disorders. In A. Martin, M. H. Bloch, & F. R. Volkmar (Eds.), *Lewis's child and adolescent psychiatry* (5th ed., pp. 473–482). Lippincott Williams & Wilkins.

Brotman, M. A., Kircanski, K., & Leibenluft, E. (2017). Irritability in children and adolescents. *Annual review of clinical psychology, 13*, 317–341. https://doi.org/10.1146/annurev-clinpsy-032816-044941

*Cattarinussi, G., Di Giorgio, A., Wolf, R. C., Balestrieri, M., & Sambataro, F. (2019). Neural signatures of the risk for bipolar disorder: A meta-analysis of structural and functional neuroimaging studies. *Bipolar Disorders, 21*(3), 215–227. https://doi.org/10.1111/bdi.12720

*Donohue, M. R., Whalen, D. J., Gilbert, K. E., Hennefield, L., Barch, D. M., & Luby, J. (2019). Preschool depression: A diagnostic reality. *Current Psychiatry Reports, 21*(12), Article 128. https://doi.org/10.1007/s11920-019-1102-4

Dwyer, J. B., Stringaris, A., Brent, D. A., & Bloch, M. H. (2020). Annual research review: Defining and treating pediatric treatment-resistant depression. *The Journal of Child Psychology and Psychiatry, 61*(3), 312–332. https://doi.org/10.1111/jcpp.13202

Estrada-Prat, X., Van Meter, A. R., Camprodon-Rosanas, E., Batlle-Vila, S., Goldstein, B. I., & Birmaher, B. (2019). Childhood factors associated with increased risk for mood episode recurrences in bipolar disorder—A systematic review. *Bipolar Disorders, 21*(6), 483–502. https://doi.org/10.1111/bdi.12785

Findling, R. L., Robb, A., McNamara, N. K., Pavuluri, M. N., Kafantaris, V., Scheffer, R., Frazier, J. A., Rynn, M., DelBello, M., Kowatch, R. A., Rowles, B. M., Lingler, J., Martz, K., Anand, R., Clemons, T. E., & Taylor-Zapata, P. (2015). Lithium in the acute treatment of bipolar I disorder: A double-blind, placebo-controlled study. *Pediatrics, 136*(5), 885–894. https://doi.org/10.1542/peds.2015-0743

*Geller, B., & Luby, J. (2019). Child and adolescent bipolar disorder: A review of the past 10 years. In S. Hyman, (Ed.), *Bipolar disorder: The science of mental health* (pp. 120–126). Routledge. https://doi.org/10.4324/9781315054308-13

Geller, B., Zimerman, B., Williams, M., Bolhofner, K., Craney, J. L., DelBello, M. P., & Soutullo, C. (2001). Reliability of the Washington University in St. Louis Kiddie Schedule for Affective Disorders and Schizophrenia (WASH-U-KSADS) mania and rapid cycling sections. *Journal of the American Academy of Child and Adolescent Psychiatry, 40*(4), 450–455. https://doi.org/10.1097/00004583-200104000-00014

*Goldstein, B. I., Birmaher, B., Carlson, G. A., DelBello, M. P., Findling, R. L., Fristad, M., Kowatch, R. A., Miklowitz, D. J., Nery, F. G., Perez-Algorta, G., Van Meter, A., Zeni, C. P., Correll, C. U., Kim, H. W.,

Wozniak, J., Chang, K. D., Hillegers, M., & Youngstrom, E. A. (2017). The International Society for Bipolar Disorders Task Force report on pediatric bipolar disorder: Knowledge to date and directions for future research. *Bipolar Disorders, 19*(7), 524–543. https://doi.org/10.1111/bdi.12556

Goldstein, T. R., Axelson, D. A., Birmaher, B., & Brent, D. A. (2007). Dialectical behavior therapy for adolescents with bipolar disorder: A 1-year open trial. *Journal of the American Academy of Child and Adolescent Psychiatry, 46*(7), 820–830. https://doi.org/10.1097/chi.0b013e31805c1613

Goodyer, I. M. (2015). Genes, environments and depressions in young people. *Archives of Disease in Childhood, 100*(11), 1064–1069. https://doi.org/10.1136/archdischild-2014-306936

Goodyer, I. M., Dubicka, B., Wilkinson, P., Kelvin, R., Roberts, C., Byford, S., Breen, S., Ford, C., Barrett, A., Leech, A., Rothwell, J., White, L., & Harrington, R. (2008). A randomised controlled trial of cognitive behaviour therapy in adolescents with major depression treated by selective serotonin reuptake inhibitors. The ADAPT trial. *Health Technology Assessment, 12*(14), iii–60. https://doi.org/10.3310/hta12140

Goodyer, I. M., Reynolds, S., Barrett, B., Byford, S., Dubicka, B., Hill, J., Holland, F., Kelvin, R., Midgley, N., Roberts, C., Senior, R., Target, M., Widmer, B., Wilkinson, P., & Fonagy, P. (2017). Cognitive behavioural therapy and short-term psychoanalytical psychotherapy versus a brief psychosocial intervention in adolescents with unipolar major depressive disorder (IMPACT): A multicentre, pragmatic, observer-blind, randomised controlled superiority trial. *The Lancet Psychiatry, 4*(2), 109–119. https://doi.org/10.1016/S2215-0366(16)30378-9

*Goodyer, I. M., & Wilkinson, P. O. (2019). Practitioner review: Therapeutics of unipolar major depressions in adolescents. *The Journal of Child Psychology and Psychiatry, 60*(3), 232–243. https://doi.org/10.1111/jcpp.12940

Hetrick, S. E., Cox, G. R., Witt, K. G., Bir, J. J., & Merry, S. N. (2016). Cognitive behavioural therapy (CBT), third-wave CBT and interpersonal therapy (IPT) based interventions for preventing depression in children and adolescents. *Cochrane Database of Systematic Reviews, 2016*(8), 1–305. https://doi.org/10.1002/14651858.CD003380.pub4

Kelberman, C., Biederman, J., Green, A., Spera, V., Maiello, M., & Uchida, M. (2021). Differentiating bipolar disorder from unipolar depression in youth: A systematic literature review of neuroimaging research studies. *Psychiatry Research: Neuroimaging, 307*, Article 111201. https://doi.org/10.1016/j.pscychresns.2020.111201

*Keren, H., O'Callaghan, G., Vidal-Ribas, P., Buzzell, G. A., Brotman, M. A., Leibenluft, E., Pan, P. M., Meffert, L., Kaiser, A., Wolke, S., Pine, D. S., & Stringaris, A. (2018). Reward processing in depression: A conceptual and meta-analytic review across fMRI and EEG studies. *American Journal of Psychiatry, 175*(11), 1111–1120. https://doi.org/10.1176/appi.ajp.2018.17101124

Kovacs, M. (1992). *Children's depression inventory*. Multi-Health Systems.

LeMoult, J., Humphreys, K. L., Tracy, A., Hoffmeister, J. A., Ip, E., & Gotlib, I. H. (2020). Meta-analysis: Exposure to early life stress and risk for depression in childhood and adolescence. *Journal of the American Academy of Child and Adolescent Psychiatry, 59*(7), 842–855. https://doi.org/10.1016/j.jaac.2019.10.011

*Lipsitz, J. D., & Markowitz, J. C. (2013). Mechanisms of change in interpersonal therapy (IPT). *Clinical Psychology Review, 33*(8), 1134–1147. https://doi.org/10.1016/j.cpr.2013.09.002

*March, J. S. (2004). Fluoxetine, cognitive-behavioral therapy, and their combination for adolescents with depression: Treatment for Adolescents with Depression Study (TADS) randomized controlled trial. *Journal of the American Medical Association, 292*(7), 807–820. https://doi.org/10.1001/jama.292.7.807

Miklowitz, D. J., George, E. L., Axelson, D. A., Kim, E. Y., Birmaher, B., Schneck, C., Beresford, C., Craighead, W. E., & Brent, D. A. (2004). Family-focused treatment for adolescents with bipolar disorder. *Journal of Affective Disorders, 82*(Suppl.), S113–S128. https://doi.org/10.1016/j.jad.2004.05.020

Miller, C. H., Hamilton, J. P., Sacchet, M. D., & Gotlib, I. H. (2015). Meta-analysis of functional neuroimaging of major depressive disorder in youth. *Journal of the American Medical Association Psychiatry, 72*(10), 1045–1053. https://doi.org/10.1001/jamapsychiatry.2015.1376

Mufson, L., Moreau, D., Weissman, M. M., & Klerman, G. L. (1993). *Interpersonal psychotherapy for depressed adolescents*. Guilford.

*Nolen-Hoeksema, S. (1991). Responses to depression and their effects on the duration of depressive episodes. *Journal of Abnormal Psychology, 100*(4), 569–582. https://doi.org/10.1037/0021-843X.100.4.569

Pavuluri, M. N., Henry, D. B., Devineni, B., Carbray, J. A., & Birmaher, B. (2006). Child mania rating scale: Development, reliability, and validity. *Journal of the American Academy of Child and Adolescent Psychiatry, 45*(5), 550–560. https://doi.org/10.1097/01.chi.0000205700.40700.50

Poznanski, E. O., & Mokros, H. B. (1996). *Children's depression rating scale-revised (CDRS-R)*. WPS.

*Roy, A. K., Lopes, V., & Klein, R. G. (2014). Disruptive mood dysregulation disorder: A new diagnostic approach to chronic irritability in youth. *The American Journal of Psychiatry*, 171(9), 918–924. https://doi.org/10.1176/appi.ajp.2014.13101301

Shanahan, L., Copeland, W. E., Costello, E. J., & Angold, A. (2011). Child-, adolescent- and young adult-onset depressions: Differential risk factors in development? *Psychological Medicine*, 41(11), 2265–2274. https://doi.org/10.1017/S0033291711000675

Solmi, M., Fornaro, M., Ostinelli, E. G., Zangani, C., Croatto, G., Monaco, F., Krinitski, D., Fusar-Poli, P., & Correll, C. U. (2020). Safety of 80 antidepressants, antipsychotics, anti-attention-deficit/hyperactivity medications and mood stabilizers in children and adolescents with psychiatric disorders: A large scale systematic meta-review of 78 adverse effects. *World Psychiatry*, 19(2), 214–232. https://doi.org/10.1002/wps.20765

*Stringaris, A., Vidal-Ribas, P., Brotman, M. A., & Leibenluft, E. (2018). Practitioner review: Definition, recognition, and treatment challenges of irritability in young people. *The Journal of Child Psychology and Psychiatry*, 59(7), 721–739. https://doi.org/10.1111/jcpp.12823

Toenders, Y. J., van Velzen, L. S., Heideman, I. Z., Harrison, B. J., Davey, C. G., & Schmaal, L. (2019). Neuroimaging predictors of onset and course of depression in childhood and adolescence: A systematic review of longitudinal studies. *Developmental Cognitive Neuroscience*, 39, 1–17. https://doi.org/10.1016/j.dcn.2019.100700

Van Meter, A., Moreira, A. L. R., & Youngstrom, E. (2019). Updated meta-analysis of epidemiologic studies of pediatric bipolar disorder. *Journal of Clinical Psychiatry*, 80(3), E1–E11. https://doi.org/10.4088/JCP.18r12180

Weisz, J. R., McCarty, C. A., & Valeri, S. M. (2006). Effects of psychotherapy for depression in children and adolescents: A meta-analysis. *Psychological Bulletin*, 132(1), 132–149. https://doi.org/10.1037/0033-2909.132.1.132

Wesselhoeft, R., Stringaris, A., Sibbersen, C., Kristensen, R. V., Bojesen, A. B., & Talati, A. (2019). Dimensions and subtypes of oppositionality and their relation to comorbidity and psychosocial characteristics. *European Child & Adolescent Psychiatry*, 28(3), 351–365. https://doi.org/10.1007/s00787-018-1199-8

West, A. E., Jacobs, R. H., Westerholm, R., Lee, A., Carbray, J., Heidenreich, J., & Pavuluri, M. N. (2009). Child and family-focused cognitive-behavioral therapy for pediatric bipolar disorder: Pilot study of group treatment format. *Journal of the Canadian Academy of Child and Adolescent Psychiatry*, 18(3), 239–245. https://pubmed.ncbi.nlm.nih.gov/19718425/

Young, R. C., Biggs, J. T., Ziegler, V. E., & Meyer, D. A. (1978). A rating scale for mania: Reliability, validity and sensitivity. *British Journal of Psychiatry*, 133(11), 429–435. https://doi.org/10.1192/bjp.133.5.429

Suggested Readings

Abright, A. R., & Grudnikoff, E. (2020). Measurement-based care in the treatment of adolescent depression. *Child and Adolescent Psychiatric Clinics of North America*, 29(4), 631–643. https://doi.org/10.1016/j.chc.2020.06.003

Asarnow, L. D., & Mirchandaney, R. (2021). Sleep and mood disorders among youth. *Child and Adolescent Psychiatric Clinics of North America*, 30(1), 251–268. https://doi.org/10.1016/j.chc.2020.09.003

Costello, E. J., & Angold, A. (1988). Scales to assess child and adolescent depression: Checklists, screens, and nets. *Journal of the American Academy of Child & Adolescent Psychiatry*, 27(6), 726–737. https://doi.org/10.1097/00004583-198811000-00011

Cuijpers, P., Karyotaki, E., Eckshtain, D., Ng, M. Y., Corteselli, K. A., Noma, H., Quero, S., & Weisz, J. R. (2020). Psychotherapy for depression across different age groups: A systematic review and meta-analysis. *JAMA Psychiatry*, 77(7), 694–702. https://doi.org/10.1001/jamapsychiatry.2020.0164

Dragioti, E., Solmi, M., Favaro, A., Fusar-Poli, P., Dazzan, P., Thompson, T., Stubbs, B., Firth, J., Fornaro, M., Tsartsalis, D., Carvalho, A. F., Vieta, E., McGuire, P., Young, A. H., Shin, J. I., Correll, C. U., & Evangelou, E. (2019). Association of antidepressant use with adverse health outcomes: A systematic umbrella review. *JAMA Psychiatry*, 76(12), 1241–1255. https://doi.org/10.1001/jamapsychiatry.2019.2859

Eckshtain, D., Kuppens, S., Ugueto, A., Ng, M. Y., Vaughn-Coaxum, R., Corteselli, K., & Weisz, J. R. (2020). Meta-analysis: 13-year follow-up of psychotherapy effects on youth depression. *Journal of the American Academy of Child and Adolescent Psychiatry*, 59(1), 45–63. https://doi.org/10.1016/j.jaac.2019.04.002

Forbes, E. E. (2020). Chasing the holy grail: Developmentally informed research on frontostriatal reward circuitry in depression. *American Journal of Psychiatry, 177*(8), 660–662. https://doi.org/10.1176/appi.ajp.2020.20060848

Luby, J. L., Gilbert, K., Whalen, D., Tillman, R., & Barch, D. M. (2020). The differential contribution of the components of parent-child interaction therapy emotion development for treatment of preschool depression. *Journal of the American Academy of Child and Adolescent Psychiatry, 59*(7), 868–879. https://doi.org/10.1016/j.jaac.2019.07.937

Miklowitz, D. J., Schneck, C. D., Walshaw, P. D., Singh, M. K., Sullivan, A. E., Suddath, R. L., Forgey Borlik, M., Sugar, C. A., & Chang, K. D. (2020). Effects of family-focused therapy vs enhanced usual care for symptomatic youths at high risk for bipolar disorder: A randomized clinical trial. *JAMA Psychiatry, 77*(5), 455–463. https://doi.org/10.1001/jamapsychiatry.2019.4520

Nielson, D. M., Keren, H., O'Callaghan, G., Jackson, S. M., Douka, I., Vidal-Ribas, P., Pornpattananangkul, N., Camp, C. C., Gorham, L. S., Wei, C., Kirwan, S., Zheng, C. Y., & Stringaris, A. (2021). Great expectations: A critical review of and suggestions for the study of reward processing as a cause and predictor of depression. *Biological Psychiatry, 89*(2), 134–143. https://doi.org/10.1016/j.biopsych.2020.06.012

Parens, E., & Johnston, J. (2010). Controversies concerning the diagnosis and treatment of bipolar disorder in children. *Child and Adolescent Psychiatry and Mental Health, 4*, 1–14. https://doi.org/10.1186/1753-2000-4-9

Somers, J. A., Borelli, J. L., & Hilt, L. M. (2020). Depressive symptoms, rumination, and emotion reactivity among youth: Moderation by gender. *Journal of Clinical Child & Adolescent Psychology, 49*(1), 106–117. https://doi.org/10.1080/15374416.2018.1466304

Stallwood, E., Monsour, A., Rodrigues, C., Monga, S., Terwee, C., Offringa, M., & Butcher, N. J. (2021). Systematic review: The measurement properties of the children's depression rating scale—revised in adolescents with major depressive disorder. *Journal of the American Academy of Child and Adolescent Psychiatry, 60*(1), 119–133. https://doi.org/10.1016/j.jaac.2020.10.009

Stringaris, A. (2017). What is depression? *The Journal of Child Psychology and Psychiatry, 58*(12), 1287–1289. https://doi.org/10.1111/jcpp.12844

Van Meter, A. R., Burke, C., Kowatch, R. A., Findling, R. L., & Youngstrom, E. A. (2016). Ten-year updated meta-analysis of the clinical characteristics of pediatric mania and hypomania. *Bipolar Disorders, 18*(1), 19–32. https://doi.org/10.1111/bdi.12358

Zhou, X., Teng, T., Zhang, Y., Del Giovane, C., Furukawa, T. A., Weisz, J. R., Li, X., Cuijpers, P., Coghill, D., Xiang, Y., Hetrick, S. E., Leucht, S., Qin, M., Barth, J., Ravindran, A. V., Yang, L., Curry, J., Fan, L., Silva, S. G., ... Xie, P. (2020). Comparative efficacy and acceptability of antidepressants, psychotherapies, and their combination for acute treatment of children and adolescents with depressive disorder: A systematic review and network meta-analysis. *The Lancet Psychiatry, 7*(7), 581–601. https://doi.org/10.1016/S2215-0366(20)30137-1

CHAPTER 15 ■ CHILDHOOD SCHIZOPHRENIA AND CHILDHOOD PSYCHOSIS

■ BACKGROUND

Interest in psychotic disorders in childhood is a relatively recent historical phenomenon. As commonly used, the term *psychotic* can itself be problematic given the changing nature of children's conceptions of reality (Volkmar, 2000; Volkmar & Tsatsanis, 2002). At one time, the term *childhood psychosis* was used quite broadly, but more recently the term and its related diagnostic concepts have been more narrowly defined. The prototypic disorder is childhood-onset schizophrenia (COS) but other psychotic conditions, much less well defined, and transient psychotic phenomena are not uncommon (Box 15.1). When present in children, schizophrenia and related psychotic conditions have the potential for serious disruption of development and hence may be more severe than in adulthood (Ordóñez & Gogtay, 2018). This chapter focuses on onset of schizophrenia in childhood and adolescence and, more briefly, children with psychosis resembling schizophrenia but not meeting current *DSM-5* criteria for the condition. Psychosis related to mood disorder is discussed in Chapter 14 and delirium and catatonia in Chapter 27.

Before age 5, psychotic phenomena are uncommon and often stress related. Hallucinations may be seen as isolated phenomena and generally are relatively much more prognostically benign. By school age, the presence of psychotic phenomena is more concerning as such symptoms may persist. Transient psychotic phenomena are less worrisome than more persistent or recurrent ones (Ordóñez & Gogtay, 2018). In this age group, potential factors such as drug exposure or other mental disorders should be considered, for example, hallucinations and psychotic phenomena may also be observed in mood disorders. By the end of middle childhood, the presence of persistent psychotic phenomena becomes much more predictive of subsequent schizophrenia (Ordóñez & Gogtay, 2018).

■ DIAGNOSIS, DEFINITION, CLINICAL FEATURES

Kraepelin's description of "dementia praecox" or what would today be termed *schizophrenia* was a watershed in psychiatric taxonomy. He explicitly noted that in some cases, onset was in childhood and a downward extrapolation of the concept to children ("dementia praecossisma") quickly followed and severe psychiatric disturbance in childhood became

---

BOX 15.1   **Case Report—Childhood-Onset Schizophrenia**

Kristine was the second of two children born to upper-middle-class parents after a term pregnancy complicated by maternal viral illness and prolonged labor. At birth, she was noted to be in good condition. She was a somewhat fussy baby whose motor and communication development appeared to proceed appropriately. She appeared to be normally related socially and enjoyed social interaction games with her parents and older sister. She was enrolled in a nursery school program at age 4 and subsequently in regular kindergarten and first-grade classes; although she was noted to be somewhat shy, no other concerns were raised about her cognitive or emotional development. At age 6 years 11 months, she exhibited an episode of acute delusions and hallucinations. This had been preceded by a period of several weeks during which she was noted to be somewhat withdrawn and occasionally talked to herself. The hallucinations were predominately auditory in nature but not very elaborate consisting mostly of single words. Delusional beliefs centered around being kidnaped. She became progressively more anxious and developed some complicated rituals apparently revolving around her delusional fears. She was hospitalized for evaluation.

Extensive medical evaluations failed to reveal an explanation for her difficulties. Various studies, including EEG, were normal. A positive family history of schizophrenia in a maternal aunt was noted. The clinician in charge of her care began a low dose of an atypical neuroleptic with partial remission of the hallucinations and delusions. Kristine remained rather withdrawn. She was seen for ongoing supportive psychotherapy and medication management.

At age 10 years, she was seen for comprehensive assessment. IQ testing revealed borderline intellectual functioning. She had some communication problems. Projective testing revealed some continued difficulties with reality testing. She had occasional hallucinations and a fairly complicated set of delusional beliefs. Her affect was relatively bland. She exhibited some unusual mannerisms.

As an adolescent, Kristine had an exacerbation of her difficulties. She became overtly suicidal, and a residential placement was arranged following hospitalization.

Comment: Early-onset schizophrenia is, as this case illustrates, often associated with relatively poor outcome. In this case, the child had a relatively prolonged period of normal development prior to onset of psychotic symptoms; this is a different pattern than that observed in autism.

Case adapted with permission from Volkmar, F. R., & Tsatsanis, K. (2002). Childhood schizophrenia. In M. Lewis (Ed.), *Child and adolescent psychiatry: A comprehensive textbook* (3rd ed., pp. 745–754). Williams & Wilkins.

equated with schizophrenia (Volkmar & Tsatsanis 2002). Kanner's description of the syndrome of infantile autism was taken, by some, as a description of the first manifestations of schizophrenia in infants and young children. However, with the pioneering work of Kolvin (1971), Rutter (1972), and others, it became clear that autism (see Chapter 7) was quite different from schizophrenia of childhood onset and the latter was, if anything, much less common than autism. As a result, a category for childhood schizophrenia was dropped and *infantile autism* officially recognized in *DSM-III* (APA, 1980). Since then, the same criteria for schizophrenia are used in children as well as in young and older adults (the much more typical period of onset). Changes made in *DSM-5* (APA, 2013) to the criteria for schizophrenia include elimination of subtypes and catatonia, and there is an emphasis on discussing current state and historical development (i.e., to better understand the progression of the disorder).

The previous emphasis on Kurt Schneider's "first-rank" symptoms[1] is replaced by a comprehensive assessment of multiple areas of functioning (reality testing, thought organization, negative symptoms, and so forth), and, for children, information can be facilitated by information from parents, teachers, and others.

An assessment covering eight domains of psychopathology—including reality distortion, negative symptoms, thought and action disorganization, cognition impairment, catatonia, and symptoms similar to those found in certain mood disorders, such as whether hallucination or mania is experienced—is recommended to help clinical decision making. In clinical literature, it is frequent to make a distinction between COS with onset between 13 and 18 years and "very early onset schizophrenia" (VEOS) with onset under 13 years (Volkmar & Tsatsanis, 2002).

Several different patterns of onset have been identified. These include a pattern of acute onset, another with gradual onset, and finally a pattern where there is gradual onset followed by acute exacerbation of symptoms. The insidious-onset pattern is more common. Sometimes symptoms emerge in a child who has previous premorbid difficulties.

Auditory hallucinations are reported most frequently (in about 80% of cases). As with adults, the content might include voices, often with persecutory content, commenting about the child. Somatic and visual hallucinations are also observed less frequently (David et al., 2011). The content of the hallucinations is usually less elaborate in children and often reflects age-appropriate concerns, for example, monsters or toys rather than more sexual themes (Volkmar & Tsatsanis, 2002).

Delusions in children with schizophrenia are often less bizarre and systematic than those observed in adults. There may be concerns with thought broadcasting, thought insertion, and thought withdrawal (Caplan et al., 2000). It is important to note that some children have psychotic features but may not exhibit more classic childhood schizophrenia (Ordóñez & Gogtay, 2018). The National Institute of Mental Health group has described these as multidimensionally impaired (see Kumra et al., 1998, and discussion of differential diagnosis later in this chapter).

■ EPIDEMIOLOGY AND DEMOGRAPHICS

Although solid epidemiologic data are critically needed, the childhood form of the disorder is probably 50 times less frequent than adult-onset schizophrenia (Ordóñez & Gogtay, 2018; Volkmar & Tsatsanis, 2002). Among school-age children, schizophrenia is relatively rare on the order of 1 in 10,000 for VEOS and around 5% in COS. The rate increases with age so that by late adolescence the condition appears to be somewhat more common in males, particularly with younger children. As with adult schizophrenia, males also appear to have an earlier onset than females. Also, as with adults, there is probably some bias for increased rates in lower socioeconomic status families. Reported rates may be somewhat underestimating the true prevalence of the condition given lack of clinical familiarity and reluctance to make the diagnosis.

■ ETIOLOGY AND PATHOGENESIS

Several factors have been associated with risk for COS. These include older paternal age (Tsuchiya et al., 2005) as well as obstetric complications (Cannon et al., 2002) and family history of the conditions (Asarnow et al., 2001). The strength of these associations has been questioned. Higher rates of cytogenetic abnormalities and potential gene associations have led to the identification of associated specific syndromes, for example, the Smith–Magenis

---

[1]These are the "positive" (i.e., present) signs of schizophrenia like auditory hallucinations, delusions, delusional perceptions, thought insertion, thought broadcasting.

syndrome (17p11.2del), 15q11-q13 deletions/duplications as well as the 22q11 deletion syndrome (22q11DS), and the velocardiofacial syndrome that is associated with a high risk for schizophrenia. Mosaic Turner syndrome has also been noted at a higher than expected rate (see Ordóñez & Gogtay, 2018 for a more extensive discussion). A number of other associations have been noted as well (e.g., Addington et al., 2004; Ambalavanan et al., 2019).

Various studies have examined the neuropsychological correlates of COS. Children with schizophrenia have more difficulty with tasks that involve greater attention, fine motor coordination, and working memory. Attentional difficulties have been explored using event-related evoked potentials showing decreased event-related potential amplitude when children are engaged in these tasks—results similar to those seen in adults.

The NIH group has looked for various risk factors associated with schizophrenia in adults within their childhood-onset sample. This group found a suggestion of difference in smooth pursuit eye movement. As with adult-onset schizophrenia, there appeared to be a significant genetic component, with higher than expected rates of schizophrenia spectrum disorders in family members. In their samples, the NIH group assessed neurocognitive functioning and found that siblings of COS cases had poor performance on a battery of neuropsychological assessments than community control. However, the rates of neuropsychological abnormalities did not differ between COS and adult-onset schizophrenia.

Neuroimaging studies have been conducted in COS and fairly consistently revealed increased volume of the lateral ventricles along with reduced gray matter but with increased volume of the basal ganglia. It should be noted that some of the observed changes may, however, relate to medication effects, but the longitudinal studies of the National Institute of Mental Health cohort of cases have documented progressive changes over a period of several years. Findings have included observation of smaller overall brain size in COS and progressive increased ventricular size compared to healthy controls (Ordóñez & Gogtay, 2018). Progressive loss of gray matter has been noted, and there is a suggestion of abnormalities in the hippocampus, cerebellum, and some other areas (Anvari et al., 2015; Arango et al., 2008) (Box 15.2).

■ COURSE

The course of COS tends, unfortunately, to resemble that of adult cases with poor outcome, that is, symptoms tend to be severe and persistent (Clemmensen et al., 2012; Volkmar & Tsatsanis, 2002). Stentebjerg-Olesen et al. (2016) noted that poorer premorbid function was associated with poorer outcome. Ross and colleagues (2006) also noted the role of the high rates of comorbidity associated with the condition as a factor related to poor outcome. Although some variability in course is noted, the most typical pattern is one with periodic acute

---

| **BOX 15.2** | **Neuroimaging Findings in Childhood-Onset Schizophrenia** |

- Increased volume of the lateral ventricles
- Reduced gray matter
- Increased volume of basal ganglia
- Smaller overall brain size
- Possible abnormalities in hippocampus, cerebellum, and other structures

Note: Some of these changes may be related to medication effects

From Ordóñez, A. E., & Gogtay, N. (2018). Childhood onset schizophrenia and other early onset psychotic disorders. In A. Martin, M. Bloch, & F. R. Volkmar (Eds.), *Lewis's child and adolescent psychiatry: A comprehensive textbook* (pp. 461–472). Wolters Kluwer.

exacerbations occurring in the context of a steady deterioration in functioning. Sometimes stabilization occurs.

Several different factors may contribute to the worsened prognosis of schizophrenia with childhood onset. These include the possibility of increased genetic risk and/or the disruption that the disorder causes for subsequent learning and development. There is some suggestion that association with more affective symptoms, acute onset, later onset, and well-differentiated symptoms are associated with better outcome.

DIFFERENTIAL DIAGNOSIS AND ASSESSMENT

Although rare, schizophrenia of childhood onset should be considered if a child, or adolescent, manifests obvious psychotic symptoms. Onset may be dramatic or more insidious. Diagnosis, particularly early onset, can be difficult if the insidious-onset pattern is exhibited. Usually, these hallucinations are mood congruent and less disorganized. The course of the disorders also provides clarification. Particularly among adolescents but even among younger children, substance abuse, various medical conditions, or even side effects of medications may lead to psychotic phenomena. Hallucinations can be seen as isolated phenomena in some conditions, for example, conduct disorders, but other symptoms of schizophrenia should not then be present. Sometimes simple techniques like drawing with the child may elicit psychotic phenomena (see Figure 15.1). Similarly, the thoughts and compulsions of obsessive-compulsive disorder may sometimes be taken to suggest schizophrenia, although careful inquiry should then fail to find the characteristic psychotic symptoms. Sometimes children with medical or substance abuse issues or delirium may present with hallucinations. Occasionally, children with autism spectrum disorder, particularly the more verbal child with Asperger's disorder, may present with eccentricities and unusual interests, although usually careful review of history and current examination will clarify the diagnosis. As noted earlier, some children exhibit psychotic features without fitting into classic syndrome patterns. Various terms have been used to refer to this group of cases; the NIH group has used the term *multidimensionally impaired* (Ordóñez & Gogtay, 2018).

Developmental issues and comorbid disorder can complicate the clinical presentation of the condition. For example, young children have normative beliefs in fantasy figures (Superman, Santa Claus, super heroes) or may even exhibit hallucinations, particularly at times of stress; these tend to be visual and tactile rather than auditory. For children under 6 years of age, problems in understanding language can complicate assessment. Piaget uses the term *magical thinking* in describing young children's gradual understanding of adult conceptions of reality (see Chapter 3). With the onset of adolescence, the diagnosis of schizophrenia becomes easier to make. Specific assessment instruments for children and adolescents have been developed (e.g., Caplan et al., 2000) and, as with adults, projective techniques can be helpful. Several medical conditions should be considered in the differential diagnosis. These include partial complex seizures (Caplan et al., 1997), substance abuse, side effects of medications, delerium in relation to physical illness, and so forth (see Chapter 27). Medical assessments including toxicology screens can be helpful.

The diagnosis of childhood schizophrenia in children with severe cognitive limitations of language disorder is particularly challenging. Other conditions can present with psychotic features, for example, adolescents with borderline personality can exhibit psychotic phenomena although these usually are less enduring and less frequently associated with thought disorder.

Evaluation of the child with possible schizophrenia should include a careful history including premorbid functioning, nature and type of onset, and family and medical history. Psychological testing may be used to document thought disorder, that is, projective testing and IQ and achievement testing may help clarify issues relevant to intervention. The mental status examination and history should be careful to include inquiry relative to both positive and negative symptoms of the conditions. Sometimes just giving the child a pencil and drawing materials is sufficient to elicit psychotic symptoms (see Figure 15.1). Any

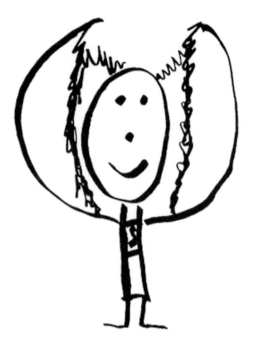

FIGURE 15.1. Drawing by a 9-year-old boy with schizophrenia. He believed a radio transmitter had been implanted in his head (see antennae). He had persecutory delusions as well. Reprinted with permission from Lewis, M., & Volkmar, F. R. (1990). *Clinical aspects of child and adolescent development* (3rd ed., Figure 29-1). Lea and Febinger.

unusual features, for example, prominent mood symptoms, should be noted. The physical examination should include consideration of conditions with a potential to cause psychosis, for example, substance abuse. EEG and neurologic consultation may be considered. It is important for the clinician to be aware that delirium may be mistaken for psychosis and schizophrenia and occasionally a child may present with catatonic symptoms (see Williams, 2018).

■ TREATMENT

Research on treatment of COS is relatively limited. This reflects several factors including the difficulty in obtaining adequate samples for well-controlled studies. The few studies available confirm that the first-generation antipsychotics are of benefit, and studies of the second-generation antipsychotics have been conducted, with the latter having a better side-effect profile. One study suggested that clozapine was more helpful than haloperidol, but use of this agent is essentially restricted to the most severe and treatment-refractory patients because of the potential for untoward side effects.

As with adult-onset schizophrenia, comorbid conditions are frequent and can be an important consideration in management. Careful use of neuroleptics may be indicated (Ross et al., 2003). Anxiety and mood disorders can significantly impact both the presentation and clinical management of cases; anxiety disorders, in particular, seem to persist over time. Treatment of additional conditions, when present, can be particularly helpful. The clinician should be careful to titrate medication doses so as to achieve a balance of control of psychotic symptoms while avoiding sedation and other side effects. The clinician should also be alert to the potential for side effects of some of the second-generation neuroleptics, for example, weight gain, neuroleptic malignant syndrome, and so forth. Supportive counseling/psychotherapy can also be used as one important aspect of a comprehensive treatment program.

Many children with schizophrenia have significant issues in learning and development that can be addressed through a comprehensive educational plan. Special education services should be provided as appropriate. Integration of the treatment program and thoughtful involvement of a clinician over time are helpful. Family involvement is important.

SUMMARY

COS and VEOS are rare conditions. Manifestations of the condition are similar to those seen in adults, although developmental level impacts expression of clinical features. At times, the diagnosis is challenging. Various factors including genetic risk appear to be implicated in the pathogenesis of the condition. Treatment must be comprehensive in nature and often includes administration of agents to help manage psychotic symptoms so that the child is more amenable to treatment. Unfortunately, outcome is frequently poor, and more research is needed to clarify best approaches to treatment and enhance our understanding of syndrome pathogenesis.

References

Addington, A. M., Gornick, M., Sporn, A. L., Gogtay, N., Greenstein, D., Lenane, M., Gochman, P., Baker, N., Balkissoon, R., Vakkalanka, R. K., Weinberger, D. R., Straub, R. E., & Rapoport, J. L. (2004). Polymorphisms in the 13q33.2 gene G72/G30 are associated with childhood-onset schizophrenia and psychosis not otherwise specified. *Biological Psychiatry, 55*(10), 976–980. https://doi.org/10.1016/j.biopsych.2004.01.024

Ambalavanan, A., Chaumette, B., Zhou, S., Xie, P., He, Q., Spiegelman, D., Dionne-Laporte, A., Bourassa, C. V., Therrien, M., Rochefort, D., Xiong, L., Dion, P. A., Joober, R., Rapoport, J. L., Girard, S. L., & Rouleau, G. A. (2019). Exome sequencing of sporadic childhood-onset schizophrenia suggests the contribution of X-linked genes in males. *American Journal of Medical Genetics. Part B, Neuropsychiatric Genetics, 180*(6), 335–340. https://doi.org/10.1002/ajmg.b.32683

American Psychiatric Association. (1980). *Diagnostic and statistical manual.* APA Press.

American Psychiatric Association. (2013). *Diagnostic and statistical manual (DSM-5)* (5th ed.). Author.

Anvari, A. A., Friedman, L. A., Greenstein, D., Gochman, P., Gogtay, N., & Rapoport, J. L. (2015). Hippocampal volume change relates to clinical outcome in childhood-onset schizophrenia. *Psychological Medicine, 45*(12), 2667–2674. https://doi.org/10.1017/S0033291715000677

Arango, C., Moreno, C., Martinez, S., Parellada, M., Desco, M., Moreno, D., Fraguas, D., Gogtay, N., James, A., & Rapoport, J. L. (2008). Longitudinal brain changes in early-onset psychosis. *Schizophrenia Bulletin, 34*(2), 341–353. https://doi.org/10.1093/schbul/sbm157

Asarnow, R. F., Nuechterlein, K. H., Fogelson, D., Subotnik, K. L., Payne, D. A., Russell, A. T., Asamen, J., Kuppinger, H., & Kendler, K. S. (2001). Schizophrenia and schizophrenia-spectrum personality disorders in the first-degree relatives of children with schizophrenia: The UCLA family study. *Archives of General Psychiatry, 58*(6), 581–588. https://doi.org/10.1001/archpsyc.58.6.581

Cannon, M., Jones, P. B., & Murray, R. M. (2002). Obstetric complications and schizophrenia: Historical and meta-analytic review. *American Journal of Psychiatry, 159*(7), 1080–1092. https://doi.org/10.1176/appi.ajp.159.7.1080

Caplan, R., Arbelle, S., Guthrie, D., Komo, S., Shields, W. D., Hansen, R., & Chayasirisobhon, S. (1997). Formal thought disorder and psychopathology in pediatric primary generalized and complex partial epilepsy. *Journal of the American Academy of Child & Adolescent Psychiatry, 36*(9), 1286–1294. https://doi.org/10.1097/00004583-199709000-00022

Caplan, R., Guthrie, D., Tang, B., Komo, S., & Asarnow, R. F. (2000). Thought disorder in childhood schizophrenia: Replication and update of concept. *Journal of the American Academy of Child & Adolescent Psychiatry, 39*(6), 771–778. https://doi.org/10.1097/00004583-200006000-00016

Clemmensen, L., Vernal, D. L., & Steinhausen, H. C. (2012). A systematic review of the long-term outcome of early onset schizophrenia. *BMC Psychiatry, 12*, 150. https://doi.org/10.1186/1471-244X-12-150

David, C. N., Greenstein, D., Clasen, L, Gochman, P., Miller, R., Tossell, J. W., Mattai, A. A., Gogtay, N., & Rapoport, J. L. (2011). Childhood onset schizophrenia: High rate of visual hallucinations. *Journal of the American Academy of Child & Adolescent Psychiatry, 50*(7), 681–686.e683. https://doi.org/10.1016/j.jaac.2011.03.020

Kolvin, I. (1971). Studies in the childhood psychoses. I. Diagnostic criteria and classification. *British Journal of Psychiatry, 118*(545), 381–384. https://doi.org/10.1192/bjp.118.545.381

Kumra, S., Jacobsen, L. K., Lenane, M., Zahn, T. P., Wiggs, E., Alaghband-Rad, J., Castellanos, F. X., Frazier, J. A., McKenna, K., Gordon, C. T., Smith, A., Hamburger, S., & Rapoport, J. L. (1998). Multidimensionally impaired disorder: Is it a variant of very early-onset schizophrenia? *Journal of the American Academy of Child & Adolescent Psychiatry, 37*(1), 91–99. https://doi.org/10.1097/00004583-199801000-00022

Ordóñez, A. E., & Gogtay, N. (2018). Childhood onset schizophrenia and other early onset psychotic disorders. In A. Martin, M. Bloch, & F. R. Volkmar (Eds.), *Lewis's child and adolescent psychiatry: A comprehensive textbook* (pp. 1530–1574). Wolters Kluwer.

Ross, R. G., Heinlein, S., & Tregellas, H. (2006). High rates of comorbidity are found in childhood-onset schizophrenia. *Schizophrenia Research, 88*(1–3), 90–95. https://doi.org/10.1016/j.schres.2006.07.006

Ross, R. G., Novins, D., Farley, G. K., & Adler, L. E. (2003). A 1-year open-label trial of olanzapine in school-age children with schizophrenia. *Journal of Child & Adolescent Psychopharmacology, 13*(3), 301–309. https://doi.org/10.1089/104454603322572633

Rutter, M. (1972). Childhood schizophrenia reconsidered. *Journal of Autism & Childhood Schizophrenia, 2*(4), 315–337. https://doi.org/10.1007/BF01537622

Stentebjerg-Olesen, M., Pagsberg, A. K., Fink-Jensen, A., Correll, C. U., & Jeppesen, P. (2016). Clinical characteristics and predictors of outcome of Schizophrenia-Spectrum Psychosis in children and adolescents: A systematic review. *Journal of Child & Adolescent Psychopharmacology, 26*(5), 410–427. https://doi.org/10.1089/cap.2015.0097

Tsuchiya, K. J., Takagai, S., Kawai, M., Matsumoto, H., Nakamura, K., Minabe, Y., Mori, N., & Takei, N. (2005). Advanced paternal age associated with an elevated risk for schizophrenia in offspring in a Japanese population. *Schizophrenia Research, 76*(2/3), 337–342. https://doi.org/10.1016/j.schres.2005.03.004

Volkmar, F. R. (2000). Childhood schizophrenia: Developmental aspects. In H. Remschmidt (Ed.), *Schizophrenia in children and adolescents (Cambridge child and adolescent psychiatry)* (pp. 60–81). Cambridge University Press.

Volkmar, F. R., & Tsatsanis, K. (2002). Psychosis and psychotic conditions in childhood and adolescence. In D. T. Marsh & M. A. Fristad (Eds.), *Handbook of serious emotional disturbance in children and adolescents* (pp. 266–283). John Wiley & Sons, Inc.

Williams, D. T. (2018). Delirium and catatonia. In A. Martin, M. Block, & F. R. Volkmar (Eds.), *Lewis's child and adolescent psychiatry: A comprehensive textbook* (pp. 604–612). Wolters Kluwer.

Suggested Readings

*Indicates Particularly Recommended

Asarnow, J. R., Tompson, M. C., & McGrath, E. P. (2004). Annotation: Childhood-onset schizophrenia: Clinical and treatment issues. *Journal of Child Psychology & Psychiatry & Allied Disciplines, 45*(2), 180–194. https://doi.org/10.1111/j.1469-7610.2004.00213.x

Asarnow, R. F., Brown, W., & Strandburg, R. (1995). Children with a schizophrenic disorder: Neurobehavioral studies. *European Archives of Psychiatry Clinical Neuroscience, 245*(2), 70–79. https://doi.org/10.1007/BF02190733

Calderoni, D., Wudarsky, M., Bhangoo, R., Dell, M. L., Nicolson, R., Hamburger, S. D., Gochman, P., Lenane, M., Rapoport, J. L., & Leibenluft, E. (2001). Differentiating childhood-onset schizophrenia from psychotic mood disorders. *Journal of the American Academy of Child & Adolescent Psychiatry, 40*(10), 1190–1196. https://doi.org/10.1097/00004583-200110000-00013

Cogulu, O., Pariltay, E., Durmaz, A. A., Aykut, A., Gunduz, C., Ozbaran, B., Aydin, H. H., Erermis, S., Aydin, C., & Ozkinay, F. (2012). Demonstration of uniparental-isodisomy on chromosome 22q11.2 in a patient with childhood schizophrenia and facial dysmorphology by whole-genome analysis. *Journal of Neuropsychiatry & Clinical Neurosciences, 24*(1), E13–E14. https://doi.org/10.1176/appi.neuropsych.11010027

Egan, M. F., Goldberg, T. E., Gscheidle, T., Weirich, M., Rawlings, R., Hyde, T. M., Bigelow, L., & Weinberger, D. R. (2001). Relative risk for cognitive impairments in siblings of patients with schizophrenia. *Biological Psychiatry, 50*(2), 98–107. https://doi.org/10.1016/s0006-3223(01)01133-7

Eggers, C., Bunk, D., & Kraus, D. (2000). Schizophrenia with onset before the age of eleven: Clinical characteristics of onset and course. *Journal of Autism and Developmental Disabilities, 30,* 29–38. https://doi.org/10.1023/A:1005408010797

Gochman, P. A., Greenstein, D., Sporn, A., Gogtay, N., Nicolson, R., Keller, A., Lenane, M., Brookner, F., & Rapoport, J. L. (2004). Childhood onset schizophrenia: Familial neurocognitive measures. *Schizophrenia Research, 71*(1), 43–47. https://doi.org/10.1016/j.schres.2004.01.012

Gogtay, N., & Rapoport, J. (2007). Childhood onset schizophrenia and other early onset disorders. In A. Martin & F. R. Volkmar (Eds.), *Lewis's child and adolescent psychiatry: A comprehensive textbook* (pp. 493–502). Wolters Kluwer.

Kumra, S., Oberstar, J. V., Sikich, L., Findling, R. L., McClellan, J. M., Vinogradov, S., & Schulz, S. C. (2008). Efficacy and tolerability of second-generation antipsychotics in children and adolescents with schizophrenia. *Schizophrenia Bulletin, 34*(1), 60–71. https://doi.org/10.1093/schbul/sbm109

Kumra, S., Wiggs, E., Bedwell, J., Smith, A. K., Arling, E., Albus, K., Hamburger, S. D., McKenna, K., Jacobsen, L. K., Rapoport, J. L., & Asarnow, R. F. (2000). Neuropsychological deficits in pediatric patients with childhood-onset schizophrenia and psychotic disorder not otherwise specified. *Schizophrenia Research, 42*(2), 135–144. https://doi.org/10.1016/s0920-9964(99)00118-8

Majeske, M., & Kellner, C. H. (2014). Consider ECT for treatment-resistant childhood schizophrenia. *American Journal of Psychiatry, 171*(9), 1000. https://doi.org/10.1176/appi.ajp.2014.14050628

Martinez, G., Alexandre, C., Mam-Lam-Fook, C., Bendjemaa, N., Gaillard, R., Garel, P., Dziobek, I., Amado, I., & Krebs, M.-O. (2018). Phenotype continuum between autism and schizophrenia: Evidence from the Movie for the Assessment of the social cognition (MASC): Corrigendum. *Schizophrenia Research, 193,* 489. https://doi.org/10.1016/j.schres.2017.12.013

Mesholam-Gately, R. I., Giuliano, A. J., Goff, K. P., Faraone, S. V., & Seidman, L. J. (2009). Neurocognition in first-episode schizophrenia: A meta-analytic review. *Neuropsychology, 23*(3), 315–336. https://doi.org/10.1037/a0014708

Murphy, K. C., Jones, L. A., & Owen, M. J. (1999). High rates of schizophrenia in adults with velo-cardio-facial syndrome. *Archives of General Psychiatry, 56*(10), 940–945. https://doi.org/10.1001/archpsyc.56.10.940

Papp-Hertelendi, R., Tenyi, T., Hadzsiev, K., Hau, L., Benyus, Z., & Csabi, G. (2018). First report on the association of SCN1A mutation, childhood schizophrenia and autism spectrum disorder without epilepsy. *Psychiatry Research, 270,* 1175–1176. https://doi.org/10.1016/j.psychres.2018.07.028

Rapoport, J. C., Addington, A. M., Frangou, S., & Psych, M. R. C. (2005). The neurodevelopmental model of schizophrenia: Update 2005. *Molecular Psychiatry, 10*(6), 434–449. https://doi.org/10.1038/sj.mp.4001642

Remschmidt, H. (2001). *Schizophrenia in children and adolescents.* Cambridge University Press.

Schaeffer, J. L., & Ross, R. G. (2002). Childhood-onset schizophrenia: Premorbid and prodromal diagnostic and treatment histories. *Journal of the American Academy of Child & Adolescent Psychiatry, 41*(5), 538–545. https://doi.org/10.1097/00004583-200205000-00011

Seese, R. R., O'Neill, J., Hudkins, M., Siddarth, P., Levitt, J., Tseng, B., Wu, K. N., & Caplan, R. (2011). Proton magnetic resonance spectroscopy and thought disorder in childhood schizophrenia. *Schizophrenia Research, 133*(1–3), 82–90. https://doi.org/10.1016/j.schres.2011.07.011

Sowell, E.R., Toga, A. W., & Asarnow, R. (2000). Brain abnormalities observed in childhood-onset schizophrenia: A review of the structural magnetic resonance imaging literature. *Mental Retardation and Developmental Disabilities Research Review, 6*(3), 180–185. https://doi.org/10.1002/1098-2779(2000)6:3<180::AID-MRDD5>3.0.CO;2-I

Sporn, A., Greenstein, D. K., Gogtay, N., Sailer, F., Hommer, D. W., Rawlings, R., Nicolson, R., Egan, M. F., Lenane, M., Gochman, P., Weinberger, D. R., & Rapoport, J. L. (2005). Childhood-onset schizophrenia: Smooth pursuit eye-tracking dysfunction in family members. *Schizophrenia Research, 73*(2–3), 243–252. https://doi.org/10.1016/j.schres.2004.07.020

Sporn, A. L., Vermani, A., Greenstein, D. K., Bobb, A. J., Spencer, E. P., Clasen, L. S., Tossell, J. W., Stayer, C. C., Gochman, P. A., Lenane, M. C., Rapoport, J. L., & Gogtay, N. (2007). Clozapine treatment of childhood-onset schizophrenia: Evaluation of effectiveness, adverse effects, and long-term outcome. *Journal of the American Academy of Child & Adolescent Psychiatry, 46*(10), 1349–1356. https://doi.org/10.1097/chi.0b013e31812eed10

Usiskin, S. I., Nicolson, R., Krasnewich, D. M., Yan, W., Lenane, M., Wudarsky, M., Hamburger, S. D., & Rapoport, J. L. (1999). Velocardiofacial syndrome in childhood-onset schizophrenia. *Journal of the American Academy of Child & Adolescent Psychiatry, 38*(12), 1536–1543. https://doi.org/10.1097/00004583-199912000-00015

CHAPTER 16 ■ TIC DISORDERS

■ BACKGROUND

Tics are sudden, repetitive movements and vocalizations that typically are brief but occur in bouts. For example, blinking, nose twitching, and rapid jerking of any part of the body are common motor tics, and throat clearing, coughing, and grunting are simple phonic tics (Leckman et al., 2013). The complexity of tics ranges from brief and meaningless to longer and seemingly purposeful behaviors. Tics can take the form of obscene movements (copropraxia) or expression of obscene words or phrases (coprolalia). Vocal tics can involve repetition of one's own words (palilalia) or the words of others (echolalia). In addition to varying in severity, tic disorders are often associated with other behavioral problems such as inattention, hyperactivity, anxiety, and irritability. Tic disorders and associated conditions have traditionally been evaluated and treated by neurologists and psychiatrists. More recently, behavior therapy known as habit reversal training (HRT) has been shown to be a helpful treatment for tic disorders, reflecting the somewhat unique way in which these conditions seem to be at the interface of "mind and body."

■ DIAGNOSIS, DEFINITION, CLINICAL FEATURES

Tics have been observed for hundreds of years and were once viewed as examples of demonic possession. The modern study of tics began in France with the work of Itard and Gilles de la Tourette in the second half of the 19th century. Regarding diagnostic criteria and features, in 1885 Gilles de la Tourette described nine patients with motor and phonic tics and noted that tics were characterized by childhood onset, lifelong duration, and a waxing and waning course. These characteristics have since been confirmed in a large number of clinical series worldwide (Lin et al., 2002; Robertson et al., 1988). Of note, coprolalia, a feature that has become engraved in the public view of Tourette's syndrome (TS) (Olson, 2004), is present only in 15% to 20% of cases in clinical samples (Freeman et al., 2009). Several types of tic disorder are presently recognized. The distinctions among these types have to do with the persistence of tics (chronic or transient) and whether vocal as well as motor tics are observed (both are seen in Tourette's disorder). A diagnosis of tic disorder is not made if the tics are caused by another medical condition (e.g., Huntington's disease or postviral encephalopathies) or physiologic effects of a substance (e.g., cocaine).

In chronic or persistent vocal or motor tic disorder, the tics (either vocal or motor but not both) have lasted for at least 1 year without a long symptom-free period. The tics wax and wane over time and can be simple or more complex with a broad range of severity. Motor tics are more common than vocal tics and usually involve the head and upper body. As with other tic disorders, the tics can be voluntarily suppressed for periods of time and are exacerbated by stress. The condition may persist into adulthood and become noticeable at times when the individual is fatigued or anxious (Box 16.1).

BOX 16.1 **Did Samuel Johnson Have Tourette's Disorder?**

Dr. Samuel Johnson, the most famous writer in 18th-century England and subject of one of the greatest biographies in the English language, may have had Tourette's disorder. His biographers have noted that throughout his life, Dr. Johnson exhibited various unusual movements and gestures as well as many verbal "eccentricities." Dr. Johnson had many different symptoms, including bouts of melancholy (depression) as well as some obsessions (e.g., with his feelings of guilt and lack of faithfulness). In his biography of Johnson, Boswell noted his "convulsive cramps" and unusual gestures as well as his tendency to talk to himself. His contemporaries commented that his unusual gestures were so extraordinary that he attracted the attention of spectators who would come to watch him. Throughout his life, Dr. Johnson feared that he might become insane, but his contemporaries regarded his difficulties as reflecting some medical illness (e.g., such as a form of seizure disorder).

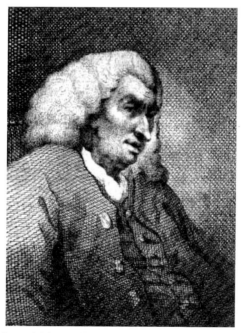

Samuel Johnson (Courtesy of Yale British Art Center.
https://collections.britishart.yale.edu/catalog/tms:53067.)

Reprinted from Volkmar, F. R., & Martin, A. (2011). *Essentials of child and adolescent psychiatry* (p. 173). Lippincott Williams & Wilkins.

If both motor and vocal tics are present, a diagnosis of Tourette's disorder is made. Tourette's disorder is the best known of the tic disorders. In Tourette's disorder, both vocal and motor tics must be present. Tourette's disorder usually has its onset in childhood with simple motor tics, often involving the head or face (e.g., eye blinking or head jerks). Gradually, tics come to involve other regions of the body, often following a "rostral to caudal" progression (i.e., head to rest of body). As motor tics persist, they may have a negative impact on the child's functioning. Typically, vocal or phonic tics usually begin after the motor tics but then have a progression from more simple manifestations (throat clearing) to much more complex forms such as echolalia and coprolalia in a minority of cases. The severity of symptoms tends to a peak in middle childhood (Figure 16.1). As noted subsequently, various other disorders may coexist with Tourette's disorder and may, in some ways, pose even greater obstacles for treatment (Boxes 16.2 and 16.3).

Transient tics are frequent in childhood but often are of brief duration. On the other hand, sometimes the onset of motor tics marks the onset of Tourette's disorder often between ages 5 and 7 years. In this condition, motor tics persist and generally progress down and away from the midline (e.g., head, neck, arms, and, last and least frequently, the lower extremities). Phonic tics usually appear after motor tics and are rare in isolation. Tic complexity changes with age, although most individuals with Tourette's disorder have a diagnosis in childhood. It is important to note that the severity of tics in Tourette's disorder waxes and wanes over time. Tics can be voluntarily suppressed for brief periods and are exacerbated by stress, fatigue, and lack of sleep. Tic episodes occur in bouts, which also often cluster. The pattern of tics is highly unique to the person. Often, as children with Tourette's disorder become older, they develop a sense that a tic is about to happen and may be able to exert some control over them, although this also serves as a source of anxiety and worry and can require much effort.

In some cases, tics are frequent and forceful, resulting in social impairment or, rarely, physical disability. However, in some individuals, tics may be frequent but may go unnoticed

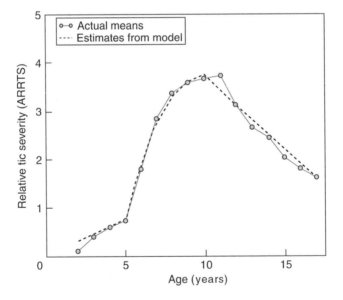

FIGURE 16.1. Plot of mean tic severity, ages 2–18 years. The *solid line* connecting the *small circles* plots the means of the annual rating of relative tic severity scores (ARRTS) recorded by the parents. The *dashed line* represents a mathematical model designed to best fit the clinical data. Two inflection points are evident that correspond to the age of tic onset and the age at worst-ever tic severity, respectively. Adapted with permission from Leckman, J. F., Zhang, H., Vitale, A., Lahnin, F., Lynch, K., Bondi, C., Kim, Y. S., & Peterson, B. S. (1998). Course of tic severity in Tourette syndrome: The first two decades. *Pediatrics, 102*(1 Pt 1), 14–19. Copyright © 1998 American Academy of Pediatrics.

and do not interfere with daily living (Coffey et al., 2004). Overall impairment, however, may not be directly related to tic severity. Some patients with TS and mild tics may be distressed and impaired, whereas some patients are seemingly unaffected by their more prominent tics. Consequently, the tic-related impairment is not part of the current diagnostic criteria for TS. However, individuals who meet some but not all criteria for TS or chronic tic disorder but present with clinically significant distress or impairment can be diagnosed with unspecified tic disorder (American Psychiatric Association, 2013).

Although TS is defined by motor and phonic tics, individuals with TS also experience premonitory urges, recurrent unpleasant sensations associated with the tics. The urges are commonly described as discomfort, pressure, or tingling localized in the muscles involved in the performance of the tics. These premonitory sensations prompt the performance of the tic, which is followed by momentary relief of the associated discomfort. Up to 90% of individuals with TS report the experience of premonitory urges (Banaschewski et al., 2003), and some describe the urges as more bothersome than the tics themselves. Tics involving head, neck, and shoulder movements are associated with particularly prominent urges (Leckman et al., 1993). It has been argued that tics may represent a voluntary response aimed at reducing the discomfort associated with premonitory urges (Lang, 1991). As with tics, the occurrences of urges vary in their frequency, intensity, and duration. The intensity of the urge can vary from fleeting and easily ignored to irresistible and inevitably leading to a tic. Despite the growing consensus that the premonitory urges trigger performance of the tics, the mechanisms of premonitory urges remain poorly understood (Leckman et al., 2006). A closely related phenomenologic aspect of TS is the often-reported capacity to suppress tics, at least temporarily. Even though tics are involuntary, they can be suppressed for minutes or even hours, which may result in uncertainty regarding the voluntary control of tics. Many patients report that the intensity of premonitory urges increases during tic suppression.

■ EPIDEMIOLOGY AND DEMOGRAPHICS

Transient tic behaviors may be seen in 2% to 10% of school-age children. The prevalence of chronic motor tics is about 1%. Estimates of the frequency of Tourette's disorder (vocal and motor tics) vary considerably depending on the age group studied and definitions used; it appears that among older adolescents and adults, the rate is on the order of 4.5 per 10,000. This number is higher for younger children, many of whom improve over time or are not impaired by the condition. The best current estimate of the prevalence of TS was reported to be 14 per 1000 children (Scahill et al., 2013). Tic disorders are 3 to 4 times more common in boys than in girls (Centers for Disease Control and Prevention, 2009).

BOX 16.2   **Case Report: Transient Tic Disorder**

Christopher is a 6-½-year-old boy who recently developed a facial tic. This occurred while he was away at summer camp, and several people and his camp counselor had commented on his unusual eye movements that included lifting his eyebrows and widening his eyes. By the time Christopher returned from camp, these movements had largely disappeared. His parents consulted with his pediatrician and were told that there was some chance the tics would return but also a good chance that these were transient in nature.

Comment: Transient tics are very common in the population. In this case, the consultant is right to note, particularly given the history, that there is some chance that the tics would return.

Adapted from Volkmar, F. R., & Martin, A. (2011). *Essentials of child and adolescent psychiatry* (pp. 175–176). Lippincott Williams & Wilkins.

 BOX 16.3   **Case Report: Chronic Motor Tic Disorder**

Rob is a 15-year-old boy with periodic tics since age 6. These included some unusual head movements, eye blinking, and occasional shoulder movements. He had recently started football, and his tics seemed to increase when he was anxious about having these movements in front of his teammates, although they were subtle and barely noticeable most of the time. He developed some compensatory strategies when tics became more prominent but overall had made a good adjustment to them, although complaining, occasionally, when they were worse. According to Rob and his parents, he had never developed vocal tics.

Comment: The differentiation between chronic motor (or vocal) tic disorder and Tourette's disorder rests on the latter including *both* vocal and motor tics. Some children begin with motor tics and then progress over time to have both vocal and motor tics. In such cases, a diagnosis of Tourette's disorder would be made. In this case, chronic motor tic disorder is the correct diagnosis, and a conservative approach (avoiding the potential side effects of medication) is warranted.

Adapted from Volkmar, F. R., & Martin, A. (2011). *Essentials of child and adolescent psychiatry* (pp. 175–176). Lippincott Williams & Wilkins.

Tics may be only one part of a constellation of problems that children with Tourette's disorder may experience. Indeed, 50% or more of referred children with Tourette's disorder are diagnosed with comorbid ADHD in clinical samples, although epidemiologic studies show a much lower rate (Figure 16.2). At least more than 40% of individuals with Tourette's disorder experience recurrent symptoms of OCD. Tourette's disorder is also associated with higher rates of mood and anxiety disorders (Coffey et al., 2000; Robertson et al., 2002), disruptive behavior (Sukhodolsky et al., 2003), and learning disabilities (Yeates & Bornstein, 1996).

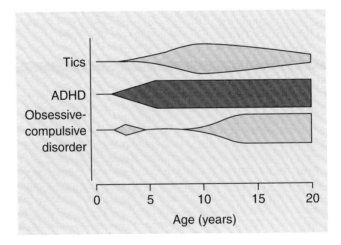

FIGURE 16.2. Age at which tics and coexisting disorders affect patients with Tourette's disorder. The width of the bars shows schematically the amount the disorder affects a patient at a particular age. Adapted from Leckman, J. F. (2002). Tourette's syndrome. *Lancet, 360*(9345), 1577–1586. https://doi .org/10.1016/S0140-6736(02)11526-1. Copyright © 2002 Elsevier. With permission.

ETIOLOGY AND PATHOGENESIS

Tic disorders have a strong genetic component. A child of a parent with Tourette's disorder has a 10% to 15% chance of having Tourette's disorder and a 20% to 30% chance of having tics. A higher risk has been shown in twin and family studies, similarly suggesting genetic factors. In monozygotic twin pairs, the concordance of Tourette's disorders is at least 50%; in dizygotic twin pairs, it is about 10%. Differences in the concordance of monozygotic and dizygotic twin pairs indicate that genetic factors play an important role in the etiology of TS and related conditions. These figures also suggest that nongenetic factors are critical in determining the nature and severity of the clinical syndrome (Bloch & Leckman, 2018).

Several studies involving segregation analysis of large multigenerational families have implicated the possible importance of single gene(s) inherited with an autosomal dominant pattern in the pathogenesis of TS (Pauls et al., 1999). Unfortunately, genetic linkage studies that have screened the entire genome have eliminated the possibility of a single gene being responsible for TS. Despite the well-established large hereditary component of TS, establishing any definitive TS genes has proven difficult. Numerous genome-wide linkage studies in TS failed to produce any consistent results. Increasingly, candidate gene approaches that identify chromosomal anomalies in patients with TS have been successful in helping us better understand the pathophysiology of the disorder.

Studies of the brain have focused on the basal ganglia and corticostriatal thalamocortical area. The basal ganglia model of TS suggests that tics are caused by the aberrantly active striatal neurons, which in turn lead to disinhibition of cortical motor areas (Albin & Mink, 2006). This model is supported by structural and functional neuroimaging studies in children and adults with Tourette's disorder. One of the largest studies to date (Peterson et al., 2003) demonstrated reduced volumes of the caudate nucleus (portion of the basal ganglia of the brain) in subjects with Tourette's disorder. Tic suppression, an act of stopping a tic, is thought to rely upon the neural circuitry that regulates response inhibition and cognitive control of motor behavior (Leckman et al., 2010). Although the causes of age-related tic reduction are unknown, it is likely to be associated with increased functional capacity of the frontal cortex subserved by an increased myelinization and compensatory increased postnatal generation of inhibitory interneurons.

DIFFERENTIAL DIAGNOSIS AND ASSESSMENT

In assessing a child with tics, it is important that the tics not overshadow other aspects of the child's life. The assessment should focus on strengths and weaknesses; the presence of comorbid medical conditions; and the impact of the condition on the family, academic performance, and peer relationships. For older individuals, there may be a long history of medication trials. Various rating scales are available and maybe useful in gaining a developmental perspective on the tics. Direct observation and videotape may be helpful in documenting tics. The medical history should pay careful attention to risk factors and movement disorders associated with other conditions.

Motor tics must be differentiated from a host of other movement difficulties, including tremor, dystonias, and akathitic movements. Movement problems are observed in certain genetic disorders (e.g., Huntington's chorea) and after infection (e.g., Sydenham's chorea). Movement problems can arise as a result of drug side effects or may be noted in myoclonic seizures. Occasionally, stereotyped movements (e.g., as in individuals with autism or severe intellectual deficiency) may be confused with tics, but usually are of earlier onset, are bilateral (not unilateral), and do not wax and wane; however, the diagnosis can sometimes be difficult. The presentation and history typically aid in the differential diagnosis. There are no specific laboratory tests. A number of psychometric instruments can be helpful for assessment of tic severity (Martino et al., 2017). The most comprehensive, valid, and reliable instrument is the Yale Global Tic Severity Scale (Leckman et al., 1989). This instrument, besides being most commonly used, has been recommended by TS international guidelines. The Yale Global Tic

Severity Scale assesses tic dimensions including frequency, intensity, complexity, distribution, as well as interference and impairment. Although relatively longer to administer, this scale highlights relevant exacerbations that can aid in treatment.

As noted earlier, various psychiatric conditions may coexist with tic disorders (e.g., ADHD, OCD, anxiety, disruptive behavior). Often, parents report attentional difficulties in the years before onset of tics. Diagnosis can be difficult given the difficulties in distinguishing the complex behaviors associated with Tourette's from other conditions. Around 40% of individuals with Tourette's disorder exhibit OCD symptoms. There is some suggestion of differences between OCD with and without a history of tics, with an earlier onset in Tourette's disorder–related OCD.

■ TREATMENT

The approach to treatment of patients with tic disorders should be comprehensive and flexible. The diagnosis may sometimes be clarified only over time (e.g., a child may initially present with simple motor tics and only sometime later develop vocal tics of Tourette's disorder). Initially, education and supportive treatment are used with drug treatments held in reserve because the severity of the condition varies among individuals and within the same individual over time. In some cases, tics are barely noticeable; in others, they are extremely disruptive. Tics may be transient, and even when chronic tics are present, they may not necessarily require specific intervention. On the other hand, as tics become more severe and disabling and when they are associated with other conditions, they may require more intensive treatment. Supportive treatment involves education of the individual and family as well as teachers. The child's self-esteem can be fostered by an understanding and supportive school environment with appropriate accommodations made for any needs for support (e.g., situations where the child is anxious will make tics more likely, and an alternative might be found for oral presentations). Helping the child and peers understand the problem is important. Many educational recommendations can be made that will be helpful.

Since the seminal work on HRT by Azrin and Nunn (1973), considerable progress has been made in developing and testing behavioral interventions for tics (McGuire et al., 2014). A treatment program entitled Comprehensive Behavioral Intervention for Tics (CBIT) (Woods et al., 2008) has received rigorous testing in two randomized controlled trials, one in children (Piacentini et al., 2010) and another in adults with TS (Wilhelm et al., 2012). Medium effect sizes (ESs) were found in both the pediatric (ES = 0.68) and the adult (ES = 0.57) trials, and based on these studies CBIT is now considered to be the first-line treatment for tics. The data from both child and adult CBIT studies were recently combined to examine moderators of treatment response. These analyses revealed that presence of co-occurring ADHD, OCD, or anxiety disorders did not moderate response to CBIT. There was a moderating effect of tic medication such that all participants showed improvement after CBIT, but the difference between CBIT and psychoeducation and supportive therapy was greater for participants who were not on tic-suppressing medication (Sukhodolsky et al., 2017).

The key component of CBIT is HRT, which involves teaching individuals with TS to detect the initial signs of tics and then performing a "competing response" instead of the tic until the urge to tic dissipates. The treatment starts with tic awareness training that entails self-monitoring of current tics while focusing on the premonitory urge or other early signs that a tic is about to occur. When the patient is able to detect the first sign of the tics, they are taught to perform voluntary behaviors that are physically incompatible with the tic (i.e., competing responses). Competing response training is different from tic suppression that many individuals may attempt on their own in that it teaches the patient to perform a specific voluntary movement when they notice that a tic is about to occur. CBIT starts with an assessment of tics that is used to create a tic hierarchy where tics are listed from most to least distressing. As a rule, more distressing tics are addressed first, although tics with more readily identifiable competing responses can be addressed first too (McGuire et al., 2015). Awareness training and competing response training are then implemented and practiced during CBIT sessions, one tic at a time. For example, a child with a neck-jerking tic may be taught to look forward with their chin slightly down while gently tensing neck muscles for 1 minute or until the urge goes away. Current guidelines suggest that the competing response does not have to be physically incompatible with the targeted tic to be effective and any voluntary movement can reduce the desire to perform the tics. This observation is consistent with the commonly reported reduction of tics during periods of goal-directed behavior, especially those that involve both focused attention and fine motor control, as occurs in musical and athletic performances.

Drug treatments are usually not the first line of intervention, and even when medications are used, the comorbid conditions (ADHD, OCD) may be the first targets of treatment. Various medications are now available, and the choice of medication should include consideration of the expected benefits and potential side effects. The most consistently effective medications include the dopamine D_2 receptor antagonists, which were first noted in the 1960s to suppress tics. Several drugs in this group have been evaluated in double-blind clinical trials, including haloperidol, pimozide, and tiapride, and the U.S. Food and Drug Administration has approved Tourette's disorder as an indication for the use of both haloperidol and pimozide. Potential side effects include dystonic reactions, sedation, depression, school and social phobia, and tardive dyskinesia. By starting with a low dose and gradually increasing it, the clinician may be able to minimize these problems. The goal of treatment is not to totally eliminate the tics but to make them less troublesome to the individual. The atypical neuroleptics hold promise given their better side-effect profile, and a few double-blind clinical trials have now been conducted for several of these agents. Although avoiding some of the difficulties of the first-generation agents, these atypical neuroleptics may be associated with weight gain or sedation (e.g., with risperidone and olanzapine) (Bloch & Leckman, 2018).

Another pharmacologic approach has used the potent α_2-receptor agonists, clonidine and guanfacine, which are presumed to decrease central noradrenergic activity. Initial, open-label studies were more favorable than subsequent double-blind studies. There can be a significant reduction in symptoms, particularly motor tics. This effect appears over some weeks. Although less effective than the neuroleptics, these agents are often better tolerated. The most frequent side effect, sedation, is observed in 10% to 20% of cases, but often abates with continued use. Other potential side effects include hypotension. It is important for parents to realize that clonidine should be tapered rather than stopped abruptly because there may be a blood pressure rebound. Guanfacine has been used particularly in individuals with Tourette's disorder and comorbid ADHD and is generally less sedating than clonidine. Drug treatments for individuals with comorbid conditions present special consideration. The use of stimulants for attentional problems in children with tic disorders remains a source of controversy. Some children do well with stimulants, but other children with attentional problems appear to develop tics for the first time after stimulant administration or stimulants may exacerbate tics. As noted previously, the α_2-agonists may be used as can be the antidepressants nortriptyline, atomoxetine, and bupropion. For individuals with tic disorders and OCD, cognitive behavioral therapies can be used alone or in combination with serotonin reuptake inhibitors, although as a group, these individuals respond less well than do patients with OCD without tics. Occasionally, small doses of haloperidol or risperidone may be added to augment the serotonin reuptake inhibitor's effect.

Other approaches to treatment include botulinum toxin injections to temporarily weaken muscle groups involved in tics; such injections may also reduce the individual's awareness ("premonitory urge") associated with the tic. Rarely, neurosurgical interventions are used when tics are severe or life threatening. Most recently, real-time fMRI neurofeedback of activity in supplemental motor area was shown to have potential for reducing tics in adolescents with Tourette's disorder (Sukhodolsky et al., 2020) (Box 16.4).

BOX 16.4   **Case Report: Tourette's Disorder**

Jeremy, a 10-year-old boy, was referred for evaluation of multiple behavioral and emotional problems. Starting at age 6, he had attentional difficulties (noted in school) that seemed initially to respond well to stimulant medications. By the time he was in second grade, he had developed an eye-blinking tic and, over time, other motor tics as well. Starting about a year ago, he began to exhibit an odd throat clearing sound, which was eventually diagnosed as a vocal tic. Both his motor and vocal tics varied over time. They virtually disappeared while he was playing videogames and could be voluntarily suppressed for short periods. His popularity at school suffered considerably with the onset of the vocal tics, as he reported being worried that children will make fun of him. In addition, Jeremy continued to struggle academically in school and had frequent arguments about homework with his parents. A reward system was instituted at school and home to attempt to help him stay on task but did not meet with success. Jeremy was treated with guanfacine for the past year but as his tics persisted, his child psychiatrist suggested a trial of a low dose of risperidone. The tics improved considerably, but Jeremy became somewhat sedated on the risperidone, and several adjustments were made to balance the benefit of the medication on the tics and the sedative effect.

Comment: In Tourette's disorder, both vocal and motor tics are present. It is common for attentional difficulties to precede the tics. Learning difficulties and oppositional behaviors are also common. Waxing and waning of the tics is characteristic, as is the ability to voluntarily suppress the tics for short periods. Medications can be helpful in controlling the tics, but side effects can be problematic.

Adapted from Volkmar, F. R., & Martin, A. (2011). *Essentials of child and adolescent psychiatry* (p. 179). Lippincott Williams & Wilkins.

COURSE

The course of tic disorders is quite variable. Transient tics are, of course, by definition just that. As noted previously, the tics in Tourette's disorder follow a developmental progression. The intensity and frequency of tics in affected individuals parallel this progression. In general, it appears that the tics of Tourette's disorder reach their peak in early adolescence (ages 10–15 years) and tend to decrease after that time to a lower level where tics come and go over time. Some individuals—more than half—with Tourette's disorder become largely asymptomatic in adulthood with some becoming symptom free (Peterson & Leckman, 1998). In other cases, the tics typically persist but are reduced in both frequency and intensity. Occasionally, tics become worse in adulthood.

The associated behavioral and emotional problems of these disorders are also important in determining outcome. By late adolescence, many individuals regard comorbid OCD, ADHD, and other behavioral or learning difficulties as more problematic than the tics. Probably 50% of children with Tourette's disorder also exhibit ADHD in clinical settings (the rate is lower in epidemiologically based samples). Having both conditions presents more of a challenge for the child, family, and clinicians. These children are particularly likely to have peer problems and social difficulties and are at increased risk for other disorders (e.g., mood and anxiety problems) later in life. There is also an increased risk for conduct problems. ADHD appears to be a powerful mediator because children with Tourette's disorder but without ADHD do substantially better even if their tics are more severe.

The symptoms of Tourette's disorder are sometimes difficult to distinguish from those of OCD and, as already noted, the two conditions may coexist. In many cases, adults with Tourette's disorder experience moderate levels of symptoms of OCD. If OCD symptoms are present in children with Tourette's disorder, they tend to persist into adulthood even more so than the tics themselves. The presence of associated attentional difficulties or learning problems may also impact outcome. Similarly, stressful and nonsupportive social environments and exposure to certain illicit drugs (e.g., cocaine) are associated with a worse prognosis.

■ SUMMARY

Tourette's disorder is a childhood-onset neurodevelopmental disorder that is diagnosed based on the presence of chronic motor and vocal tics. The severity of the disorder and associated impairments can vary dramatically among affected individuals and require competent and comprehensive evaluations. There has been considerable progress in developing behavioral and pharmacologic treatments for tics over the past 20 years. However, more work is needed to develop treatments for more severe and refractory forms of the disorder. Lastly, the neural basis of the disorder remains to be an area of active investigations looking at genetic and molecular mechanisms of Tourette's disorder and associated conditions.

References

*Indicates Particularly Recommended

Albin, R. L., & Mink, J. W. (2006). Recent advances in Tourette syndrome research. *Trends in Neurosciences, 29*(3), 175–182. https://doi.org/10.1016/j.tins.2006.01.001

American Psychiatric Association. (2013). *Diagnostic and statistical manual of mental disorders (DSM-5)* (5th ed.). American Psychiatric Publishing.

Azrin, N. H., & Nunn, R. G. (1973). Habit reversal: A method of eliminating nervous habits and tics. *Behaviour Research and Therapy, 11*(4), 619–628. https://doi.org/10.1016/0005-7967(73)90119-8

Banaschewski, T., Woerner, W., & Rothenberger, A. (2003). Premonitory sensory phenomena and suppressibility of tics in Tourette syndrome: Developmental aspects in children and adolescents. *Developmental Medicine and Child Neurology, 45*(10), 700–703. http://www.ncbi.nlm.nih.gov/entrez/query.fcgi?cmd=Retrieve&db=PubMed&dopt=Citation&list_uids=14515942

*Bloch, M. H., & Leckman, J. F. (2018). Tic disorders. In A. Martin, M. H. Bloch, & F. R. Volkmar (Eds.), *Lewis's child and adolescent psychiatry: A comprehensive textbook* (5th ed., pp. 534–548). Wolters Kluwer.

Centers for Disease Control and Prevention. (2009). Prevalence of diagnosed Tourette syndrome in persons aged 6–17 years—United States, 2007. *MMWR. Morbidity and Mortality Weekly Report, 58*(21), 581–585. http://www.ncbi.nlm.nih.gov/entrez/query.fcgi?cmd=Retrieve&db=PubMed&dopt=Citation&list_uids=19498335

Coffey, B. J., Biederman, J., Geller, D., Frazier, J., Spencer, T., Doyle, R., Gianini, L., Small, A., Frisone, D. F., Magovcevic, M., Stein, N., & Faraone, S. V. (2004). Reexamining tic persistence and tic-associated impairment in Tourette's disorder findings from a naturalistic follow-up study. *Journal of Nervous and Mental Disease, 192*(11), 776–780. https://doi.org/10.1097/01.nmd.0000144696.14555.c4

Coffey, B. J., Biederman, J., Geller, D. A., Spencer, T. J., Kim, G. S., Bellordre, C. A., Frazier, J. A., Cradock, K., & Magovcevic, M. (2000). Distinguishing illness severity from tic severity in children and adolescents with Tourette's disorder. *Journal of the American Academy of Child and Adolescent Psychiatry, 39*(5), 556–561. http://www.ncbi.nlm.nih.gov/entrez/query.fcgi?cmd=Retrieve&db=PubMed&dopt=Citation&list_uids=10802972

Freeman, R. D., Zinner, S. H., Müller-Vahl, K. R., Fast, D. K., Burd, L. J., Kano, Y., Rothenberger, A., Roessner, V., Kerbeshian, J., & Stern, J. S. (2009). Coprophenomena in Tourette syndrome. *Developmental Medicine and Child Neurology, 51*(3), 218–227. https://doi.org/10.1111/j.1469-8749.2008.03135.x

Lang, A. (1991). Patient perception of tics and other movement disorders. *Neurology, 41*(2, Pt 1), 223–228. http://www.scopus.com/inward/record.url?eid=2-s2.0-0026101003&partnerID=40

*Leckman, J. F., Bloch, M. H., Scahill, L., & King, R. A. (2006). Tourette syndrome: The self under siege. *Journal of Child Neurology, 21*(8), 642–649. http://www.scopus.com/scopus/inward/record.url?eid=2-s2.0-33748059851&partnerID=40&rel=R5.6.0

Leckman, J. F., Bloch, M. H., Smith, M. E., Larabi, D., & Hampson, M. (2010). Neurobiological substrates of Tourette's disorder. *Journal of Child and Adolescent Psychopharmacology, 20*(4), 237–247. http://www.ncbi.nlm.nih.gov/entrez/query.fcgi?cmd=Retrieve&db=PubMed&dopt=Citation &list_uids=20807062

*Leckman, J. F., Bloch, M. H., Sukhodosky, D. G., Scahill, L., & King, R. A. (2013). Phenomenology of tics and sensory urges: The self under siege. In D. Martino & J. F. Leckman (Eds.), *Tourette syndrome* (pp 3–25). Oxford University Press.

Leckman, J. F., Riddle, M. A., Hardin, M. T., Ort, S. I., Swartz, K. L., Stevenson, J., & Cohen, D. J. (1989). The Yale Global Tic Severity Scale: Initial testing of a clinician-rated scale of tic severity. *Journal of the American Academy of Child and Adolescent Psychiatry, 28*(4), 566–573. http://www.ncbi.nlm.nih.gov/ entrez/query.fcgi?cmd=Retrieve&db=PubMed&dopt=Citation&list_uids=2768151

Leckman, J. F., Walker, D. E., & Cohen, D. J. (1993). Premonitory urges in Tourette's syndrome. *American Journal of Psychiatry, 150*(1), 98–102. http://www.ncbi.nlm.nih.gov/entrez/query .fcgi?cmd=Retrieve&db=PubMed&dopt=Citation&list_uids=8417589

Lin, H., Yeh, C. B., Peterson, B. S., Scahill, L., Grantz, H., Findley, D. B., Katsovich, L., Otka, J., Lombroso, P. J., King, R. A., & Leckman, J. F. (2002). Assessment of symptom exacerbations in a longitudinal study of children with Tourette's syndrome or obsessive-compulsive disorder. *Journal of the American Academy of Child and Adolescent Psychiatry, 41*(9), 1070–1077. http://www.ncbi.nlm.nih.gov/entrez/ query.fcgi?cmd=Retrieve&db=PubMed&dopt=Citation&list_uids=12218428

*Martino, D., Pringsheim, T. M., Cavanna, A. E., Colosimo, C., Hartmann, A., Leckman, J. F., Luo, S., Munchau, A., Goetz, C. G., Stebbins, G. T., & Martinez-Martin, P. (2017). Systematic review of severity scales and screening instruments for tics: Critique and recommendations. *Movement Disorders, 32*(3), 467–473. https://doi.org/10.1002/mds.26891

McGuire, J. F., Piacentini, J., Brennan, E. A., Lewin, A. B., Murphy, T. K., Small, B. J., & Storch, E. A. (2014). A meta-analysis of behavior therapy for Tourette syndrome. *Journal of Psychiatric Research, 50*(1), 106–112. http://www.scopus.com/inward/record.url?eid=2-s2.0-84892550980&partnerID=40 &md5=0e39879306265aef73668aedc0b673fa

McGuire, J. F., Piacentini, J., Scahill, L., Woods, D. W., Villarreal, R., Wilhelm, S., Walkup, J. T., & Peterson, A. L. (2015). Bothersome tics in patients with chronic tic disorders: Characteristics and individualized treatment response to behavior therapy. *Behaviour Research and Therapy, 70*, 56–63. https://doi .org/10.1016/j.brat.2015.05.006

Olson, S. (2004). Neurobiology. Making sense of Tourette's. *Science, 305*, 1390–1392. https://doi .org/10.1126/science.305.5689.1390

Pauls, D. L., Alsobrook, J. P., II, Gelernter, J., & Leckman, J. F. (1999). Genetic vulnerability. In J. F. Leckman & D. J. Cohen (Eds.), *Tourette's syndrome—Tics, obsessions, compulsions: Developmental psychopathology and clinical care* (pp. 194–212). John Wiley & Sons, Inc.

Peterson, B. S., & Leckman, J. F. (1998). The temporal dynamics of tics in Gilles de la Tourette syndrome. *Biological Psychiatry, 44*(12), 1337–1348. http://www.ncbi.nlm.nih.gov/entrez/query .fcgi?cmd=Retrieve&db=PubMed&dopt=Citation&list_uids=9861477

Peterson, B. S., Thomas, P., Kane, M. J., Scahill, L., Zhang, H., Bronen, R., King, R. A., Leckman, J. F., & Staib, L. (2003). Basal Ganglia volumes in patients with Gilles de la Tourette syndrome. *Archives of General Psychiatry, 60*(4), 415–424. http://www.ncbi.nlm.nih.gov/entrez/query .fcgi?cmd=Retrieve&db=PubMed&dopt=Citation&list_uids=12695320

Piacentini, J., Woods, D. W., Scahill, L., Wilhelm, S., Peterson, A. L., Chang, S., Ginsburg, G. S., Deckersbach, T., Dziura, J., Levi-Pearl, S., & Walkup, J. T. (2010). Behavior therapy for children with Tourette disorder: A randomized controlled trial. *JAMA, 303*(19), 1929–1937. http://www.ncbi.nlm .nih.gov/entrez/query.fcgi?cmd=Retrieve&db=PubMed&dopt=Citation&list_uids=20483969

Robertson, M. M., Banerjee, S., Eapen, V., & Fox-Hiley, P. (2002). Obsessive compulsive behaviour and depressive symptoms in young people with Tourette syndrome. A controlled study. *European Child and Adolescent Psychiatry, 11*(6), 261–265. http://www.ncbi.nlm.nih.gov/entrez/query .fcgi?cmd=Retrieve&db=PubMed&dopt=Citation&list_uids=12541004

Robertson, M. M., Trimble, M. R., & Lees, A. J. (1988). The psychopathology of the Gilles de la Tourette syndrome. A phenomenological analysis. *British Journal of Psychiatry, 152*, 383–390. http://www.ncbi .nlm.nih.gov/entrez/query.fcgi?cmd=Retrieve&db=PubMed&dopt=Citation&list_uids=3167374

Scahill, L., Dalsgaard, S., & Bradbury, K. (2013). The prevalence of Tourette Syndrome and its relationship to clinical features. In D. Martino & J. F. Leckman (Eds.), *Tourette syndrome* (pp. 121–136). Oxford University Press.

Sukhodolsky, D. G., Scahill, L., Zhang, H., Peterson, B. S., King, R. A., Lombroso, P. J., Katsovich, L., Findley, D., & Leckman, J. F. (2003). Disruptive behavior in children with Tourette's syndrome: Association with ADHD comorbidity, tic severity, and functional impairment. *Journal of the American Academy of Child & Adolescent Psychiatry, 42*(1), 98–105. https://doi.org/10.1097/00004583-200301000-00016

Sukhodolsky, D. G., Walsh, C., Koller, W. N., Eilbott, J., Rance, M., Fulbright, R. K., Zhao, Z., Bloch, M. H., King, R., Leckman, J. F., Scheinost, D., Pittman, B., & Hampson, M. (2020). Randomized, sham-controlled trial of real-time functional magnetic resonance imaging neurofeedback for tics in adolescents with Tourette syndrome. *Biological Psychiatry, 87*(12), 1063–1070. https://doi .org/10.1016/j.biopsych.2019.07.035

*Sukhodolsky, D. G., Woods, D. W., Piacentini, J., Wilhelm, S., Peterson, A. L., Katsovich, L., Dziura, J., Walkup, J. T., & Scahill, L. (2017). Moderators and predictors of response to behavior therapy for tics in Tourette syndrome. *Neurology, 88*(11), 1029–1036. https://doi.org/10.1212/WNL.0000000000003710

Wilhelm, S., Peterson, A. L., Piacentini, J., Woods, D. W., Deckersbach, T., Sukhodolsky, D. G., Chang, S., Liu, H., Dziura, J., Walkup, J. T., & Scahill, L. (2012). Randomized trial of behavior therapy for adults with Tourette's disorder. *Archives of General Psychiatry, 69*(8), 795–803. https://doi.org/10.1001/ archgenpsychiatry.2011.1528

Woods, D. W., Piacentini, J. C., Chang, S. W., Deckersbach, T., Ginsburg, G. S., Peterson, A. L., Scahill, L., Walkup, J. T., & Wilhelm, S. (2008). *Managing Tourette syndrome: A behavioral intervention.* Oxford University Press.

Yeates, K. O., & Bornstein, R. A. (1996). Neuropsychological correlates of learning disability subtypes in children with Tourette's syndrome. *Journal of the International Neuropsychological Society, 2*(5), 375–382. http://www.ncbi.nlm.nih.gov/entrez/query.fcgi?cmd=Retrieve&db=Pub Med&dopt=Citation&list_uids=9375162

Suggested Readings

*Cappi, C., Oliphant, M. E., Péter, Z., Zai, G., Conceição do Rosário, M., Sullivan, C. A. W., Gupta, A. R., Hoffman, E. J., Virdee, M., Olfson, E., Abdallah, S. B., Willsey, A. J., Shavitt, R. G., Miguel, E. C., Kennedy, J. L., Richter, M. A., & Fernandez, T. V. (2020). De novo damaging DNA coding mutations are associated with obsessive-compulsive disorder and overlap with Tourette's disorder and autism. *Biological Psychiatry, 87*(12), 1035–1044. https://doi.org/10.1016/j.biopsych.2019.09.029

DeLong, M. R., & Wichmann, T. (2007). Circuits and circuit disorders of the basal ganglia. *Archives of Neurology, 64*(1), 20–24. https://doi.org/10.1001/archneur.64.1.20

Graybiel, A. M. (2008). Habits, rituals, and the evaluative brain. *Annual Review of Neuroscience, 31*, 359–387. https://doi.org/10.1146/annurev.neuro.29.051605.112851

*Groth, C., Mol Debes, N., Rask, C. U., Lange, T., & Skov, L. (2017). Course of Tourette syndrome and comorbidities in a large prospective clinical study. *Journal of the American Academy of Child and Adolescent Psychiatry, 56*(4), 304–312. https://doi.org/10.1016/j.jaac.2017.01.010

Isaacs, D., & Riordan, H. (2020). Sensory hypersensitivity in Tourette syndrome: A review. *Brain and Development, 42*(9), 627–638. https://doi.org/10.1016/j.braindev.2020.06.003

Kushner, H. I. (1999). *A cursing brain? The histories of Tourette syndrome.* Harvard University Press.

Martino, D. (2020). Update on the treatment of tics in Tourette syndrome and other chronic tic disorders. *Current Treatment Options in Neurology, 22*(4). https://doi.org/10.1007/s11940-020-0620-z

Sacks, O. (Ed.). (1995). A surgeon's life. In *An anthropologist on Mars: Seven paradoxical tales.* Random House.

Sukhodolsky, D. G., Landeros-Weisenberger, A., Scahill, L., Leckman, J. F., & Schultz, R. T. (2010). Neuropsychological functioning in children with Tourette syndrome with and without attention-deficit/hyperactivity disorder. *Journal of the American Academy of Child and Adolescent Psychiatry, 49*(11), 1155–1164.e1. https://doi.org/10.1097/00004583-201011000-00009

Sukhodolsky, D. G., Vitulano, L. A., Carroll, D. H., McGuire, J., Leckman, J. F., & Scahill, L. (2009). Randomized trial of anger control training for adolescents with Tourette's Syndrome and disruptive behavior. *Journal of the American Academy of Child & Adolescent Psychiatry, 48*(4), 413–421. https:// doi.org/10.1097/CHI.0b013e3181985050

Tudor, M. E., Bertschinger, E., Piasecka, J., & Sukhodolsky, D. G. (2018). Cognitive behavioral therapy for anger and aggression in a child with Tourette's syndrome. *Clinical Case Studies, 17*(4), 220–232. https://doi.org/10.1177/1534650118782438

Wolicki, S. B., Bitsko, R. H., Holbrook, J. R., Danielson, M. L., Zablotsky, B., Scahill, L., Walkup, J. T., Woods, D. W., & Mink, J. W. (2020). Treatment use among children with Tourette syndrome living in the United States, 2014. *Psychiatry Research, 293*, 113400. https://doi.org/10.1016/j .psychres.2020.113400

Woods, D. W., Piacentini, J. C., Chang, S. W., Deckersbach, T., Ginsburg, G. S., Peterson, A. L., Scahill, L., Walkup, J. T., & Wilhelm, S. (2008). *Managing Tourette syndrome: A behavioral intervention.* Oxford University Press.

CHAPTER 17 ■ EATING AND FEEDING DISORDERS

■ BACKGROUND

Eating is of obvious and critical importance to the development, health, and, indeed, the survival of children. Eating is among the very earliest of the behaviors that make up the behavioral repertoire of infants and develops rapidly as babies grow into children and then adolescents. Problems with the consumption and retention of food are a source of acute concern for parents and can pose serious risk for the child. Indeed, serious eating disorders are life-threatening and among the most fatal of all mental health problems (Arcelus et al., 2011; Franko et al., 2013; Smink et al., 2014; van Son et al., 2010).

Eating problems have been recognized for centuries, with descriptions of restricted eating, binge behavior, and the purging of consumed food through use of vomiting and laxatives dating back to at least the Middle Ages (Bell, 1985). Numerous descriptions of medieval saints, for example, portray either self-starvation or bingeing episodes (or both). Similar descriptions can be found consistently in historical documents from the intervening centuries, such as those described by John Reynolds and Richard Morton in the 17th century and those of Marcé, Gull, and Laséque in the 19th century. Over the years, different terms were used to describe these behavioral patterns, reflecting the understanding and values of the time. In the Middle Ages, the term *anorexia mirabilis* reflected the association of self-starvation with spiritual purity and other penitential practices; in the 17th century, the term *nervous atrophy* described a condition with psychological roots and a "morbid state of the spirits"; in the 19th century, the term *hypochondriacal delusion* was used to describe a psychological condition characterized by food refusal. During the first half of the 20th century, mental health problems were being more rigorously studied as medical conditions. In this period, the two prevailing theories were endocrinologic (centered around dysfunction of the pituitary) and psychoanalytic (centered around the defense against unconscious wishes for impregnation) (Eissler, 1943; Masserman, 1941; Meyer & Weinroth, 1957).

The latter half of the 20th century saw the introduction of formal systems for the classification of psychological disorders and the establishment of agreed-upon criteria for their diagnosis. The first iteration of the *DSM* in the 1950s (American Psychiatric Association, 1952) recognized anorexia nervosa as a "neurotic illness," and by the second version of *DSM*, pica and rumination were also recognized, with bulimia nervosa added in the next version (American Psychiatric Association, 1968). The next major revision to *DSM* added the broad category of *Eating Disorder Not Otherwise Specified* to capture all eating disorders apart from anorexia and bulimia. Finally, the latest iteration of the *DSM*, *DSM-5*, recognizes several eating disorders grouped together under the category of feeding and eating disorders (American Psychiatric Association, 2013). These include, in addition to anorexia and bulimia, binge eating disorder (in acknowledgment of data indicating that binge behavior can occur in the absence of weight loss behaviors), pica, rumination disorder, and avoidant/restrictive food intake disorder (ARFID). *DSM-5* also maintains the diagnostic classifications for other specified eating or feeding disorder and unspecified eating or feeding disorder.

■ DIAGNOSIS, DEFINITION, AND CLINICAL FEATURES

Table 17.1 summarizes the key diagnostic features of each of the eating or feeding disorders classified under *DSM-5*.

■ ANOREXIA NERVOSA

The three criteria for establishing a diagnosis of anorexia nervosa relate to restricted energy intake leading to low body weight, intense fear of gaining weight or becoming fat, and the perception of one's body shape or weight.

TABLE 17.1

Key Diagnostic Features of Eating/Feeding Disorders in *DSM-5*

Condition	Key Diagnostic Features
Anorexia nervosa	Restricted energy intake leading to abnormally low body weight
	Intense fear of gaining weight or becoming fat
	Distorted perception of body weight or shape; body weight or shape unduly influences self-evaluation, not recognizing the seriousness of current low weight.
Bulimia nervosa	Recurrent binge eating episodes
	Compensatory behaviors to prevent weight gain
	Body weight or shape unduly influences self-evaluation.
Binge eating disorder	Recurrent episodes of distressing binge eating
	Binge eating is not associated with compensatory behaviors to prevent weight gain.
Pica	Persistent eating of nonnutritive nonfoods
	The eating of nonfoods is abnormal for the cultural and social context.
Rumination disorder	Frequent regurgitation of food
	The regurgitation does not occur exclusively during another eating disorder and is not attributable to a gastrointestinal or other medical condition.
ARFID	Avoidance or selectivity of foods leads to inappropriate nutritional or energy intake.
	No distortion in perception of body weight or shape

ARFID, avoidant/restrictive food intake disorder.

> **BOX 17.1   Case Report: Anorexia Nervosa**
>
> Linda, a 16-year-old high school sophomore, was evaluated at the insistence of her parents who were concerned about her high levels of exercise and weight loss. Although 5 feet 6 inches tall, her greatest weight, of 105 lb, had been achieved a year ago. At that time, a friend had commented unfavorably on her weight and she had begun a program of diet and exercise. Over the next 6 months, she had lost 25 lb through vigorous exercise. She had become obsessed with food, spending much time planning elaborate meals that she barely ate. She became more irritable and her grades began to suffer. Even with her weight loss, she remained unsatisfied with her appearance and believed she needed to lose more weight. She had stopped having her period several months previously.
>
> A multimodal treatment program was begun that included education and CBT as well as treatment with an SSRI and a program designed to help her achieve a reasonable weight. Although her initial course was rocky, she was able to achieve what she, her family, and therapists agreed was a reasonable goal weight.

Reprinted with permission from Volkmar, F. R., & Martin, A. (2011). *Essentials of Lewis's child and adolescent psychiatry* (1st ed., p. 188). Lippincott Williams & Wilkins/Wolters Kluwer.

The first criterion, of restricted energy intake leading to low body weight, is not very specific and how to define "significantly low weight" remains a question. The *DSM* states that weight should be *less than minimally normal or expected*, but there is no consensus on how to calculate weight loss or on the boundaries of minimally normal. One strategy relies on the body mass index (BMI), which is calculated as one's weight in kilograms divided by one's height in meters squared. The World Health Organization views a BMI of 18.5 kg/m² as the lower threshold for normal body weight (in adults), and this definition does not vary for different locations or cultures. In the United States, the Centers for Disease Control and Prevention views a BMI below the 5th percentile, using their calculator, as underweight.

The second criterion, of intense fear of becoming fat or gaining weight, or behaviors that interfere with weight gain despite low actual weight, is more straightforward but relies heavily on patients' self-disclosure. This poses a challenge as it is not uncommon for patients with anorexia to be less than forthcoming about their symptoms. Likewise, the third criterion of distorted perception of body weight or shape, or undue influence of body weight or shape on self-evaluation, or lack of recognition of the current unhealthy body weight, relies on subjective information provided by the patient. Distortions in the perception of body weight and shape in patients with anorexia can vary a great deal. In some cases, the distortion can relate to the entire body, with a sense of simply being fat overall, whereas in other cases it may be more specific to particular parts of the body such as the arms, thighs, or abdomen (Box 17.1).

Anorexia nervosa is further divided into two subtypes, restricting and binge-purge. Certain behavioral patterns, including impulsive behaviors, suicidal behavior, and substance abuse, are more commonly associated with the binge-purge subtype of anorexia, as are a history of obesity and some medical complications.

BULIMIA NERVOSA

The essential criteria for establishing a diagnosis of bulimia are the recurring presence of episodes of binge eating, compensatory behaviors aimed at preventing weight gain, and a self-image that is unduly influenced by body shape and weight. Binge eating episodes are discrete periods of time (*DSM* suggests 2 hours as an example) during which an unusually

Case Report—Bulimia Nervosa

Nancy, an 18-year-old senior in high school, was referred for evaluation by her parents because of binge eating. She had begun to binge periodically in her junior year—often when anxious and studying for her classes. She had been urged by her parents to take a challenging course load in hopes of getting her into the most advanced AP classes this year. The binges included a range of what she called "junk" food—typically, high-calorie foods were consumed. At these times, she described herself as having lost control over eating and she would feel disgusted with herself afterward. As her weight started to increase, she began to self-induce vomiting and also used laxatives in an attempt to keep her weight down. At the time of this referral, she was not overweight although her recurrent vomiting had begun to cause some dental problems. The parents had been largely unaware of these behaviors until the dentist spoke with them about his concern. At the time of referral, Nancy reported that she was typically vomiting several times a week and had been doing so for most of the past year. On examination, Nancy was noted to be depressed and somewhat anxious. Intervention included a number of different components including work with the family, individual work with Nancy, careful monitoring of her eating, and an explicit focus on the link between anxiety/depression and her eating.

Reprinted with permission from Volkmar, F. R., & Martin, A. (2011). *Essentials of Lewis's child and adolescent psychiatry* (1st ed., p. 190). Lippincott Williams & Wilkins/Wolters Kluwer.

large amount of food is consumed, along with a lack of control over the eating. The loss of control is critical to the diagnosis and must be subjectively endorsed by the patient for a diagnosis to be established.

The most common form of compensatory behavior aimed at preventing weight gain is self-induced vomiting. However, other compensatory behaviors can occur instead of or in addition to vomiting, such as fasting or the use of laxatives (Box 17.2).

BINGE EATING DISORDER

Binge eating disorder is defined by the presence of binge eating episodes (as in bulimia nervosa) and distress relating to the binge eating. *DSM* also includes some more specific descriptive criteria surrounding the binge eating, such as eating rapidly or until uncomfortably full, eating alone because of embarrassment about the quantity of food, and feeling disgusted with oneself or guilty about the binge eating.

Importantly, concerns relating to weight loss or appearance do not make up part of the diagnosis of binge eating disorder, and this is the most important distinction between binge eating disorder and bulimia nervosa. Extensive research demonstrating that the pattern of binge eating without such weight and shape concerns does occur supported the addition of binge eating disorder to the latest iteration of the *DSM*.

PICA

Pica refers to the consumption of nonfood, nonnutritive substances. The essential criteria for diagnosing pica per *DSM-5* are the consumption of nonfoods for at least a month in a manner that is abnormal for the individual's age, development, and cultural context. When other physical or mental health problems are present, for example, during pregnancy or in the context of autism spectrum disorder, pica is only diagnosed when the consumption of the nonfoods represents a hazard to the physical health of the individual. Individuals who eat nonnutritive substances that can be considered "food," such as ice or artificial sweeteners, are not diagnosed with pica. Among the substances consumed by individuals with pica are chalk, powdery substances such as talcum powder or makeup, and feces.

The age of the patient must be considered, as it is not uncommon for very young children to suck on or swallow nonfoods, and thus pica is generally not diagnosed before 2 years of age. Likewise, cultural context must be taken into consideration. Some cultures and religious practices include the consumption of nonfoods for spiritual or medicinal purposes; when the behavior matches the cultural context, pica is not diagnosed. Pica is also not diagnosed when the eating behavior is intended to serve a specific purpose such as appetite suppression or as a means of self-mutilation, or when it is the manifestation of a psychotic delusion.

Pica is often associated with intellectual and developmental disabilities and may also occur in obsessive-compulsive spectrum disorders, such as the consumption of pulled hair in trichotillomania. The clear concern in individuals with pica is that the nonfoods will cause physical harm, injuries, disease, or even death.

■ RUMINATION DISORDER

Rumination disorder is diagnosed based on frequent regurgitation of swallowed food, meaning that previously swallowed food is brought back up into the mouth. Regurgitated food may be spat out or swallowed again. The regurgitation must be frequent, occurring several times per week, and often daily or even consistently at almost every meal. Regurgitation is not the result of nausea and is distinct from vomiting, in which retching occurs and regurgitated food is acidic. The behavior must also be distinct from compensatory weight loss behaviors, as in anorexia or bulimia nervosa. Individuals with rumination disorder typically describe the behavior as habitual or uncontrollable, rather than as a completely voluntary action (Box 17.3).

Regurgitation is most common in individuals with intellectual disability and can occur at any age, starting in infancy. The persistent regurgitation can lead to medical complications, such as malnutrition, and to social impairment. Individuals with rumination disorder may come to avoid eating in the presence of others because of social discomfort associated with the regurgitation.

BOX 17.3 **Case Report—Rumination Disorder**

Steven was seen for evaluation at 7 months of age by his pediatrician because his grandmother was concerned that he was not eating well. Steven had been born to his 16-year-old mother following an unexpected pregnancy. Labor and delivery were unremarkable. His maternal grandmother assumed care on a day-to-day basis but worked much of the time, and a series of relatives provided much of his care. One month previously, he had been regurgitating food following feeding. At first, this was occasional but now routine. He continued to gain weight but his grandmother was concerned about the regurgitation. On examination, he was alert but somewhat apathetic and less interested in people and the environment than would be typical. Observation of him following a feeding did demonstrate regurgitation and rechewing of his food. Consultation with a behavioral psychologist recommended several steps to interrupt the regurgitation. In addition, arrangements were made for placement in a stable family day care setting. Both interventions resulted in relatively prompt resolution of the symptom.

Reprinted with permission from Volkmar, F. R., & Martin, A. (2011). *Essentials of Lewis's child and adolescent psychiatry* (1st ed., p. 184). Lippincott Williams & Wilkins/Wolters Kluwer.

AVOIDANT/RESTRICTIVE FOOD INTAKE DISORDER

ARFID is a newly established diagnosis under *DSM-5* and replaces a subset of diagnoses previously categorized under *Feeding or Eating Disorder of Infancy or Early Childhood* in the previous version of the *DSM*. The essential criterion for establishing a diagnosis of ARFID is the failure to meet appropriate nutritional or energy needs because of lack of interest in eating, avoidance of foods based on their sensory characteristics, or concern about negative consequences of eating. The disturbed eating pattern must result in significant weight loss or low weight, nutritional deficiency, dependence on enteral eating or supplements, and/or marked interference in psychosocial functioning. An emerging consensus in the field is that ARFID diagnoses should not be limited only to children with nutritional deficits or low weight, and that marked psychosocial impairment, stemming from the restricted eating, is sufficient for the diagnosis to be established. In contrast to the previous characterization of this problem as a disorder of infancy or early childhood, ARFID, per *DSM-5*, may set in and be diagnosed later in development.

ARFID cannot be diagnosed if present only during episodes of anorexia or bulimia, and individuals with ARFID do not present with distorted perceptions of their body weight or shape and do not restrict their eating as a weight loss strategy.

Because sensory sensitivity and picky eating are common phenomena, in particular in young children, it is important that the ARFID be abnormal and cause physical or psychosocial impairment for a diagnosis to be established.

As described in the main diagnostic criterion, three not mutually exclusive subtypes of ARFID have been recognized based on the functional motivation of the avoidant or restricted eating. The first subtype describes individuals with low interest in food and eating. This pattern tends to emerge early in life, during infancy, but can persist throughout development. The second subtype relates to restricted eating based on the sensory characteristics of foods. For example, a child may avoid foods that feel too hard, too soft, or too wet, or they may avoid foods of certain colors or shapes. This subtype tends to emerge during the first decade of life, but also can persist into later adolescence and adulthood. The third subtype describes avoidance or restriction of food because of fears of negative consequences of eating. Fear of choking is a common example of this kind of fear. This subtype is less closely linked to any particular development epoch and can arise at any age. In some cases, a frightening or traumatic event (such as choking) can trigger the fear and lead to ARFID (Box 17.4).

EPIDEMIOLOGY AND DEMOGRAPHICS

Estimating the prevalence of eating disorders is challenging, as much of the research in this area has focused on specific populations rather than on population-based sampling (Halmi, 2018). In the United States, the lifetime prevalence of anorexia nervosa in youth aged 13–18 was estimated at 0.3% (Swanson et al., 2011), whereas a study of Dutch youth found a lifetime prevalence rate of 1.7% for females aged 11–19 and 0.1% for males (Smink et al., 2014). For bulimia nervosa, a lifetime prevalence rate of 1.6% was reported for females up to age 20 in the United States (Stice et al., 2009), and a point prevalence rate of 0.6% was reported in Australian 14-year-olds (Allen et al., 2009). The challenges in estimating prevalence rates are compounded by the changing diagnostic criteria with successive iterations of the *DSM*. It is safe to say that anorexia nervosa and bulimia nervosa, although very serious disorders, are not exceedingly common, likely affecting one in several thousand individuals at any given time, and females more often than males.

The lifetime prevalence of binge eating disorder in the United States is estimated at 3.5% for women and 2% for men (Hudson et al., 2007, 2012). However, these estimates are across the entire lifespan and not for youth alone. A representative sample of American adolescents found lifetime prevalence rates of 2.3% for females and 0.8% for males (Swanson et al., 2011).

| BOX 17.4 | Case Report—ARFID |

Sandor was 9 years old and had an overall normal development, having achieved all developmental milestones within normal time ranges. He had no history of significant physical or psychological problems, but his parents described him as being high in sensory sensitivity. For example, he always asked his parents to remove labels from his clothes because they bothered him and he preferred to wear loose clothing, saying that tighter clothes were uncomfortable.

Sandor's eating had long been a source of some challenge and frustration for his parents. As a toddler, he had been highly selective about food, eating only simple foods such as mac and cheese, mashed potatoes, and other things of soft texture that did not require a lot of chewing. His parents hoped that this would change as he matured, and, for a while, it seemed to be improving. However, over the past year his eating had regressed significantly. Sandor began avoiding many foods saying they either tasted "bad" or were uncomfortable in his mouth. He also avoided foods with strong smells and recently had completely limited his food intake to only a small number of items. Sandor ate only at home or food that his parents prepared at home, and this was causing some difficulties in social situations. He avoided going to play dates or parties because of the worry that he would not have anything to eat there; the family felt unable to eat out at restaurants because Sandor would be visibly upset and would end up eating nothing at the restaurant.

Sandor's parents tried to accommodate his difficulties by always serving him his preferred foods and by bringing food with them if they were forced to eat outside. They tried to encourage him to eat, or at least to try, additional items, even offering "bribes" such as rewards and prizes for trying a new food. But their efforts had not yielded any positive results and they were concerned that the list of foods that Sandor was willing to eat was only shrinking instead of growing.

Based on recent examinations and blood work, Sandor was healthy, but his weight was low for his age and height. His parents feared that if the situation continued, he would have medical complications and his growth might be affected.

Following an initial consultation, a two-pronged treatment approach was formulated. Sandor would work directly with a therapist on gradual exposure to unfamiliar and nonpreferred foods. His parents would work with the therapist to learn how to modify their own behavior, including gradually reducing the accommodations they had been making because of Sandor's food-related restrictions.

Pica appears to be more common than other eating disorders, but actual prevalence rates are not really known and studies report widely varying prevalence rates, based in part on different inclusion and exclusion criteria. For example, studies that include the eating of ice as a nonnutritive substance report higher prevalence rates than studies that exclude ice eating as a symptom of pica. What is clear is that pica is more commonly reported in samples of individuals with intellectual disabilities, in particular those who require residential and institutional care. In such samples, prevalence rates for pica have ranged from 10% to 25% (Ali, 2001; Coniglio & Thomas, 2018). Prevalence rates for rumination disorder are also not known for the general population. One study in Swiss elementary schoolchildren found that approximately 4% of children endorsed clinically elevated rumination symptoms (Murray et al., 2018). However, the study relied on self-report questionnaires rather than on formal diagnostic evaluation. Another study of youth in Sri Lanka reported a prevalence rate of 5.1% for adolescents (Rajindrajith et al., 2012).

ARFID is the newest eating disorder included in *DSM*, and as such, studies estimating its prevalence using the most current diagnostic criteria remain scarce. Furthermore, some degree of picky eating is normative over the course of development and should not be viewed as pathologic. One study found a prevalence rate of 1.5% in a sample of pediatric patients (Eddy et al., 2015), whereas a community study reported a prevalence rate of 3.2% (Kurz et al., 2015).

ETIOLOGY AND PATHOGENESIS

The etiology of eating disorders remains not well understood and prevailing theories emphasize both environmental and individual variables as risk factors (Striegel-Moore & Bulik, 2007). Anorexia and bulimia are thought to commonly emerge through a process that begins with dieting behavior, which is itself spurred by individual and cultural factors, and then escalates as the dieting behavior increases and physiologic changes occur. Among the individual variables that increase vulnerability to eating disorders is female sex. In studies of both anorexia and bulimia, girls consistently outnumber boys by considerable margins (Currin et al., 2005; Hudson et al., 2007; Swanson et al., 2011). This difference is less pronounced, and not consistently found, in other eating disorders. White females are also more likely to be diagnosed with eating disorders than are members of minority ethnicities, but biases in research samples and different attitudes toward seeking mental health services in different racial and ethnic groups lower the confidence in actual prevalence rates (Javier et al., 2016; Lydecker & Grilo, 2016). Stressful life events, including trauma and physical, sexual, and emotional abuse, may also contribute to the risk of anorexia and bulimia nervosa (Becker & Grilo, 2011; Chen et al., 2010; Jaite et al., 2011; Racine & Wildes, 2015; Steiger et al., 2010). Psychological traits such as anxiety, perfectionism, and high harm avoidance have all been linked to greater risk of developing an eating disorder (Atiye et al., 2015; Grucza et al., 2007; Halmi et al., 2000; Wonderlich et al., 2015).

Genetic differences may also play an important role in the etiology of eating disorders (Thornton et al., 2011; Trace et al., 2013). Twin and family studies have pointed to considerable heritability, but the specific genes implicated in eating disorders remain a focus of ongoing research (Bulik et al., 2006; Javaras et al., 2008; Klump et al., 2009; Strober et al., 2000). The serotonergic system is implicated in both mood and appetite regulation, and as such, genes that impact this system have been identified as potentially contributing to the etiology of eating disorders (Bergen et al., 2003; Bulik et al., 2003). Epigenetic and gene by environment interactions are also plausible and supported by research (Frieling et al., 2008, 2010). For example, environmental factors may predispose to dieting, with certain genotypes making it more likely for the behavior to escalate to the point of an eating disorder.

Among the environmental factors that may contribute to eating disorders, much research has focused on the culture of thinness and the objectification of the female form (Katzman et al., 2004; Pike & Borovoy, 2004; Wardle & Watters, 2004). The idealization of thinness can be internalized and lead to dissatisfaction with the actual self, and in turn to dieting and other maladaptive eating-related behaviors. Weight loss can provide powerful reinforcement, including praise from others and a sense of control over one's life, especially when other stressors produce feelings of helplessness or loss of control. Fasting can also increase secretion of corticotropin-releasing hormone, which further assists in avoiding eating. Likewise, exercise can stimulate the release of endogenous opioids, which can serve as powerful reinforcers for the behavior. As such, neuroendocrinologic abnormalities in eating disorders often reflect the result of the abnormal eating, rather than its cause.

Neurocircuitry research has revealed differences in brain function in patients with eating disorder (e.g., increased activation in anterior cingulate and medial prefrontal cortical regions in response to food images), but here too it is not clear to what extent these differences reflect biologic vulnerabilities and risk factors, or the presence of the disorder itself (Bailer et al., 2005; Bailer & Kaye, 2011; Frank et al., 2011).

Familial factors that may influence the development of eating disorders include history of parental psychiatric problems and family or parenting style (Barona et al., 2016; Bould et al., 2015; Micali et al., 2014). For example, parental psychological control has been implicated in adolescent eating problems, as have both pressures to eat and food restriction (Berge et al., 2014). Likewise, parental attitudes about eating, body weight, and body shape and intraparental conflict are linked with greater risk of eating disorders in youth (Ciao et al., 2015; George et al., 2014; Palfreyman et al., 2015; White et al., 2014).

For pica, both biologic and behavioral etiologies have been proposed. Physiologic theories emphasize micronutrient deficiencies that may spur the eating behavior, whereas behavioral theories emphasize learned behaviors that may be most likely to emerge in environments with low social interaction, or even neglect (McNaughten et al., 2017).

Research on the etiology of ARFID is scarce and focuses primarily on behavioral factors. Children who experience a frightening event while eating, such as choking, may develop fears of certain foods and seek to eat only foods that they perceive as safe. Biologic differences may also contribute to the development of ARFID, however. Children with heightened sensory sensitivity may be particularly prone to eating only limited foods and to avoiding many others (Dovey et al., 2019). The three subtypes of ARFID described earlier may have distinct etiologies, though risk factors may also be shared across these presentations of the disorder.

■ ASSESSMENT AND DIFFERENTIAL DIAGNOSIS WITH EATING DISORDERS

Assessing the presence, presentation, and severity of eating disorders is challenging and should include a comprehensive multifaceted strategy (Anderson et al., 2004). One factor that complicates the assessment and poses a significant challenge to developing an accurate formulation is the tendency of patients with eating disorders to be reluctant to disclose the full extent of their symptoms. Dissembling and concealing are not uncommon and should be expected to some degree, especially in adolescent patients and those with anorexia nervosa and bulimia nervosa.

The scope of the assessment should cover symptoms and motivations of the patient, as well as a physical examination and in many cases blood work, to determine body weight and nutritional deficiencies. In young children and adolescents, assessment should include an examination of family patterns, including intrafamily relationships and interactions, current or past eating disorders of family members, and household eating patterns. It is also important for the assessor to gain an understanding of the cultural context of the patient and family, especially as it relates to eating expectations and weight or shape perceptions (Treasure et al., 2008). In most cases, a multidisciplinary effort is required for comprehensive assessment, usually including a psychiatrist, psychologist, pediatrician, and dietitian.

Clinical interviewing can be structured or unstructured. The Eating Disorder Examination is a validated semistructured interview schedule appropriate for children as young as 9 years (Cooper & Fairburn, 1987). For younger children, a developmentally appropriate version called the "Children's Eating Disorder Examination" (Watkins et al., 2005) exists.

Self-report questionnaires can also be administered such as the Eating Disorder Examination—Self Report Questionnaire (Luce & Crowther, 1999), the Children's Eating Attitudes Test (Smolak & Levine, 1994), and the Eating Disorders Inventory (Rosen et al., 1988) for children for anorexia, bulimia, and binge eating, and the Nine Item Avoidant/Restrictive Food Intake Screener for ARFID (Zickgraf & Ellis, 2018).

■ TREATMENT AND OUTCOME

When not treated successfully, eating disorders carry significant risk, including risk of mortality. Anorexia nervosa is associated with the highest mortality rate, and a significant proportion of deaths are from suicide (Arcelus et al., 2011; Franko et al., 2013; Smink et al., 2014; van Son et al., 2010).

Treatment for eating disorders usually involves a multidisciplinary effort including primary care, psychiatry, psychology/social work, and nutrition. The level of care is suited to the severity of the case, with outpatient treatment provided when possible, including family-based intervention, and in-patient care provided when necessary.

Family therapy is among the best established treatment interventions for anorexia and aims to promote effective parental management of weight restoration and healthier family dynamics relating to food and eating (Lock & Le Grange, 2012). Additional treatment protocols that have garnered empirical support include family systems therapy and individual adolescent-focused therapy (Agras et al., 2014; Fitzpatrick et al., 2010; Lock et al., 2010).

A central aim of treatment for anorexia nervosa is weight restoration, given the risks of serious nutritional deficits and the impact of being underweight on physical, emotional, and cognitive functions. Low weight is associated with poor mood, attention problems, anger, and over-preoccupation with food. Thus, food intake is usually monitored closely, alongside other cognitive and behavioral components of treatment.

Achieving normal weight in anorexia nervosa also requires medical management, including assessment of vital signs, electrolytes, and other physical indicators. Food supplements may be used to facilitate weight gain, particularly early in treatment. And, in life-threatening circumstances, nasal gastric feeding may be required. However, forceful feeding should be limited to severe cases in which the patient refuses to collaborate with treatment and the risks are acute. Medications can also be adjunct to other treatment components, but their efficacy is limited, and they do not represent a primary treatment strategy for anorexia.

Cognitive-behavioral therapy (CBT) is the best established treatment for bulimia nervosa and binge eating disorder, with numerous controlled trials demonstrating its efficacy in adults, but few in youth (Le Grange et al., 2015; Schmidt et al., 2007). Treatment focuses on maladaptive cognitions relating to food, body image, and weight and aims to disrupt the cycle of bingeing and purging behavior. Some CBT protocols for bulimia also include a focus on perfectionism, relationships, and other associated factors. Medications, primarily antidepressants, have also been found to be efficacious in reducing bingeing behavior in bulimia nervosa and binge eating disorder (Guerdjikova et al., 2008; McElroy et al., 2000, 2003).

Treatments for childhood ARFID include family-based treatment, CBT, and behavioral parent training (Eddy et al., 2019; Sharp et al., 2017; Shimshoni & Lebowitz, 2020). Treatment is most often carried out in an outpatient setting, with in-patient treatment used when nutritional deficiencies are severe and weight restoration is an acute need. Family-based treatment promotes increased food intake and variety by providing parents with tools for better eating management, whereas CBT focuses on cognitive restructuring and systematic exposure to various avoided foods. Completely parent-based interventions for childhood ARFID have also been developed. SPACE-ARFID is an adaptation of SPACE, a parent-based treatment for childhood anxiety and obsessive-compulsive disorder (Shimshoni & Lebowitz, 2020; Shimshoni et al., 2020). SPACE-ARFID promotes greater food-related flexibility in the child by reducing stress surrounding eating, increasing supportive parental responses to child symptoms, and reducing family accommodation of the disorder.

There are no well-established treatments for pica and rumination disorder. In rumination disorder, clinicians may employ diaphragmatic breathing to reduce regurgitation. In pica, functional analysis and applied behavioral analysis can be used to identify the antecedents of the eating behavior and a behavioral system of rewards can be implemented to reduce it.

SUMMARY

Eating and feeding disorders are a diverse group of conditions that present important treatment challenges. Clinically, they occupy an interesting niche at the intersection of medicine and mental health and thus present many challenges for management. A growing body of work on the treatment of these conditions in the past decades has enhanced and informed clinical intervention strategies. Additional work is clearly also needed.

Another condition at the intersection of medicine and mental health that also presents significant challenges is obesity. The marked increase in obesity levels over the past decades is a source of considerable concern, and although this increase may be slowing in recent years there is no evidence of decreased obesity levels. Although obesity was ultimately not included in *DSM-5* as a mental health disorder, the *DSM* workgroup considered the inclusion of obesity or an overeating disorder and called for additional research to inform such a potential diagnosis in the future.

The overlap between currently recognized diagnostic categories and the fact that not all patients will fit neatly into one of them indicate the need for additional research to inform the evolving understanding of the nosology of eating problems.

Greater public, and professional, awareness may help facilitate early diagnosis and treatment. The role of neurobiologic factors, including genetics, remains an important area for future research.

References

*Indicates Particularly Recommended

*Agras, W. S., Lock, J., Brandt, H., Bryson, S. W., Dodge, E., Halmi, K. A., Jo, B., Johnson, C., Kaye, W., Wilfley, D., & Woodside, B. (2014). Comparison of 2 family therapies for adolescent anorexia nervosa: A randomized parallel trial. *JAMA Psychiatry*, 71(11), 1279–1286. https://doi.org/10.1001/jamapsychiatry.2014.1025

Allen, K. L., Byrne, S. M., Forbes, D., & Oddy, W. H. (2009). Risk factors for full-and partial-syndrome early adolescent eating disorders: A population-based pregnancy cohort study. *Journal of the American Academy of Child and Adolescent Psychiatry*, 48(8), 800–809. https://doi.org/10.1097/CHI.0b013e3181a8136d

Ali, Z. (2001). Pica in people with intellectual disability: A literature review of aetiology, epidemiology and complications. *Journal of Intellectual and Developmental Disability*, 26(3), 205–215. https://doi.org/10.1080/13668250020054486

American Psychiatric Association. (1952). *Diagnostic and statistical manual of mental disorders*. Author.

American Psychiatric Association. (1968). *Diagnostic and statistical manual of mental disorders* (2nd ed.). Author.

American Psychiatric Association. (2013). *Diagnostic and statistical manual of mental disorders* (5th ed.). American Psychiatric Publishing.

Anderson, D. A., Lundgren, J. D., Shapiro, J. R., & Paulosky, C. A. (2004). Assessment of eating disorders: Review and recommendations for clinical use. *Behavior Modification*, 28(6), 763–782. https://doi.org/10.1177/0145445503259851

*Arcelus, J., Mitchell, A. J., Wales, J., & Nielsen, S. (2011). Mortality rates in patients with anorexia nervosa and other eating disorders: A meta-analysis of 36 studies. *Archives of General Psychiatry*, 68(7), 724–731. https://doi.org/10.1001/archgenpsychiatry.2011.74

Atiye, M., Miettunen, J., & Raevuori-Helkamaa, A. (2015). A meta-analysis of temperament in eating disorders. *European Eating Disorders Review*, 23(2), 89–99. https://doi.org/10.1002/erv.2342

Bailer, U. F., Frank, G. K., Henry, S. E., Price, J. C., Meltzer, C. C., Weissfeld, L., Mathis, C. A., Drevets, W. C., Wagner, A., Hoge, J., Ziolko, S. K., McConaha, C. W., & Kaye, W. H. (2005). Altered brain serotonin 5-HT1A receptor binding after recovery from anorexia nervosa measured by positron emission tomography and [carbonyl11C]WAY-100635. *Archives of General Psychiatry*, 62(9), 1032–1041. https://doi.org/10.1001/archpsyc.62.9.1032

Bailer, U. F., & Kaye, W. H. (2011). Serotonin: Imaging findings in eating disorders. *Current Topics in Behavior Neuroscience*, 6, 59–79. https://doi.org/10.1007/7854_2010_78

Barona, M., Nybo Andersen, A. M., & Micali, N. (2016). Childhood psychopathology in children of women with eating disorders. *Acta Psychiatrica Scandinavica*, 134(4), 295–304. https://doi.org/10.1111/acps.12616

Becker, D. F., & Grilo, C. M. (2011). Childhood maltreatment in women with binge-eating disorder: Associations with psychiatric comorbidity, psychological functioning, and eating pathology. *Eating and Weight Disorders*, 16(2), e113–e120. https://doi.org/10.1007/BF03325316

Bell, R. M. (1985). *Holy anorexia*. University of Chicago Press.

Berge, J. M., Wall, M., Larson, N., Eisenberg, M. E., Loth, K. A., & Neumark-Sztainer, D. (2014). The unique and additive associations of family functioning and parenting practices with disordered eating behaviors in diverse adolescents. *Journal of Behavior Medicine*, 37(2), 205–217. https://doi.org/10.1007/s10865-012-9478-1

Bergen, A. W., van den Bree, M. B. M., Yeager, M., Welch, R., Ganjei, J. K., Haque, K., Bacanu, S., Berrettini, W. H., Grice, D. E., Goldman, D., Bulik, C. M., Klump, K., Fichter, M., Halmi, K., Kaplan, A., Strober, M., Treasure, J., Woodside, B., & Kaye, W. H. (2003). Candidate genes for anorexia nervosa in the 1p33-36 linkage region: Serotonin 1D and delta opioid receptor loci exhibit significant association to anorexia nervosa. *Molecular Psychiatry, 8*(4), 397–406. https://doi.org/10.1038/sj.mp.4001318

Bould, H., Koupil, I., Dalman, C., DeStavola, B., Lewis, G., & Magnusson, C. (2015). Parental mental illness and eating disorders in offspring. *International Journal of Eating Disorders, 48*(4), 383–391. https://doi.org/10.1002/eat.22325

Bulik, C. M., Devlin, B., Bacanu, S. A., Thornton, L., Klump, K. L., Fichter, M. M., Halmi, K. A., Kaplan, A. S., Strober, M., Woodside, D. B., Bergen, A. W., Ganjei, J. K., Crow, S., Mitchell, J., Rotondo, A., Mauri, M., Cassano, G., Keel, P., Berrettini, W. H., & Kaye, W. H. (2003). Significant linkage on chromosome 10p in families with bulimia nervosa. *American Journal of Human Genetics, 72*(1), 200–207. https://doi.org/10.1086/345801

Bulik, C. M., Sullivan, P. F., Tozzi, F., Furberg, H., Lichtenstein, P., & Pedersen, N. L. (2006). Prevalence, heritability, and prospective risk factors for anorexia nervosa. *Archive of General Psychiatry, 63*(3), 305–312. https://doi.org/10.1001/archpsyc.63.3.305

Chen, L. P., Murad, M. H., Paras, M. L., Colbenson, K. M., Sattler, A. L., Goranson, E. N., Elamin, M. B., Seime, R. J., Shinozaki, G., Prokop, L. J., & Zirakzadeh, A. (2010). Sexual abuse and lifetime diagnosis of psychiatric disorders: Systematic review and meta-analysis. *Mayo Clinic Proceedings, 85*(7), 618–629. https://doi.org/10.4065/mcp.2009.0583

Ciao, A. C., Accurso, E. C., Fitzsimmons-Craft, E. E., Lock, J., & Le Grange, D. (2015). Family functioning in two treatments for adolescent anorexia nervosa. *International Journal of Eating Disorders, 48*(1), 81–90. https://doi.org/10.1002/eat.22314

*Coniglio, K. A., & Thomas, J. J. (2018). Pica, rumination disorder, and avoidant/restrictive food intake disorder. In A. Martin, M. H. Bloch, & F. R. Volkmar (Eds.), *Lewis's child and adolescent psychiatry: A comprehensive textbook* (5th ed.). Wolters Kluwer.

Cooper, Z., & Fairburn, C. (1987). The eating disorder examination: A semi-structured interview for the assessment of the specific psychopathology of eating disorders. *International Journal of Eating Disorders, 6*(1), 1–8. https://doi.org/10.1002/1098-108X(198701)6:1<1::AID-EAT2260060102>3.0.CO;2-9

Currin, L., Schmidt, U., Treasure, J., & Jick, H. (2005). Time trends in eating disorder incidence. *The British Journal of Psychiatry, 186*(2), 132–135. https://doi.org/10.1192/bjp.186.2.132

Dovey, T. M., Kumari, V., Blissett, J., & Mealtime Hostage Parent Science Gang. (2019). Eating behaviour, behavioural problems and sensory profiles of children with avoidant/restrictive food intake disorder (ARFID), autistic spectrum disorders or picky eating: Same or different? *Euopean Psychiatry, 61*, 56–62. https://doi.org/10.1016/j.eurpsy.2019.06.008

Eddy, K. T., Thomas, J. J., Hastings, E., Edkins, K., Lamont, E., Nevins, C. M., Patterson, R. M., Murray, H. B., Byrant-Waugh, R., & Becker, A. E. (2015). Prevalence of *DSM-5* avoidant/restrictive food intake disorder in a pediatric gastroenterology healthcare network. *International Journal of Eating Disorders, 48*(5), 464–470. https://doi.org/10.1002/eat.22350

Eddy, K. T., Harshman, S. G., Becker, K. R., Bern, E., Bryant-Waugh, R., Hilbert, A., Katzman, D. K., Lawson, E. A., Manzo, L. D., Menzel, J., Micali, N., Ornstein, R., Sally, S., Serinsky, S. P., Sharp, W., Stubbs, K., Walsh, B. T., Zickgraf, H., … Thomas, J. J. (2019). Radcliffe ARFID Workgroup: Toward operationalized research diagnostic criteria and directions for the field. *International Journal of Eating Disorders, 52*(4), 361–366. https://doi.org/10.1002/eat.23042

Eissler, K. R. (1943). Some psychiatric aspects of anorexia nervosa, demonstrated by a case report. *Psychoanalytic Review, 30*, 121–145.

Fitzpatrick, K. K., Moye, A., Hoste, R., Lock, J., & le Grange, D. (2010). Adolescent focused psychotherapy for adolescents with anorexia nervosa. *Journal of Contemporary Psychotherapy: On the Cutting Edge of Modern Developments in Psychotherapy, 40*(1), 31–39. https://doi.org/10.1007/s10879-009-9123-7

Frank, G. K., Reynolds, J. R., Shott, M. E., & O'Reilly, R. C. (2011). Altered temporal difference learning in bulimia nervosa. *Biological Psychiatry, 70*(8), 728–735. https://doi.org/10.1016/j.biopsych.2011.05.011

Franko, D. L., Keshaviah, A., Eddy, K. T., Krishna, M., Davis, M. C., Keel, P. K., & Herzog, D. B. (2013). A longitudinal investigation of mortality in anorexia nervosa and bulimia nervosa. *The American Journal of Psychiatry, 170*(8), 917–925. https://doi.org/10.1176/appi.ajp.2013.12070868

Frieling, H., Bleich, S., Otten, J., Römer, K. D., Kornhuber, J., de Zwaan, M., Jacoby, G. E., Wilhelm, J., & Hillemacher, T. (2008). Epigenetic downregulation of atrial natriuretic peptide but not vasopressin mRNA in females with eating disorders is related to impulsivity. *Neuropsychopharmacology, 33*(11), 2605–2609. https://doi.org/10.1038/sj.npp.1301662

Frieling, H., Römer, K. D., Scholz, S., Mittelbach, F., Wilhelm, J., De Zwaan, M., Jacoby, G. E., Kornhuber, J., Hillemacher, T., & Bleich, S. (2010). Epigenetic dysregulation of dopaminergic genes in eating disorders. *International Journal of Eating Disorders, 43*(7), 577–583. https://doi.org/10.1002/eat.20745

George, M. W., Fairchild, A. J., Mark Cummings, E., & Davies, P. T. (2014). Marital conflict in early childhood and adolescent disordered eating: Emotional insecurity about the marital relationship as an explanatory mechanism. *Eating Behaviors, 15*(4), 532–539. https://doi.org/10.1016/j.eatbeh.2014.06.006

Grucza, R. A., Przybeck, T. R., & Cloninger, C. R. (2007). Prevalence and correlates of binge eating disorder in a community sample. *Comprehensive Psychiatry, 48*(2), 124–131. https://doi.org/10.1016/j.comppsych.2006.08.002

Guerdjikova, A. I., McElroy, S. L., Kotwal, R., Welge, J. A., Nelson, E., Lake, K., Alessio, D. D., Keck, P. E. Jr., & Hudson, J. I. (2008). High-dose escitalopram in the treatment of binge-eating disorder with obesity: A placebo-controlled monotherapy trial. *Human Psychopharmacology: Clinical and Experimental, 23*(1), 1–11. https://doi.org/10.1002/hup.899

*Halmi, K. (2018). Anorexia nervosa, bulimia nervosa, and binge eating disorder. In A. Martin, M. H. Bloch, & F. R. Volkmar (Eds.), *Lewis's child and adolescent psychiatry: A comprehensive textbook* (5th ed., pp. 548–562). Wolters Kluwer.

Halmi, K. A., Sunday, S. R., Strober, M., Kaplan, A., Woodside, D. B., Fichter, M., Treasure, J., Berrettini, W. H., & Kaye, W. H. (2000). Perfectionism in anorexia nervosa: Variation by clinical subtype, obsessionality, and pathological eating behavior. *The American Journal of Psychiatry, 157*(11), 1799–1805. https://doi.org/10.1176/appi.ajp.157.11.1799

Hudson, J. I., Coit, C. E., Lalonde, J. K., & Pope, H. G. (2012). By how much will the proposed new DSM-5 criteria increase the prevalence of binge eating disorder? *International Journal of Eating Disorders, 45*(1), 139–141. https://doi.org/10.1002/eat.20890

*Hudson, J. I., Hiripi, E., Pope, H. G., Jr., & Kessler, R. C. (2007). The prevalence and correlates of eating disorders in the national comorbidity survey replication. *Biological Psychiatry, 61*(3), 348–358. https://doi.org/10.1016/j.biopsych.2006.03.040

Jaite, C., Schneider, N., Hilbert, A., Pfeiffer, E., Lehmkuhl, U., & Salbach-Andrae, H. (2011). Etiological role of childhood emotional trauma and neglect in adolescent anorexia nervosa: A cross-sectional questionnaire analysis. *Psychopathology, 45*(1), 61–66. https://doi.org/10.1159/000328580

Javaras, K. N., Laird, N. M., Reichborn-Kjennerud, T., Bulik, C. M., Pope, H. G., Jr., & Hudson, J. I. (2008). Familiality and heritability of binge eating disorder: Results of a case-control family study and a twin study. *International Journal of Eating Disorders, 41*(2), 174–179. https://doi.org/10.1002/eat.20484

Javier, S. J., Moore, M. P., & Belgrave, F. Z. (2016). Racial comparisons in perceptions of maternal and peer attitudes, body dissatisfaction, and eating disorders among African American and White women. *Women & Health, 56*(6), 615–633. https://doi.org/10.1080/03630242.2015.1118721

Katzman, M. A., Hermans, K. M. E., Van Hoeken, D., & Hoek, H. W. (2004). Not your "typical island woman": Anorexia nervosa is reported only in subcultures in curacao. *Culture, Medicine, and Psychiatry: An International Journal of Cross-Cultural Health Research, 28*(4), 463–492. https://doi.org/10.1007/s11013-004-1065-7

Klump, K. L., Suisman, J. L., Burt, S. A., McGue, M., & Iacono, W. G. (2009). Genetic and environmental influences on disordered eating: An adoption study. *Journal of Abnormal Psychology, 118*(4), 797–805. https://doi.org/10.1037/a0017204

Kurz, S., van Dyck, Z., Dremmel, D., Munsch, S., & Hilbert, A. (2015). Early-onset restrictive eating disturbances in primary school boys and girls. *European Child & Adolescent Psychiatry, 24*(7), 779–785. https://doi.org/10.1007/s00787-014-0622-z

Le Grange, D., Lock, J., Agras, W. S., Bryson, S. W., & Jo, B. (2015). Randomized clinical trial of family-based treatment and cognitive-behavioral therapy for adolescent bulimia nervosa. *Journal of the American Academy of Child and Adolescent Psychiatry, 54*(11), 886–894.e2. https://doi.org/10.1016/j.jaac.2015.08.008

Lock, J., & Le Grange, D. (2012). *Treatment manual for anorexia nervosa: A family-based approach* (2nd ed.). Guilford Press.

Lock, J., Le Grange, D., Agras, W. S., Moye, A., Bryson, S. W., & Jo, B. (2010). Randomized clinical trial comparing family-based treatment with adolescent-focused individual therapy for adolescents with anorexia nervosa. *Archives of Generaly Psychiatry, 67*(10), 1025–1032. https://doi.org/10.1001/archgenpsychiatry.2010.128

Luce, K. H., & Crowther, J. H. (1999). The reliability of the Eating Disorder Examination-Self-Report Questionnaire Version (EDE-Q). *International Jouranl of Eating Disorders, 25*(3), 349–351. https://doi.org/10.1002/(sici)1098-108x(199904)25:3<349::aid-eat15>3.0.co;2-m

Lydecker, J. A., & Grilo, C. M. (2016). Different yet similar: Examining race and ethnicity in treatment-seeking adults with binge eating disorder. *Journal of Consulting and Clinical Psychology, 84*(1), 88–94. https://doi.org/10.1037/ccp0000048

Masserman, J. H. (1941). Psychodynamisms in anorexia nervosa and neurotic vomiting. *The Psychoanalytic Quarterly, 10*(2), 211–242. https://doi.org/10.1080/21674086.1941.11925457

McElroy, S. L., Casuto, L. S., Nelson, E. B., Lake, K. A., Soutullo, C. A., Keck, P. E., Jr., & Hudson, J. I. (2000). Placebo-controlled trial of sertraline in the treatment of binge eating disorder. *The American Journal of Psychiatry, 157*(6), 1004–1006. https://doi.org/10.1176/appi.ajp.157.6.1004

McElroy, S. L., Hudson, J. I., Malhotra, S., Welge, J. A., Nelson, E. B., & Keck, P. E., Jr. (2003). Citalopram in the treatment of binge-eating disorder: A placebo-controlled trial. *The Journal of Clinical Psychiatry, 64*(7), 807–813. https://doi.org/10.4088/JCP.v64n0711

McNaughten, B., Bourke, T., & Thompson, A. (2017). Fifteen-minute consultation: The child with pica. *Archives of Disease in Childhood—Education and Practice, 102*(5), 226–229. https://doi.org/10.1136/archdischild-2016-312121

Meyer, B. C., & Weinroth, L. A. (1957). Observations on psychological aspects of anorexia nervosa: Report of a case. *Psychosomatic Medicine, 19*(5), 389–398. https://doi.org/10.1097/00006842-195709000-00006

Micali, N., Stahl, D., Treasure, J., & Simonoff, E. (2014). Childhood psychopathology in children of women with eating disorders: Understanding risk mechanisms. *Journal of Child Psychology and Psychiatry, 55*(2), 124–134. https://doi.org/10.1111/jcpp.12112

Murray, H. B., Thomas, J. J., Hinz, A., Munsch, S., & Hilbert, A. (2018). Prevalence in primary school youth of pica and rumination behavior: The understudied feeding disorders. *International Journal of Eating Disorders, 51*(8), 994–998. https://doi.org/10.1002/eat.22898

Palfreyman, Z., Haycraft, E., & Meyer, C. (2015). Parental modelling of eating behaviours: Observational validation of the Parental Modelling of Eating Behaviours scale (PARM). *Appetite, 86*, 31–37. https://doi.org/10.1016/j.appet.2014.08.008

Pike, K. M., & Borovoy, A. (2004). The rise of eating disorders in Japan: Issues of culture and limitations of the model of "Westernization". *Culture, Medicine, and Psychiatry: An International Journal of Cross-Cultural Health Research, 28*(4), 493–531. https://doi.org/10.1007/s11013-004-1066-6

Racine, S. E., & Wildes, J. E. (2015). Emotion dysregulation and anorexia nervosa: An exploration of the role of childhood abuse. *International Journal of Eating Disorders, 48*(1), 493–531. https://doi.org/10.1002/eat.22364

Rajindrajith, S., Devanarayana, N. M., & Crispus Perera, B. J. (2012). Rumination syndrome in children and adolescents: A school survey assessing prevalence and symptomatology. *BMC Gastroenterology, 12*, 163. https://doi.org/10.1186/1471-230X-12-163

Rosen, J. C., Silberg, N. T., & Gross, J. (1988). Eating attitudes test and eating disorders inventory: Norms for adolescent girls and boys. *Journal of Consulting and Clinical Psychology, 56*(2), 305–308. https://doi.org/10.1037/0022-006X.56.2.305

Schmidt, U., Lee, S., Beecham, J., Perkins, S., Treasure, J., Yi, I., Winn, S., Robinson, P., Murphy, R., Keville, S., Johnson-Sabine, E., Jenkins, M., Frost, S., Dodge, L., Berelowitz, M., & Eisler, I. (2007). A randomized controlled trial of family therapy and cognitive behavior therapy guided self-care for adolescents with bulimia nervosa and related disorders. *American Journal of Psychiatry, 164*(4), 591–598. https://doi.org/10.1176/ajp.2007.164.4.591

* Sharp, W. G., Volkert, V. M., Scahill, L., McCracken, C. E., & McElhanon, B. (2017). A systematic review and meta-analysis of intensive multidisciplinary intervention for pediatric feeding disorders: How standard is the standard of care? *The Journal of Pediatrics, 181*, 116–124.e114. https://doi.org/10.1016/j.jpeds.2016.10.002

*Shimshoni, Y., & Lebowitz, E. R. (2020). Childhood avoidant/restrictive food intake disorder: Review of treatments and a novel parent-based approach. *Journal of Cognitive Psychotherapy, 34*(3), 200–224. https://doi.org/10.1891/JCPSY-D-20-00009

Shimshoni, Y., Silverman, W. K., & Lebowitz, E. R. (2020). SPACE-ARFID: A pilot trial of a novel parent-based treatment for avoidant/restrictive food intake disorder. *International Journal of Eating Disorders, 53*(10), 1623–1635. https://doi.org/10.1002/eat.23341

Smink, F. R. E., van Hoeken, D., Oldehinkel, A. J., & Hoek, H. W. (2014). Prevalence and severity of DSM-5 eating disorders in a community cohort of adolescents. *International Journal of Eating Disorders, 47*(6), 610–619. https://doi.org/10.1002/eat.22316

Smolak, L., & Levine, M. P. (1994). Psychometric properties of the Children's Eating Attitudes Test. *International Journal of Eating Disorders, 16*(3), 275–282. https://doi.org/10.1002/1098-108x(199411)16:3<275::aid-eat2260160308>3.0.co;2-u

Steiger, H., Richardson, J., Schmitz, N., Israel, M., Bruce, K. R., & Gauvin, L. (2010). Trait-defined eating-disorder subtypes and history of childhood abuse. *International Journal of Eating Disorders, 43*(5), 428–432. https://doi.org/10.1002/eat.20711

Stice, E., Marti, C. N., Shaw, H., & Jaconis, M. (2009). An 8-year longitudinal study of the natural history of threshold, subthreshold, and partial eating disorders from a community sample of adolescents. *Journal of Abnormal Psychology, 118*(3), 587–597. https://doi.org/10.1037/a0016481

Striegel-Moore, R. H., & Bulik, C. M. (2007). Risk factors for eating disorders. *American Psychologist, 62*(3), 181–198. https://doi.org/10.1037/0003-066X.62.3.181

Strober, M., Freeman, R., Lampert, C., Diamond, J., & Kaye, W. (2000). Controlled family study of anorexia nervosa and bulimia nervosa: Evidence of shared liability and transmission of partial syndromes. *The American Journal of Psychiatry, 157*(3), 393–401. https://doi.org/10.1176/appi.ajp.157.3.393

Swanson, S. A., Crow, S. J., Le Grange, D., Swendsen, J., & Merikangas, K. R. (2011). Prevalence and correlates of eating disorders in adolescents: Results from the national comorbidity survey replication adolescent supplement. *Archives of General Psychiatry, 68*(7), 714–723. https://doi.org/10.1001/archgenpsychiatry.2011.22

Thornton, L. M., Mazzeo, S. E., & Bulik, C. M. (2011). The heritability of eating disorders: Methods and current findings. In R. Adan & W. Kaye (Eds.), *Behavioral neurobiology of eating disorders. Current topics in behavioral neurosciences* (Vol. 6, pp. 141–156). Springer-Verlag. https://doi.org/10.1007/7854_2010_91

Trace, S. E., Baker, J. H., Penas-Lledo, E., & Bulik, C. M. (2013). The genetics of eating disorders. *Annual Review of Clinical Psychology, 9*, 589–620. https://doi.org/10.1146/annurev-clinpsy-050212-185546

Treasure, J., Sepulveda, A. R., MacDonald, P., Whitaker, W., Lopez, C., Zabala, M., Kyriacou, O., & Todd, G. (2008). The assessment of the family of people with eating disorders. *European Eating Disorders Review, 16*(4), 247–255. https://doi.org/10.1002/erv.859

van Son, G. E., van Hoeken, D., van Furth, E. F., Donker, G. A., & Hoek, H. W. (2010). Course and outcome of eating disorders in a primary care-based cohort. *International Journal Eating Disorders, 43*(2), 130–138. https://doi.org/10.1002/eat.20676

Wardle, J., & Watters, R. (2004). Sociocultural influences on attitudes to weight and eating: results of a natural experiment. *International Journal Eating Disorders, 35*(4), 589–596. https://doi.org/10.1002/eat.10268

Watkins, B., Frampton, I., Lask, B., & Bryant-Waugh, R. (2005). Reliability and validity of the child version of the eating disorder examination: A preliminary investigation. *International Journal Eating Disorders, 38*(2), 183–187. https://doi.org/10.1002/eat.20165

White, J., Shelton, K. H., & Elgar, F. J. (2014). Prospective associations between the family environment, family cohesion, and psychiatric symptoms among adolescent girls. *Child Psychiatry & Human Development, 45*(5), 544–554. https://doi.org/10.1007/s10578-013-0423-5

Wonderlich, J. A., Lavender, J. M., Wonderlich, S. A., Peterson, C. B., Crow, S. J., Engel, S. G., Le Grange, D., Mitchell, J. E., & Crosby, R. D. (2015). Examining convergence of retrospective and ecological momentary assessment measures of negative affect and eating disorder behaviors. *The International Journal of Eating Disorders, 48*(3), 305–311. https://doi.org/10.1002/eat.22352

Zickgraf, H. F., & Ellis, J. M. (2018). Initial validation of the Nine Item Avoidant/Restrictive Food Intake disorder screen (NIAS): A measure of three restrictive eating patterns. *Appetite, 123*, 32–42. https://doi.org/10.1016/j.appet.2017.11.111

Suggested Readings

Baker, J. H., Maes, H. H., Lissner, L., Aggen, S. H., Lichtenstein, P., & Kendler, K. S. (2009). Genetic risk factors for disordered eating in adolescent males and females. *Journal of Abnormal Psychology, 118*(3), 576–586. https://doi.org/10.1037/a0016314

Bemporad, J. R. (1997). Cultural and historical aspects of eating disorders. *Theoretical Medicine, 18*(4), 401–420. https://doi.org/10.1023/A:1005721808534

Bliss, E., & Branch, C. H. (1960). *Anorexia nervosa: Its history, psychology and biology.* Hoeber.

Bohon, C., & Stice, E. (2012). Negative affect and neural response to palatable food intake in bulimia nervosa. *Appetite, 58*(3), 964–970. https://doi.org/10.1016/j.appet.2012.02.051

Burns, E. E., Fischer, S., Jackson, J. L., & Harding, H. G. (2012). Deficits in emotion regulation mediate the relationship between childhood abuse and later eating disorder symptoms. *Child Abuse and Neglect, 36*(1), 32–39. https://doi.org/10.1016/j.chiabu.2011.08.005

Frank, G. K. W., Shott, M. E., Hagman, J. O., & Yang, T. T. (2013). Localized brain volume and white matter integrity alterations in adolescent anorexia nervosa. *Journal of the American Academy of Child and Adolescent Psychiatry, 52*(10), 1066–1075.e5. https://doi.org/10.1016/j.jaac.2013.07.007

Gentile, K., Raghavan, C., Rajah, V., & Gates, K. (2007). It doesn't happen here: Eating disorders in an ethnically diverse sample of economically disadvantaged, urban college students. *Eating Disorders, 15*(5), 405–425. https://doi.org/10.1080/10640260701667904

Gull, W. (1888). Anorexia nervosa. *Lancet, 47*, 516–517. https://doi.org/10.1016/S0140-6736(00)48519-3

Halmi, K. A., Tozzi, F., Thornton, L. M., Crow, S., Fichter, M. M., Kaplan, A. S., Keel, P., Klump, K. L., Lilenfeld, L. R., Mitchell, J. E., Plotnicov, K. H., Pollice, C., Rotondo, A., Strober, M., Woodside, D. B., Berrettini, W. H., Kaye, W. H., & Bulik, C. M. (2005). The relation among perfectionism, obsessive-compulsive personality disorder and obsessive-compulsive disorder in individuals with eating disorders. *International Journal of Eating Disorders, 38*(4), 371–374. https://doi.org/10.1002/eat.20190

Harris, J. C. (2014). Anorexia nervosa and anorexia mirabilis: Miss K. R—and St Catherine of Siena. *JAMA Psychiatry, 71*(11), 1212–1213. https://doi.org/10.1001/jamapsychiatry.2013.2765

Hopwood, C. J., Ansell, E. B., Fehon, D. C., & Grilo, C. M. (2011). The mediational significance of negative/depressive affect in the relationship of childhood maltreatment and eating disorder features in adolescent psychiatric inpatients. *Eating and Weight Disorders, 16*(1), e9–e16. https://doi.org/10.1007/BF03327515

Hoste, R. R., Lebow, J., & Le Grange, D. (2015). A bidirectional examination of expressed emotion among families of adolescents with bulimia nervosa. *International Journal of Eating Disorders, 48*(2), 249–252. https://doi.org/10.1002/eat.22306

Keski-Rahkonen, A., Raevuori, A., Bulik, C. M., Hoek, H. W., Rissanen, A., & Kaprio, J. (2014). Factors associated with recovery from anorexia nervosa: A population-based study. *International Journal of Eating Disorders, 47*(2), 117–123. https://doi.org/10.1002/eat.22168

Kluck, A. S. (2010). Family influence on disordered eating: The role of body image dissatisfaction. *Body Image, 7*(1), 8–14. https://doi.org/10.1016/j.bodyim.2009.09.009

Marce, L. (1860). On a form of hypochondriacal delirium occurring consecutive to dyspepsia, and characterized by refusal of food. *Journal of Psychological Medicine and Mental Pathology, 13*, 264–266.

Quick, V. M., & Byrd-Bredbenner, C. (2014). Disordered eating, socio-cultural media influencers, body image, and psychological factors among a racially/ethnically diverse population of college women. *Eating Behaviors, 15*(1), 37–41. https://doi.org/10.1016/j.eatbeh.2013.10.005

Rotella, F., Fioravanti, G., Godini, L., Mannucci, E., Faravelli, C., & Ricca, V. (2015). Temperament and emotional eating: a crucial relationship in eating disorders. *Psychiatry Research, 225*(3), 452–457. https://doi.org/10.1016/j.psychres.2014.11.068

Schmidt, R., Tetzlaff, A., & Hilbert, A. (2015). Perceived expressed emotion in adolescents with binge-eating disorder. *Journal of Abnormal Child Psychology, 43*(7), 1369–1377. https://doi.org/10.1007/s10802-015-0015-x

Shott, M. E., Pryor, T. L., Yang, T. T., & Frank, G. K. W. (2016). Greater insula white matter fiber connectivity in women recovered from anorexia nervosa. *Neuropsychopharmacology, 41*(2), 498–507. https://doi.org/10.1038/npp.2015.172

Soundy, T. J., Lucas, A. R., Suman, V. J., & Melton, L. J. (1995). Bulimia nervosa in Rochester, Minnesota from 1980 to 1990. *Psychological Medicine, 25*(5), 1065–1071. https://doi.org/10.1017/S0033291700037557

Vrabel, K. R., Hoffart, A., Ro, O., Martinsen, E. W., & Rosenvinge, J. H. (2010). Co-occurrence of avoidant personality disorder and child sexual abuse predicts poor outcome in long-standing eating disorder. *Journal of Abnormal Psychology, 119*(3), 623–629. https://doi.org/10.1037/a0019857

Wilson, G. T., & Fairburn, C. G. (1993). Cognitive treatments for eating disorders. *Journal of Consulting and Clinical Psychology, 61*(2), 261–269. https://doi.org/10.1037/0022-006X.61.2.261

Zerwas, S., Lund, B. C., Von Holle, A., Thornton, L. M., Berrettini, W. H., Brandt, H., Crawford, S., Fichter, M. M., Halmi, K. A., Johnson, C., Kaplan, A. S., La Via, M., Mitchell, J., Rotondo, A., Strober, M., Woodside, D. B., Kaye, W. H., & Bulik, C. M. (2013). Factors associated with recovery from anorexia nervosa. *Journal of Psychiatric Research, 47*(7), 972–979. https://doi.org/10.1016/j.jpsychires.2013.02.011

CHAPTER 18 ■ SOMATIC SYMPTOMS AND SOMATOFORM DISORDERS

■ BACKGROUND

Persistent somatic symptoms and complaints are present in many children and adolescents and cause both suffering and functional impairment (Dell & Campo, 2011; Marwah et al., 2016). In many cases, no clear physical cause for the complaints can be established. For example, many children experience chronic head or abdominal pain, even in the absence of any identifiable and diagnosable physical illness. In other cases, the somatic complaints are more easily understood to be the symptoms of a recognized illness or condition.

The dualism between that which is "physical" and that which is "mental" that held sway for much of Western history, and influenced beliefs about health and functioning, exerted great influence on attitudes toward poorly understood somatic symptoms. Indeed, patients who present with such symptoms have in the past been viewed as "neurotic," "hysterical," and in some cases as lacking in morality. In 1895, Freud and Breuer published *Studies in Hysteria*, a seminal book that described unexplained neurologic symptoms as resulting from psychological forces, and in particular from sexual incidents in the patient's history. The book presented five case studies, the most famous of which is that of Anna O (Bertha Pappenheim), who suffered from partial paralysis; impaired vision, hearing, and speech; and hallucinations. Freud and Breuer suggested that these symptoms were rooted in unresolved feelings relating to her father's illness and death. This case, along with the others described in the book, is credited with laying the foundation for the development of Freud's psychoanalytic theories and treatment approach.

Dualism has given way in more modern times to a unitary view of health as a biopsychosocial construct and to the recognition that physical and mental health are not discrete categories. Nonetheless, dualism continues to exert influence on both attitudes and medical services. Although somatic symptoms that are clearly tied to underlying pathophysiology of disease are generally accepted as "valid" and "real," symptoms that are not linked to a disease are often met with considerable doubt and skepticism. Such symptoms (often termed *functional somatic symptoms*) are still frequently questioned for both their validity (do they actually exist?) and their implications (why does the child have them?). This kind of skepticism can amplify the child's suffering and leave parents feeling bewildered, confused, and angry with the child, the doctor, or both. Statements such as "It's all in her head" remain not uncommon and are often perceived, or even intended, as disparaging.

These negative attitudes on the part of physicians confronted with unexplained somatic symptoms can reflect the sense of helplessness that can stem from a problem that appears outside of their domain of expertise, but which they are expected to be able to address. Although many mental health problems remain largely "unexplained," as no clear pathophysiology has been determined for the most common mental health problems, these disorders have achieved a greater validity in the lay and professional thinking through the establishment of clear diagnostic categories. The development of clearer nosologic categories for somatic symptoms may be useful in reducing stigma and confusion around somatic symptoms as well.

In its most recent iteration, the *Diagnostic and Statistical Manual of Mental Disorders* (*DSM-5*) (American Psychiatric Association, 2013) has taken further steps toward establishing a unitary approach to somatic symptoms. One important shift is deemphasizing the "unexplained" nature of somatic symptoms. Instead, *DSM-5* focuses on the presence of somatic symptoms (whether explained or not) and on the distress and impairment caused by the symptoms. As such, somatic symptom disorder, the primary somatic diagnostic category under *DSM-5*, can include both symptoms that are "unexplained" and those that are more clearly linked to a known physical cause. This shift not only changes significantly the actual diagnostic criteria but also implicitly acknowledges that symptoms that are unexplained at one point in time may be understood differently at another. Grouping the somatic symptoms together, with no requirement that they be unexplained, recognizes that lack of a known physical cause is not in and of itself evidence of a root mental cause. Furthermore, the shift away from a focus on unexplained symptoms allows for a focus on other features that are clearly present. Thus, instead of basing the diagnosis on what is not present (a clear medical explanation for the symptoms), *DSM-5* focuses more on patterns of maladaptive cognitive, emotional, and behavioral functioning that clearly are.

Another diagnosis that highlights the inextricable link between physical and mental health is that of psychological factors affecting medical conditions. This refers to situations in which a nonmental condition is present, and psychological or behavioral factors are adversely impacting the medical condition or hampering or delaying its treatment.

Alongside these diagnoses, *DSM-5* also recognizes several other diagnoses characterized by somatic complaints or a focus on physical well-being. Illness anxiety, newly introduced in *DSM-5*, refers to excessive preoccupation with being or becoming seriously ill. Conversion disorder (functional neurological symptom disorder) is diagnosed in patients who present with abnormal motor or sensory function that is not compatible with known neurologic conditions. As such, conversion disorder retains the focus on the seemingly unexplained nature of the symptoms. And factitious disorder refers to the deliberate falsification of symptoms in oneself or in others.

◼ DIAGNOSIS, DEFINITION, AND CLINICAL FEATURES

The currently recognized somatic diagnoses and their key diagnostic features are summarized in Table 18.1 and include Somatic Symptom Disorder, Illness Anxiety Disorder, Conversion Disorder (Functional Neurological Symptom Disorder), Psychological Factors Affecting Other Medical Conditions, and Factitious Disorder, as well as Other Specified Somatic Symptom and Related Disorder and Unspecified Somatic Symptom and Related Disorder.

Somatic Symptom Disorder

The key diagnostic criteria for establishing a diagnosis of somatic symptom disorder are that somatic symptoms are persistently present, cause distress or impairment, and excessive thoughts, feelings, or behaviors are devoted to them or to related health concerns. The specific somatic symptoms may vary and change over time, but some symptoms will be present for a period of typically at least 6 months. The diagnosis is further classified according to the current severity and number of the somatic symptoms, and according to whether or not the

TABLE 18.1

Main Diagnostic Categories for Somatic Disorders in *DSM-5* and Key Criteria

Diagnosis	Key Diagnostic Criteria
Somatic symptom disorder	• Persistent somatic symptoms • Symptoms cause distress and/or functional impairment • Excessive thoughts, feelings, or behaviors related to the symptoms or to health
Illness anxiety	• Excessive preoccupation with having or developing an illness • Anxiety about health • Performing excessive health-related behaviors or avoiding medical procedures • Somatic symptoms are not present or are mild and not the source of impairment
Conversion disorder	• Sensory or motor symptoms that are incompatible with neurologic conditions
Psychological factors affecting other medical conditions	• A physical medical condition is adversely affected by psychological or behavioral factors (e.g., the condition is exacerbated or recovery impeded) • The psychological factors are exerting a clear negative impact on the medical condition
Factitious disorder	• Deliberate falsification of physical or psychological symptoms • Can include exaggeration of real symptoms and/or fabrication of symptoms or medical signs • In some cases, the deliberate induction of illness or injury • Can be imposed on the self—individual falsifies their own symptoms • Can be imposed on another—individual falsifies symptoms of another person (e.g., a parent falsifies symptoms of a child)

symptoms predominantly involve pain. When symptoms are severe and persistent (more than 6 months), the diagnosis is also classified as "persistent."

Importantly, the somatic symptoms in somatic symptom disorder may, or may not, be associated with another medical condition. For example, a child who underwent a medical procedure and experiences persistent somatic symptoms following the procedure may meet criteria for the diagnosis, despite the link to the medical procedure, if all other criteria are met.

Children with somatic symptom disorder are typically chronically worried about their health. They may interpret their somatic symptoms as signs of a serious medical condition and fear grave illness or death. In severe cases, the concerns around the somatic symptoms may take on a central focus of the child's identify and life. The child may view themselves as "sick," require many medical examinations, and avoid activities because of fear of becoming more ill or of exacerbating their symptoms. This concern can appear to be immune to any reassurance that is provided by adults and experts in the child's life. For example, a visit to the doctor, with a reassuring message that the child is not seriously ill, may provide only very temporary relief, which is soon replaced by renewed anxiety and worry. Furthermore, the preoccupation with health and somatic symptoms may make the child more likely to notice any small physical experience and perceive it as another indication of the seriousness of their overall condition. It is common for somatic symptoms to accumulate, for example, for a child with chronic complaints of abdominal discomfort, to also develop headaches, leading to further impairment.

Although any somatic symptom can be present in somatic symptom disorder, headache, abdominal distress or pain, fatigue, and chest pain are among the most common complaints. The somatic symptoms, and the anxiety they cause, can lead to serious impairment in a child's ability to function normally. School attendance is a major challenge, and absenteeism is common.

Illness Anxiety Disorder

The central features and diagnostic criteria of illness anxiety disorder are preoccupation with having or developing an illness, high levels of anxiety about health, and the performance of excessive health-related behaviors or the avoidance of health-related procedures and situations. Somatic symptoms are either not present in illness anxiety disorder or are present but are mild. And the impairment in illness anxiety disorder is not caused by the presence of the somatic symptoms, although such symptoms can contribute to the anxiety about becoming sick. When illness anxiety is diagnosed in a person who also suffers from a diagnosable medical condition, the anxiety is excessive in relation to the severity of the medical condition. For example, a child with a benign and nondangerous heart murmur may be excessively preoccupied with the risk of heart failure, in a manner that is not proportionate to the realistic risk.

Children with illness anxiety disorder may exhibit high interest in news or information relating to health and disease. Hearing about another person, such as a grandparent, becoming ill can trigger severe anxiety in the child, leading them to seek out additional information and potentially perpetuating a cycle of elevated anxiety. For some children with illness anxiety, the preoccupation with health and disease will be extensive enough to interfere with most other interests and activities. Dinner table conversations may repeatedly center around health-related topics, for example, causing frustration and exasperation to other family members. The child may also engage in frequent self-checks, examining parts of their body for signs of illness. For example, the child may frequently take their temperature, search for signs of hair loss, or attempt to inspect their own throat in the mirror. The child may also pressure their parents to take them to frequent medical check-ups, and parents who are attempting to reassure the child may accommodate by arranging such visits. Reassurance from the medical professional, however, is unlikely to relieve the anxiety for more than a brief period of time.

Conversion Disorder

Conversion disorder (functional neurological symptom disorder) is diagnosed when a patient presents with sensory or motor symptoms that are not compatible with established neurologic or medical conditions. Symptoms can include muscle weakness or paralysis, tremors, abnormal posture or gait, and reduced skin sensation. Some symptoms of conversion disorder appear similar to seizures, as when a patient appears to shake or twitch and lose consciousness, but neurologic examination will not be consistent with seizure. Speech and vision can also be abnormal or altered. For example, a child may report seeing double or may show difficulty articulating words.

An important note is that the absence of neurologic findings to support a diagnosis compatible with the symptoms is not in and of itself sufficient to establish a diagnosis of conversion disorder. That is to say, a child who presents with symptoms that are strange and remarkable or a child whose symptoms are not clearly aligned with any established neurologic condition should not be diagnosed with conversion disorder based solely on the fact that no known condition matches their symptoms. Rather, the diagnosis should only be established when there is clear evidence of actual incompatibility between the symptoms and neurologic conditions. One example of such *incompatibility* is the presence of tremors that cease when the child is distracted by some other action. The tremor entrainment test is a procedure in which a patient who presents with a tremor on one side of the body, for example, in the right hand, is asked to follow the doctor's rhythmic motions with their left hand. When the tremor in the right hand changes as a result (e.g., the child begins to make the same motion with the right hand as well), this would be incompatible with "true" neurologic tremor behavior. This guideline on diagnosing conversion disorder only when there is clear evidence of incompatibility with neurologic conditions is important, because not adhering to it could lead to misdiagnosis of conversion disorder in children who may later be found to be suffering from an as-yet undiagnosed condition.

The diagnosis also does not rest upon ascertaining that the child is not deliberately producing (or misreporting) their symptoms. This is a difficult judgment to make and is not required. Likewise, although secondary gains (i.e., external rewards derived by the child from the symptoms) may be present, they are not part of the diagnostic considerations. In some cases of conversion disorder, patients exhibit a seeming lack of interest or concern about the symptoms (sometimes referred to as *la belle indifférence*).

Psychological Factors Affecting Other Medical Conditions

This diagnosis is appropriate when a patient has a medical condition or symptom (not a mental health disorder) and psychological or behavioral factors are adversely affecting that condition. The psychological factors could be exacerbating the condition, hampering recovery, or interfering with treatment of the condition. The diagnosis is specified as mild when the psychological factors are increasing medical risk, moderate when they are aggravating the underlying medical condition, severe when they result in hospital visits or stays, and extreme when they pose a life-threatening risk.

Examples of psychological and behavioral factors that could contribute to this diagnosis are distress that exacerbates the physical condition, engaging in maladaptive health-related behaviors, lack of adherence to treatment protocols, and denial of symptoms. A child with asthma or migraines, for example, may experience more symptoms due to anxiety. Another example is a youth with diabetes who manipulates their insulin intake with the aim of losing weight, leading to poorer treatment of the diabetes and potentially dangerous blood sugar fluctuations.

This diagnosis should only be conferred when the psychological or behavioral factors are exerting a clear and negative effect on the medical condition. Psychological problems that emerge in response to the medical condition but are not adversely impacting its course or treatment do not meet this criterion. Thus, for example, a child who is diagnosed with a serious illness and develops depression, without evidence that the depression is impacting the illness, may meet criteria for an adjustment disorder, but would not be diagnosed with psychological factors affecting other medical conditions. Likewise, when a medical condition directly causes psychological symptoms (as when a hormonal imbalance leads to a deterioration in mood), a diagnosis of mental disorder due to another medical condition may be appropriate, rather than psychological factors affecting other medical conditions.

Factitious Disorder

Factitious disorder refers to the deliberate falsification of physical or psychological symptoms, or to the deliberate induction of illness or injury. The factitious behavior must be present even in the absence of obvious external rewards that may be gained by performing it.

Factitious disorder is divided into two subtypes: factitious disorder imposed on self, in which the person falsifies their own symptoms or causes themselves illness or injury, and factitious disorder imposed on another, in which the person falsifies the symptoms of another person or deliberately causes them illness or injury (this is the syndrome formerly referred to as *Munchausen by proxy*). In both cases, the diagnosis should specify whether a single episode of factitious behavior is known or whether multiple episodes have occurred.

Falsifying symptoms could include exaggeration of actual symptoms, simulation of physical signs, and lying about the presence of symptoms. When the factitious behavior occurs in the context of an actual physical illness, it causes the patient to be perceived as more sick or impaired and has the potential to lead to unnecessary medical interventions.

For children, the most common scenario for a diagnosis of factitious disorder imposed on another is when parents or caregivers are falsifying the child's symptoms or causing them deliberate harm and seeking medical attention. In all cases, the diagnosis is conferred on the person enacting the factitious behavior, not on the child victim of the behavior. Such behavior may also be criminal on the part of the caregiver. The diagnosis, however, does not address the forensic aspect or the motivations of the perpetrator, beyond establishing that the behavior is not clearly motivated by external rewards. Thus, a parent who lies about a child's symptoms to protect themselves from legal liability (an external reward) would not meet criteria for this diagnosis unless the falsification was clearly beyond what is necessary for the legal protection. This condition is also discussed in detail in Chapter 24 on child abuse and neglect.

EPIDEMIOLOGY AND DEMOGRAPHICS

Somatic symptoms are very common in children and adolescents (Perquin et al., 2000), but the prevalence of somatic symptoms disorder is less clear. Most research focuses on the presence of particular symptoms and group of symptoms, rather than on the diagnosis, and many studies have focused on adults rather than children.

In both clinical and community samples, some somatic symptoms are reported by as many as half of all youth, and many report the presence of multiple somatic symptoms (Domenech-Llaberia et al., 2004; Saps, 2017). Indeed, the presence of one somatic symptom consistently predicts the presence of at least one, and often multiple, additional complaints (Alfven, 1993). Furthermore, the presence of somatic symptoms at one point in time predicts future somatic symptoms, which could be a recurrence of the same symptom, a different symptom, or both. Particularly common in youth are complaints of pain symptoms, including headache, stomach ache, and musculoskeletal pain, with headache being the most common of all (Perquin et al., 2000; Shanahan et al., 2015).

Headaches can be further classified into subtypes, with migraines being the most impairing. Migraines are headaches that are often felt on only one side of the head, have a pulsating quality, are aggravated by physical activity, sounds, and light, and are accompanied by nausea and vomiting, although not all these characteristics are necessarily present in each case. Headaches that lack all (or all but one) of the features of migraines are most often grouped together under the category of tension headaches.

Abdominal pain is also common in youth and is responsible for a considerable proportion of all pediatric doctor visits (Reust, 2018). Among very young children of preschool age, abdominal pain is even more commonly reported than headaches (Domenech-Llaberia et al., 2004). Likewise, gastrointestinal distress without pain, including nausea, vomiting, and problems with bowel movements, are common in children. Less common than headache and abdominal or gastrointestinal pain or distress, but still common, are chest pains and respiratory issues, other muscle pains, and fatigue (Lipsitz et al., 2004; Meyer, 2019).

Somatic symptoms are more commonly reported by females than by males, especially postpuberty (Dell & Campo, 2011), and the prevalence of somatic symptom disorder may also be higher in females. As noted, however, data on actual prevalence rates for the disorder remain scant.

Illness anxiety disorder is a new diagnosis in *DSM-5* and its prevalence is also not well established (Brakoulias, 2014; Scarella, 2019). Most patients who formerly met criteria for a diagnosis of hypochondriasis would currently be diagnosed with illness anxiety disorder under *DSM-5*, though some may be better classified as having somatic symptom disorder. Illness anxiety is likely less prevalent in young children than in adolescents, and less common in youth overall than in adults. Unlike somatic symptom disorder, rates may be similar for males and for females.

Conversion disorder is also less common in youth than in adults and prevalence rates may vary considerably across cultures (Lieb et al., 2002; Pehlivanturk & Unal, 2002). Community samples usually find low rates of conversion disorder, but among clinical samples rates can be higher (Ani et al., 2013). In particular, among pediatric neurologic patients presenting at specialty centers, nonepileptic seizures and other sensory and motor symptoms are to be found with greater frequency. These commonly resolve favorably within a few months (Pehlivanturk & Unal, 2002). In preschool age children, conversion is rare and should be diagnosed only with a high degree of caution and confidence (De Cos Milas et al., 2016).

The deception that is inherent to factitious disorder, whether of the self or of others, makes it extremely challenging to estimate the prevalence of this disorder. It has been estimated that approximately 1% of all hospitalizations in the United States involve factitious behavior, but research is very limited.

ETIOLOGY AND PATHOGENESIS

The exact pathogenesis of the physical complaints in somatic symptom disorder is by definition unknown. However, certain individual and cultural characteristics have been associated with higher risk for these disorders. Females are more likely than males to have persistent somatic complaints past young childhood (Dell & Campo, 2011; Sirri et al., 2015). The degree to which this reflects an actual difference in the rates of the somatic symptoms or a tendency for females to report their symptoms more commonly and to seek medical assistance more frequently is not well established (Perquin et al., 2000). Although some somatic symptoms, such as chronic fatigue, have historically been thought of as problems of "luxury" and believed to be more common in patients from higher socioeconomic status, empirical data do not consistently support this view. Indeed, chronic fatigue may actually be more common among children who experience deprivation than among those who do not (Crawley, 2014).

Anxiety and its disorders and depression are linked to the presence of somatic symptoms (Egger et al., 1999; Shanahan et al., 2015) (see also Chapter 12). This association holds in both directions. That is to say, children with anxiety or depression are more likely to report the presence of somatic symptoms, and the presence of such symptoms are predictive of concurrent or future anxiety and depressive disorders (Campo et al., 2004). Likewise, temperamental traits that are linked to anxiety and depression, such as behavioral inhibition, neuroticism, and harm avoidance, are also linked to the risk of somatic symptom disorders.

Exposure to adversity, negative life events, and trauma are also associated with somatic symptoms (Bonvanie et al., 2015; Lieb et al., 2002). Most children with somatic symptoms will not have a history of trauma, abuse, neglect, or maltreatment, but all of these predict somatic symptoms. Children presenting with somatic symptoms should be carefully assessed to rule out any history of such negative life events.

Family factors and genetic and nongenetic heritability can also play a role in the risk for somatic symptoms. Family styles that emphasize somatic issues and concerns may reinforce somatization in children, as can the provision of rewards or reinforcements for children's somatic complaints. For example, some children may gain parental attention through somatic symptoms or may be excused from responsibilities and functional demands that they find challenging. Some parents respond to children's physical complaints with overly protective behavior, reinforcing a child's view of somatic symptoms as "dangerous" and disproportionately important. And family therapy theorists have posited that a child's physical symptoms may serve a familial function, helping the family to avoid other issues such as marital stress (Levy et al., 2001; Wood, 2001).

Genetic heritability of somatic symptoms is poorly understood but may play a role. Temperamental traits that increase the risk of somatic symptoms are at least partially heritable. Some specific genetic variations have been linked to both somatic symptoms and traits such as neuroticism and anxiety, but considerably more research is required before the genetics of somatic symptoms become clear (Kendler et al., 1995; Levy et al., 2001).

COURSE

Somatic symptom disorders can be chronic and tend to recur after remitting (Lieb et al., 2002). Children with somatic symptoms in early childhood are at significant risk of future somatic problems later on in development, including into and throughout adulthood (Borge et al., 1994). Furthermore, somatic symptoms in childhood also predict later mental health problems such as anxiety and depression. Conversion disorder and factitious disorder are more episodic, often coming and going through multiple episodes rather than persisting more chronically like somatic symptom disorder.

Somatic symptom disorders in youth tend to be relatively stable. In one study conducted in Germany, for example (Lieb et al., 2002), youth with somatic symptom disorders were as likely as not to still have at least one somatic disorder up to 4 years later, although the specific physical complaints often changed. The somatic symptom disorders were particularly stable and chronic in females and in those with anxiety or substance use problems.

DIFFERENTIAL DIAGNOSIS AND ASSESSMENT

Assessment and diagnosis of somatic symptom disorders pose several important challenges. The lack of a clear medical explanation for the symptoms can be confusing to clinicians and providers alike. The tendency to disbelieve the "reality" of the child's symptoms can represent an empathic failure on the part of the clinician and can alienate children and parents; messages such as "it's all in their head" are likely to be perceived as disparaging or as trivializing what can be a major problem for the family; and the reliance on subjective reports by the patient makes it difficult to feel confident about the frequency and severity of the symptoms.

Parents of children with somatic symptoms may present with high levels of anxiety about the child's health and may fear that the child's symptoms are indicative of a serious underlying condition that could be missed by a clinician who does not take them seriously enough. Many parents will have had frustrating experiences with seeking medical answers to the unexplained symptoms and may approach the encounter with a high degree of skepticism and suspicion. Furthermore, the classification of somatic symptoms and related disorders as mental health problems, and referrals to mental health providers, can be interpreted as suggesting that the child is either "crazy" or lying.

In light of these challenges, assessment depends on forging a strong therapeutic alliance with the child and their caregivers. This alliance may only be achievable through an accepting and empathetic communication style. The symptoms should be treated as "real" by the clinician unless considerable evidence for fabrication exists. A child whose head or stomach hurts without a clearly identified medical cause suffers no less than a child whose symptoms are linked to a medical diagnosis and known etiology.

The assessment generally comprises a team effort, including providers from the areas of mental health and physicians with expertise in the relevant body systems. To the extent it is possible, the use of multiple informants and of objective measures can increase the accuracy of diagnosis. For example, teachers may be able to provide information on how the child functions and appears in the school setting and sports coaches can provide insight into physical functioning outside of the home. And self-report and parent report instruments can be used, including the Children's Somatization Inventory (Garber et al., 1991; Walker et al., 2009) and the Functional Disability Inventory (Walker & Greene, 1991), which query the presence, severity, and related impairment of children's somatic symptoms.

Physical examination and laboratory tests can be used to rule out potential physical illnesses and conditions that may be causing the child's somatic symptoms. But it is important to note that somatic symptoms can coexist alongside physical conditions, even when not directly caused by them. Once a diagnosis of somatic symptom disorder or illness anxiety disorder has been clearly established, further physical examinations and laboratory tests may be counterproductive, serving to reinforce the maladaptive behavioral patterns and not revealing any new medical information. Such tests should usually only be conducted when a meaningful change in symptoms or some new information arises.

When clear evidence of fabrication, simulation, or exaggeration exists, a diagnosis of factitious disorder may be appropriate. This should be considered with a high level of caution and is exceedingly rare in very young children before puberty. When diagnosing factitious disorder, the distinction from malingering should also be kept in mind. The factitious behavior in factitious disorder is not enacted in order to achieve an external reward and is more closely linked to the desire to be viewed and treated as a patient. In malingering, the fabrication of symptoms is aimed at achieving some external reward or reinforcement, whether functional, financial, or other.

▮▮ TREATMENT

Treatment of somatic symptom disorders includes both management of the actual physical complaints and therapeutic interventions aimed at the mental health aspects of the problem. For both of these, treatment can include pharmacologic and psychosocial intervention strategies. The treatment team may need to include representatives from multiple disciplines and areas of expertise, including medical, social work, psychology, psychiatry, and in some cases physiotherapy and others. Rigorous clinical trial research of somatic symptom disorders in children and adolescents is scarce however, and there is need for better empirical evidence to support the efficacy of treatments and to inform treatment guidelines.

Treatment usually includes a focus on function and rehabilitation (Campo & Fritz, 2001). In contrast to a view by which normal function can only resume or be maintained after the somatic symptoms have been accurately explained and successfully treated, the rehabilitation approach encourages maintaining function as much as possible even while symptoms persist. The view that normal function must necessarily follow successful remission of the somatic symptoms increases the risk of long-term disability and accumulating problems, as the symptoms may defy treatment for considerable time and the lack of function may even exacerbate them. As such, it is often important to reassure both child and parents that engaging in normal behavior will not increase risk and that the symptoms are not life threatening.

A child can be encouraged to view themselves as "heroic" by continuing to function normally despite significant challenges and discomfort, and this view is more likely to be acceptable to the child than one that trivializes or downplays their suffering. Emphasizing coping, rather than rest or recuperation, can help the child to mitigate the potential risks of enduring disability. And parents should be encouraged to view their child as fundamentally healthy and capable, rather than as inherently weak, vulnerable, or disabled. Excessive accommodation of the somatic symptoms by parents, for example, by excusing the child from functional expectations or encouraging unnecessary bedrest, should be explained as a risk factor (Garralda & Chalder, 2005). In particular, school attendance should be maintained whenever possible and is likely to prove a superior strategy to home schooling or frequent absences.

Psychosocial therapies that may be helpful in the treatment of somatic symptoms include cognitive-behavioral therapy (CBT) and family-based therapy. CBT can target unrealistic thoughts and beliefs and maladaptive behavioral patterns (Powers et al., 2013). The use of rewards and contingencies, managed by parents, can incentivize adaptive functioning in the child, but the use of punishments for somatic symptoms and the behaviors they elicit are discouraged. Interventions that focus on physical regulation such as biofeedback and yoga, and treatments that promote greater acceptance such as mindfulness-based therapy may also be helpful (Rutten et al., 2015) (Box 18.1).

Medications can also be one component in the treatment of somatic symptom disorder, but significantly more research with high-quality randomized controlled trials is needed. It is not uncommon for parents, and even physicians, to advocate the use of a "sham" or placebo medication for the child, in the hopes of rapidly improving their functioning. This strategy, however, may be ill advised. Introducing a placebo medication (e.g., by providing the child with

| BOX 18.1 | **Somatic Symptom Disorder—Clinical Vignette** |

Emma is a 12-year-old girl with a typical developmental history apart from suffering from repeated ear infections in toddlerhood. At age 11, Emma began to complain frequently about headaches and abdominal pains. The pains occurred most often during the morning hours, but sometimes would last the entire day. Emma's pains caused her to miss numerous school days or to arrive to school late. Emma's parents had consulted first with her pediatrician and then with a number of medical experts who conducted various tests and examinations. All the medical procedures failed to provide an explanation for Emma's pains, and her parents were told by one doctor, "it's all in her head." Emma's parents believed that Emma genuinely experienced the pains she described but were at a loss as to how to help her. Over the course of the past year, Emma became increasingly concerned that her pains were the symptoms of a serious medical condition. She feared that she had cancer or another life-threatening disease and begged her parents to take her to more and more doctors.

Ultimately, Emma received psychotherapy from a cognitive-behavioral therapist who helped her to challenge her anxious beliefs and to focus on coping with daily life rather than on the fear of illness or on the discomfort her symptoms caused. Emma told her parents that she was able to talk with her therapist because the therapist believed her "unlike some of those other doctors."

vitamins and telling them they are pain or nausea medications), apart from being deceptive and potentially harming the child's trust over time, may reinforce the child's self-image as a "sick" child and strengthening their belief that normal function can only follow successful medical intervention to reduce the physical complaints. "Real" pain medication may be useful, for example, the use of acetaminophen or ibuprofen for headaches and migraines.

The common co-occurrence of anxiety and depression alongside somatic symptoms has led to some research on the use of antidepressants, mostly in adults thus far (Kleinstauber et al., 2014). Research in children is inconclusive, but some studies of antidepressants in somatic symptom disorders have shown promise.

SUMMARY

Although the prevalence of somatic symptom disorders is not yet well established, somatic symptoms are common in youth and cause significant distress and impairment to the child and the family. Children with somatic complaints should be believed and not dismissed, even when no clear medical cause can be attributed to the symptoms.

Somatic symptom disorders can be highly chronic, persisting over long periods of time. Psychosocial problems including anxiety and mood disorders and history of adverse experiences can contribute to the risk of somatic symptom disorders.

However, there is need for considerably more research to inform both etiology and treatment. Current treatments include CBT and family therapy and can be helpful in a significant proportion of cases.

References

*Indicates Particularly Recommended

Alfven, G. (1993). The covariation of common psychosomatic symptoms among children from socio-economically differing residential areas. An epidemiological study. *Acta Paediatrica, 82*(5), 484–487. https://doi.org/10.1111/j.1651-2227.1993.tb12728.x

American Psychiatric Association. (2013). *Diagnostic and statistical manual of mental disorders* (5th ed.). American Psychiatric Publishing.

Ani, C., Reading, R., Lynn, R., Forlee, S., & Garralda, E. (2013). Incidence and 12-month outcome of non-transient childhood conversion disorder in the U.K. and Ireland. *British Journal of Psychiatry, 202,* 413–418. https://doi.org/10.1192/bjp.bp.112.116707

Bonvanie, I. J., van Gils, A., Janssens, K. A., & Rosmalen, J. G. (2015). Sexual abuse predicts functional somatic symptoms: An adolescent population study. *Child Abuse and Neglect, 46,* 1–7. https://doi.org/10.1016/j.chiabu.2015.06.001

Borge, A. I., Nordhagen, R., Moe, B., Botten, G., & Bakketeig, L. S. (1994). Prevalence and persistence of stomach ache and headache among children. Follow-up of a cohort of Norwegian children from 4 to 10 years of age. *Acta Paediatrica, 83*(4), 433–437. https://doi.org/10.1111/j.1651-2227.1994.tb18137.x

Brakoulias, V. (2014). DSM-5 bids farewell to hypochondriasis and welcomes somatic symptom disorder and illness anxiety disorder. *The Australian and New Zealand Journal of Psychiatry, 48*(7), 688. https://doi.org/10.1177/0004867414525844

Campo, J. V., Bridge, J., Ehmann, M., Altman, S., Lucas, A., Birmaher, B., Lorenzo, C. D., Iyengar, S., & Brent, D. A. (2004). Recurrent abdominal pain, anxiety, and depression in primary care. *Pediatrics, 113*(4), 817–824. https://doi.org/10.1542/peds.113.4.817

Campo, J. V., & Fritz, G. (2001). A management model for pediatric somatization. *Psychosomatics, 42*(6), 467–476. https://doi.org/10.1176/appi.psy.42.6.467 11815681

Crawley, E. (2014). The epidemiology of chronic fatigue syndrome/myalgic encephalitis in children. *Archives of Disease and Children, 99*(2), 171–174. https://doi.org/10.1136/archdischild-2012-302156

De Cos Milas, A., Moreno, M. G., Macías, V. G., Chinchurreta de Lora, N. E., Criado, N. R., & Sánchez, B. S. (2016). Conversion disorder in adolescents: A review and case report. *European Psychiatry, 33*(Suppl 1), S349–S350. https://doi.org/10.1016/j.eurpsy.2016.01.1235

Dell, M. L., & Campo, J. V. (2011). Somatoform disorders in children and adolescents. *Psychiatric Clinics of North America, 34*(3), 643–660. https://doi.org/10.1016/j.psc.2011.05.012

Domenech-Llaberia, E., Jane, C., Canals, J., Ballespi, S., Esparo, G., & Garralda, E. (2004). Parental reports of somatic symptoms in preschool children: Prevalence and associations in a Spanish sample. *Journal of American Academy of Child and Adolescent Psychiatry, 43*(5), 598–604. https://doi.org/10.1097/00004583-200405000-00013

Egger, H. L., Costello, E. J., Erkanli, A., & Angold, A. (1999). Somatic complaints and psychopathology in children and adolescents: Stomach aches, musculoskeletal pains, and headaches. *Journal of American Academy of Child and Adolescent Psychiatry, 38*(7), 852–860. https://doi.org/10.1097/00004583-199907000-00015

Garber, J., Walker, L. S., & Zeman, J. (1991). Somatization symptoms in a community sample of children and adolescents: Further validation of the Children's Somatization Inventory. *Psychological Assessment, 3*(4), 588–595. https://doi.org/10.1037/1040-3590.3.4.588

Garralda, M. E., & Chalder, T. (2005). Practitioner review: Chronic fatigue syndrome in childhood. *Journal of Child Psychology and Psychiatry, 46*(11), 1143–1151. https://doi.org/10.1111/j.1469-7610.2005.01424.x

Kendler, K. S., Walters, E. E., Truett, K. R., Heath, A. C., Neale, M. C., Martin, N. G., & Eaves, L. J. (1995). A twin-family study of self-report symptoms of panic-phobia and somatization. *Behaviour Genetics, 25*(6), 499–515. https://doi.org/10.1007/BF02327574

Kleinstauber, M., Witthoft, M., Steffanowski, A., van Marwijk, H., Hiller, W., & Lambert, M. J. (2014). Pharmacological interventions for somatoform disorders in adults. *Cochrane Database of Systematic Reviews,* (11), CD010628. https://doi.org/10.1002/14651858.CD010628.pub2

Levy, R. L., Jones, K. R., Whitehead, W. E., Feld, S. I., Talley, N. J., & Corey, L. A. (2001). Irritable bowel syndrome in twins: Heredity and social learning both contribute to etiology. *Gastroenterology, 121*(4), 799–804. https://doi.org/10.1053/gast.2001.27995

Lieb, R., Zimmermann, P., Friis, R. H., Hofler, M., Tholen, S., & Wittchen, H. U. (2002). The natural course of *DSM-IV* somatoform disorders and syndromes among adolescents and young adults: A prospective-longitudinal community study. *European Psychiatry, 17*(6), 321–331. https://doi.org/10.1016/s0924-9338(02)00686-7

Lipsitz, J. D., Masia-Warner, C., Apfel, H., Marans, Z., Hellstern, B., Forand, N., Levenbraun, Y., & Fyer, A. J. (2004). Anxiety and depressive symptoms and anxiety sensitivity in youngsters with noncardiac chest pain and benign heart murmurs. *Journal of Pediatric Psychology, 29*(8), 607–612. https://doi.org/10.1093/jpepsy/jsh062

Marwah, A., Swami, M. K., & Kumar, M. (2016). Childhood somatoform disorders and its associated stressors. *Paediatric Oncall Journal, 13,* 62–65. https://doi.org/10.7199/ped.oncall.2016.42

Meyer, R. M. L. (2019). Somatization, fatigue, and quality of life in children and adolescents with chronic pain. *Journal of Child and Family Studies, 29*(5), 1293–1300. https://doi.org/10.1007/s10826-019-01624-0

Pehlivanturk, B., & Unal, F. (2002). Conversion disorder in children and adolescents: A 4-year follow-up study. *Journal of Psychosomatic Research, 52*(4), 187–191. https://doi.org/10.1016/S0022-3999(01)00306-3

Perquin, C. W., Hazebroek-Kampschreur, A. A., Hunfeld, J. A., Bohnen, A. M., van Suijlekom-Smit, L. W., Passchier, J., & van der Wouden, J. C. (2000). Pain in children and adolescents: A common experience. *Pain, 87*(1), 51–58. https://doi.org/10.1016/S0304-3959(00)00269-4

Powers, S. W., Kashikar-Zuck, S. M., Allen, J. R., LeCates, S. L., Slater, S. K., Zafar, M., Kabbouche, M. A., O'Brien, H. L., Shenk, C. E., Rausch, J. R., & Hershey, A. D. (2013). Cognitive behavioral therapy plus amitriptyline for chronic migraine in children and adolescents: A randomized clinical trial. *JAMA, 310*(24), 2622–2630. https://doi.org/10.1001/jama.2013.282533

Reust, C. (2018). Recurrent abdominal pain in children. *American Family Physician, 97*(12), 785–793. https://www.aafp.org/afp/2018/0615/p785.html

Rutten, J. M., Korterink, J. J., Venmans, L. M., Benninga, M. A., & Tabbers, M. M. (2015). Nonpharmacologic treatment of functional abdominal pain disorders: A systematic review. *Pediatrics, 135*(3), 522–535. https://doi.org/10.1542/peds.2014-2123

Saps, M. (2017). A nationwide study on the prevalence of functional gastrointestinal disorders in school-children. *Boletin Medico del Hospital Infantil de Mexico, 74*(6), 407–412. https://doi.org/10.1016/j.bmhimx.2017.05.005

Scarella, T. M. (2019). Illness anxiety disorder: Psychopathology, epidemiology, clinical characteristics, and treatment. *Psychosomatic Medicine, 81*(5), 398–407. https://doi.org/10.1097/PSY.0000000000000691

Shanahan, L., Zucker, N., Copeland, W. E., Bondy, C. L., Egger, H. L., & Costello, E. J. (2015). Childhood somatic complaints predict generalized anxiety and depressive disorders during young adulthood in a community sample. *Psychological Medicine, 45*(8), 1721–1730. https://doi.org/10.1017/S0033291714002840

Sirri, L., Ricci Garotti, M. G., Grandi, S., & Tossani, E. (2015). Adolescents' hypochondriacal fears and beliefs: Relationship with demographic features, psychological distress, well-being and health-related behaviors. *Journal of Psychosomatic Research, 79*(4), 259–264. https://doi.org/10.1016/j.jpsychores.2015.07.002

Walker, L. S., Beck, J. E., Garber, J., & Lambert, W. (2009). Children's somatization inventory: Psychometric properties of the revised form (CSI-24). *Journal of Pediatric Psychology, 34*(4), 430–440. https://doi.org/10.1093/jpepsy/jsn093

Walker, L. S., & Greene, J. W. (1991). The functional disability inventory: Measuring a neglected dimension of child health status. *Journal of Pediatric Psychology, 16*(1), 39–58. https://doi.org/10.1093/jpepsy/16.1.39

Wood, B. L. (2001). Physically manifested illness in children and adolescents. A biobehavioral family approach. *Child and Adolescent Psychiatric Clinics of North America, 10*(3), 543–562. https://doi.org/10.1016/S1056-4993(18)30045-2

Suggested Readings

Breuer, J., & Freud, S. (1966). *Freud & Breuer: Studies in hysteria*. Avon Books.

*Campo, J. V., Dell, M. L., & Fritz, G. K. (2018). Functional somatic symptoms and disorders. In A. Martin, M. H. Bloch, & F. R. Volkmar (Eds.), *Lewis's child and adolescent psychiatry: A comprehensive textbook* (5th ed., pp. 591–603). Wolters Kluwer.

Scamvougeras, A., & Howard, A. (2018). *Understanding and managing somatoform disorders—A guide for clinicians*. AJKS Publishing.

Shapiro, E. G. (1998). *The somatizing child: Diagnosis and treatment of conversion and somatization disorders*. Springer.

Vesterling, C., & Koglin, U. (2020). The relationship between attachment and somatoform symptoms in children and adolescents: A systematic review and meta-analysis. *Journal of Psychosomatic Research, 130*, 109932. https://doi.org/10.1016/j.jpsychores.2020.109932

*Williams, S. E., & Zahka, N. E. (2017). *Treating somatic symptoms in children and adolescents*. Guilford Press.

Woolfolk, R. L., & Allen, L. A. (2006). *Treating somatization: A cognitive-behavioral approach*. Guilford Press.

CHAPTER 19 ■ DISORDERS OF ELIMINATION: ENURESIS AND ENCOPRESIS

BACKGROUND

Helping children acquire bowel and bladder control is, of course, a long-standing problem to parents throughout history (Glicklich, 1951). Typically, this is accomplished by around 3 years of age. The process often begins around 18 months of age and boys are usually slightly later than girls in acquiring good toileting skills. There are some cultural differences in practice and age at which independent toileting is expected (Mikkelsen, 2018).

This entire process goes best for all concerned if parents are supportive and consistent. From the point of view of the child, it is helpful if (1) the child understands what is wanted; (2) has the motor ability to participate; (3) and has the motivation to comply and please caregivers. If any of these factors are not present, toilet training goes much less smoothly (although it can still be accomplished). Piaget (1954) noted that the child may not understand the meaning of toileting, for example, might see the elimination product as alive in some way/sense and hence be anxious when it is flushed away! Inconsistency from the parents and/or a harsh approach can lead to difficulties quickly. These issues have, of course, been of great concern to parents for millennia.

ENURESIS

Diagnosis, Definition, and Clinical Features

The word *enuresis* itself comes from the Greek word for voiding and interest in the condition can be traced to ancient times. Usually, a distinction is made between primary enuresis (the child has never been dry) versus secondary enuresis (the child had the skill but lost it). Nighttime enuresis is most common whereas daytime enuresis less so (once the ability to void properly is acquired) (Shaffer et al., 1984). In *DSM-5* (APA, 2013), the condition is defined based on involuntary voiding (in bed or clothes) that happens twice weekly for a period of several months after age 5 (or equivalent developmental level). The problem must not be due to a medical problem or drug and must be a source of distress or impairment. This approach is largely consistent with earlier definition. Distinctions can be made between primary or secondary enuresis (or both). For secondary enuresis, the child is usually only said to have the condition after at least one year of being dry (Mikkelsen, 2018). The child must be at least 5 years of age or at that developmental level (a potential problem for more cognitively impaired individuals who can, and should, be toilet trained). By definition, wetting due to use of a drug or substance or medical condition is excluded. The usual distinction between primary and secondary is made.

Epidemiology and Demographics

Longitudinal studies provide rather similar rates of the condition, and it varies dramatically with age (Feehan et al., 1990). Occasional bed-wetting is fairly common and decreases as children become older. Boys are at increased risk. There may be a positive family history (in fathers). Children with developmental delays may achieve continence later than other children (Mikkelsen, 2018). By age 6, about 90% of children are dry at night. Over time, this number continues to decrease so that by age 14 about 1% of boys and 0.5% of girls are having enuretic episodes at least once a week. Risk is increased in the context of ongoing mental health problems; stress and socioeconomic disadvantage also contribute to increased risk (Rutter et al., 1973, Rutter, 1989).

Etiology and Pathogenesis

Numerous theoretical models have been developed and range from the anatomic and neurologic to neuropsychological and psychodynamic (Mikkelsen, 2018). Overall developmental delay is associated with later toilet training (Matson & LoVullo, 2009). There has been some suggestion of association with specific sleep phases, but this is unclear (Neveus et al., 1999) (Box 19.1).

BOX 19.1 Enuresis: Case Report

Tyler, a 7-½-year-old boy, had never been fully toilet trained at night. He sometimes wet the bed once a week, but more typically 2 or 3 nights a week. His parents had expressed concern to the pediatrician when he was 5 but a medical evaluation had failed to show any medical condition that might account for the problem. His pediatrician had discussed both the bell and pad and medication, but the parents had decided to forgo treatment in hopes that the problem would correct itself over time. Tyler now is frustrated by the problem—he is invited to sleepovers but almost never goes because of his worry about wetting. His mother reports that his self-image has begun to suffer. Tyler is doing well in school, is popular, and otherwise seems to be developing well.

After some discussion, the parents and Tyler elected a trial of DDAVP. They chose this over the bell and pad method because of a new baby in the home and the general feeling of all concerned that they did not want an alarm going off at night. Tyler responded to a relatively small dose and had only the occasional accident. He and his family also restricted his fluid intake before bedtime. After 9 months of treatment, the family and Tyler agreed to taper his medication. At that point, he remained dry and has subsequently.

Comment: This case illustrates the fact that enuresis often will resolve over time but either drug treatment or behavioral intervention may be needed, particularly if the child's self-esteem begins to suffer. In this case, the family elected a pharmacologic treatment although, in general, the bell and pad method is more likely to have last benefit and, often, the symptom returns once DDAVP is discontinued.

Reprinted with permission from Volkmar, F. R., & Martin, A. (2011). *Essentials of Lewis's child and adolescent psychiatry* (1st ed., p. 234). Lippincott Williams & Wilkins/Wolters Kluwer.

There are associations with psychosocial stress, and clearly, psychosocial factors can contribute to delayed toilet training or loss of skills (Joinson et al., 2007). The interrelationships of behavioral and developmental difficulties with enuresis are difficult to disentangle, although it does appear that, at least in some cases, a strong genetic component is present (von Gontard et al., 2001, 2006). In one study, positive family history was related to better outcome.

Course

Spontaneous remission of bed-wetting is common, particularly between the ages of 5 and 7 and again in adolescence. In a given year, about 15% of children experience a spontaneous remission of the condition. As noted in the ensuing section, both psychological and pharmacologic treatments are available. As the condition is resolved, self-concept may improve (Moffatt et al., 1987).

Differential Diagnosis and Assessment

Urinalysis is an obvious first step in evaluation of enuresis, for example, to rule out urinary tract infection as a cause. In general, invasive studies do not have a particularly high yield and are not needed unless other indications are present. Children who have problems during both night AND daytime may be more likely to exhibit structural or other problems of the urinary tract. Ultrasound evaluation is less invasive than past procedures. At times, enuresis may be seen in association with other medical conditions and physical examination should look for potentially treatable underlying conditions. Associations with other factors, for example, nocturnal enuresis that follows administration of a new medication, should be explored as relevant.

Treatment

Historically, two rather different approaches have been used with success in treatment of enuresis: behavioral and pharmacologic approaches (Mikkelsen, 2018; Reiner, 2008; Robson, 2008). Behavioral treatments have a long history and have the important advantage of avoiding potential side effects of pharmacologic ones. It is important to note that there is some potential for parents or the child to view use of behavioral techniques as somehow suggesting that the condition is, at least in part, volitional. The bell and pad method has a long history of use, and essentially combines principles of both classical and operant conditions in helping the child to learn to avoid nighttime awakening and thus stay dry. In this approach, the child sleeps on a pad that, when wet, rings a bell arousing the child from sleep. This method has a reasonably high success rate (as many as two-thirds of children will respond) and response is maintained in many (50% of cases) after the treatment is discontinued. Lower levels of family stress and an absence of other psychiatric problems in the child are associated with higher success rates. Some studies have investigated the impact of bladder capacity and response to this treatment. New behavioral approaches continue to be developed and behavioral approaches can be combined with pharmacologic ones.

Drug treatments include the use of imipramine, and, more recently, DDAVP. The tricyclic antidepressant imipramine has been used for treatment of nighttime bed-wetting for many decades and a series of double-blind studies have confirmed its usefulness. ECG should be obtained at baseline. Given the high rate of remission, regular attempts should be made to evaluate the continued need for medication, for example, a slow taper every 3–4 months allows the medication to be increased if wetting returns. Some children have a transient response and for these individuals, the periodic use of the agent, for example, at summer camp, may be an option. Given the potential for side effects, careful education of child and parents is needed,

TABLE 19.1

Factors to Consider When Constructing a Treatment Algorithm for Primary Nocturnal Enuresis

- Age of child
- Medical cause has been ruled out
- Rate of spontaneous remission (approximately 14%–16% per year)
- Behavioral conditioning with bell and pad or similar methodology
  - Equally effective as pharmacologic treatment
  - Lower rate of relapse than with pharmacologic treatment
  - Safer than pharmacologic treatment
- Most commonly used pharmacologic intervention is desmopressin acetate (DDAVP).
- Imipramine is no longer a first-line choice for pharmacologic treatment, but can be used for refractory individuals.
- Combination of behavioral and pharmacologic treatment can be considered for refractory enuresis.

Adapted and reprinted with permission from Mikkelson, E. (2018). Elimination disorders: Enuresis and encopresis. In A. Martin, M. H. Bloch, & F. R. Volkmar (Eds.), *Lewis's child and adolescent psychiatry: A comprehensive textbook* (5th ed., p. 659). Wolters Kluwer.

for example, to avoid a child taking "extra" medication. There appears to be some correlation between blood level and therapeutic effect, although as a practical matter side effects like dry mouth may be a simpler way to be sure that an adequate level has been obtained. The mechanism of action of this agent remains unclear, but it does not simply appear to relate to its antidepressant properties. It is now less commonly used.

Desmopressin acetate (DDAVP) is a synthetic analogue of the pituitary hormone 8-arginine vasopressin (ADH), which affects renal water conservation. It now has a substantial evidence base and many children who do not respond to other approaches may respond to it (Vande Walle et al., 2007). The most frequent side effects include headache, flushing, and abdominal pain. The medication should not be used to treat enuresis resulting from a specific medical condition causing increased urination.

One major follow-up study compared imipramine, DDAVP, and the bell and pad method along with an observation-only group. Treatment was discontinued after 6 months and patients then followed. Six months later, 16% of the observation-only cases were continent compared to 16% of the imipramine-treated group, 10% of the DDAVP group, and 56% of the behavioral treatment group. Accordingly, behavioral treatments should be regarded as the first line of intervention, with DDAVP and then imipramine available for children who do not respond to the behavioral intervention.

In the distant past, psychotherapy was a mainstay of treatment but now is viewed as being indicated for any associated behavioral or mental health problem rather than having a primary impact on enuresis itself. Given the high rates of spontaneous remission (as much as 20% of cases), it is hard to evaluate the impact of longer term psychosocial interventions. However, if stressful events, negative self-image, or other comorbid problems are present, psychotherapy may be indicated. Practice guidelines for treatment are available (Fritz et al. 2004) (See Table 19.1).

ENCOPRESIS

Diagnosis, Definition, and Clinical Features

The definition of encopresis in *DSM-5* is largely consistent with the *DSM-IV* definition of the condition. It includes "repeated passage" of feces in inappropriate places. This can be voluntary or involuntary but must happen at least once a month for 3 months. The definition requires mental and chronologic age of at least 4 years. The distinction between primary (never

---

BOX 19.2 | **Encopresis: Case Report**

Shirley is an 8-year-old girl whose parents were going through a bitter divorce and later separated. The parents had been fighting for much of the previous year. During this time, Shirley was noted to become more anxious and have trouble sleeping. Although previously toilet trained, she had particular trouble in using the bathroom in her father's new home, and eventually began to have difficulties at her mother's home as well. She had become quite constipated and was regularly having overflow incontinence. This was a source of embarrassment to her and a further source of tension with the parents. A medical evaluation had revealed significant constipation but some simple medical interventions and a behavioral reward system instituted by the pediatrician were not successful—in part because the parents fought over this as well. Shirley started to refuse to go to school because of her concern about soiling. A referral was made to a child psychiatrist.

Interviews with the parents focused on their troubled relationship as it related to their inability to parent adequately. Individual sessions with Shirley focused on her anxiety as well as her frustration at her own lack of control of the situation with her parents. In addition to various medical steps taken to reduce constipation, a behavioral program was put in place with both parents agreeing to support it. Although their marriage was ending, they were able to agree to focus on Shirley and her needs and be supportive of each other as parents. Over the course of 3 months of work, tension between the parents significantly decreased and Shirley was able to re-establish regular bowel control and her anxiety symptoms lessened.

Comment: Often, simple medical procedures and a behavioral intervention program are sufficient to help children return to being fully continent. However, as in this case, the presence of major psychological problems in the child or family can make this effort more complicated. In this instance, encopresis was one part of a broader array of difficulties. Lessened tension between the parents enabled them to function more effectively and helped Shirley return to continence.

Reprinted with permission from Volkmar, F. R., & Martin, A. (2011). *Essentials of Lewis's child and adolescent psychiatry* (1st ed., p. 236). Lippincott Williams & Wilkins/Wolters Kluwer.

---

fully trained) and secondary (once trained but then lost the ability) is made. Physical problems accounting for the condition should be ruled out. It provides for differentiation of encopresis based on whether there is constipation and overflow incontinence or not (Box 19.2).

This definition may present some challenges for severely cognitively impaired children, many of whom can in fact be helped to be continent. For the child with the capacity for bowel control, the encopresis may have important psychological meaning.

Epidemiology and Demographics

In the Isle of Wight study, Rutter and colleagues (1973), Rutter (1989) reported that 1.3% of boys and 0.3% of girls between the ages of 10 and 12 experienced soiling at least once a month. In younger children, the rate is higher; for example, in one large study in the Netherlands, the prevalence was 4.1% in the 5–6 year age range (van der Wal et al., 2005). Encopresis is sometimes observed with daytime enuresis as well as with attention deficit/hyperactivity disorder and anxiety disorders. Most studies continue to report that boys are more frequently affected than girls.

Etiology and Pathogenesis

Many factors can lead to encopresis. Chronic constipation is frequent and can itself arise for psychological and/or physiologic reasons. Chronic constipation can contribute to fecal impaction and diminished sensation and awareness. Stress and trauma can also be associated with encopresis and various psychodynamic explanations have been formulated.

Primary encopresis is more frequently associated with developmental delays and other forms of psychopathology. In this group, associated enuresis is frequent. Children with secondary encopresis are more likely to have experienced stress and conduct problems.

Course

About 75% of children respond well to a supportive approach with attention to educational, behavioral, and physiologic aspects. As with enuresis, there is a steady decrease in rates of the condition as children grow older. It is very unusual for the condition to persist after age 16.

Differential Diagnosis and Assessment

Probably only the most severe cases are seen for psychiatric assessment, that is, primary care providers likely deal with many cases. Careful review of systems and physical examination are indicated. A plain abdominal x-ray may be useful in showing fecal retention.

The history should include a developmental history and review of the nature of the difficulties with parents and child, for example, frequency, context of the soiling, and so forth. Children with significant developmental delay (intellectual disability) may present special challenges for toilet training, but various resources including consultation with a behavior specialist may be helpful. Associations with other psychiatric problems, for example, enuresis, should be noted as should associations of the problem with acute or chronic stress.

Treatment

Typically, treatment will include multiple modalities including education of the child and parent as well as behavioral and psychological approaches (Borowitz et al., 2002). In the situation of chronic constipation, often an initial bowel clean out is undertaken with subsequent interventions designed to assist the child gain greater control. This can include modification of diet (with additional fiber), increased exercise and water, and so forth. Behavioral approaches will vary depending on the context but might including frequent trips to the bathroom, particularly after meals, use of positive reinforcements for success, etc.

The presence of comorbid conditions and psychopathology or stress may require specific psychotherapeutic treatment. For some children, low self-esteem is an important target for treatment. Parent/family engagement can be particularly helpful. Table 19.2 summarizes approaches to treatment.

■ SUMMARY

Enuresis has been much more extensively studied than encopresis in part because of the advent of drug treatments. There has long been awareness of a potential role of genetics, and advances in this area may lead to a better understanding of potential subgroups and, hopefully, new treatments. Both enuresis and encopresis provide an opportunity to understand the complex interaction of biologic, psychological, and social factors in developmental psychopathology.

TABLE 19.2

Factors to Consider When Constructing a Treatment Algorithm for Encopresis

- Subtypes of encopresis
  - Retentive (most common)
  - Nonretentive
  - Volitional (least frequent)
- A thorough history that documents frequency, nature, and circumstances of event is essential.
- First line of treatment for retentive subtype usually includes the following:
  - Education about bowel functioning with both parents and child;
  - Physiologic treatment with laxatives or mineral oil;
  - Behavioral component with time intervals on toilet and positive reinforcement.
- Extensive research into biofeedback:
  - Not proven to be more effective than traditional interventions;
  - May be a consideration in refractory cases.
- Psychodynamic assessment for those with volitional encopresis

Adapted and reprinted with permission from Mikkelson, E. (2018). Elimination disorders: Enuresis and encopresis. In A. Martin, M. H. Bloch, & F. R. Volkmar (Eds.), *Lewis's child and adolescent psychiatry: A comprehensive textbook* (5th ed., p. 664). Wolters Kluwer.

References

*Indicates Particularly Recommended

American Psychiatric Association. (2013). *Diagnostic and statistical manual of mental disorders* (5th ed.). APA Press.

*Borowitz, S. M., Cox, D. J., Sutphen, J. L., & Kovatchev, B. (2002). Treatment of childhood encopresis: A randomized trial comparing three treatment protocols. *Journal of Pediatric Gastroenterology and Nutrition, 34,* 378–384. https://doi.org/10.1097/00005176-200204000-00012

Feehan, M., McGee, R., Stanton, W., & Silva, P. A. (1990). A six-year follow-up of childhood enuresis: Prevalence in adolescence and consequences for mental health. *Journal of Pediatric Child Health, 26*(2), 75–79. https://doi.org/10.1111/j.1440-1754.1990.tb02390.x

Fritz, G., Rockney, R., & The Work Group on Quality Issues. (2004). Practice parameter for the assessment and treatment of children and adolescents with enuresis. *Journal of American Academy of Child and Adolescent Psychiatry, 43*(12), 1540–1550. https://doi.org/10.1097/01.chi.0000142196.41215.cc

Glicklich, L. B. (1951). A historical account of enuresis. *Pediatrics, 8,* 859–876.

Joinson, C., Heron, J., Emond, A., & Butler, R. (2007). Psychological problems in children with bedwetting and combined (day and night) wetting: A UK population-based study. *Journal of Pediatric Psychology, 32*(5), 605–616. https://doi.org/10.1093/jpepsy/jsl039

Matson, J. L., & LoVullo, S. V. (2009). Encopresis, soiling and constipation in children and adults with developmental disability. *Research in Developmental Disabilities, 30*(4), 799–807. https://doi.org/10.1016/j.ridd.2008.12.001

Mikkelsen, E. (2018). Elimination disorders: Encopresis and enuresis. In A. Martin, M. Bloch, & F. R. Volkmar (Eds.), *Lewis's child and adolescent psychiatry: A comprehensive textbook* (5th ed. pp. 655–669). Wolters Kluwer Health/Lippincott Williams & Wilkins.

Moffatt, M. E., Kato, C., & Pless, I. B. (1987). Improvements in self-concept after treatment of nocturnal enuresis: Randomized controlled trial. *Journal of Pediatrics, 110,* 647–652. https://doi.org/10.1016/S0022-3476(87)80572-3

Neveus, T., Hetta, J., Cnattingius, S., Tovemo, T., Läckgren, G., Olsson, U., & Stenberg, A. (1999). Depth of sleep and sleep habits among enuretic and incontinent children and incontinent children. *Acta Paediatrica, 88*(7), 748–752. https://doi.org/10.1111/j.1651-2227.1999.tb00036.x

Piaget, J. (1954). *The construction of reality in the child.* Basic Books.

Reiner, W. G. (2008). Pharmacotherapy in the management of voiding and storage disorders, including enuresis and encopresis. *Journal of American Academy of Child Adolescent Psychiatry, 47*(5), 491–498. https://doi.org/10.1097/CHI.0b013e31816774c5

Robson, W. L. M. (2008). Current management of nocturnal enuresis. *Current Opinion in Urology, 18*(4), 425–430. https://doi.org/10.1097/MOU.0b013e3282fcea9c

Rutter, M. (1989). Isle of Wight revisited: Twenty-five years of child psychiatric epidemiology. *Journal of American Academy of Child Adolescent Psychiatry, 28,* 633–653. https://doi .org/10.1097/00004583-198909000-00001

Rutter, M. L., Yule, W., & Graham, P. J. (1973). Enuresis and behavioral deviance: Some epidemiological considerations. *Development of Clinical Medicine, 48*(49), 137–147.

Shaffer, D., Gardner, A., & Hedge, B. (1984). Behavior and bladder disturbance of enuretic children: A rational classification of a common disorder. *Developmental Medicine & Child Neurology, 26,* 781–792. https://doi.org/10.1111/j.1469-8749.1984.tb08172.x

Van der Wal, M. F., Benninga, M. A., & Hirasing, P. A. (2005). The prevalence of encopresis in a multicultural population. *Journal of Pediatric Gastroenterology and Nutrition, 40*(Suppl 3), 345–348. https://doi.org/10.1097/01.MPG.0000149964.77418.27

Vande Walle, J., Stockner, M., Raes, A., & Nørgaard, J. P. (2007). Desmopressin 30 years in clinical use: A safety review. *Current Drug Safety, 2*(3), 232–238. https://doi.org/10.2174/157488607781668891

Von Gontard, A., Freitag, C. M., Seifen, S., Pukrop, R., & Rühling, D. (2006). Neuromotor development in nocturnal enuresis. *Developmental Medicine & Child Neurology, 48*(9), 744–750. https://doi .org/10.1017/S0012162206001599

Von Gontard, A., Schaumburg, H., Hollmann, E., Eiberg, H., & Rittig, S. (2001). The genetics of enuresis: a review. *Journal of Urology, 166,* 2438–2443. https://doi.org/10.1016/S0022-5347(05)65611-X

Suggested Readings

Akdemir, D., Cengel Kultur, S. E., Saltik Temizel, I. N., Zeki, A., & Senses Dinc, G. (2015). Familial psychological factors are associated with encopresis. *Pediatrics International, 57*(1), 143–148. https:// doi.org/10.1111/ped.12427

Call, N. A., Mevers, J. L., McElhanon, B. O., & Scheithauer, M. C. (2017). A multidisciplinary treatment for encopresis in children with developmental disabilities. *Journal of Applied Behavior Analysis, 50*(2), 332–344. https://doi.org/10.1002/jaba.379

Kuwertz-Broking, E., & von Gontard, A. (2018). Clinical management of nocturnal enuresis. *Pediatric Nephrology, 33*(7), 1145–1154. https://doi.org/10.1007/s00467-017-3778-1

Nield, L. S., Nease, E. K., & Grossman, O. K. (2018). Enuresis management in the primary care pediatrics clinic. *Pediatric Annals, 47*(10), e390–e395. https://doi.org/10.3928/19382359-20180920-01

Perrin, N., Sayer, L., & While, A. (2015). The efficacy of alarm therapy versus desmopressin therapy in the treatment of primary mono-symptomatic nocturnal enuresis: A systematic review. *Primary Health Care Research & Development, 16*(1), 21–31. https://doi.org/10.1017/S146342361300042X

Shepard, J. A., Poler, J. E., Jr., & Grabman, J. H. (2017). Evidence-based psychosocial treatments for pediatric elimination disorders. *Journal of Clinical Child & Adolescent Psychology, 46*(6), 767–797. https://doi.org/10.1080/15374416.2016.1247356

von Gontard, A., & Equit, M. (2015). Comorbidity of ADHD and incontinence in children. *European Child & Adolescent Psychiatry, 24*(2), 127–140. https://doi.org/10.1007/s00787-014-0577-0

Walker, R. A. (2019). Nocturnal enuresis. *Primary Care; Clinics in Office Practice, 46*(2), 243–248. https:// doi.org/10.1016/j.pop.2019.02.005

CHAPTER 20 ■ GENDER DISORDERS AND GENDER DYSPHORIA

BACKGROUND

Gender identity refers to a person's fundamental sense of their own gender. For most children, an awareness of core gender identity (one's sense of inner sexual identity) begins to develop early in life and is usually firmly in place by 3 years of age. For other children, this sense may not develop in the same way or may become clear only with age. Gender identity is distinct from sexual orientation, gender expression, and gender role. Genetic sex is determined at the moment of conception, although, as noted in the following section, even this can be complex. Once they are born, babies start to tell men and women apart from early in life. The term *gender identity* is used for the child's personal sense of their own gender, although gender expression does not always mirror this sense. Even when gender expression differs from gender identity, this may not reflect the core gender sense or their gender role. Some of the terms used with reference to gender identity and gender roles are defined in Table 20.1.

Historically, interest in sexual development and its patterns of growth had a major impetus from the work of Freud and his theories of sexuality (1905/1962), particularly when it was repressed and resulting in the pathogenesis of mental illness. Although variations of sexual attraction were widely recognized and accepted in ancient times, more recent Western views, until recently, regarded nontraditional patterns of sexual attraction as a mental disorder and/or as a criminal act. Indeed, until 1973, when it was removed from the *DSM*, the American Psychiatric Association regarded homosexuality as a disorder (Drescher, 2015). This removal followed the pioneering work of Kinsey and colleagues (2003/1948, 1953) showing more flexibility in sexual roles than previously had been appreciated. Increased activism on the part of the LGBTQ community followed the Stonewall riots (Duberman, 1993) and began the movement toward increased acceptance for a range of sexual expression. Greater acceptance also began to reflect important contributions of scholarship on cultural, sociological, and psychological aspects of sexuality (Foucault, 1979/1976), the growing work on women's studies (Friedan, 1963), as well as an interesting body of work on patterns of gender identity and role development that are discussed subsequently.

In the late 1940s and early 1950s, the work of Kinsey on the sexual development of males and females began to question the simplistic dichotomy views of sexual orientation. John Money (1988) was a pioneer in the field of gender studies. Money introduced concepts like gender roles, sexual orientation, and gender identity. He studied the development of

TABLE 20.1

Terminology

Term	Definition
Gender assigned at birth/natal sex/birth sex	Gender assigned to an infant at birth, generally based on physical characteristics (genitalia, etc.)
Experienced gender/gender identity	An individual's psychological understanding of one's own gender
Affirmed gender	An individual's psychological understanding of one's own gender, typically referring to one who lives socially as that understood gender
Sexuality/sexual orientation	Refers to the types of individuals toward whom one is romantically and/or sexually attracted
Transgender	Refers to an individual whose gender identity is incongruent with that of one's gender assigned at birth. Sometimes also used as a term for an individual whose gender identity is binary opposite one's gender assigned at birth.
Gender dysphoria	Refers to psychological distress in relationship to one's experienced gender; is also the classification used in the *DSM-5* (requiring fulfillment of certain clinical criteria)
Cisgender	Refers to an individual whose experienced gender matches that of one's gender assigned at birth
Gender nonconforming/gender variant	Refers to variation from developmental norms in gender role behavior that may be considered as nongender stereotypical. This may include identifying as both genders or identifying with neither gender, among others.
Transsexual	Typically used to refer to individuals who desire medical interventions to align their physiologies with the gender identities. This term is used synonymously with transgender by some and has largely fallen out of favor (though it was used commonly in the past).
Nonbinary	Gender identification in which the individual may identify with more than one gender, no gender, other gendered, or fluid in their gender identity.
Genderqueer	Gender identification as both male and female or somewhat in between

Adapted and reprinted with permission from de Vries, T. Z. (2018). Gender dysphoria and gender incongruence. In A. Martin, M. H. Bloch, & F. R. Volkmar (Eds.), *Lewis's child and adolescent psychiatry: A comprehensive textbook* (5th ed., p. 633). Wolters Kluwer.

children born with ambiguous genitalia because of medical or biological factors and the impact of rearing as a male or female in contravention to biological gender. He also was an early investigator of the impact of gender change through surgery. There became a broader awareness of psychological, sociological, and cultural factors in sexual roles and identity; greater acceptance of the range of sexual orientations and identifications began to develop. By the end of 1990s, there was growing interest in the issue of supporting treatments (including hormonal treatments and surgical approaches) for individuals desiring to change their gender identity through medical means. It is important to note that sexual identity and gender identity are distinct concepts. *Gender identity* refers to the person's sense of self as female,

male, neither, or both whereas *sexual identity* refers to whom one is sexually attracted, that is, sexual orientation identity.

DIAGNOSIS, DEFINITION, AND CLINICAL FEATURES

The conceptualization and classification of gender-related issues have significantly evolved in the various editions of *DSM*. By the time of the *DSM-IV-TR* (APA, 2000), the concept of gender dysphoria was explicitly recognized as a disorder; this recognition was, in part, used to justify insurance coverage of medical/surgical treatments for individuals who desired gender change. Criteria for the condition as a disorder (*gender identity disorder*) in *DSM-IV-TR* included cross-gender identification that was "strong and persistent" and not simply a result of some presumed advantage to being the other sex. This identification was also associated with continued discomfort about the person's assigned gender/gender role as well as impairment/distress. The condition was not diagnosed if a physical intersex condition was present. For children with this diagnosis, multiple features of gender identity had to be present (cross-dressing, a stated desire, participation in stereotyped activities of other sex, persistent choice of other sex role in play, etc.).

In contrast to the *DSM-IV-TR*, in *DSM-5* (APA, 2013) the condition was renamed *gender dysphoria* (rather than disorder) and moved to its own category (i.e., out of the sex disorders group). The new name was meant to destigmatize the condition. A separate category for children was included and meant to reflect the presumption of a lesser degree of certainty in developing children about their gender identification. Again, intersex individuals were excluded from this diagnosis, although many would actually receive a diagnosis of unspecified gender dyphoria. Criteria for the category of gender dysphoria in adolescents and adults require at least two of a series of five features, all of which have to do with incongruence between the person's experience and their sexual characteristics, desire for the sexual characteristics of the other gender, and strong feelings that one's reactions are more consistent with those of the other gender. It is common for individuals with gender dysphoria to identify as transgender. Some individuals object to this feeling because it tends to be an overly simplistic approach to gender classification. Some groups have suggested the use of terms like *gender diversity, nonbinary,* or *genderqueer* to convey the complexity of classification of gender.

EPIDEMIOLOGY AND DEMOGRAPHICS

Given the various changes in diagnosis and classification, epidemiologic data are rather limited. Often data are derived from work with adults seeking medical treatment. One meta-analysis of this group found rates of 6.8 for transwomen per 100,000 and 2.0 per 100,000 for transmen (Arcelus et al., 2015). One study reported overall rates of about 0.6% of adults who identify as transgender (Turban et al., 2018). In studies of children, this number is larger: between 1% and 2% typically identify as either transgender or unsure (Clark et al., 2014; Shields et al., 2013).

ETIOLOGY AND PATHOGENESIS

The early focus on psychological and sociocultural factors has shifted over time to a broader focus including neurobiology and other factors. A strong heritability component has been suggested by studies comparing fraternal and identical twins. These suggested a very strong genetic component—usually on the order of 60% to 70% of variance accounted for (Coolidge et al., 2002) and some environmental contribution as well. Differences in brain structure and function relative to behavior have also been shown in animals, and in humans in cisgender males and females (Hines, 2020). Differences are observed in overall brain volumes with males having greater volume and females having more gray matter when this volume difference is taken into context (Giedd et al., 2012; Guillamon et al., 2016; Ruigrok et al., 2014). The sexual differentiation hypothesis has posited a difference in transgender individuals suggesting that their brain structures and function may be more like that of the gender they experience (Swaab & Garcia-Falgueras, 2009). Results of neuroimaging studies have been mixed, although functional neuroimaging has suggested similarities to experienced gender (Turban et al., 2018). Sex hormones have an important role both prenatally and during puberty on development of the physical body as well as of brain structures. In animals, there are very clear effects of prenatal testosterone on behavior (Hines, 2011). In humans, there is some suggestion of higher levels of gender dysphoria and cross-gender identification in relation to specific medical problems (Jürgensen et al., 2013).

Genetic females with congenital adrenal hyperplasia have higher rates of gender dysphoria and cross-gender identification (Pasterski et al., 2015), although most of those reared as females develop a female gender identity (Dessens et al., 2005). Individuals who are XY but have complete androgen insensitivity develop a female gender identity in most cases underscoring the role of testosterone in male gender identity (Mazur, 2005).

Although there is clearly some role for environmental (social and psychological) factors, the literature on this topic has provided mixed and somewhat conflicting results (Zucker & Bradley, 1995), and in any case the topic remains controversial.

COURSE

Understanding the clinical course of children who are transgender or gender nonconforming is an area of very active research (Olson, 2016). Much of the follow-up data available are based on earlier concepts of gender issues (particularly binary gender identification with almost no research on nonbinary identification) that were used prior to the *DSM-5* view, thus complicating the interpretation of available data in light of current diagnostic models. Important questions remain to be answered; for example, data on whether or not those who are gender nonconforming as children persist with this identification are somewhat contradictory with some showing differences between males and females whereas others do not (Turban et al., 2018). Several factors have been related to persistent gender nonconformity (Green, 1987; Steensma et al., 2013; Zucker et al., 2012). These complexities make it tremendously difficult to provide simple generalization for the individual as to whether or not cross-gender identification will persist from childhood into adolescence and beyond (Steensma et al., 2013). The data are reasonably clear that persistence of transgender identification from adolescence into adulthood is usual (Cohen-Kettenis & Pfäfflin, 2003). Many children go on to identify as cisgender and gay, although again it is important to emphasize that gender identification is not the same as sexual orientation. Most of these children will grow up to become adults who have an identity as cisgender persons and will have a same-sex or bisexual orientation (Green, 1987; Wallen & Cohen-Kettenis, 2008). Children growing up with gender incongruence exhibit higher rates of both internalizing and externalizing problems. It is important to note the relevance of the gender minority stress model that underscores the experiences of stressful experiences in the lives of children, youth, and adults who are trans and gender diverse people (Tan et al., 2020). For example, rates of bullying are high and peer problems predict associated behavioral and mental health difficulties (McGuire et al., 2010; Steensma et al., 2014). Anxiety problems appear to be particularly common followed by mood and disruptive disorder (de Vries et al., 2016). Higher rates of suicide and self-harm have also been noted (Olson et al., 2015). There is also some suggestion of increased number of transgender individuals in youth with autism spectrum disorder (ASD)—perhaps as many as 10% to 20% of those with ASD (Jones et al., 2012; Pasterski et al., 2014)—although this has been much debated. Several potential explanations for this have been proposed (Strang et al., 2018; van der Miesen et al., 2016). Clinical management and diagnostic issues can be complicated in the ASD population given social-communication problems and rigidities in thinking and behavior (Parkinson, 2014). Some studies have focused more exclusively on children and youth presenting to specialized gender identity clinical programs and these typically have noted even higher rates of psychiatric comorbidities, particularly mood and anxiety problems, and, to a lesser extent, disruptive behavior disorder (Skagerberg & Carmichael, 2013). Clearly, awareness of potentially associated problems is an important part of clinical management.

■ INTERVENTIONS

In recent years, there has been considerable disagreement about best approaches to treatment of children and youth with gender dysphoria (Drescher and Byne, 2012; Turban et al., 2018). There are three common approaches. The first treatment approach seeks to directly or indirectly reduce cross identification, for example, by psychotherapy or by parents on a daily basis. This has been termed the *therapeutic model* (Zucker et al., 2012). A second approach sometimes referred to as *watchful waiting* allows the child to engage in cross-gender behavior but avoids early efforts to assist with gender transition. The third approach sometimes referred to as the *affirmative model* allows children who desire to gender transition to do so with thoughtful assessment and counseling. These approaches are reviewed in detail elsewhere (see Adelson, 2012; Turban et al., 2018).

The therapeutic model essentially seeks reduction in cross-gender identification. A variety of methods are encompassed within this approach ranging from psychotherapy, behavior therapy, parental guidance, and interventions at home (Turban et al., 2018). This approach assumes flexibility in childhood sexual identification and its potential to be altered through various psychosocial interventions and treatments. Past the implicit and not insignificant value judgment it is the case that this model avoids potentially costly and lengthy medical treatment like gender-affirming/changing surgery. However, it makes judgments for the child and has now moved out of favor and some states now prohibit attempts to change a child or adolescent's gender identity. Indeed, this approach has been viewed as a thinly veiled attempt to promote a same-sex sexual orientation and might, of course, contribute to mental health problems as a child's beliefs are being opposed by parents, family, and others (Adelson, 2012).

The watchful waiting approach strives for a middle position in that it does not recommend rapid gender transition, but does not constrain the child's behavior or attempt to modify gender identification. Sometimes the "only at home" approach is suggested to avoid risks for the child of transgender expression in the community (Hill & Menvielle, 2009). Although described as watchful waiting, children are allowed to pursue their own interests so that by the time many later seek services in specialized clinical settings they will have established a strong gender identity. Allowing for more flexibility may encourage the child to more fully reflect on their own identification and feelings. It is, however, important to realize that delaying decisions until after puberty complicates further medical interventions.

Finally, the third affirmative model approach is based on the notion that no specific judgment need be made about the child's gender identification and that early acceptance and transition may foster longer term mental health outcomes (Turban et al., 2018). In this model, children are allowed to live and dress as they like. The child is supported in their choices and helped to gain an understanding of the issues involved and of the supports and obstacles within the community. In this model, the child is allowed to transition back (de Vries et al., 2016) if that becomes desired or to delay puberty and allow more time for a decision on other interventions. At least one study shows that early efforts at transition are associated with persistent chosen gender identity (Steensma et al., 2013). Within this model, there is no judgment of whether persistence is to be desired; rather, the emphasis is on accepting all forms of gender identity and in supporting the youth with regard to their own decision. Data on mental health related issues associated with these models are sparse. One study suggested positive mental health outcomes when children were allowed to socially transition early (Olson et al., 2016). The issue of who (parent or child or both) is best and most able to make these important decisions (and when in life they are made) remains an area of controversy.

Adolescence

For most children entering adolescence, transgender identity will persist and medical intervention can be implemented. Typically, this begins with suppression of puberty that is then often (but not always) followed by cross-hormone treatment and surgery. Some parents are reluctant to start puberty suppression because they do not understand that it does not necessarily lead to cross-hormone treatment and surgery. Data on efficacy are mixed (de Vreis et al., 2011, 2014). Clearly, more work is needed to establish the generalizability of these findings to other populations. The Endocrine Society Guidelines (Wylie et al., 2009) suggest use of hormone-based intervention with the onset of puberty. They also require that the criteria/guidelines for gender dysphoria (termed *gender identity disorder* in the 2009 guidelines) be met and that the youth is experiencing negative feelings about early pubertal changes. Additionally, the child must have sufficient social and psychological supports and a good understanding of the potential risks and benefits of treatment as well of those entailed in not pursing treatment. Certain psychiatric comorbidities are seen as a contraindication, particularly if they might interfere with treatment. Specialized clinics usually include a mental health consultant as part of the team and as a person who can establish a long-term relationship with the child and family (Simons et al., 2013). Some adolescents will want to explore their range of options and for some with comorbid problems, special considerations may arise, for example, the youth with ASD or severe anxiety or depression (de Vries et al., 2011). Clearly, appropriate intervention for any psychiatric comorbidities is important (Kaltiala et al., 2020). Aspects of treatment are summarized in Table 20.2.

Fully reversible pharmacologic interventions can be undertaken to block puberty. Gonadotropin-releasing hormone is produced in the hypothalamus at lower levels before puberty. Once puberty has begun, the cyclic release of this hormone leads the pituitary to release follicle-stimulating hormone and luteinizing hormone that then initiate the production of sex hormones (estrogen in natal women and testosterone in natal men). The use of gonadotropin-releasing hormone analogs (GnRHa) (by any of several methods including drug implant) prevents the initiation of this process so that the child does not enter puberty with development of secondary sex characteristics (Costa et al., 2015). This method allows a

TABLE 20.2

Treatment of Transgender Youth

Timing	Intervention
Prepubertal	No endocrine intervention recommended. Patient should have regular psychotherapy to discuss gender identity and assess possible future need for hormonal intervention.
Early signs of puberty	Pubertal blockade with gonadotropin-releasing hormone analogs to prevent the development of secondary sex characteristics and provide additional time for psychotherapy and consideration regarding partially reversible interventions.
Age 14+ or 16+, depending on the center	Cross-sex hormonal therapy with estrogen or testosterone. Less frequently with other endocrine-acting medications that have less favorable side-effect profiles.
Age 18 for most centers	Gender-affirming surgeries may be considered. Note that some surgeries may be performed earlier for select patients (generally mastectomies for transgender males).

Reprinted with permission from de Vries, T. Z. (2018). Gender dysphoria and gender incongruence. In A. Martin, M. H. Bloch, & F. R. Volkmar (Eds.), *Lewis's child and adolescent psychiatry: A comprehensive textbook* (5th ed., p. 636). Wolters Kluwer.

longer period for decisions to be made and is readily reversible. For those who choose not to pursue further treatments, puberty can resume and the treatment period may thus function as an extended diagnostic phase. There are some side effects on bone density, but generally this approach appears safe and effective.

Another approach may be employed as the adolescent nears later adolescence when cross-hormonal therapy can be begun and elicit the secondary sex characteristics desired. It is possible to allow for reproduction of biologic children through preservation of sperm or egg, although this requires that puberty be allowed to have its onset and is expensive and not commonly used. Cross-hormonal treatments result in some irreversible changes (such as voice change and increased body hair growth in the case of testosterone) and have more potential side effects. Close follow-up is needed (Turban et al., 2018).

The irreversible gender-affirming surgeries are usually undertaken as the youth become a young adult. These can include a range of interventions such as vaginoplasty, phalloplasty, scrotoplasty, breast augmentation/reduction, facial reconstruction, and hysterectomy. The most common surgical procedure is bilateral mastectomy with chest reconstruction for trans males. Some surgical interventions may be considered earlier in the course of treatment. The issue of adult fertility remains a relatively less explored topic. Many adolescents are less concerned with this issue, but some adults do express concern regarding the issue. Clearly, careful discussion with patients is always needed.

■ SUMMARY

Greater acceptance of diverse gender identification has facilitated the ability of individuals with nontraditional identifications to be more open regarding their preferences. In the past, and in some areas today, lack of acceptance of gender-incongruent and gender-dysphoric youth has led to a number of psychiatric comorbidities including a range of psychiatric problems and suicidal thinking and behavior. Individuals now have the possibility of delaying any decision by delaying puberty and having a longer period to consider other less reversible interventions. The latter can include medical and surgical interventions for those youth who maintain strong cross-gender identification. These interventions may improve mental health outcomes. Clearly, more work on adult outcome is needed (Cooper et al., 2020). More education on the part of the general medical community (Howard, 2020) and of the public at large (Jackman et al., 2018) clearly is also needed (Telingator, Boyum, Daniolos, 2018).

References and Suggested Readings

*Indicates Particularly Recommended

*Adelson, S. L. (2012). Practice parameter on gay, lesbian, or bisexual sexual orientation, gender nonconformity, and gender discordance in children and adolescents. *Journal of the American Academy of Child and Adolescent Psychiatry, 51*, 957–974. https://doi.org/10.1016/j.jaac.2012.07.004

American Psychiatric Association. (2000). *Diagnostic and statistical manual of mental disorders (DSM-IV)* (4th ed.). Author.

American Psychiatric Association. (2013). *Diagnostic and statistical manual (DSM-5)* (5th ed.). Author.

Arcelus, J., Bouman, W. P., Van Den Noortgate, W., Claes, L., Witcomb, G., & Fernandez-Aranda, F. (2015). Systematic review and meta-analysis of prevalence studies in transsexualism. *European Psychiatry, 30*, 807–815. https://doi.org/10.1016/j.eurpsy.2015.04.005

Berglund, H., Lindstrom, P., Dhejne-Helmy, C., & Savic, I. (2008). Male-to-female transsexuals show sex-atypical hypothalamus activation when smelling odorous steroids. *Cerebral Cortex, 18*, 1900–1908. https://doi.org/10.1093/cercor/bhm216

Clark, T. C., Lucassen, M. F., Bullen, P., Denny, S. J., Fleming, T. M., Robinson, E. M., & Rossen, F. V. (2014). The health and well-being of transgender high school students: Results from the New Zealand adolescent health survey (Youth'12). *Journal of Adolescent Health, 55*, 93–99. https://doi.org/10.1016/j.jadohealth.2013.11.008

Cohen-Kettenis, P. T., & Pfäfflin, F. (2003). *Transgenderism and intersexuality in childhood and adolescence: Making choices.* Sage Publishing.

Coolidge, F. L., Thede, L. L., & Young, S. E. (2002). The heritability of gender identity disorder in a child and adolescent twin sample. *Behavior Genetics, 32*(4), 251–257. https://doi.org/10.1023/a:1019724712983

*Cooper, K., Russell, A., Mandy, W., & Butler, C. (2020). The phenomenology of gender dysphoria in adults: A systematic review and meta-synthesis. *Clinical Psychology Review, 80,* 101875. https://doi.org/10.1016/j.cpr.2020.101875

Costa, R., Dunsford, M., Skagerberg, E., Holt, V., Carmichael, P., & Colizzi, M. (2015). Psychological support, puberty suppression, and psychosocial functioning in adolescents with gender dysphoria. *The Journal of Sexual Medicine, 12,* 2206–2214. https://doi.org/10.1111/jsm.13034

de Vries, A. L., Doreleijers, T. A., Steensma, T. D., & Cohen-Kettenis, P. T. (2011). Psychiatric comorbidity in gender dysphoric adolescents. *Journal of Child Psychology and Psychiatry, 52,* 1195–1202. https://doi.org/10.1111/j.1469-7610.2011.02426.x

de Vries, A. L., McGuire, J. K., Steensma, T. D., Wagenaar, E. C., Doreleijers, T. A., & Cohen-Kettenis, P. T. (2014). Young adult psychological outcome after puberty suppression and gender reassignment. *Pediatrics, 134,* 696–704. https://doi.org/10.1542/peds.2013-2958

de Vries, A. L., Steensma, T. D., Cohen-Kettenis, P. T., VanderLaan, D. P., & Zucker, K. J. (2016). Poor peer relations predict parent- and self-reported behavioral and emotional problems of adolescents with gender dysphoria: A cross-national, cross-clinic comparative analysis. *European Child & Adolescent Psychiatry, 25*(6), 579–588. https://doi.org/10.1007/s00787-015-0764-7

de Vries, A. L., Steensma, T. D., Doreleijers, T. A., & Cohen-Kettenis, P. T. (2011). Puberty suppression in adolescents with gender identity disorder: A prospective follow-up study. *Journal of Sexual Medicine, 8,* 2276–2283. https://doi.org/10.1111/j.1743-6109.2010.01943.x

Dessens, A. B., Slijper, F. M., & Drop, S. L. (2005). Gender dysphoria and gender change in chromosomal females with congenital adrenal hyperplasia. *Archives of Sexual Behavior, 34,* 389–397. https://doi.org/10.1007/s10508-005-4338-5

Drescher, J. (2015). Out of *DSM*: Depathologizing homosexuality. *Behavioral Sciences (Basel, Switzerland), 5*(4), 565–575. https://doi.org/10.3390/bs5040565

Drescher, J., & Byne, W. (2012). Introduction to the special issue on "The treatment of gender dysphoric/gender variant children and adolescents." *Journal of Homosexuality, 59,* 295–300. https://doi.org/10.1080/00918369.2012.653299

Duberman, M. (1993). *Stonewall: The definitive story of the LGBTQ rights uprising that changed America.* Random House.

Foucault, M. (1979/1976). *The history of sexuality. Volume 1: An introduction.* Allen Lane.

Freud, S. (1905/1962). *Three essays on the theory of sexuality* (James Strachey, Trans.). Basic Books.

Friedan, B. (1963). *The feminine mystique mass market paperback.* W. W. Norton & Co.

Giedd, J. N., Raznahan, A., Mills, K. L., & Lenroot, R. K. (2012). Magnetic resonance imaging of male/female differences in human adolescent brain anatomy. *Biology of Sex Differences, 3*(1), 19. https://doi.org/10.1186/2042-6410-3-19

Green, R. (1987). *The "Sissy Boy Syndrome" and the development of homosexuality.* Yale University Press.

Guillamon, A., Junque, C., & Gomez-Gil, E. (2016). A review of the status of brain structure research in transsexualism. *Archives of Sexual Behavior, 45,* 1615–1648. https://doi.org/10.1007/s10508-016-0768-5

Hill, D. B., & Menvielle, E. (2009). You have to give them a place where they feel protected and safe and loved: The views of parents who have gender-variant children and adolescents. *Journal of LGBT Youth, 6,* 243–271. https://doi.org/10.1080/19361650903013527

Hines, M. (2011). Gender development and the human brain. *Annual Review of Neuroscience, 34,* 69–88. https://doi.org/10.1146/annurev-neuro-061010-113654

Hines, M. (2020). Neuroscience and sex/gender: looking back and forward. *The Journal of Neuroscience: The Official Journal of the Society for Neuroscience, 40*(1), 37–43. https://doi.org/10.1523/JNEUROSCI.0750-19.2019

Holt, V., Skagerberg, E., & Dunsford, M. (2016). Young people with features of gender dysphoria: Demographics and associated difficulties. *Clinical Child Psychology and Psychiatry, 21,* 108–118. https://doi.org/10.1177/1359104514558431

Howard, S. (2020). The struggle for GPs to get the right care for patients with gender dysphoria. *BMJ, 368,* m215. https://doi.org/10.1136/bmj.m215

Jackman, K. B., Dolezal, C., Levin, B., Honig, J. C., & Bockting, W. O. (2018). Stigma, gender dysphoria, and nonsuicidal self-injury in a community sample of transgender individuals. *Psychiatry Research, 269,* 602–609. https://doi.org/10.1016/j.psychres.2018.08.092

Jones, R. M., Wheelwright, S., Farrell, K., Martin, E., Green, R., Di Ceglie, D., & Baron-Cohen, S. (2012). Female-to-male transsexual people and autistic traits. *Journal of Autism and Developmental Disorders, 42,* 301–306. https://doi.org/10.1007/s10803-011-1227-8

Jürgensen, M., Kleinemeier, E., Lux, A., Steensma, T. D., Cohen-Kettenis, P. T., Hiort, O., Thyen, U., Köhler, B., & DSD Network Working Group. (2013). Psychosexual development in adolescents and adults with disorders of sex development—Results from the German Clinical Evaluation Study. *The Journal of Sexual Medicine, 10*(11), 2703–2714. https://doi.org/10.1111/j.1743-6109.2012.02751.x

Kaltiala, R., Heino, E., Tyolajarvi, M., & Suomalainen, L. (2020). Adolescent development and psychosocial functioning after starting cross-sex hormones for gender dysphoria. *Nordic Journal of Psychiatry, 74*(3), 213–219. https://doi.org/10.1080/08039488.2019.1691260

Khatchadourian, K., Amed, S., & Metzger, D. L. (2014). Clinical management of youth with gender dysphoria in Vancouver. *Journal of Pediatrics, 164*(4), 906–911. https://doi.org/10.1016/j.jpeds.2013.10.068

Kinsey, A. C., Pomeroy, W. R., & Martin, C. E. (2003/1948). Sexual behavior in the human male. *American Journal of Public Health, 93*(6), 894–898. https://doi.org/10.2105/AJPH.93.6.894

Kinsey, A. C., Pomeroy, W. R., Martin, C. E., & Gebhard, P. (1953). *Sexual behavior in the human female.* Saunders.

Mazur, T. (2005). Gender dysphoria and gender change in androgen insensitivity or micropenis. *Archives of Sexual Behavior, 34,* 411–421. https://doi.org/10.1007/s10508-005-4341-x

McGuire, J. K., Anderson, C. R., Toomey, R. B., & Russell, S. T. (2010). School climate for transgender youth: A mixed method investigation of student experiences and school responses. *Journal of Youth and Adolescence, 39,* 1175–1188. https://doi.org/10.1007/s10964-010-9540-7

Money, J. (1988). *Gay, straight, and in-between: The sexology of erotic orientation.* Oxford University Press.

Olson, K. R. (2016). Prepubescent transgender children: What we do and do not know. *Journal of the American Academy of Child and Adolescent Psychiatry, 55,* 155–156. https://doi.org/10.1016/j.jaac.2015.11.015

Olson, J., Schrager, S. M., Belzer, M., Simons, L. K., & Clark, L. F. (2015). Baseline physiologic and psychosocial characteristics of transgender youth seeking care for gender dysphoria. *Journal of Adolescent Health, 57,* 374–380. https://doi.org/10.1016/j.jadohealth.2015.04.027

Olson, K. R., Durwood, L., DeMeules, M., & McLaughlin, K. A. (2016). Mental health of transgender children who are supported in their identities. *Pediatrics, 137*(3), e20153223. https://doi.org/10.1542/peds.2015-3223

Parkinson, J. (2014). Gender dysphoria in Asperger's syndrome: A caution. *Australasian Psychiatry, 22,* 84–85. https://doi.org/10.1177/1039856213497814

Pasterski, V., Gilligan, L., & Curtis, R. (2014). Traits of autism spectrum disorders in adults with gender dysphoria. *Archives of Sexual Behavior, 43,* 387–393. https://doi.org/10.1007/s10508-013-0154-5

Pasterski, V., Zucker, K. J., Hindmarsh, P. C., Hughes, I. A., Acerini, C., Spencer, D., Neufeld, S., & Hines, M. (2015). Increased cross-gender identification independent of gender role behavior in girls with congenital adrenal hyperplasia: Results from a standardized assessment of 4- to 11-year-old children. *Archives of Sexual Behavior, 44,* 1363–1375. https://doi.org/10.1007/s10508-014-0385-0

Ruigrok, A. N., Salimi-Khorshidi, G., Lai, M. C., Baron-Cohen, S., Lombardo, M. V., Tait, R. J., & Suckling, J. (2014). A meta-analysis of sex differences in human brain structure. *Neuroscience & Biobehavioral Reviews, 39,* 34–50. https://doi.org/10.1016/j.neubiorev.2013.12.004

Schoning, S., Engelien, A., Bauer, C., Kugel, H., Kersting, A., Roestel, C., Zwitserlood, P., Pyka, M., Dannlowski, U., Lehmann, W., Heindel, W., Arolt, V., & Konrad, C. (2010). Neuroimaging differences in spatial cognition between men and male-to-female transsexuals before and during hormone therapy. *The Journal of Sexual Medicine, 7,* 1858–1867. https://doi.org/10.1111/j.1743-6109.2009.01484.x

Shields, J. P., Cohen, R., Glassman, J. R., Whitaker, K., Franks, H., & Bertolini, I. (2013). Estimating population size and demographic characteristics of lesbian, gay, bisexual, and transgender youth in middle school. *Journal of Adolescent Health, 52,* 248–250. https://doi.org/10.1016/j.jadohealth.2012.06.016

Simons, L., Schrager, S. M., Clark, L. F., Belzer, M., & Olson, F. (2013). Parental support and mental health among transgender adolescents. *Journal of Adolescent Health, 53,* 791–793. https://doi.org/10.1016/j.jadohealth.2013.07.019

Skagerberg, E., & Carmichael, P. (2013). Internalizing and externalizing behaviors in a group of young people with gender dysphoria. *International Journal of Transgenderism, 14,* 105–112. https://doi.org/10.1080/15532739.2013.822340

Spack, N. P., Edwards-Leeper, L., Feldman, H. A., Leibowitz, S., Mandel, F., Diamond, D. A., & Vance, S. R. (2012). Children and adolescents with gender identity disorder referred to a pediatric medical center. *Pediatrics, 129,* 418–425. https://doi.org/10.1542/peds.2011-0907

Steensma, T. D., McGuire, J. K., Kreukels, B. P. C., Beekman, A. J., & Cohen-Kettenis, P. T. (2013). Factors associated with desistence and persistence of childhood gender dysphoria: A quantitative follow-up study. *Journal of the American Academy of Child and Adolescent Psychiatry, 52*, 582–590. https://doi .org/10.1016/j.jaac.2013.03.016

Steensma, T. D., Zucker, K. J., Kreukels, B. P., VanderLaan, D. P., Wood, H., Fuentes, A., & Cohen-Kettenis, P. T. (2014). Behavioral and emotional problems on the Teacher's Report Form: A cross-national, cross-clinic comparative analysis of gender dysphoric children and adolescents. *Journal of Abnormal Child Psychology, 42*, 635–647. https://doi.org/10.1007/s10802-013-9804-2

*Strang, J. F., Meagher, H., Kenworthy, L., de Vries, A. L. C., Menvielle, E., Leibowitz, S., Janssen, A., Cohen-Kettenis, P., Shumer, D. E., Edwards-Leeper, L., Pleak, R. R, Spack, N., Karasic, D. H., Schreier, H., Balleur, A., Tishelman, A., Ehrensaft, D., Rodnan, L., Kuschner, E. S., … Anthony, L. G. (2018). Initial clinical guidelines for co-occurring autism spectrum disorder and gender dysphoria in adolescents. *Journal of Clinical Child & Adolescent Psychology, 47*(1), 105–115. https://doi.org/10.1080/153744 16.2016.1228462

Swaab, D. F., & Garcia-Falgueras, A. (2009). Sexual differentiation of the human brain in relation to gender identity and sexual orientation. *Functional Neurology, 24*(1), 17–28.

Tan, K., Treharne, G. J., Ellis, S. J., Schmidt, J. M., & Veale, J. F. (2020). Gender minority stress: A critical review. *Journal of Homosexuality, 67*(10), 1471–1489. https://doi.org/10.1080/00918369.2019.1591789

*Telingator, C. J., Boyum, E. M., & Daniolos, P. T. (2018). Sexual minority youth: Identity role and orientation. In A. Martin, M. BLoch, and F. R. Volkmar (Eds.), *Lewis's child and adolescent psychiatry* (pp. 138–148). Wolters Kluwer.

*Turban, J., de Vries, A. L., & Zucker, K. J. (2018). Gender dysphoria and gender incongruence. In A. Martin, M. Bloch, & F. R. Volkmar (Eds.), *Lewis's child and adolescent psychiatry: A comprehensive textbook* (5th ed., pp. 632–643). Wolters Kluwer.

van Beijsterveldt, C. E., Hudziak, J. J., & Boomsma, D. I. (2006). Genetic and environmental influences on cross-gender behavior and relation to behavior problems: A study of Dutch twins at ages 7 and 10 years. *Archives of Sexual Behavior, 35*, 647–658. https://doi.org/10.1007/s10508-006-9072-0

van der Miesen, A. I., Hurley, H., & de Vries, A. L. (2016). Gender dysphoria and autism spectrum disorder: A narrative review. *International Review of Psychiatry, 28*, 70–80. https://doi.org/10.3109/0 9540261.2015.1111199

VanderLaan, D. P., Leef, J. H., Wood, H., Hughes, S. K., & Zucker, K. J. (2015). Autism spectrum disorder risk factors and autistic traits in gender dysphoric children. *Journal of Autism and Developmental Disorders, 45*, 1742–1750. https://doi.org/10.1007/s10803-014-2331-3

Wallen, M. S., & Cohen-Kettenis, P. T. (2008). Psychosexual outcome of gender-dysphoric children. *Journal of the American Academy of Child and Adolescent Psychiatry, 47*, 1413–1423. https://doi .org/10.1097/CHI.0b013e31818956b9

Wylie, C. H., Cohen-Kettenis, P. T., Delemarre-van de Waal, H., Gooren, L. J., Meyer, W. J., Spack, N. P., Tangpricha, V., & Montori, V. M. (2009). Endocrine treatment of transsexual persons: An endocrine society clinical practice guideline. *The Journal of Clinical Endocrinology and Metabolism, 94*, 3132–3154. https://doi.org/10.1210/jc.2009-0345

Zucker, K. J., & Bradley, S. J. (1995). *Gender identity disorder and psychosexual problems in children and adolescents.* Guilford Press.

Zucker, K. J., Bradley, S. J., Owen-Anderson, A., Kibblewhite, S. J., Wood, H., Singh, D., & Choi, K. (2012). Demographics, behavior problems, and psychosexual characteristics of adolescents with gender identity disorder or transvestic fetishism. *Journal of Sex & Marital Therapy, 38*, 151-89. https://doi .org/10.1080/0092623X.2011.611219

CHAPTER 21 ■ SLEEP AND SLEEP DISORDERS

■ BACKGROUND

There have been major advances in understanding sleep and sleep problems in both children and adults over the past several decades. This began with the advent of polysomnographic (PSG) sleep recording in the 1950s and the description of the rapid eye movement (REM) and non–rapid eye movement (NREM) sleep (see Table 21.1). Sleep Disorders Medicine has now been recognized in its own right and includes a pediatric section. Consensus on nosology and classification and the development of both sleep laboratories and clinical training programs have advanced the field (Baroni & Anders, 2018).

■ THE ORGANIZATION OF SLEEP: DEVELOPMENTAL ASPECTS

The organization of sleep–wake patterns has marked developmental aspects. Adults spend about 80% of their sleep time in NREM sleep (20% in REM). In contrast, newborn infants spend about half of their time in REM sleep. By adolescence, children achieve the pattern of sleep organization seen in adults (see Table 21.1). Other differences include the pattern of sleep. Thus when adults begin to sleep they typically start in stage 4 of NREM sleep and spend a considerable initial period in this sleep stage before the REM–NREM cycles recur, at intervals of about 90 minutes, during the night. Proportionally most of the REM sleep occurs in the latter part of the sleep cycle in adults. Interestingly infants have sleep patterns associated with an initial REM period and with REM and NREM sleep alternating through much of the night. The gradual reorganization of the sleep cycles begins early in life as central timing mechanisms become more active.

For the developing infant (and for the parents) the regulation of sleep–wake cycles and the ability to sleep through the night are important tasks that provide important opportunities for interaction and set the stage for other aspects of self-regulation. Difficulties in this process thus typically require some assessment of psychosocial and parent–child issues that might be having an impact. Factors important in this include the infant's temperament and background of the caregivers, their supports, etc. Cultural, family, and other environmental influences may be important as are other potential variables such as physical condition of the infant and mother. There are frequently complicated interactions between the infant's sleep pattern and the entire family's ability to sleep through the night. In clinical practice all possible permutations and combinations are seen, for example, some infants may sleep/nap better in

TABLE 21.1

Features of NREM Sleep and REM Sleep

NREM Sleep	REM Sleep
EEG: synchronized, slower frequencies and higher voltages than wakefulness and REM	EEG: desynchronized, mixed, low-amplitude fast frequencies, similar to wakefulness
Reduced metabolic activity	Increased metabolic activity
Autonomic slowing	Autonomic activation
Maintained thermoregulation	Altered thermoregulation: poikilothermia
Episodic, involuntary movements	Skeletal muscle atonia
Slow rolling eye movements	Rapid eye movements
Few penile erections or little vaginal lubrication	Partial or full penile erections or significant vaginal lubrication
Limited mentation/dreaming	Dreaming
Defined as quiet sleep in infants	Defined as active sleep in infants
Sleepwalking and sleep terrors arise from NREM sleep	Nightmares arise from REM sleep

EEG, electroencephalogram; NREM, non–rapid eye movement; REM, rapid eye movement.
Reprinted with permission from Baroni, A., & Anders, T. F. (2018). Sleep disorders. In A. Martin, M. H. Bloch, & F. R. Volkmar (Eds.), *Lewis's child and adolescent psychiatry: A comprehensive textbook* (5th ed., p. 581). Wolters Kluwer.

TABLE 21.2

Differences Between Sleep in Infants and Adults

	Infants	Adults
NREM/REM %	50/50	80/20
Ultradian Cycle Length	50–60 min	90 min
Circadian Cycle	Polyphasic	Diurnal
Temporal Distribution of NREM/REM During the Night	Equi-distributed	First third/last third
Sleep Stages	Quiet Sleep (NREM) Active Sleep (REM)	NREM (N1–N2–N3) REM

NREM, non–rapid eye movement; REM, rapid eye movement.
Reprinted with permission from Baroni, A., & Anders, T. F. (2018). Sleep disorders. In A. Martin, M. H. Bloch, & F. R. Volkmar (Eds.), *Lewis's child and adolescent psychiatry: A comprehensive textbook* (5th ed., p. 581). Wolters Kluwer.

day care or with a nanny than with the parents. Occasionally, infants will sleep better with one parent or the other.

Table 21.2 summarizes some of the differences between sleep in infants and adults, and Table 21.3 summarizes changes in sleep duration over the course of development. As Baroni and Anders (2018) note, the sleep–wake cycle has two important elements. One is more homeostatic and sleep dependent and varies with the awake time that precedes sleep, whereas

TABLE 21.3

Sleep Durations in Childhood and Adolescence

	Mean Nighttime Sleep Duration (hours)	Mean Daytime Sleep Duration (hours)
6 mos old	14.2	3.4
3 yrs old	12.5	1.7
6 yrs old	11	—
10 yrs old	9.9	—
12 yrs old	9.3	—
15 yrs old	8.5	—

Reprinted with permission from Baroni, A., & Anders, T. F. (2018). Sleep disorders. In A. Martin, M. H. Bloch, & F. R. Volkmar (Eds.), *Lewis's child and adolescent psychiatry: A comprehensive textbook* (5th ed., p. 582). Wolters Kluwer.

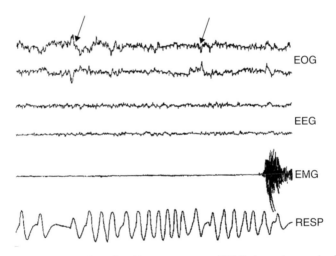

FIGURE 21.1. Polygraphic recording of rapid eye movement (REM) sleep. An epoch of REM sleep in a newborn infant characterized by a low-voltage, fast electroencephalogram (EEG); active rapid eye movements (arrows); an inhibited electromyograph (EMG); and rapid irregular respirations (RESP). EOG, electrooculogram. Reprinted with permission from Anders, T. F. (2007). Sleep disorders. In A. Martin & F. R. Volkmar (Eds.), *Lewis's child and adolescent psychiatry: A comprehensive textbook* (4th ed., p. 630). Lippincott Williams & Wilkins.

the second process has more to do with circadian rhythms reflecting both internal central nervous system (CNS) factors and the body's internal clock and the day–night light cycle.

The electroencephalogram (EEG) pattern during REM sleep is characterized by fast, low-voltage activity similar to that observed while the individual is awake. During REM sleep, there are bursts of eye movements and rapid, irregular breathing and heart rate patterns. Dreams are reported during REM sleep. Thus while the individual appears to be sleeping, significant CNS activity is noted. This is observed in infants where it is sometimes referred to as "active sleep." In contrast to the apparent activation during REM sleep, the pattern during NREM sleep is one associated with inhibition, for example, slow and regular heart and breathing rate with EEG activity showing slower frequencies. In babies, this stage is also referred to as quiet sleep. Figures 21.1 and 21.2 illustrated PSG recordings during REM and NREM sleep.

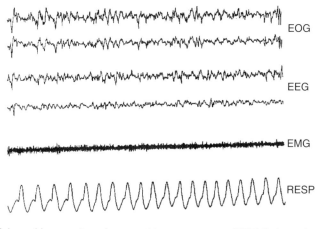

FIGURE 21.2. Polygraphic recording of non–rapid eye movement (NREM) sleep. An epoch of NREM sleep characterized by high-voltage, slow waves on the electroencephalogram (EEG); an absence of rapid eye movements; a tonic electromyograph (EMG) pattern; and slowed, regular respirations (RESP). EOG, electrooculogram. Reprinted with permission from Anders, T. F. (2007). Sleep disorders. In A. Martin & F. R. Volkmar (Eds.), *Lewis's child and adolescent psychiatry: A comprehensive textbook* (4th ed., p. 630). Lippincott Williams & Wilkins.

CLASSIFICATION OF SLEEP DISORDERS IN CHILDREN AND ADOLESCENTS

There are two separate major approaches to diagnosis: they are largely, but not entirely, overlapping. One in the *International Classification of Sleep Disorders, Third Edition* (*ICSD-3*) (Mindell et al., 2006) and the second approach is that of *Diagnostic and Statistical Manual of Mental Disorders, 5th Edition* (*DSM-5*; American Psychiatric Association [APA], 2013). The former is oriented more for use by sleep specialists and the latter to general use; there are some differences in the two systems. To further complicate issues of diagnosis for younger children, there is yet another approach, which is the Diagnostic Classification: Zero to Three, Revised (DC 0–3R); this includes sleep disorders as well (Zero To Three Press, 2005). An important strength of *DSM-5* is that it makes it possible to denote sleep disorders that are concurrent with mental health disorders—if this is justified, that is, if the sleep problem is not simply secondary to the mental health disturbance. The main categories of sleep disorder in the *DSM-5* and *ICSD-3* are summarized in Table 21.4. There are some differences and many similarities. The *DSM-5* includes idiopathic hypersomnia and hypersomnia associated with a mental disorder. The *DSM-5* approach is, of course, not limited solely to sleep. This discussion here follows the *DSM-5* classification.

It is important to note that sleep disorders clearly vary with age. Infants have the most trouble with falling asleep and then with night awakening, whereas older children may have sleeping walking and adolescents are more likely to have insufficient sleep and circadian rhythm disorders (Baroni & Anders, 2018).

SPECIFIC SLEEP DISORDERS

Insomnia

Difficulties in going to bed or falling asleep and staying asleep as well as frequent nighttime awakening are the most frequent features of childhood insomnia. The child may, for example,

TABLE 21.4

Main Categories of Sleep Disorders in *DSM-5* and *ICSD-3*

Category	Description
Insomnia	• Persistent difficulties sleeping • Adequate opportunity for sleep • Daytime impairment (e.g., chronic insomnia)
Sleep-related breathing disorders	• Irregular breathing during sleep, possibly accompanied by sleep disruption (e.g., obstructive sleep apnea)
Hypersomnolence disorder and narcolepsy	• Excessive daytime sleepiness, in spite of adequate sleep (e.g., narcolepsy, hypersomnolence disorder)
Circadian rhythm disorders	• Misalignment of circadian rhythms and social requirement (e.g., delayed sleep phase)
Parasomnias	• Abnormal physical and emotional experiences during sleep or sleep–wake transitions (e.g., sleepwalking, nightmares)
Sleep-related movement disorders	• Presence of movements that delay sleep onset or disrupt sleep (e.g., restless leg syndrome)

DSM-5, Diagnostic and Statistical Manual of Mental Disorders, 5th Edition; ICSD-3, International Classification of Sleep Disorders, Third Edition.
Reprinted with permission from Baroni, A., & Anders, T. F. (2018). Sleep disorders. In A. Martin, M. H. Bloch, & F. R. Volkmar (Eds.), *Lewis's child and adolescent psychiatry: A comprehensive textbook* (5th ed., p. 585). Wolters Kluwer.

only want to fall asleep with the caregiver rather than on their own. The child may resist bedtime. As Baroni and Anders (2018) note, these have had various terminologies and classifications in the past.

Daytime difficulties can include a range of problems including irritability, behavioral difficulties, overactivity, and chronic tiredness (Reid et al., 2009). Although this can start at any age, it is not typically diagnosed until after children are 6 months or so of age when more typical sleep patterns are established (Reid et al., 2009). Rates of 20%–30% are reported in community samples (Honaker & Meltzer, 2014). For adolescents, this number is somewhat reduced. Other factors in the child, for example, developmental difficulties like autism spectrum disorder (ASD), can substantially increase sleep problems (Won et al., 2019).

Although mechanisms of pathogenesis are unclear, most research suggest that a combination of factors including child, parent, family, and other variables is important. Temperamental difficulties are also a risk factor. Treatments have to do with helping parents of younger children establish better sleep patterns. Behavioral methods may help significantly (Reid et al., 2009). Most of this literature has focused on young children and there has been less work on older children and adolescents as well as those with special needs (Buckley et al., 2020; Durand, 2014; Meltzer & Mindell, 2014). For younger children, behavioral treatments are very effective. These include unmodified or graduated extinction (total or phased-out parental attention after lights out); this can be difficult for parents to do.

Helping parents understand good bedtime practices like using the bed only for sleep and the use of calming bedtime routines is important. Parents should be reassured that behavioral interventions have not been associated with negative outcomes (Baroni & Anders, 2018; Meltzer & Mindell, 2014; Taylor & Roane, 2010). Having phones, TVs, computers, etc., outside the bedroom is also helpful.

The addition of medications should be considered only after behavioral approaches have been attempted. There are no Food and Drug Administration (FDA)-approved medications for pediatric insomnia. Medications may be used at times of stress or illness (see Baroni & Anders, 2018). Many of the agents used have potential for "paradoxical" reactions (i.e., making the child more agitated). Melatonin is frequently used given its efficacy and relatively few side effects. Typical doses range from 1 to 3 mg (see Baroni & Anders, 2018). Other medications like clonidine or guanfacine are sometimes used particularly for children who have attention-deficit hyperactivity disorder (ADHD) (see Chapter 10), in particular, given how frequently these children have insomnia (Owens & Moturi, 2009). There are more risks with these agents. Although some of the antihistamines such as diphenhydramine are frequently used by pediatricians, there are limited data to support their efficacy, and these agents also have some important side effects.

Obstructive Sleep Apnea

Obstructive sleep apnea (OSA) is a well-known but frequently unrecognized condition and should be considered in any child where snoring is reported. Overall, it has a prevalence of 1%–5% but becomes much more common in children who are obese or who have medical problems and habitual snoring (Marcus et al., 2012). Parents may not report snoring unless they are specifically asked. Even in the absence of OSA, snoring may have some of its features and consequences (Brockmann et al., 2012).

In addition to chronic snoring, the clinical features of OSA include labored breathing as well as gasping or choking during sleep. Apnea (breathing pauses) may be present and observed by parents. OSA can be associated with nocturnal enuresis (see Chapter 19). Unlike adults, excessive sleepiness in the daytime is less frequent in children. However, children are at risk for a number of other behavioral problems (Marcus et al., 2012; Mindell & Owens, 2015).

To establish the diagnosis of OSA, PSG is needed to help to determine the severity of the condition. During PSG, the children will be noted to exhibit episodes of apnea, hypopnea, and brief periods of cortical arousals due to the intermittent upper respiratory obstructions. The latter frequently is associated with enlarged tonsils and adenoids. Other factors like obesity as well as muscular problems and craniofacial problems can also contribute. It is important to inquire as to whether children snore—particularly in those with ADHD. Neurodevelopmental conditions like Prader–Willi and Down syndrome also are frequently associated with OSA. If untreated, OSA can lead to difficulties with cognitive functioning, behavioral, growth, and other problems (Marcus et al., 2012).

The primary treatment for OSA is adenotonsillectomy in children. This usually results in improved sleep, behavior, and cognitive function. Sometimes residual OSA persists after adenotonsillectomy, particularly in obese children.

Parasomnias

In these sleep disorders, problematic behaviors or affective–emotional reactions are noted during sleep or at sleep transitions. The parasomnias are classified as REM or NREM (or other) depending on when they occur in the sleep cycle. Sleep walking and sleep terrors are examples of NREM parasomnias. The parasomnias that are REM-related include nightmare disorder, REM behavior disorder, and recurrent sleep paralysis. Enuresis is viewed as an "other parasomnia" (American Academy of Sleep Medicine [AASM], 2014) (see Chapter 19). A key diagnostic feature is the association of sleep and wakefulness, for example, as in sleep walking.

Sleep Walking and Sleep Terrors

In these conditions, motor behavior along with arousal and/or autonomic activation while a child is asleep (or only partial aroused) are key features (Avidan & Kaplish, 2010). Typically the child has complete amnesia for the event unless the child is awakened. These is some danger of inadvertent injury to the child during the event (Petit et al., 2015). In a sleep walking episode, the child will move out of the bed and can wander, even possibly leaving the house. The child will appear confused and only have limited response to physical or verbal stimulation. Sometimes the family will become aware of this when the child is found awakening in a different location than their bed in the morning. It is typically the case that sleep walking is brief but can last up to half an hour (Baroni & Anders, 2018).

During a night terror, the child has a period of intense, sudden arousal and autonomic activation usually accompanied by loud screaming and some simple vocalizations. The child may be unresponsive to verbal or visual cues or directions and may seem to stare without actually seeing. These episodes are brief—30 seconds to 5 minutes in length but sometimes longer. The episodes decrease with age.

These NREM parasomnias are frequent in children. Sleep terrors may affect one-third of children below age 2. Sleep walking similarly affects about 30% of children at some point—usually between the ages of 6 and 12 (Avidan & Kaplish, 2010; Petit et al., 2015). In a small number of instances, the disorders persist into adulthood (Avidan & Kaplish, 2010; Baroni & Anders, 2018). There are no sex differences in rates. There is a strong familial component. There is also some suggestion of overlap of the two conditions, with perhaps one-third of children who have sleep terrors going on to have sleep walking (36). Sleep deprivation and factors that interfere with sleep in general can serve as triggers for both night terrors and sleep walking (Petit et al., 2015).

As Baroni and Anders (2018) note, these events occur during slow-wave sleep and therefore the individual will have amnesia and not be dreaming (despite the apparent distress—unlike a nightmare). Given the association with slow-wave sleep, these events are more frequent in the first third of the night (when slow-wave sleep is most common).

Differential diagnosis includes nocturnal frontal lobe epilepsy, although in this condition episodes are usually brief and don't cluster in the beginning of the night. In contrast to night terrors, nightmares are more frequent in the last part of the night and will have dream content and can be remembered when the child awakens in the morning. A PSG is useful if nocturnal epilepsy is a consideration or if episodes are very frequent and problematic (see Table 21.5 for nonrespiratory indications for PSG). Baroni and Anders (2018) discuss some of the safety considerations, for example, relative to access to the stove, leaving the house, etc.

TABLE 21.5

Common Nonrespiratory Indications for Polysomnography and Multiple Sleep Latency Test in Children

Evaluation of Hypersomnolence and Narcolepsy	Unexplained excessive daytime sleepiness should be assessed with PSG followed by multiple sleep latency test (MSLT)
Parasomnias	In the presence of frequent or potentially injurious parasomnias, to differentiate parasomnia from nocturnal epilepsy, in case of enuresis, or if there is suspicion for parasomnia comorbid with sleep-disordered breathing or periodic limb movement disorder
Suspicion for Periodic Limb Movement Disorder and Possibly for Supportive Data for Restless Leg Syndrome (RLS)	For children with RLS who also complain of poor sleep or those symptoms suggestive of periodic limb movement disorder

Reprinted with permission from Baroni, A., & Anders, T. F. (2018). Sleep disorders. In A. Martin, M. H. Bloch, & F. R. Volkmar (Eds.), *Lewis's child and adolescent psychiatry: A comprehensive textbook* (5th ed., p. 587). Wolters Kluwer.

Nightmares

Children start to remember and report their dreams (and nightmares) at around age 3 (Foulkes, 1982). Baroni and Anders (2018) note a standard definition is lacking, but generally nightmares are characterized by having negative emotional content that awakens the child (Levin & Nielsen, 2007). "Bad dreams" also have disturbing content that does not, however, awaken the child from sleep. Nightmares and bad dreams are likely part of a continuum and may be the focus of clinical attention if they cause distress. Nightmares usually are associated with REM sleep. Once the child is awakened, they will be fully oriented and able to describe dream content (unlike in night terrors). Given the association with REM sleep, these tend to occur in the latter part of the night. Dream content with younger children is usually simple and becomes more involved and elaborate over time. Both nightmares and disturbing "bad" dreams are more frequent in children who have experienced stress, anxiety disorders, or suicidal ideation (Gauchat et al., 2014). Nightmares and bad dreams are frequent in children, with rates 3–4 fold higher than adults; their frequency peaks around ages 10–12 and then progressively diminishes (Gauchat et al., 2014; Levin & Nielsen, 2007). There may be some gender differences, with girls having more nightmares in early adolescence (Gauchat et al., 2014).

Hypersomnia Disorders and Narcolepsy

These conditions are characterized by excessive daytime sleepiness. The *DSM-5* (APA, 2013) divides these into two groups: (1) hypersomnia and (2) narcolepsy. The International Classification System further subdivided narcolepsy (see Barateau & Dauvilliers, 2019; Baroni & Anders, 2018).

Hypersomnia

This condition (excessive sleepiness not associated with epilepsy) is characterized by excessive sleepiness during the daytime not due to sleep deprivation. Typically individuals will complain of a need for frequent naps or dozing off and need a long night of restorative sleep. Some have trouble with awakening in the morning or are confused on awakening. Sometimes other problems are noted as well including difficulties with memory and focus, headache, and gastrointestinal (GI) problems (Billiard & Sonka, 2015).

The pathophysiologic mechanism of the condition has yet to be clearly established (Billiard & Sonka, 2015). Prevalence rates are between 0.5% and 1% in the general population (Billiard & Sonka, 2015). The onset is usually during adolescence or young adulthood. The condition may be associated with mood problems and affective disorder. As Baroni and Anders (2018) note, differential diagnosis is complex and should be done by a sleep specialist (Billiard & Sonka, 2015).

Narcolepsy

In this condition, there is severe hypersomnolence with the brief intrusions of REM sleep–like states during wakefulness. It is these REM sleep intrusions that appear to be the cause for most of the associated symptoms including cataplexy, hypnagogic hallucination, and sleep paralysis. As Baroni and Anders (2018) note, cataplexy is an essential feature and often follows some strong, often positive, affect; slurred speech and decreased muscle tone particularly involving the muscles of the face and neck are often observed. Usually episodes last a few minutes and recovery is complete. In children the period of decreased muscle tone can be longer (Scammell, 2015). There is memory of the episode. Episodes may happen a few times a day or only a few times a year. The sleep paralysis observed is a function of the atonia that occurs with REM sleep incursion that has intruded into wakefulness. Dreaming can be reported as can be complex hallucinations of short duration. Common associated features include obesity and depression. Rates in the general population are on the order of 1 in 2000, although missed diagnosis is not uncommon. Usually the onset is in adolescence (Scammell, 2015). Sleep studies confirm the diagnosis.

Treatment includes both behavioral and drug interventions. Children and youth should be encouraged to keep to a regular sleep–wake cycle, engage in physical activity (to avoid weight gain), and use regular short (20–30 minutes) daytime naps.

The daytime sleepiness can be treated with stimulants and cataplexy can be treated with stimulant venlafaxine and tricyclic antidepressants. Other treatments are available as well (see Baroni & Anders, 2018).

Patients with narcolepsy frequently have trouble adjusting to this condition as the latter causes problems both in school and with peer relations. Accordingly, behavioral and emotional support and counseling are indicated.

Circadian Rhythm Sleep Disorder — Delayed Sleep Phase Type

The usual circadian rhythms are one of the major physiologic regulators of the sleep–wake cycle. The sleep–wake cycle can be advanced or delayed if the sleep–wake times occur earlier or later than is usual. Sometimes this change in sleep–wake cycle causes academic or other problems and becomes a circadian rhythm disorder. It is common for adolescents to have some sleep phase delay (falling to sleep and then awakening later). The adolescent may have difficulty remaining awake in the morning and may miss or be late for school. Adolescents often build up "sleep debt" as they go to bed later and get up earlier without a sufficient night's sleep.

Probably at least 7% of adolescents have a delayed sleep phase disorder (APA, 2013). Various etiologic factors including genetic ones as well as social factors, light sensitivity, and other issues contribute (Mindell & Owens, 2015). Given the presence of daytime sleepiness the differential diagnosis includes narcolepsies and insomnia. But unlike those with insomnia there is no difficulty in falling asleep or with their sleep pattern. Sleep diaries can be helpful and will usually show delays in wake-up times over weekends.

Treatment includes setting a strict sleep cycle, avoiding light-emitting tablets/computers in the 2 hours prior to sleep, and avoiding the long periods of sleeping on weekends. Melatonin can be helpful (Kotagal & Chopra, 2012; Morgenthaler et al., 2007).

Restless Leg Syndrome

In restless leg syndrome (RLS), as defined in *DSM-5* (APA, 2013), there is a persistent and uncomfortable sensation of "creepy-crawlies" and feeling of burning or tingling in the leg with a concurrent wish to move the leg. The feelings often start in the soles of the feet and then gradually move upward and often start at bedtime. The feelings can be temporarily relieved by movement or rubbing of the feet and legs. The condition disrupts sleep and leads to delayed sleep onset and daytime fatigue. Asking the child or adolescent about whether their legs bother them or whether they kick at night is an excellent screen for the disorder (Baroni & Anders, 2018). Estimates of the prevalence of the condition in the United States range from 2% to 4%, but misdiagnosis is common, that is, it is written off to "growing pains" (Baroni & Anders, 2018). Restlessness of the legs and the other associated features are required diagnostically (Gonzalez-Latapi & Malkani, 2019).

Difficulty falling asleep is a major consequence of RLS along with fatigue, inattentiveness, or sleepiness. Simple questions such as "Do your legs want to kick at night?" and "Do your legs bother you at night?" can be good screening probes for the disorder. During PSG, periodic limb jerks are noted and associated with sleep disruption. The condition is highly familial, and several genes have now been associated with the condition (Picchietti et al., 2013). As Baroni and Anders (2018) note, the pathophysiology of RLS is unclear but appears related to iron and dopamine metabolism; the iron is a cofactor for tyrosine hydroxylase, the latter being needed for dopamine synthesis. Thus, ferritin, a measure of iron storage, should be routinely assessed in children with RLS. Oral iron supplementation should be considered depending on ferritin levels. There is some association with ADHD in children. Children with the condition should be referred to specialists for treatment.

SLEEP DIFFICULTIES AND OTHER MENTAL HEALTH PROBLEMS

As noted, one of the strengths of the *DSM-5* (APA, 2013) approach is the opportunity to observe association between sleep disorder and other problems in children and adolescents. The last decade has seen a remarkable upsurge in interest in these relatively common associations. Groups at risk for sleep difficulties include children living in institution, those with ASD (see Chapter 7), as well as those with ADHD (see Chapter 10). The sleep difficulties in ADHD are particularly noteworthy and can include RLS (Cortese et al., 2010). Differences in sleep are also noted in adolescents with depression, although research is needed to clarify similarities and differences from adult depression (Pigeon et al., 2012). Children and youth with anxiety problems also have sleep problems. It should also be noted that some of the drugs that are the focus of abuse (see Chapter 22) can disrupt the sleep cycle as can various psychotropic and other medications.

SLEEP PROBLEM ASSESSMENT

Assessment of sleep problems can be done with clinical interviews along with questionnaires and sleep diaries. Depending on the situation, more specific and objective methods such as actigraphy and PSG have an important role in assessment of specific disorders of sleep (Aurora et al., 2012) (see Tables 21.5 and 21.6).

Screening tools as described earlier are very helpful in detecting sleep disorders. The use of screening tools increases the detection of sleep disorders even if sleep problems are not the primary complaint (Owens & Dalzell, 2005). Given the challenges many clinicians face in understanding approaches to sleep conditions, the acronym BEARS is helpful to keep in mind. It reminds the care provider to assess: (1) Bedtime (including problems with insomnia), (2) Excessive sleepiness in daytime, (3) Awakening or abnormal behaviors during the time asleep, (4) Regulation of sleep duration, and (5) Snoring (see Table 24.5). Problems can then be explored in more detail along with physical examination to look for potential contributing factors related to body mass, tonsils, etc. Baroni and Anders (2018) provide a list of questions that can be included in a sleep interview.

Data from sleep diaries can help. These have good reliability when compared to more objective sleep measures (Werner et al., 2008). Both parents and children should complete a daily entry for a period of 1 or 2 weeks. Sleep problems can be recorded (e.g., nightmares) as well as duration, latency to sleep, etc. The diaries are available online from the Academy of Pediatrics.

EDUCATION AND PREVENTION OF SLEEP PROBLEMS

It is important that both parents and children be educated relative to healthy sleep practices—starting when the child is an infant (Hoanker & Meltzer, 2014; Mindell & Owens, 2015; Mindell et al., 2006). This helps improve later sleep patterns and includes a regular and daily sleep schedule, avoiding stimulant foods or screen time/TV in the period prior to bed, having age-appropriate naps, windows that are open to the sunlight in the morning, etc. (see Baroni & Ander, 2018). Having a consistent pattern is important. Maintaining good sleep patterns

TABLE 21.6

BEARS Form Circle or Highlight Any Question You Would Answer Yes

	Toddler/Preschool (3–5 yrs)	School-Aged (6–12 yrs)	Adolescent (13–18 yrs)
1. Bedtime Problems	Does your child have any problems going to bed? Falling asleep?	Does your child have any problems at bedtime (fights, complaints, fears)? Does your child have difficulties falling asleep?	Does your teenager have any problems falling asleep at bedtime?
2. Excessive Daytime Sleepiness	Does your child seem overtired or sleepy a lot during the day? Do they still take naps?	Does your child have difficulty waking in the morning, or seem sleepy during the day or take naps during the day?	Does your teenager have difficulty waking in the morning, seem sleepy during the day, or take naps during the day? More than average?
3. Awakenings During the Night	Does your child wake up a lot at night? Night terrors? Sleep walking?	Does your child seem to wake up a lot at night? Any sleepwalking or nightmares? Bedwetting?	Does your teenager wake up a lot at night? Does your teenager have trouble getting back to sleep in the middle of the night? Any sleepwalking or nightmares?
4. Regularity and Duration of Sleep	Does your child have difficulties maintaining a regular bedtime and wake time (falling asleep/waking up at different times)?	Does your child have difficulties maintaining a regular bedtime and wake time during school days? During weekends? Do you think they are not getting enough sleep?	Does your teenager have difficulties maintaining a regular bedtime and wake time during school days? During weekends?
5. Snoring	Does your child snore a lot or have difficulty breathing at night?	Does your child have loud or nightly snoring or any breathing difficulties at night?	Does your teenager snore loudly or nightly? Does your teenager ever stop breathing during the night?

Reprinted with permission from Baroni, A., & Anders, T. F. (2018). Sleep disorders. In A. Martin, M. H. Bloch, & F. R. Volkmar (Eds.), *Lewis's child and adolescent psychiatry: A comprehensive textbook* (5th ed., p. 583). Wolters Kluwer.

has, unfortunately, become more challenging in the modern era, but having a good bedtime routine and avoiding arousal in the period leading to sleep are important.

As Baroni and Anders (2018) point out, bedtime routines vary with age and they also note that using the bedroom for "time out" is particularly complicated for younger children. The latter may need things like transitional objects and more parental involvement in the bedtime ritual than older children. Children with developmental difficulties can experience special problems relative to sleep and may need more extensive behavioral and other supports (Buckley et al., 2020; Durand, 2014).

When indicated, clinical sleep studies in the sleep laboratory will include a range of measures. These include measures of peripheral muscle tone, eye movements, and an EEG as well as other measures of cardiac, respiratory, and peripheral motor activity. Typically, these measures are obtained from nighttime recordings in a sleep laboratory. In some cases, several nights of recording are required, particularly for children, given the potential for the various sensors and unfamiliar setting to disrupt usual sleep patterns. Increasingly there is potential for both home-based and 24 hours recording approaches, which have particularly value for children.

■ SUMMARY

Considerable progress has been made in our understanding of sleep–wake cycles in children and adolescents. Many sleep disorders can now be effectively treated. In some areas, knowledge remains limited. Clearly, sleep problems can have important negative effects on the growing child. Available research on sleep disorders varies with the age of the child, and the nature of sleep problems in relation to both general medical and psychiatric disorders remains controversial. Larger scale treatment studies are needed to establish the efficacy of commonly recommended treatments, although increasingly effective treatments are available.

References

American Academy of Sleep Medicine. (2014). *International classification of sleep disorders*. Author.

American Psychiatric Association. (2013). *Diagnostic and statistical manual of mental disorders (DSM-5)*. Author.

Aurora, R. N., Lamm, C. I., Zak, R. S., Kristo, D. A., Bista, S. R., Rowley, J. A., & Casey, K. R. (2012). Practice parameters for the non-respiratory indications for polysomnography and multiple sleep latency testing for children. *Sleep, 35*(11), 1467–1473. https://doi.org/10.5665/sleep.2190

Avidan, A. Y., & Kaplish, N. (2010). The parasomnias: Epidemiology, clinical features, and diagnostic approach. *Clinics in Chest Medicine, 31*(2), 353–370. https://doi.org/10.1016/j.ccm.2010.02.015

Barateau, L., & Dauvilliers, Y. (2019). Recent advances in treatment for narcolepsy. *Therapeutic Advances in Neurological Disorders, 12*, 1–12. https://doi.org/10.1177/1756286419875622

Baroni, A., & Anders, T. F. (2018). Sleep disorders. In A. Martin, M. Bloch, & F. R. Volkmar, (Eds.), *Lewis's child and adolescent psychiatry: A comprehensive textbook* (5th ed., pp. 580–591). Wolters Kluwer.

Billiard, M., & Sonka, K. (2015). Idiopathic hypersomnia. *Sleep Medicine Reviews, 29*, 23–33. https://doi.org/10.1016/j.smrv.2015.08.007

Brockmann, P. E., Urschitz, M. S., Schlaud, M., & Poets, C. F. (2012). Primary snoring in school children: Prevalence and neurocognitive impairments. *Sleep & Breathing, 16*(1), 23–29. https://doi.org/10.1007/s11325-011-0480-6

Buckley, A. W., Hirtz, D., Oskoui, M., Armstrong, M. J., Batra, A., Bridgemohan, C., Coury, D., Dawson, G., Donley, D., Findling, R. L., Gaughan, T., Gloss, D., Gronseth, G., Kessler, R., Merillat, S., Michelson, D., Owens, J., Pringsheim, T., Sikich, L., … Ashwal, S. (2020, March). Practice guideline: Treatment for insomnia and disrupted sleep behavior in children and adolescents with autism spectrum disorder: Report of the guideline development, dissemination, and implementation subcommittee of the American Academy of Neurology [literature review; systematic review]. *Neurology, 94*(9), 392–404. https://doi.org/10.1212/WNL.0000000000009033

Cortesi, F., Giannotti, F., Ivanenko, A., & Johnson, K. (2010). Sleep in children with autistic spectrum disorder. *Sleep medicine, 11*(7), 659–664. https://doi.org/10.1016/j.sleep.2010.01.010

Durand, V. M. (2014). *Sleep better: A guide to improving sleep for children with special needs* (Rev. ed.). Brooks Publishing.

Foulkes D. (1982). A cognitive-psychological model of REM dream production. *Sleep, 5*(2), 169–187. https://doi.org/10.1093/sleep/5.2.169

Gauchat, A., Seguin, J. R., & Zadra, A. (2014). Prevalence and correlates of disturbed dreaming in children. *Pathologie Biologie (Paris), 62*(5), 311–318. https://doi.org/10.1016/j.patbio.2014.05.016

Gonzalez-Latapi, P., & Malkani, R. (2019). Update on restless legs syndrome: From mechanisms to treatment. *Current Neurology and Neuroscience Reports, 19*(8), 54. https://doi.org/10.1007/s11910-019-0965-4

Honaker, S. M., & Meltzer, L. J. (2014). Bedtime problems and night wakings in young children: An update of the evidence. *Paediatric Respiratory Reviews*, 15(4), 333–339. https://doi.org/10.1016/j.prrv.2014.04.011

Kotagal, S., & Chopra, A. (2012). Pediatric sleep-wake disorders. *Neurologic Clinics*, 30(4), 1193–1212. https://doi.org/10.1016/j.ncl.2012.08.005

Levin, R., & Nielsen, T. A. (2007). Disturbed dreaming, posttraumatic stress disorder, and affect distress: A review and neurocognitive model. *Psychological Bulletin*, 133(3), 482–528. https://doi.org/10.1037/0033-2909.133.3.482

Marcus, C. L., Brooks, L. J., Draper, K. A., Gozal, D., Halbower, A. C., Jones, J., Schechter, M. S., Ward, S. D., Sheldon, S. H., Shiffman, R. N., Lehmann, C., Spruyt, K., & American Academy of Pediatrics. (2012). Diagnosis and management of childhood obstructive sleep apnea syndrome. *Pediatrics*, 130(3), e714–e755. https://doi.org/10.1542/peds.2012-1672

Meltzer, L. J., & Mindell, J. A. (2014). Systematic review and meta-analysis of behavioral interventions for pediatric insomnia. *Journal of Pediatric Psychology*, 39(8), 932–948. https://doi.org/10.1093/jpepsy/jsu041

Mindell, J. A., Kuhn, B., Lewin, D. S., Meltzer, L. J., Sadeh, A., & American Academy of Sleep Medicine. (2006). Behavioral treatment of bedtime problems and night wakings in infants and young children. *Sleep*, 29(10), 1263–1276.

Mindell, J. A., & Owens, J. A. (2015). *A clinical guide to pediatric sleep: Diagnosis and management of sleep problems*. Lippincott Williams & Wilkins.

Morgenthaler, T. I., Lee-Chiong, T., Alessi, C., Friedman, L., Nisha Aurora, R., Boehlecke, B., Brown, T., Chesson., A. L., Jr., Kapur, V., Maganti, R., Owens, J., Pancer, J., Swick, T. J., Zak, R., & Standards of Practice Committee of the AASM. (2007). Practice parameters for the clinical evaluation and treatment of circadian rhythm sleep disorders: An American Academy of Sleep Medicine Report. *Sleep*, 30(11), 1445–1459. https://doi.org/10.1093/sleep/30.11.1445

Owens, J. A., & Moturi, S. (2009). Pharmacologic treatment of pediatric insomnia. *Child and Adolescent Psychiatric Clinics of North America*, 18(4), 1001–1016. https://doi.org/10.1016/j.chc.2009.04.009

Petit, D., Pennestri, M.-H., Paquet, J., Desautels, A., Zadra, A., Vitaro, F., Tremblay, R. E., Boivin, M., & Montplaisir, J. (2015). Childhood sleepwalking and sleep terrors: A longitudinal study of prevalence and familial aggregation. *JAMA Pediatrics*, 169(7), 653–658. https://doi.org/10.1001/jamapediatrics.2015.127

Picchietti, D. L., Bruni, O., de Weerd, A., Durmer, J. S., Kotagal, S., Owens, J. A., Simakajornboon, N., & International Restless Legs Syndrome Study Group (IRLSSG). (2013). Pediatric restless legs syndrome diagnostic criteria: An update by the International Restless Legs Syndrome Study Group. *Sleep Medicine*, 14(12), 1253–1259. https://doi.org/10.1016/j.sleep.2013.08.778

Pigeon, W. R., Pinquart, M., & Conner, K. (2012). Meta-analysis of sleep disturbance and suicidal thoughts and behaviors. *The Journal of clinical psychiatry*, 73(9), e1160–e1167. https://doi.org/10.4088/JCP.11r07586

Reid, G. J., Huntley, E. D., & Lewin, D. S. (2009). Insomnias of childhood and adolescence. *Child and Adolescent Psychiatric Clinics of North America*, 18(4), 979–1000. https://doi.org/10.1016/j.chc.2009.06.002

Scammell T. E. (2015). Narcolepsy. *The New England Journal of Medicine*, 373(27), 2654–2662. https://doi.org/10.1056/NEJMra1500587

Taylor, D. J., & Roane, B. M. (2010). Treatment of insomnia in adults and children: A practice-friendly review of research. *Journal of Clinical Psychology*, 66(11), 1137–1147. https://doi.org/10.1002/jclp.20733

Werner, H., Molinari, L., Guyer, C., & Jenni, O. G. (2008). Agreement rates between actigraphy, diary, and questionnaire for children's sleep patterns. *Archives of Pediatrics & Adolescent Medicine*, 162(4), 350–358. https://doi.org/10.1001/archpedi.162.4.350

Won, D. C., Feldman, H. M., & Huffman, L. C. (2019, January). Sleep problem detection and documentation in children with autism spectrum disorder and attention-deficit/hyperactivity disorder by developmental-behavioral pediatricians: A DBPNet study. *Journal of Developmental and Behavioral Pediatrics*, 40(1), 20–31. https://doi.org/10.1097%2FDBP.0000000000000624

Zero To Three Press. (2005). *Diagnostic classification of mental health and developmental disorders of infancy and early childhood: Revised edition (DC: 0-3R)*. Zero To Three Press.

Suggested Readings

Bernier, A., Belanger, M.-E., & Tetreault, E. (2019). The hand that rocks the cradle: The family and parenting context of children's sleep. In B. H. Fiese, M. Celano, K. Deater-Deckard, E. N. Jouriles, & M. A. Whisman, (Eds.), *APA handbook of contemporary family psychology: Applications and broad impact of family psychology APA handbooks in psychology* (Vol. 2, pp. 137–151). American Psychological Association. https://doi.org/10.1037/0000100-009

Brown, W. J., Wilkerson, A. K., Boyd, S. J., Dewey, D., Mesa, F., & Bunnell, B. E. (2018). A review of sleep disturbance in children and adolescents with anxiety. *Journal of sleep research, 27*(3), e12635. https://doi.org/10.1111/jsr.12635

Carter, K. A., Hathaway, N. E., & Lettieri, C. F. (2014). Common sleep disorders in children. *American Family Physician, 89*(5), 368–377.

Gonzalez-Latapi, P., & Malkani, R. (2019). Update on restless legs syndrome: From mechanisms to treatment. *Current Neurology and Neuroscience Reports, 19*(8), 54. https://doi.org/10.1007/s11910-019-0965-4

Goodlin-Jones, B. L., Sitnick, S. L., Tang, K., Liu, J., & Anders, T. F. (2008). The children's sleep habits questionnaire in toddlers and preschool children. *Journal of Developmental & Behavioral Pediatrics, 29*(2), 82–88. https://doi.org/10.1097/dbp.0b013e318163c39a

Gregory, A. M., & Sadeh, A. (2015). Annual research review: Sleep problems in childhood psychiatric disorders—A review of the latest science. *Journal of Child Psychology and Psychiatry, 57*(3), 296–317. https://doi.org/10.1111/jcpp.12469

Johnson, C. R., & Malow, B. A. (2019). Parent training for sleep disturbances in autism spectrum disorder. In C. R. Johnson, E. M. Butter, & L. Scahill, (Eds.), *Parent training for autism spectrum disorder: Improving the quality of life for children and their families* (pp. 149–172). American Psychological Association. https://doi.org/10.1037/0000111-007

Klingelhoefer, L., Bhattacharya, K., & Reichmann, H. (2016). Restless legs syndrome. *Clinical Medicine (London), 16*(4), 379–382. https://doi.org/10.7861/clinmedicine.16-4-379

McDonagh, M. S., Holmes, R., & Hsu, F. (2019). Pharmacologic treatments for sleep disorders in children: A systematic review. *Journal of Child Neurology, 34*(5), 237–247. https://doi.org/10.1177/0883073818821030

Meltzer, L. J., & McLaughlin Crabtree, V. (2015a). *Pediatric sleep problems: A clinician's guide to behavioral interventions.* American Psychological Association. https://doi.org/10.1037/14645-000

Meltzer, L. J., & McLaughlin Crabtree, V. (2015b). *Typical sleep across development and healthy sleep habits. A clinician's guide to behavioral interventions.* American Psychological Association. https://doi.org/10.1037/14645-002

Picchietti, M. A., & Picchietti, D. L. (2010). Advances in pediatric restless legs syndrome: Iron, genetics, diagnosis and treatment. *Sleep Medicine, 11*(7), 643–651. https://doi.org/10.1016/j.sleep.2009.11.014

CHAPTER 22 ■ SUBSTANCE USE DISORDERS

■ BACKGROUND

Use and abuse of alcohol and narcotic substances have occurred throughout history. Advances in chemistry during the 19th and 20th centuries led to the formulation of more potent preparations as active ingredients were identified and then used to search for other agents. At one time, cocaine and opiates were widely prescribed and readily available, often being included in various elixirs and tonics. By 1914, an awareness of the potential for abuse led to federal regulation so that opiates and cocaine could only be prescribed by physicians. Similarly, the advent of Prohibition meant that alcohol was no longer freely available; as a result (until the repeal of Prohibition in 1933), there was an extensive black market in alcohol, as there now is in other substances (see Musto, 1999, for an historical review). With the creation of the U.S. Federal Bureau of Narcotics (now the Drug Enforcement Administration) in 1930, the federal government took a more active role in regulating substances with potential for abuse. Throughout the second half of the 20th century and to the present time, there have been major societal shifts in the acceptance and use of various substances—including marijuana, alcohol, and tobacco.

Pharmacologic advances have improved our understanding of brain processes and the mechanisms that may underlie substance abuse. Until recently, most of the research on substance abuse and substance dependence has come from work with adults. There has been less research on children and adolescents. Unsurprisingly, adolescents who abuse drugs or alcohol have high risk for developing dependence in adulthood (Hopfer et al., 2018).

■ DEFINITIONS

Drug addiction refers to a group of chronic and relapsing disorders that are characterized by compulsion to seek and take a drug, loss of control in limiting drug use, and experience of negative emotional states, such as dysphoria, anxiety, or irritability, when access to the drug is prevented (Koob & Volkow, 2016).

The Diagnostic and Statistical Manual of Mental Disorders, Fifth Edition (DSM-5; American Psychiatric Association, 2013) combined what was previously conceptualized as two separate disorders—substance abuse and substance dependence—into one category of substance use disorders. Substance use disorders are defined by the presence of cognitive, behavioral, and physiologic symptoms and indicate that a person continues to use a substance despite experiencing significant problems. Substance use disorders are also classified by severity based on the number of symptoms endorsed and by course specifiers. The criteria for these diagnoses are described in Table 22.1.

The second category of substance-related and addictive disorders in the current edition of the *DSM* is substance-induced disorders. This category includes intoxication, withdrawal, and other disorders such as substance-induced depression or substance-induced psychotic disorder. Substances of potential abuse are divided into ten classes of known drugs: alcohol, caffeine, cannabis, stimulants, hallucinogens, inhalants, nicotine, opioids, phencyclidine, sedative-hypnotic, and other (or unknown) categories. As a practical matter, in children and adolescents, substance use disorders are more frequently encountered than substance-induced disorders that are characterized by withdrawal syndromes (Hopfer et al., 2018).

The various substances of abuse vary in both their physiologic effects and potential for addiction. A person's individual factors (e.g., genetic risk for substance abuse) as well as route

TABLE 22.1

Criteria for Substance Use Disorder, Intoxication, and Withdrawal

Substance Use Disorder: Two or more within a 12-month period
Impaired Control
1. Taken in larger amounts or over a longer period than intended 2. Persistent desire or unsuccessful effort to cut down or control use 3. Great deal of time spent to obtain, use, or recover from substance 4. Craving, or strong desire or urge to use
Social Impairment
1. Failure to fulfill major role obligations 2. Continued use despite social or interpersonal problems 3. Reduction in important social, occupational, or recreational activities
Risky Use
1. Recurrent use in physically hazardous situations 2. Continued use despite knowledge of physical or psychological problem
Pharmacologic Effect
1. Tolerance (need for increased amount or diminished effect) 2. Withdrawal (withdrawal syndrome or use to relieve/avoid withdrawal)
Intoxication
A. Recent ingestion B. Problematic behavior or psychological changes C. One or more sign or symptom attributable to the substance D. Not attributable to another medical condition, mental disorder, or substance
Withdrawal
A. Cessation or reduction in heavy, prolonged use B. Two or more signs or symptoms attributable to cessation or reduction in use C. Clinically significant distress or impairment in important areas of functioning D. Not attributable to another medical condition, mental disorder, or substance

Reprinted with permission from Hopfer, C., Hinckley, J. D., & Riggs, P. (2018). Substance use disorders. In A. Martin, M. H. Bloch, & F. R. Volkmar (Eds.), *Lewis's child and adolescent psychiatry: A comprehensive textbook* (5th ed., p. 569). Wolters Kluwer.

of administration (e.g., intravenously), can all be important in determining how rapidly one may develop a substance dependency.

Alcohol is often the first substance adolescents use and accounts for much of adolescent substance use and abuse (e.g., group drinking at parties). According to national surveys, about 6% of adolescents met criteria for alcohol abuse or dependence in the previous year. Acute alcohol intoxication is characterized by sedation, slurred speech, decreased heart rate, poor coordination, and reduced blood pressure. Repeated drinking can lead to tolerance and, occasionally, adolescents can even experience alcohol withdrawal states. As with adults, alcohol withdrawal may require emergency medical management. Severe alcohol intoxication can also be an emergent medical problem and can lead to death at high levels. Impaired judgment and coordination also contribute to accidental death and injuries.

Nicotine in tobacco products can lead to dependency and is associated with a number of medical problems. The effects of nicotine are prompt after inhalation or ingestion (e.g., from chewing) and include central nervous system (CNS) stimulation followed by symptoms of withdrawal. The mechanism of nicotine on acetylcholine receptors is well known. With a half-life of several hours, nicotine can accumulate in the body over the course of the day. Cessation of use can result in irritability, characteristic craving, and problems in mood and concentration. One of the major concerns about tobacco use is its potential for serving as an entry to use of other substances. Over the past two decades, there has been a considerable decline in adolescent cigarette smoking. The nationwide percentage of 12th-grade students who reported ever smoking a cigarette dropped dramatically from 65% to 24%. Rates dropped among younger students, as well, from 55% to 20% in 10th graders, and 41% to 9% in eighth graders (Miech et al., 2020). In contrast, nicotine vaping among U.S. adolescents has increased at a record pace from 2017 to 2019, prompting new national policies to reduce access to flavors of vaping products preferred by youth. Vaping has decreased since 2020 in response to decreased accessibility of vaping products and increased awareness of health risks. However, nicotine vaping remains highly prevalent in adolescents, with 40% lifetime prevalence rates in latest surveys (Miech et al., 2021).

Marijuana is the most frequently used illicit drug by adolescents, and marijuana dependence is the most frequently cited reason for adolescent admissions to substance abuse treatment. The mechanisms of the active ingredient Δ-9 tetrahydrocannabinol (THC) have been increasingly studied. This agent binds to the cannabinoid receptor (CNR1), which is widely distributed in the brain. Effects on anxiety, appetite, and pain are reported, as are analgesic effects and enhancement of appetite. Hallucinogenic effects can also be noted. Cannabis withdrawal syndrome, which is now recognized in *DSM-5*, consists of symptoms including irritability, anger, aggression, anxiety, sleep disturbance, restlessness, and depressed mood (Hasin, 2018).

Abuse of heroin and prescription opiates has increased over the past decade and has become a source of increasing national concern. The opioid epidemic has gained public awareness within the past two decades, with nonmedical prescription opioid use emerging as a national crisis and declared a public health emergency. A recent survey suggests that as many as 1 in 20 twelfth graders in high school reported using prescription opioids illicitly (Carmona et al., 2020). Frequent nonmedical opioid use is the most significant risk factor for heroin use (Compton et al., 2016). The price of heroin has decreased over the years, and the use of various routes of administration of purer heroin, including smoking and snorting, has likely contributed to this increase. Heroin has a very significant potential for addiction, and its use is associated with a range of problems impacting adolescents at home and in school.

Cocaine has various psychological effects, including a sense of mental clarity and lack of fatigue. Physical effects include increased heart rate, temperature, and blood pressure, as well as dilated pupils. The route of administration leads to major differences in the duration of cocaine's effects (e.g., smoking leads to a more intense but shorter high than snorting). About 6% of users become dependent within 1 year (Hopfer et al., 2018).

Amphetamines have a long history of legitimate use in medicine, including in the treatment of attention-deficit disorders. Various street names for methamphetamine include *ice*, *speed*, *crystal*, *glass*, and *crank*. This agent can be used in a host of ways, including injection, inhalation, and smoking. Similar to cocaine, dependence can develop quickly and is associated with a rapid decline in functioning. Associated effects can include psychotic behavior, aggression, and various neuropsychological deficits, such as memory loss. Appetite suppression is common, as is decreased need for sleep. Euphoria is often noted. Physical effects include hyperthermia, increased respiration, and increased risk for seizures.

MDMA (3,4-methylenedioxymethamphetamine) ("Ecstasy") is another frequently abused agent with both stimulant and psychedelic effects. Taken orally, the psychedelic effects of the agent last for several hours. Mental status changes can include anxiety, paranoia, depression, and sleeplessness. Physical symptoms can include blurred version, a sense of muscle/body tension, nausea, and sweating; occasionally, severe hyperthermia develops. Available data suggest that most users stop use of the agent in young adulthood, although some who become dependent continue.

GHB (γ-hydroxybutyrate), known colloquially as *G*, *grievous bodily harm*, or *liquid Ecstasy*, was originally used as a muscle growth agent and sold in health food stores before its effects on the CNS were recognized. A CNS depressant, many of the effects of GHB are similar to those of alcohol. Effects last for several hours. Dependence can develop along with a withdrawal syndrome similar to that sometimes seen with benzodiazepines. About 2% of high school seniors report use of this agent in the previous year (Hopfer et al., 2018).

Approximately 5% of U.S. high school students report having tried inhalants at least once in the past year; however, rates of inhalant abuse or dependence are much lower, as only 0.1% of adolescents report abuse or dependence on inhalants (Hopfer et al., 2018). Inhalants are volatile organic compounds that include many gases and fumes that are deliberately taken in order to achieve intoxication. These organic fumes and gases are more frequently abused by younger adolescents probably because of greater accessibility. These compounds can be sprayed into the mouth or inhaled either through putting the material into a cloth and inhaling it ("huffed") or via a bag ("bagged"). Psychological effects include euphoria and disorientation. A period of drowsiness or confusion may follow. A variety of materials are inhaled. They have the potential for causing relatively rapid neurologic features and changes in cognition. Their continued use can lead to neurotoxicity, making detection and treatment important public health problems.

Approximately 0.6% to 2.0% of male U.S. high school students report having used anabolic steroids within the past year, down by approximately half among younger adolescents over the past decade (Hopfer et al., 2018). The main goal of steroid use is building muscle mass, so intrinsically, abuse of these agents differs from that of other substances in which the desired effect is psychological. There are many different medical sequelae, including stopping growth prematurely and testicular shrinkage, and psychological problems that can include pronounced mood swings and even psychosis.

■ EPIDEMIOLOGY AND DEMOGRAPHICS

There have been major changes in adolescent drug use over the past decade in the United States. As noted in Table 22.1, there have been some fluctuations in patterns of substance abuse, although the most consistently used substances in adolescents have included alcohol, tobacco, and marijuana. About one-third of high school seniors report use of some illegal substance (apart from marijuana) at some point in their lives. Variations in patterns of substance abuse are noteworthy but not always well understood. There has been a noteworthy decrease in smoking in adolescents during the past two decades. Despite substantial long-term declines in alcohol use, there has been some increase in the prevalence of binge drinking over the past 2 years (2019–2020). By the end of high school, nearly two out of three students (61.5%) have consumed alcohol, and a quarter of students (26%) had done so by the eighth grade (Johnston et al., 2021).

Age-related data from publicly funded substance abuse treatment programs are also presented in Table 22.2. For younger adolescents, marijuana is most frequently cited as the primary substance of abuse, but for the oldest adolescents and young adults, marijuana combined with alcohol continues to be a major problem along with a variety of other substances.

TABLE 22.2

Primary Admitting Substance of Abuse (% of Total Admissions), by Age, from the Treatment Episode Data Set

Substance	Age 12–14 (%)	Age 15–17 (%)	Age 18–19 (%)	Age 20–24 (%)
Other/none	5.9	2.7	2.5	1.9
Alcohol only	6.9	4.3	9.0	11.1
Alcohol + secondary drug	6.4	8.3	11.7	12.3
Opioids, heroin	0.3	2.0	15.3	25.9
Opioids, other	0.8	1.7	6.9	12.1
Cocaine, smoked	0.2	0.2	0.6	1.0
Cocaine, other route	0.2	0.4	0.9	1.3
Marijuana	77.0	75.5	44.2	24.4
Methamphetamine/ amphetamine	1.4	3.7	7.1	8.3
Tranquilizers	0.3	0.5	1.0	1.0
Sedatives	0.1	0.1	0.2	0.1
Hallucinogens	0.2	0.4	0.5	0.2
Phencyclidine	<0.05	<0.05	0.1	0.2
Inhalants	0.4	0.1	0.1	0.1
Total percent	100	100	100	100
(Total, N)	(17,842)	(83,823)	(54,509)	(244,893)

From TEDS. (2005). *Treatment episode data set: 2003 highlights. National Admissions to Substance Abuse Treatment Services.* DASIS Series: S-27. DHHS Publication No. SMA 05-4043. Department of Health and Human Services, with permission. https://wwwdasis.samhsa.gov/dasis2/teds_pubs/2003_teds_highlights_rpt.pdf

Boys and young men are more likely to engage in substance abuse and also are more likely to meet criteria for substance use disorders in late adolescence, particularly for alcohol and marijuana. Girls and young women are more likely to report nicotine dependence. Rates of substance use disorders are high in the mental health setting and even more so in the juvenile justice setting, where a majority of individuals meet lifetime criteria for substance use disorders.

Risk appears to increase with early onset of substance use. It remains unclear why this is so, although animal studies have suggested greater potential for vulnerability to drug sensitization during the adolescent period. It may also be that early use of substances arises as a result of more general risk factors.

■ ETIOLOGY

Various risk factors are associated with substance abuse disorders in adolescents. Obviously, development of these disorders depends on ready access to substances. However, even when these substances are widely available, only a small number of adolescents develop substance use disorders. Attempts have been made to understand genetic and environmental factors using twin and adoption studies. Genetic factors become more apparent if environments support their expression (Waaktaar et al., 2018). Genetic mechanisms can involve a direct impact on the ability to metabolize or react to substances (Ducci & Goldman, 2012). Effects may also be more indirect (e.g., by impacting other aspects of development or behavior). It is clear that family history of substance abuse or dependence is a powerful predictor of risk.

Risk for substance abuse and dependence is increased in association with a number of other conditions. For example, the various externalizing disorders are a major risk factor for initiation of substance use (Zellers et al., 2020). Because of their frequent association with each other, disentangling contributions of these conditions is complicated, but it is clear that conduct disorder is a major risk factor for substance use, and the less severe oppositional defiant disorder (ODD) and even attention-deficit/hyperactivity disorder (ADHD) also increase risk (Molina & Pelham, 2014). In addition, parenting, home environment, neighborhood factors such as alcohol and drug availability, and peer influence have all been shown to impact substance use onset and outcomes (Buu et al., 2009). The aggregation of substance use or abuse in families has genetic and environmental components. Clearly, use or abuse of substances by parents or older siblings increases risk. Peer effects are also important, although the notion that "peer pressure" leads directly to substance abuse is overly simplistic.

Various models have been developed to understand the pattern and progression of substance abuse. Stage theory suggests that alcohol or tobacco is first used followed by marijuana before the adolescent goes on to use other substances (Kandel et al., 1992). A similar notion, the "gateway hypothesis," views marijuana as the key to the adolescent going on to use other drugs. Various explanations have been used to account for this mechanism.

Animal studies have demonstrated chronic behavioral, neurobiologic, and physiologic effects of substance use and abuse. Loss of the substance leads the dependent animal into a pattern of craving and dysphoria similar to that seen in humans. The current view of the neurobiology of addiction conceptualizes addiction as a three-stage cycle of intoxication, withdrawal/negative affect, and preoccupation/anticipation (craving) that involve changes in the brain systems of reward, stress, and executive functioning (Volkow & Boyle, 2018).

■ DIFFERENTIAL DIAGNOSIS AND ASSESSMENT

Typically, information on substance use is obtained through direct interview of the adolescent, as well as through parents, teachers, and other sources. An adolescent with a substance abuse problem often minimizes it. In general, the clinician should try to foster rapport with the patient using a nonjudgmental, empathetic, but honest approach designed to build a therapeutic relationship. The clinician should be clear about confidentiality and its limits. The adolescent should understand that, within certain limits, rules of confidentiality do apply with important exceptions relating to dangerous behaviors (see Hopfer et al., 2018). Assuring the adolescent of confidentiality (within stated limitations) generally encourages honest reporting of substance abuse problems. Relevant information from the adolescent will include the nature and extent of substance use or abuse, its onset and persistence, and association with other relevant factors in the adolescent's life (e.g., relation to stress, depression, impulse control problems). Often, the initial interview is best done with both the adolescent and parents present so that rules for the evaluation can be heard by all parties concerned.

The interview with parents should complement the interview with the adolescent in order to help the clinician understand relevant factors from history and current functioning of the child and family. The interview with the adolescent can then follow. As is often true with adolescents, beginning the interview with more affective neutral topics (e.g., developmental history) before moving to more sensitive ones is often helpful.

As noted previously, the differential diagnosis is complicated by significant potential for comorbidity to be present; in adolescents, comorbidity is present more than half the time and, in at least one study, almost 75% of the time. In addition, the clinician must determine whether substance abuse or substance dependence is present. Both externalizing disorders (ODD, conduct, ADHD) and internalizing disorders (anxiety, mood disorders) can be present,

---

| **BOX 22.1** | **Case Report: Adolescent Substance Abuse** |

Timmy, a 15-year-old boy, was seen for evaluation at the request of his parents, who were concerned about a noteworthy decline in academic skills over the past months (since starting high school) associated with increasing behavioral difficulties at home. The latter took the form of an apparent lack of engagement alternating, at times, with angry confrontations with parents and family members. Until about 1 year prior, he had been reported to be a solid academic student who was deeply engaged in several sports. On moving into high school (in the sophomore year), he had become involved with a new group of friends. His mother suspected that he had been drinking on several occasions when he came home late; she also discovered cigarettes and, recently, found a joint of marijuana in his clothing. When confronted about this, Timmy denied any problems and complained that his parents were hounding him. He reported that school was now boring. In the interview with his parents, it appeared that several stressors had contributed to both parents being less involved with Timmy over the past several years; this included a serious medical illness in a younger sibling and the onset of marital problem partly related to the younger sibling's repeated hospitalizations. They also noted that several relatives had a strong history of substance abuse, mostly involving alcohol.

During the interview, Timmy inquired about confidentiality. Although seemingly disinterested at first, he became more involved in the interview and disclosed a history of polysubstance abuse extending back over about 18 months, starting with cigarettes and an occasional beer and progressing to marijuana use. He had recently moved on to try a range of other street drugs, including amphetamines. Several of his new friends at school used drugs extensively. It appeared that with the beginning of high school and a heavier academic demand and increased demands by coaches, he began to use substances in combination, often drinking and smoking pot. As he became more engaged in the assessment, both significant anxiety and depression were noted. Treatment included family support, cognitive behavior therapy (CBT), examination of his school program, and provision of some academic supports. At follow-up 1 year later, he was doing well.

Comment: This case illustrates several features relatively typical in adolescents with substance use problems. Timmy began to use nicotine and alcohol, gradually adding other substances. Family stress and lack of supervision combined with anxiety and some degree of depression with regard to both his family situation and school demands also contributed to his problems. As is often the case, treatment was multimodal. It is somewhat less typical for adolescents to have depression and anxiety problems; externalizing difficulties (in this case possibly including the angry outbursts) are more frequent.

Reprinted with permission from Volkmar, F. R., & Martin, A. (2011). *Essentials of Lewis's child and adolescent psychiatry* (1st ed., p. 203). Lippincott Williams & Wilkins/Wolters Kluwer.

although it is somewhat more likely for externalizing disorders to coexist with substance abuse problems.

Laboratory studies, particularly urine toxicology screening, have assumed increased importance in screening for substance abuse. It is important, however, to realize that some substances are more readily detected or are only detectable for brief periods (e.g., inhalants are difficult to detect in urine, and alcohol is quickly eliminated). In most clinical settings, a standard panel of tests is available that is focused on the most commonly used substance. Detection times are summarized in Table 22.3. Alcohol levels can be assessed using a breathalyzer, and to detect hallucinogens, MDMA, and GHB, specialized tests are required.

TABLE 22.3

Urine Substance Detection Periods (Typical)

Substance	Urine Detection Time
Alcohol	After absorption, decreases by –0.02 g%/hour
Amphetamine	24–72 hours
Barbiturates	1–2 days
Benzodiazepines	3 days for therapeutic dose
Cannabis (single use)	1–3 days
Cannabis (moderate use)	3–5 days
Cannabis (heavy use)	10 days
Cocaine	24–96 hours
Codeine/morphine	24–72 hours
Heroin	24–72 hours
Methamphetamine	24–72 hours
PCP	14–30 days
LSD	1.5–5 days

LSD, lysergic acid diethylamide; PCP, phencyclidine.
Reprinted with permission from Hopfer, C., Hinckley, J. D., & Riggs, P. (2018). Substance use disorders. In A. Martin, M. H. Bloch, & F. R. Volkmar (Eds.), *Lewis's child and adolescent psychiatry: A comprehensive textbook* (5th ed., p. 572). Wolters Kluwer.

TREATMENT

Given the complex nature of substance abuse problems and frequent associations with other conditions, treatment planning should be flexible and based on an awareness of the chronicity of these conditions and the potential for relapse. Often, the adolescent is not the person complaining, and motivation, or lack thereof, for treatment is important to assess. Initial efforts typically focus on eliminating or reducing substance use, addressing the various needs of the adolescent, and preventing relapse. Various evidence-based treatment approaches are now available. In selected cases, the judicious use of psychopharmacologic interventions (e.g., to address comorbid problems) may be useful (Hopfer et al., 2018).

Screening and brief intervention in primary care usually consist of one or two sessions that can be conducted by primary care providers to address adolescent alcohol and cannabis use. The advantage of this approach is that it can be administered in a variety of settings including primary health care clinics, schools, emergency departments, and outpatient mental health settings. This approach can also enable early detection that is consistent with early intervention and prevention approaches and has demonstrated effectiveness in this capacity (Steele et al., 2020). However, this approach has limited utility as a standalone treatment for adolescents meeting criteria for substance use disorders who require more comprehensive treatments (Gray & Squeglia, 2018).

A wide range of school-based prevention and intervention programs have been studied and demonstrated small but meaningful effects on knowledge and attitudes (Stockings et al., 2016). Overall, interventions that focus on general psychosocial development and life skills may be more effective than substance-specific treatments (Foxcroft & Tsertsvadze, 2011a, 2011b). Interventions that target awareness of illicit drug harm generally do not change drug use behavior in young people. However, skill-based interventions that explicitly address social competences and refusal have been shown to have effects, albeit small, on tobacco smoking onset and cannabis use in adolescents (Thomas et al., 2013). A major limitation of school-based programs is that they do not include students who are often absent or have left school and who can be most at risk for substance use. Family and community-based interventions encourage improved monitoring and better parent–child communication. This type of program has been shown to delay the onset of alcohol and tobacco and prevent illicit drug use in both low- and high-risk youth (Stockings et al., 2016).

Motivational enhancement techniques help establish a treatment alliance and initial engagement. This set of empirically based techniques increases motivation to change by systematically focusing on "change talk" and behavioral changes. These techniques can be particularly useful for adolescents, who often have, at best, ambivalence about treatment. These methods can also be combined with family or other individual treatment approaches (Jensen et al., 2011).

CBT has also been systematically studied, and there is evidence that this modality can be helpful for reducing tobacco (Bryant et al., 2011) and cannabis use disorders (Dennis et al., 2004). CBT is also an effective treatment for anxiety and depression disorders that often co-occur with substance use. These structured treatments are usually time limited, lasting from 5 to 16 weeks. The treatments focus on cognitive distortions and learned behaviors associated with substance abuse, combined with methods to teach more effective coping strategies (e.g., in dealing with stress and drug cravings). These methods also focus on social and communication skills.

Various family-based treatment approaches have been used in the management of adolescents with substance abuse problems. These treatments have the advantage of focusing more broadly on the context of the substance abuse and have demonstrated efficacy. Multisystemic therapy uses frequent home visits and ready accessibility to therapists and has been highly effective in ensuring that adolescents remain in treatment. Less intensive approaches include brief strategic family therapy and multidimensional family therapy (Liddle et al., 2018). Small but significant effects on high-risk and harmful behaviors have been identified in several well-designed studies (Baldwin et al., 2012).

When comorbid conditions are present, pharmacotherapy may be a relevant consideration (Hopfer et al., 2018). Despite the availability of potentially helpful treatments, many adolescents who enter treatment for substance use often do not complete recommended programs or continue to require ongoing support and treatment (Passetti et al., 2016).

■ COURSE

The prognosis of substance abuse disorders depends on the nature of the substance used, the severity of the problem, and the presence of comorbid conditions. In general, earlier onset is associated with more severe difficulties, comorbidity, and worse outcome. Unfortunately, substance abuse problems are often chronic with periods of better control followed by relapse.

■ SUMMARY

Adolescents, and sometimes children, who abuse substances present important challenges for mental and public health. In adolescents, abuse, rather than dependence, is more frequently encountered. A range of different substances are abused, often in combination with each other. Adolescent substance abuse can lead to substance dependence in adulthood. Substance use problems are particularly frequent in juvenile justice and mental health settings. Adolescents who abuse substances of various types often have associated psychopathology, particularly externalizing disorders.

References

*Indicates Particularly Recommended

American Psychiatric Association. (2013). *Diagnostic and statistical manual of mental disorders (DSM-5)* (5th ed.). American Psychiatric Publishing.

Baldwin, S. A., Christian, S., Berkeljon, A., & Shadish, W. R. (2012). The effects of family therapies for adolescent delinquency and substance abuse: A meta-analysis. *Journal of Marital and Family Therapy*, 38(1), 281–304. https://doi.org/10.1111/j.1752-0606.2011.00248.x

Bryant, J., Bonevski, B., Paul, C., McElduff, P., & Attia, J. (2011). A systematic review and meta-analysis of the effectiveness of behavioural smoking cessation interventions in selected disadvantaged groups. *Addiction*, 106(9), 1568–1585. https://doi.org/10.1111/j.1360-0443.2011.03467.x

Buu, A., DiPiazza, C., Wang, J., Puttler, L. I., Fitzgerald, H. E., & Zucker, R. A. (2009). Parent, family, and neighborhood effects on the development of child substance use and other psychopathology from preschool to the start of adulthood. *Journal of Studies on Alcohol and Drugs*, 70(4), 489–498. https://doi.org/10.15288/jsad.2009.70.489

*Carmona, J., Maxwell, J. C., Park, J. Y., & Wu, L. T. (2020). Prevalence and health characteristics of prescription opioid use, misuse, and use disorders among U.S. adolescents. *Journal of Adolescent Health*, 66(5), 536–544. https://doi.org/10.1016/j.jadohealth.2019.11.306

Compton, W. M., Jones, C. M., & Baldwin, G. T. (2016). Relationship between nonmedical prescription-opioid use and heroin use. *New England Journal of Medicine*, 374(2), 154–163. https://doi.org/10.1056/NEJMra1508490

*Dennis, M., Godley, S. H., Diamond, G., Tims, F. M., Babor, T., Donaldson, J., Liddle, H., Titus, J. C., Kaminer, Y., Webb, C., Hamilton, N., & Funk, R. (2004). The Cannabis Youth Treatment (CYT) study: Main findings from two randomized trials. *Journal of Substance Abuse Treatment*, 27(3), 197–213. https://doi.org/10.1016/j.jsat.2003.09.005

Ducci, F., & Goldman, D. (2012). The genetic basis of addictive disorders. *Psychiatric Clinics of North America*, 35(2), 495–519. https://doi.org/10.1016/j.psc.2012.03.010

Foxcroft, D. R., & Tsertsvadze, A. (2011a). Universal family-based prevention programs for alcohol misuse in young people. *Cochrane Database of Systematic Reviews*, (9), CD009308. https://doi.org/10.1002/14651858.CD009308

Foxcroft, D. R., & Tsertsvadze, A. (2011b). Universal school-based prevention programs for alcohol misuse in young people. *Cochrane Database of Systematic Reviews*, (5), CD009113. https://doi.org/10.1002/14651858.CD009113

*Gray, K. M., & Squeglia, L. M. (2018). Research review: What have we learned about adolescent substance use? *Journal of Child Psychology and Psychiatry*, 59(6), 618–627. https://doi.org/10.1111/jcpp.12783

*Hasin, D. S. (2018). US epidemiology of cannabis use and associated problems. *Neuropsychopharmacology*, 43(1), 195–212. https://doi.org/10.1038/npp.2017.198

*Hopfer, C., Hinckley, J. D., & Riggs, P. (2018). Substance use disorders. In A. Martin, M. H. Bloch, & F. R. Volkmar (Eds.), *Lewis's child and adolescent psychiatry* (5th ed., pp. 568–580). Lippincott Williams & Wilkins.

*Jensen, C. D., Cushing, C. C., Aylward, B. S., Craig, J. T., Sorell, D. M., & Steele, R. G. (2011). Effectiveness of motivational interviewing interventions for adolescent substance use behavior change: A meta-analytic review. *Journal of Consulting and Clinical Psychology*, 79(4), 433–440. https://doi.org/10.1037/a0023992

*Johnston, L. D., Miech, R. A., O'Malley, P. M., Bachman, J. G., Schulenberg, J. E., & Patrick, M. E. (2021). *Monitoring the future national survey results on drug use 1975–2020: Overview, key findings on adolescent drug use*. Institute for Social Research, University of Michigan. Retrieved February 28, 2021, from http://www.monitoringthefuture.org/pubs/monographs/mtf-overview2020.pdf

Kandel, D. B., Yamaguchi, K., & Chen, K. (1992). Stages of progression in drug involvement from adolescence to adulthood: Further evidence for the gateway theory. *Journal of Studies on Alcohol*, 53(5), 447–457. https://doi.org/10.15288/jsa.1992.53.447

*Koob, G. F., & Volkow, N. D. (2016). Neurobiology of addiction: A neurocircuitry analysis. *The Lancet Psychiatry*, 3(8), 760–773. https://doi.org/10.1016/S2215-0366(16)00104-8

Liddle, H. A., Dakof, G. A., Rowe, C. L., Henderson, C., Greenbaum, P., Wang, W., & Alberga, L. (2018). Multidimensional family therapy as a community-based alternative to residential treatment for adolescents with substance use and co-occurring mental health disorders. *Journal of Substance Abuse Treatment*, 90, 47–56. https://doi.org/10.1016/j.jsat.2018.04.011

*Miech, R., Keyes, K. M., O'Malley, P. M., & Johnston, L. D. (2020). The great decline in adolescent cigarette smoking since 2000: Consequences for drug use among US adolescents. *Tobacco Control*, 29(6), 638–643. https://doi.org/10.1136/tobaccocontrol-2019-055052

*Miech, R., Leventhal, A., Johnston, L., O'Malley, P. M., Patrick, M. E., & Barrington-Trimis, J. (2021). Trends in use and perceptions of nicotine vaping among US youth from 2017 to 2020. *JAMA Pediatrics, 175*(2), 185–190. https://doi.org/10.1001/jamapediatrics.2020.5667

Molina, B. S. G., & Pelham, W. E., Jr. (2014). Attention-deficit/hyperactivity disorder and risk of substance use disorder: Developmental considerations, potential pathways, and opportunities for research. *Annual Review of Clinical Psychology, 10*, 607–639. https://doi.org/10.1146/annurev-clinpsy-032813-153722

Musto, D. F. (1999). *The American disease: Origins of narcotic control* (3rd ed.). Oxford University Press.

Passetti, L. L., Godley, M. D., & Kaminer, Y. (2016). Continuing care for adolescents in treatment for substance use disorders. *Child and Adolescent Psychiatric Clinics of North America, 25*(4), 669–684. https://doi.org/10.1016/j.chc.2016.06.003

*Steele, D. W., Becker, S. J., Danko, K. J., Balk, E. M., Adam, G. P., Saldanha, I. J., & Trikalinos, T. A. (2020). Brief behavioral interventions for substance use in adolescents: A meta-analysis. *Pediatrics, 146*(4), e20200351. https://doi.org/10.1542/peds.2020-0351

Stockings, E., Hall, W. D., Lynskey, M., Morley, K. I., Reavley, N., Strang, J., Patton, G., & Degenhardt, L. (2016). Prevention, early intervention, harm reduction, and treatment of substance use in young people. *The Lancet Psychiatry, 3*(3), 280–296. https://doi.org/10.1016/S2215-0366(16)00002-X

Thomas, R. E., McLellan, J., & Perera, R. (2013). School-based programmes for preventing smoking. *Cochrane Database of Systematic Reviews, 2017* (12), CD001293. https://doi.org/10.1002/14651858 .CD001293.pub3

*Volkow, N. D., & Boyle, M. (2018). Neuroscience of addiction: Relevance to prevention and treatment. *American Journal of Psychiatry, 175*(8), 729–740, 17101174. https://doi.org/10.1176/appi.ajp.2018

*Waaktaar, T., Kan, K. J., & Torgersen, S. (2018). The genetic and environmental architecture of substance use development from early adolescence into young adulthood: A longitudinal twin study of comorbidity of alcohol, tobacco and illicit drug use. *Addiction, 113*(4), 740–748. https://doi .org/10.1111/add.14076

Zellers, S. M., Corley, R., Thibodeau, E., Kirkpatrick, R., Elkins, I., Iacono, W. G., Hopfer, C., Hewitt, J. K., McGue, M., & Vrieze, S. (2020). Adolescent externalizing psychopathology and its prospective relationship to marijuana use development from age 14 to 30: Replication across independent longitudinal twin samples. *Behavior Genetics, 50*(3), 139–151. https://doi.org/10.1007/s10519-020-09994-8

Suggested Readings

Degenhardt, L., Stockings, E., Patton, G., Hall, W. D., & Lynskey, M. (2016). The increasing global health priority of substance use in young people. *The Lancet Psychiatry, 3*(3), 251–264. https://doi .org/10.1016/S2215-0366(15)00508-8

Haberstick, B. C., Zeiger, J. S., Corley, R. P., Hopfer, C. J., Stallings, M. C., Rhee, S. H., & Hewitt, J. K. (2011). Common and drug-specific genetic influences on subjective effects to alcohol, tobacco and marijuana use. *Addiction, 106*(1), 215–224. https://doi.org/10.1111/j.1360-0443.2010.03129.x

Hall, W. D., & Lynskey, M. (2005). Is cannabis a gateway drug? Testing hypotheses about the relationship between cannabis use and the use of other illicit drugs. *Drug and Alcohol Review, 24*(1), 39–48. https:// doi.org/10.1080/09595230500126698

Henderson, C. E., Dakof, G. A., Greenbaum, P. E., & Liddle, H. A. (2010). Effectiveness of multidimensional family therapy with higher severity substance-abusing adolescents: Report from two randomized controlled trials. *Journal of Consulting and Clinical Psychology, 78*(6), 885–897. https:// doi.org/10.1037/a0020620

Li, L., Zhu, S., Tse, N., Tse, S., & Wong, P. (2016). Effectiveness of motivational interviewing to reduce illicit drug use in adolescents: A systematic review and meta-analysis. *Addiction, 111*(5), 795–805. https://doi.org/10.1111/add.13285

Norberg, M. M., Kezelman, S., & Lim-Howe, N. (2013). Primary prevention of cannabis use: A systematic review of randomized controlled trials. *PLoS One, 8*(1), e53187. https://doi.org/10.1371/journal .pone.0053187

O'Connor, E., Thomas, R., Senger, C. A., Perdue, L., Robalino, S., & Patnode, C. (2020). Interventions to prevent illicit and nonmedical drug use in children, adolescents, and young adults: Updated evidence report and systematic review for the US Preventive Services Task Force. *JAMA, 323*(20), 2067–2079. https://doi.org/10.1001/jama.2020.1432

Spirito, A., Hernandez, L., Cancilliere, M. K., Graves, H. R., Rodriguez, A. M., Operario, D., Jones, R., & Barnett, N. P. (2018). Parent and adolescent motivational enhancement intervention for substance-using, truant adolescents: A pilot randomized trial. *Journal of Clinical Child & Adolescent Psychology, 47*(Suppl. 1), S467-S479. https://doi.org/10.1080/15374416.2017.1399402

Squeglia, L. M., Fadus, M. C., McClure, E. A., Tomko, R. L., & Gray, K. M. (2019). Pharmacological treatment of youth substance use disorders. *Journal of Child and Adolescent Psychopharmacology*, 29(7), 559–572. https://doi.org/10.1089/cap.2019.0009

Tanner-Smith, E. E., & Lipsey, M. W. (2015). Brief alcohol interventions for adolescents and young adults: A systematic review and meta-analysis. *Journal of Substance Abuse Treatment*, 51, 1–18. https://doi.org/10.1016/j.jsat.2014.09.001

Tanner-Smith, E. E., Steinka-Fry, K. T., Hennessy, E. A., Lipsey, M. W., & Winters, K. C. (2015). Can brief alcohol interventions for youth also address concurrent illicit drug use? Results from a meta-analysis. *Journal of Youth and Adolescence*, 44(5), 1011–1023. https://doi.org/10.1007/s10964-015-0252-x

Trucco, E. M. (2020). A review of psychosocial factors linked to adolescent substance use. *Pharmacology Biochemistry and Behavior*, 196, 172969. https://doi.org/10.1016/j.pbb.2020.172969

Wilens, T. E., Martelon, M., Joshi, G., Bateman, C., Fried, R., Petty, C., & Biederman, J. (2011). Does ADHD predict substance-use disorders? A 10-year follow-up study of young adults with ADHD. *Journal of the American Academy of Child and Adolescent Psychiatry*, 50(6), 543–553. https://doi.org/10.1016/j.jaac.2011.01.021

CHAPTER 23 ■ POSTTRAUMATIC STRESS DISORDER AND EFFECTS OF TRAUMA

Trauma-Related Disorders is a category of psychiatric disorders in which exposure to a traumatic event is listed explicitly as a diagnostic criterion. Although, historically, these diagnoses were classified as Anxiety Disorders, the *DSM-5* now contains a section of trauma- and stressor-related disorders including posttraumatic stress disorder (PTSD), reactive attachment disorder (RAD), disinhibited social engagement disorder (DSED), acute stress disorder, adjustment disorders, and other unspecified trauma-related disorders. These diagnoses are distinct from other disorders in the *DSM* in that their etiology is specifically linked to adverse life experiences. Children and adolescents who suffer abuse, neglect, or trauma are at increased risk for a range of mental health difficulties. Psychological symptoms following exposure to a traumatic event can vary among individuals and include a number of emotional and behavioral reactions that present similarly to fear or anxiety. However, the heterogenous group of emotional or behavioral symptoms following an identifiable stressor may be best captured by the diagnosis of an adjustment disorder.

Attachment disorders can follow periods of severe abuse or neglect during the critical development period (see Chapter 24 for more details). In the current diagnostic classification, attachment disorders and PTSD are discussed in the chapter on trauma- and stress-related disorders to underscore the common etiologic feature of exposure to traumatic events. RAD has also been formally distinguished from DSED in *DSM-5* to clearly recognize the difference between grossly underdeveloped attachment to caregivers and socially disinhibited behavior with relative strangers. However, both disorders require a developmental age of at least 9 months and duration of symptoms of more than 12 months. However, children with RAD demonstrate a consistent pattern of inhibition or emotional withdrawal around adult caregivers as well as significant negative emotional regulation and limited reciprocity. Specifically, children with RAD do not seek comfort from an attachment figure when distressed and are not calmed when comfort is offered. These difficulties in social or affective interactions may present as minimal social or emotional responsiveness to other people, a lack of positive affect, and periods of sadness, distress, or irritability that do not seem to be related to typical triggers. In DSED, children exhibit pervasive social disinhibition. In novel situations, these children are overly familiar with strangers. They do not demonstrate social reticence when meeting new adults, they tend not to check back with a caregiver in new situations, and caregivers report the child might go off with a stranger. In addition to physical intrusiveness, preschool children may exhibit verbal intrusiveness, asking overly personal questions of unfamiliar adults. These behaviors are often experienced by others as excessive and inappropriate rather than social or friendly. Although some of these features may be seen in children with other disorders, it is their presentation in the context of a lack of attachment patterns that distinguishes RAD and DSED from other disorders (Nelson et al., 2014).

Chapter 24 provides further details on the diagnosis and treatment of attachment disorders. When appropriate care is provided, infants usually rapidly develop new attachments (Wade et al., 2020). The Bucharest Early Intervention Project demonstrated that young children who were randomly selected to be removed from institutions and placed in foster care showed an early and substantial decrease in signs of RAD compared to children who remained institutionalized for longer periods of time. Children who remained in institutional care the longest had the most persistently high signs of RAD over time. In other studies of children adopted out of institutions, there have been no cases of RAD in follow-ups conducted months to years after adoption (Croft et al., 2007).

POSTTRAUMATIC STRESS DISORDER

Terms such as *shell shock* and *battle fatigue* began to be used in the early 1900s to describe the difficulties experienced by soldiers in war time. Although these problems had, in some ways, been noted for many years (e.g., during the Civil War), they became particularly noteworthy after the protracted, highly stressful trench warfare of World War I. But soldiers were not the only victims of wartime trauma. The experience of children in London suffering through World War II led Anna Freud to consider the nature of traumatic experience in children (Midgley, 2007). In Freud's original theories of neurosis, he had speculated about the role of traumatic events in producing neurotic phenomena. Anna Freud's work was concerned with the impact of stress on children and the potential, in some cases, for children to find alternative comfort figures to mitigate the effects of stressful events. In children and adolescents, violence within the family is the most common source of PTSD, although it can also emerge in the context of natural disaster, accidents, terrorism, war, and other stresses (Hoover & Kaufman, 2018).

Diagnosis, Definition, and Clinical Features

Various changes have been made to the criteria for PTSD since its inclusion in the *DSM-III* in 1980. These changes related to emerging data on the duration of symptoms, the level of trauma required, and so forth. Adoption of a minimum duration criterion (i.e., for symptoms to be present for at least 1 month) created some difficulties because a diagnosis and potential intervention were thus delayed. This was dealt with in *DSM-IV* by including a new *acute stress disorder* category. *DSM-5* criteria for PTSD added a new symptom cluster—negative alteration of cognition and mood symptom cluster and the reckless and the self-destructive behavior item in the hyperarousal symptom cluster (American Psychiatric Association, 2013). The diagnosis in children over age 6 and in adults requires at least one reexperiencing, one avoidance, two negative alteration of cognition and mood, and two hyperarousal symptoms. For the diagnosis of acute stress disorder, the child must exhibit symptoms for at least 3 days up to a maximum of 1 month after the traumatic event; at that time, continued symptoms would require that the diagnosis be changed to PTSD. The differentiation between the two conditions rests largely on the time course. In acute stress disorder, the problems last for at least 3 days and up to 1 month, but in PTSD, the symptoms have lasted more than 1 month. It is also possible for a child *not* to exhibit an acute stress disorder right away but to develop PTSD sometime after the event.

For both conditions, exposure to a traumatic event is required (this can include experience of a traumatic event personally or witnessing it); the response to the traumatic event includes intense feelings of fear, helplessness, and horror. For acute stress disorder, three or more dissociative symptoms (feelings of derealization or depersonalization, absent or detached emotional response, or even amnesia) must be present, and the traumatic event must be reexperienced (e.g., as flashbacks). In PTSD, the traumatic event is reexperienced in some way (e.g., with recurrent recollections or, in children, repetitive play, in dreams, or flashbacks with feelings of reliving the event). In both conditions, avoidance of stimuli that might trigger memories of the event is present (this is more marked in PTSD). Other symptoms in both conditions may include problems with irritability, anxiety, and exaggerated startle response. In both conditions, significant distress or impairment must be present (Smith et al., 2019).

The exposure and reexperiencing criteria for PTSD are essentially unchanged from the adult and older child criteria. However, the diagnosis of PTSD in children ages 6 and younger requires only one symptom from a combined set of items including the two avoidance symptoms and four of the seven symptoms included in the adult and older child negative alteration of cognition and mood symptom items. Symptoms that pertain to exaggerated negative beliefs, distorted cognitions, and an inability to remember events are not required for the diagnosis of PTSD in young children because of limitations in young children's ability to describe nuanced internal experiences. The *DSM* also allows for developmental differences in the presentation of symptoms in children. For example, nightmares need not be specifically trauma focused in children. Symptoms might present in children through repetitive play rather than repeated verbalization. Similarly, traumatic reenactment may be observed (e.g., inappropriate sexual behavior in sexually abused children). Despite these important changes, problems can arise in making the diagnosis in children, particularly in very young children.

Epidemiology and Demographics

In the National Comorbidity Survey for Adolescents, out of 6400 participants the rate of trauma exposure was 60%, and the lifetime prevalence of PTSD was 4.7% (McLaughlin et al., 2013). Two-thirds of adolescents in the Great Smoky Mountains Study cohort ($N = 1420$) had been exposed to trauma by the age of 16, but the point prevalence estimate for PTSD in this study was <0.5% (Copeland et al., 2007). Although the incidence of PTSD varies across studies, recent reviews estimate that approximately 16% of trauma-exposed children develop PTSD and children with symptoms of PTSD that do not reach the threshold for diagnosis may still show distress and impairment (Smith et al., 2019). Of note, trauma-exposed children are also at much greater risk of developing disorders other than PTSD. For example, in a recent epidemiologic study, prevalence rates of depression were reported to be as high as 30% and rates of conduct disorder as high as 23% (Lewis et al., 2019).

Etiology and Pathogenesis

A growing body of work on traumatic stress in children and adults has identified several important psychosocial and biologic risk factors of PTSD. These include temperamental risk factors such as early childhood emotional problems and environmental factors such as lower socioeconomic status and lack of social support. Neurobiologic characteristics including reduced volume of the hippocampus, the ventromedial prefrontal cortex, may possibly be a potential source of vulnerability (Boccia et al., 2016). Genetic factors can explain why some children exposed to trauma develop PTSD and others do not, although these genetic markers are likely to predispose individuals to a wide range of psychopathology rather than one specific disorder (Montalvo-Ortiz et al., 2016). The type of traumatic events as well as the severity and chronicity of exposure to trauma are among the most researched predictors of onset and severity of PTSD (Brewin et al., 2000).

Differential Diagnosis and Assessment

Competent assessment of PTSD or exposure to traumatic events requires collection of information from multiple sources. Incidents of sexual or physical abuse are frequently denied by parents and children. Domestic violence is the form of violence exposure reported most frequently by parents. There is considerable potential for traumatic exposures to be missed if only one or two sources are relied on for reporting. Several excellent measures are available to help assess childhood trauma. For example, the Clinician Administered PTSD Scale for Children and Adolescents (CAPS-CA) is a structured interview for diagnostic assessment of PTSD in 8 to 15-year-old children. It is one of the most frequently used interviews in research studies and was recently updated to accommodate the *DSM-5* diagnoses (Pynoos et al., 2015) (Table 23.1). The Child PTSD Symptom Scale (CPSS) (Foa et al., 2018) is widely used measure for 8-to-15-year-old children.

A number of issues can arise during assessment of potential trauma in children. At times, children may deny the experience of a traumatic event that is well documented. In such instances, the child can be carefully informed of what is known from other sources and inquiry can be made regarding PTSD symptoms without necessarily asking for a detailed review of their experience of the event. The discussion can start with symptoms related to overarousal before moving on to the avoidance symptoms and finally to reexperiencing symptoms that are most challenging for children to talk about. The clinician should be particularly aware of symptoms that are less likely to be noted by parents, foster parents, or other caregivers. For example, "acting out" or disruptive behavior symptoms are more likely to be noticed by third parties than internalizing symptoms.

Comorbid psychiatric difficulties also commonly develop over the course of time in individuals with PTSD; additional conditions frequently include major depression and other mood disorders as well as substance abuse. Diagnosis can be complicated because symptoms of both disorders can be simultaneously present. The symptoms of major depression should,

TABLE 23.1

DSM-5 Criteria for Acute Stress Disorder and Posttraumatic Stress Disorder

Acute Stress Disorder	Posttraumatic Stress Disorder
A. Exposure to actual or threatened death, serious injury, or sexual violence in one or more of the following ways: 1. Directly experiencing the traumatic event(s). 2. Witnessing, in person, the event(s) as it occurred to others. 3. Learning that the traumatic event(s) occurred to a close family member or close friend. In cases of actual or threatened death of a family member or friend, the event(s) must have been violent or accidental. 4. Experiencing repeated or extreme exposure to aversive details of the traumatic event(s) (e.g., first responders collecting human remains; police officers repeatedly exposed to details of child abuse). *Note:* Criterion A4 does not apply to exposure through electronic media, television, movies, or pictures, unless this exposure is work related.	A. Exposure to actual or threatened death, serious injury, or sexual violence in one or more of the following ways: 1. Directly experiencing the traumatic event(s). 2. Witnessing, in person, the event(s) as it occurred to others. 3. Learning that the traumatic event(s) occurred to a close family member or close friend. In cases of actual or threatened death of a family member or friend, the event(s) must have been violent or accidental. 4. Experiencing repeated or extreme exposure to aversive details of the traumatic event(s) (e.g., first responders collecting human remains; police officers repeatedly exposed to details of child abuse). *Note:* Criterion A4 does not apply to exposure through electronic media, television, movies, or pictures, unless this exposure is work related.

(continued)

TABLE 23.1

DSM-5 **Criteria for Acute Stress Disorder and Posttraumatic Stress Disorder** (***Continued***)

Acute Stress Disorder	Posttraumatic Stress Disorder
B. Presence of nine (or more) of the following symptoms: Intrusion Symptoms: 　1. Recurrent, involuntary, and intrusive distressing memories of the traumatic event(s). 　　*Note:* In children, repetitive play may occur in which themes or aspects of the traumatic event(s) are expressed. Also, in children <6 years of age, spontaneous and intrusive memories may not appear distressing. 　2. Recurrent distressing dreams in which the content and/or effect of the dream are related to the traumatic event(s). 　　*Note:* In children, there may be frightening dreams without recognizable content. 　3. Dissociative reactions (e.g., flashbacks) in which the individual feels or acts as if the traumatic event(s) were recurring. (Such reactions may occur on a continuum, with the most extreme expression being a complete loss of awareness of present surroundings.) 　　*Note:* In children, trauma-specific reenactment may occur in play. 　4. Intense or prolonged psychological distress or marked physiologic reactions at exposure to internal or external cues that symbolize or resemble an aspect of the traumatic event(s).	B. Presence of one (or more) of the following intrusion symptoms associated with the traumatic event(s), beginning after the traumatic event(s) occurred: 　1. Recurrent, involuntary, and intrusive distressing memories of the traumatic event(s). 　　*Note:* In children, repetitive play may occur in which themes or aspects of the traumatic event(s) are expressed. Also, in children <6, spontaneous and intrusive memories may not appear distressing. 　2. Recurrent distressing dreams in which the content and/or effect of the dream are related to the traumatic event(s). 　　*Note:* In children, there may be frightening dreams without recognizable content. 　3. Dissociative reactions (e.g., flashbacks) in which the individual feels or acts as if the traumatic event(s) were recurring. (Such reactions may occur on a continuum, with the most extreme expression being a complete loss of awareness of present surroundings.) 　　*Note:* In children, trauma-specific reenactment may occur in play. 　4. Intense or prolonged psychological distress at exposure to internal or external cues that symbolize or resemble an aspect of the traumatic event(s). 　5. Marked physiologic reactions to internal or external cues that symbolize or resemble an aspect of the traumatic event(s).
C. Avoidance Symptoms: 　1. Efforts to avoid distressing memories, thoughts, or feelings about or closely associated with the traumatic event(s). 　2. Efforts to avoid external reminders (people, places, conversations, activities, objects, situations) that arouse distressing memories, thoughts, or feelings about or closely associated with the traumatic event(s).	C. Persistent avoidance of stimuli associated with the traumatic event(s), beginning after the traumatic event(s) occurred, as evidenced by one or both of the following: 　1. Avoidance of or efforts to avoid distressing memories, thoughts, or feelings about or closely associated with the traumatic event(s). 　2. Avoidance of or efforts to avoid external reminders (people, places, conversations, activities, objects, situations) that arouse distressing memories, thoughts, or feelings about or closely associated with the traumatic event(s).

TABLE 23.1

DSM-5 **Criteria for Acute Stress Disorder and Posttraumatic Stress Disorder** (*Continued*)

Acute Stress Disorder	Posttraumatic Stress Disorder
D. Negative Mood and Dissociative Symptoms: 1. Persistent inability to experience positive emotions (e.g., inability to experience happiness, satisfaction, or loving feelings). 2. Inability to remember an important aspect of the traumatic event(s) (typically due to dissociative amnesia and not due to other factors such as head injury, alcohol, or drugs). 3. An altered sense of the reality of one's surroundings or oneself (e.g., seeing oneself from another's perspective, being in a daze, time slowing).	D. Negative alterations in cognitions and mood associated with the traumatic event(s), beginning or worsening after the traumatic event(s) occurred, as evidenced by two (or more) of the following: 1. Persistent inability to experience positive emotions (e.g., inability to experience happiness, satisfaction, or loving feelings). 2. Inability to remember an important aspect of the traumatic event(s) (typically due to dissociative amnesia and not due to other factors such as head injury, alcohol, or drugs). This item is not included in the criteria for children of age 6 and below. 3. Persistent and exaggerated negative beliefs or expectations about oneself, others, or the world (e.g., "I am bad," "No one can be trusted," "The world is completely dangerous," "My whole nervous system is permanently ruined"). This item is not included in the criteria for children of age 6 and below. 4. Persistent, distorted cognitions about the cause or consequences of the traumatic event(s) that lead the individual to blame themselves or others. This item is not included in the criteria for children of age 6 and below. 5. Persistent negative emotional state (e.g., fear, horror, anger, guilt, or shame). 6. Markedly diminished interest or participation in significant activities. 7. Feelings of detachment or estrangement from others. This item is behaviorally anchored as "socially withdrawn" for children of age 6 and below. *Note:* For children of age 6 and below, only one symptom is required from the combined set of items included in criterion C and criterion D.

(*continued*)

TABLE 23.1

DSM-5 Criteria for Acute Stress Disorder and Posttraumatic Stress Disorder (Continued)

Acute Stress Disorder	Posttraumatic Stress Disorder
E. Arousal Symptoms: 　1. Irritable behavior and angry outbursts (with little or no provocation) typically expressed as verbal or physical aggression toward people or objects. 　2. Hypervigilance. 　3. Exaggerated startle response. 　4. Problems with concentration. 　5. Sleep disturbance (e.g., difficulty falling or staying asleep or restless sleep).	E. Marked alterations in arousal and reactivity associated with the traumatic event(s), beginning or worsening after the traumatic event(s) occurred, as evidenced by two (or more) of the following: 　1. Irritable behavior and angry outbursts (with little or no provocation) typically expressed as verbal or physical aggression toward people or objects. 　2. Reckless or self-destructive behavior. This item is not included in the criteria for children of age 6 and below. 　3. Hypervigilance. 　4. Exaggerated startle response. 　5. Problems with concentration. 　6. Sleep disturbance (e.g., difficulty falling or staying asleep or restless sleep).
F. Duration of the disturbance (criteria B, C, D, and E) is more than 1 month.	F. The duration of the disturbance (symptoms in criterion B) is 3 days to 1 month after trauma exposure.

Reprinted with permission from Hoover, D., & Kaufman, J. (2018). Posttraumatic stress disorder. In A. Martin, M. H. Bloch, & F. R. Volkmar (Eds.), *Lewis's child and adolescent psychiatry: A comprehensive textbook* (5th ed., pp. 652–653). Wolters Kluwer.

for example, include at least some features unique to it rather than to PTSD. Hallucinations are sometimes observed in children who have suffered abuse, but usually other features suggestive of psychotic disorders are absent. These hallucinations also typically resolve with appropriate intervention.

Although clinical diagnosis of PTSD can be assigned with a high degree of confidence with a careful evaluation and a large number of valid and reliable assessment tools, an important difference between prospective and retrospective reports of maltreatment has been documented in a recent meta-analysis. This review aggregated data from 16 studies with 25,471 participants who reported on their maltreatment both prospectively, when they were children, and retrospectively, when adults were asked about maltreatment earlier in their lives. On average, 52% of individuals with prospective reports of childhood maltreatment did not retrospectively report it; similarly, 56% of individuals retrospectively reporting childhood maltreatment did not have concordant prospective observations in adulthood. The study concluded that children identified prospectively as having experienced maltreatment represent a different group of individuals with different risk pathways to mental illness than adults who report childhood maltreatment retrospectively (Baldwin et al., 2019) (Box 23.1).

Course and Prognosis

Various factors contribute to the risk for developing PTSD and its subsequent course. Most individuals who experience trauma do not go on to develop PTSD. Strong social support and psychological resilience (Feldman, 2020; Rutter, 2013) can mitigate adverse effects of trauma

---

| **BOX 23.1** | **Case Report: Posttraumatic Stress Disorder** |

Lucy, an 8-year-old girl, witnessed her father shoot and kill her mother in the family home. The parents had a stormy relationship, and the mother had recently obtained a court order to keep her husband out of the home. Lucy's older sister was out of the home at the time of the shooting. In the weeks immediately following the event, Lucy appeared to be preoccupied with themes of violence and loss in her play but seemed to be unable to recall many details of the actual event. Her maternal aunt, with whom she now resided, reported that periodically she would be very upset and anxious but was unable to talk about her emotions. Lucy was also more withdrawn from other children in school and seemed to have lost interest in activities that she used to enjoy at home such as playing with her sister. She had difficulties falling asleep and had frequent nightmares; during at least one of the nightmares, she appeared to be talking to her mother. Treatment was initiated shortly after the event and included supportive and play therapy modalities aimed at improving sleep and reducing anxiety at first, and over time, helping Lucy process deep feelings of horror and grief that she continued to suffer after witnessing the violent death of her mother.

Comment: After exposure to trauma, most children show transient symptoms such as being tearful and withdrawn and have difficulty concentrating and sleeping. PTSD is a diagnosis based on more persistent and severe symptoms including intrusive memories of traumatic events, frightening dreams, and persistent negative emotional states. Children may suffer periods of disorganized or agitated behavior. Their stress-related symptoms may be seen immediately after the event or sometime later. Treatment options can vary depending on the child's age and type and severity of traumatic event.

Adapted from Volkmar, F. R., & Martin, A. (2011). *Essentials of child and adolescent psychiatry* (p. 258). Lippincott Williams & Wilkins.

---

on mental health and developmental outcomes. The risk factors for worse outcomes include preexisting psychiatric difficulties in the child or family history of psychiatric problems. The degree to which the psychosocial environment is a supportive one after the traumatic event is also a major predictor of response; the absence of a supportive environment in conjunction with psychosocial adversity increases risk.

Treatment

A number of treatment models for childhood PTSD have now been proposed and trauma-focused psychotherapies are considered the first line of treatment (Smith et al., 2019). The National Child Traumatic Stress Network (NCTSN, https://www.nctsn.org/) maintains a listing of validated interventions. All share a major initial concern with ensuring the child's safety, providing psychosocial support (including through supporting primary caregivers), and identifying the events that trigger increases in symptoms. Trauma-focused cognitive behavior therapy (Cohen et al., 2004) has been well studied. It includes an emphasis on narrative exposure, encouraging expressing feelings, education, and stress management techniques. It provides gradual exposure with joint child–caregiver sessions that support the child's increased ability to confront reminders of the traumatic experience and gain some perspective on the experience. Treatment is usually accomplished over 10 to 18 sessions. Parents as well as children benefit, and the benefits appear to persist over time. Group therapy approaches have been developed, and other models have been proposed in the treatment of younger children (Shein-Szydlo et al., 2016; Stein et al., 2003). Shorter interventions such as the four-session Child and Family Traumatic Stress Intervention (CFTSI) with emphasis on psychological education and improving family communication have been shown to help children with PTSD symptoms (Berkowitz et al., 2011). Eye movement desensitization and reprocessing (EMDR) is a promising treatment for PTSD in young people who may be unable to engage in CBT. During EMDR, clients are asked to recall a traumatic event while simultaneously focusing on an external stimulus such as making lateral eye movement and tapping finger (Shapiro, 2001). Although the mechanisms of this treatment are not clearly understood, several studies suggest that it could reduce symptoms of PTSD in children (Smith et al., 2019).

■ SUMMARY

Children have suffered from the effects of abuse, neglect, and trauma since antiquity. Over the past century, and with an increasingly rapid pace over the past several decades, advances have been made in recognizing abuse, neglect, and trauma and their significant impact on children's development. There also has been increased recognition of the importance of several risk factors, including the major role of psychosocial adversity, in increasing risk for the child and family. As a result of studies of children who are neglected and deprived, there has been an increasing recognition of the importance of stable parent-child relationships to foster attachment and long-term development. Advances have been made in the recognition of significant effects of trauma on children and ways these effects can be either prevented or lessened and treated when they occur. Several treatment models have been developed. Challenges remain, including the need for better methods of dealing with underlying psychosocial adversity, models that treat perpetrators and victims (often members of the same family), and more integrated adult–child treatment models.

References

*Indicates Particularly Recommended

American Psychiatric Association. (2013). *Diagnostic and statistical manual of mental disorders (DSM-5)* (5th ed.). American Psychiatric Publishing.
*Baldwin, J. R., Reuben, A., Newbury, J. B., & Danese, A. (2019). Agreement between prospective and retrospective measures of childhood maltreatment: A systematic review and meta-analysis. *JAMA Psychiatry, 76*(6), 584–593. https://doi.org/10.1001/jamapsychiatry.2019.0097
Berkowitz, S. J., Stover, C. S., & Marans, S. R. (2011). The child and family traumatic stress intervention: Secondary prevention for youth at risk of developing PTSD. *Journal of Child Psychology and Psychiatry and Allied Disciplines, 52*(6), 676–685. https://doi.org/10.1111/j.1469-7610.2010.02321.x
Boccia, M., D'Amico, S., Bianchini, F., Marano, A., Giannini, A. M., & Piccardi, L. (2016). Different neural modifications underpin PTSD after different traumatic events: An fMRI meta-analytic study. *Brain Imaging and Behavior, 10*(1), 226–237. https://doi.org/10.1007/s11682-015-9387-3
Brewin, C. R., Andrews, B., & Valentine, J. D. (2000). Meta-analysis of risk factors for posttraumatic stress disorder in trauma-exposed adults. *Journal of Consulting and Clinical Psychology, 68*(5), 748–766. https://doi.org/10.1037/0022-006X.68.5.748
Cohen, J. A., Deblinger, E., Mannarino, A. P., & Steer, R. A. (2004). A multisite, randomized controlled trial for children with sexual abuse-related PTSD symptoms. *Journal of the American Academy of Child and Adolescent Psychiatry, 43*(4), 393–402. https://doi.org/10.1097/00004583-200404000-00005
*Copeland, W. E., Keeler, G., Angold, A., & Costello, E. J. (2007). Traumatic events and posttraumatic stress in childhood. *Archives of General Psychiatry, 64*(5), 577–584. https://doi.org/10.1001/archpsyc.64.5.577
Croft, C., Beckett, C., Rutter, M., Castle, J., Colvert, E., Groothues, C., Hawkins, A., Kreppner, J., Stevens, S. E., & Sonuga-Barke, E. J. S. (2007). Early adolescent outcomes of institutionally-deprived and non-deprived adoptees. II: Language as a protective factor and a vulnerable outcome. *Journal of Child Psychology and Psychiatry and Allied Disciplines, 48*(1), 31–44. https://doi.org/10.1111/j.1469-7610.2006.01689.x
*Feldman, R. (2020). What is resilience: An affiliative neuroscience approach. *World Psychiatry, 19*(2), 132–150. https://doi.org/10.1002/wps.20729
*Foa, E. B., Asnaani, A., Zang, Y., Capaldi, S., & Yeh, R. (2018). Psychometrics of the child PTSD symptom scale for *DSM-5* for trauma-exposed children and adolescents. *Journal of Clinical Child and Adolescent Psychology, 47*(1), 38–46. https://doi.org/10.1080/15374416.2017.1350962

Hoover, D., & Kaufman, J. (2018). Posttraumatic stress disorder. In A. Martin, M. H. Bloch, & F. R. Volkmar (Eds.), *Lewis's child and adolescent psychiatry: A comprehensive textbook* (5th ed., pp. 651–658). Wolters Kluwer.

*Lewis, S. J., Arseneault, L., Caspi, A., Fisher, H. L., Matthews, T., Moffitt, T. E., Odgers, C. L., Stahl, D., Teng, J. Y., & Danese, A. (2019). The epidemiology of trauma and post-traumatic stress disorder in a representative cohort of young people in England and Wales. *The Lancet Psychiatry, 6*(3), 247–256. https://doi.org/10.1016/S2215-0366(19)30031-8

McLaughlin, K. A., Koenen, K. C., Hill, E. D., Petukhova, M., Sampson, N. A., Zaslavsky, A. M., & Kessler, R. C. (2013). Trauma exposure and posttraumatic stress disorder in a national sample of adolescents. *Journal of the American Academy of Child and Adolescent Psychiatry, 52*(8), 815–830. e814. https://doi.org/10.1016/j.jaac.2013.05.011

*Midgley, N. (2007). Anna Freud: The Hampstead war nurseries and the role of the direct observation of children for psychoanalysis. *International Journal of Psychoanalysis, 88*(4), 939–959. https://doi .org/10.1516/V28R-J334-6182-524H

Montalvo-Ortiz, J. L., Gelernter, J., Hudziak, J., & Kaufman, J. (2016). RDoC and translational perspectives on the genetics of trauma-related psychiatric disorders. *American Journal of Medical Genetics, Part B: Neuropsychiatric Genetics, 171*(1), 81–91. https://doi.org/10.1002/ajmg.b.32395

*Nelson, C. A., Fox, N. A., & Zeanah, C. H. (2014). *Romania's abandoned children: Deprivation, brain development and the struggle for recovery*. Harvard University Press.

*Pynoos, R., Weathers, F., Steinberg, A., Marx, B., Layne, C., Kaloupek, D., & Kriegler, J. (2015). *Clinician-administered PTSD scale for DSM-5—Child/adolescent version*. National Center for PTSD. https:// www.ptsd.va.gov/professional/assessment/child/caps-ca.asp#:~:text=Description,adolescents%20 ages%207%20and%20above.&text=Similar%20to%20the%20CAPS%2D5,questions%20and%20 probes%20are%20provided

Rutter, M. (2013). Annual research review: Resilience—Clinical implications. *Journal of Child Psychology and Psychiatry and Allied Disciplines, 54*(4), 474–487. https://doi.org/10.1111/j.1469-7610.2012.02615.x

Shapiro, F. (2001). *Eye movement desensitization and reprocessing: Basic principles, protocols, and procedures*. Guilford Press.

Shein-Szydlo, J., Sukhodolsky, D. G., Kon, D. S., Tejeda, M. M., Ramirez, E., & Ruchkin, V. (2016). A randomized controlled study of cognitive–behavioral therapy for posttraumatic stress in street children in Mexico City. *Journal of Traumatic Stress, 29*(5), 406–414. https://doi.org/10.1002/jts.22124

Smith, P., Dalgleish, T., & Meiser-Stedman, R. (2019). Practitioner review: Posttraumatic stress disorder and its treatment in children and adolescents. *Journal of Child Psychology and Psychiatry and Allied Disciplines, 60*(5), 500–515. https://doi.org/10.1111/jcpp.12983

Stein, B. D., Tu, W., Elliott, M. N., Jaycox, L. H., Kataoka, S. H., Fink, A., & Wong, M. (2003). A mental health intervention for school children exposed to violence: A randomized controlled trial. *Journal of the American Medical Association, 290*(5), 603–611. https://doi.org/10.1001/jama.290.5.603

*Wade, M., Zeanah, C. H., Fox, N. A., & Nelson, C. A. (2020). Social communication deficits following early-life deprivation and relation to psychopathology: A randomized clinical trial of foster care. *Journal of Child Psychology and Psychiatry and Allied Disciplines, 61*(12), 1360–1369. https://doi .org/10.1111/jcpp.13222

Suggested Readings

American Psychiatric Association. (2013). *Diagnostic and statistical manual of mental disorders (DSM-5)* (5th ed.). American Psychiatric Publishing.

Baldwin, J. R., Reuben, A., Newbury, J. B., & Danese, A. (2019). Agreement between prospective and retrospective measures of childhood maltreatment: A systematic review and meta-analysis. *JAMA Psychiatry, 76*(6), 584–593. https://doi.org/10.1001/jamapsychiatry.2019.0097

Berkowitz, S. J., Stover, C. S., & Marans, S. R. (2011). The child and family traumatic stress intervention: Secondary prevention for youth at risk of developing PTSD. *Journal of Child Psychology and Psychiatry and Allied Disciplines, 52*(6), 676–685. https://doi.org/10.1111/j.1469-7610.2010.02321.x

Boccia, M., D'Amico, S., Bianchini, F., Marano, A., Giannini, A. M., & Piccardi, L. (2016). Different neural modifications underpin PTSD after different traumatic events: An fMRI meta-analytic study. *Brain Imaging and Behavior, 10*(1), 226–237. https://doi.org/10.1007/s11682-015-9387-3

Brewin, C. R., Andrews, B., & Valentine, J. D. (2000). Meta-analysis of risk factors for posttraumatic stress disorder in trauma-exposed adults. *Journal of Consulting and Clinical Psychology, 68*(5), 748–766. https://doi.org/10.1037/0022-006X.68.5.748

Cohen, J. A., Mannarino, A. P., Deblinger, E., & Steer, R. A. (2004). A multisite, randomized controlled trial for children with sexual abuse-related PTSD symptoms. *Journal of the American Academy of Child and Adolescent Psychiatry, 43*(4), 393–402. https://doi.org/10.1097/00004583-200404000-00005

Copeland, W. E., Keeler, G., Angold, A., & Costello, E. J. (2007). Traumatic events and posttraumatic stress in childhood. *Archives of General Psychiatry, 64*(5), 577–584. https://doi.org/10.1001/archpsyc.64.5.577

Croft, C., Beckett, C., Rutter, M., Castle, J., Colvert, E., Groothues, C., Hawkins, A., Kreppner, J., Stevens, S. E., & Sonuga-Barke, E. J. S. (2007). Early adolescent outcomes of institutionally-deprived and non-deprived adoptees. II: Language as a protective factor and a vulnerable outcome. *Journal of Child Psychology and Psychiatry and Allied Disciplines, 48*(1), 31–44. https://doi.org/10.1111/j.1469-7610.2006.01689.x

Feldman, R. (2020). What is resilience: An affiliative neuroscience approach. *World Psychiatry, 19*(2), 132–150. https://doi.org/10.1002/wps.20729

Foa, E. B., Asnaani, A., Zang, Y., Capaldi, S., & Yeh, R. (2018). Psychometrics of the child PTSD symptom scale for *DSM-5* for trauma-exposed children and adolescents. *Journal of Clinical Child and Adolescent Psychology, 47*(1), 38–46. https://doi.org/10.1080/15374416.2017.1350962

Hoover, D., & Kaufman, J. (2018). Posttraumatic stress disorder. In A. Martin, M. H. Bloch, & F. R. Volkmar (Eds.), *Lewis's child and adolescent psychiatry: A comprehensive textbook* (5th ed., pp. 651–658). Wolters Kluwer.

Lehmann, S., Monette, S., Egger, H., Breivik, K., Young, D., Davidson, C., & Minnis, H. (2020). Development and examination of the reactive attachment disorder and disinhibited social engagement disorder assessment interview. *Assessment, 27*(4), 749–765. https://doi.org/10.1177/1073191118797422

Lewis, S. J., Arseneault, L., Caspi, A., Fisher, H. L., Matthews, T., Moffitt, T. E., Odgers, C. L., Stahl, D., Teng, J. Y., & Danese, A. (2019). The epidemiology of trauma and post-traumatic stress disorder in a representative cohort of young people in England and Wales. *The Lancet Psychiatry, 6*(3), 247–256. https://doi.org/10.1016/S2215-0366(19)30031-8

McLaughlin, K. A., Koenen, K. C., Hill, E. D., Petukhova, M., Sampson, N. A., Zaslavsky, A. M., & Kessler, R. C. (2013). Trauma exposure and posttraumatic stress disorder in a national sample of adolescents. *Journal of the American Academy of Child and Adolescent Psychiatry, 52*(8), 815–830. e814. https://doi.org/10.1016/j.jaac.2013.05.011

Midgley, N. (2007). Anna Freud: The Hampstead war nurseries and the role of the direct observation of children for psychoanalysis. *International Journal of Psychoanalysis, 88*(4), 939–959. https://doi.org/10.1516/V28R-J334-6182-524H

Montalvo-Ortiz, J. L., Gelernter, J., Hudziak, J., & Kaufman, J. (2016). RDoC and translational perspectives on the genetics of trauma-related psychiatric disorders. *American Journal of Medical Genetics, Part B: Neuropsychiatric Genetics, 171*(1), 81–91. https://doi.org/10.1002/ajmg.b.32395

Pynoos, R., Weathers, F., Steinberg, A., Marx, B., Layne, C., Kaloupek, D., & Kriegler, J. (2015). *Clinician-administered PTSD scale for DSM-5—Child/adolescent version*. National Center for PTSD. https://www.reactionindex.com/tools_measures/

Rutter, M. (2013). Annual research review: Resilience—Clinical implications. *Journal of Child Psychology and Psychiatry and Allied Disciplines, 54*(4), 474–487. https://doi.org/10.1111/j.1469-7610.2012.02615.x

Shapiro, F. (2001). *Eye movement desensitization and reprocessing: Basic principles, protocols, and procedures*. Guilford Press.

Shein-Szydlo, J., Sukhodolsky, D. G., Kon, D. S., Tejeda, M. M., Ramirez, E., & Ruchkin, V. (2016). A randomized controlled study of cognitive–behavioral therapy for posttraumatic stress in street children in Mexico City. *Journal of Traumatic Stress, 29*(5), 406–414. https://doi.org/10.1002/jts.22124

Smith, P., Dalgleish, T., & Meiser-Stedman, R. (2019). Practitioner review: Posttraumatic stress disorder and its treatment in children and adolescents. *Journal of Child Psychology and Psychiatry and Allied Disciplines, 60*(5), 500–515. https://doi.org/10.1111/jcpp.12983

Stein, B. D., Tu, W., Elliott, M. N., Jaycox, L. H., Kataoka, S. H., Fink, A., & Wong, M. (2003). A mental health intervention for schoolchildren exposed to violence: A randomized controlled trial. *Journal of the American Medical Association, 290*(5), 603–611. https://doi.org/10.1001/jama.290.5.603

SECTION III ▪ SPECIAL SITUATIONS

CHAPTER 24 ▪ ABUSE AND NEGLECT

Child abuse and neglect is an important phenomenon with a long and complex history. The Bible refers to the near sacrifice of Jacob by Abraham. Throughout much of history, children were treated as chattels (movable property), with them being bought and sold. Given the lack of birth control, infanticide and child abandonment were common (see Chapter 1). Foundling hospitals were equipped to accept infants or children who otherwise would have been abandoned. In the Middle Ages, attempts were made by the Church to provide alternatives to abandonment, for example, the anonymous Rota (see Figure 24.1), where a child could be placed in a rotating device in a monastery or convent—the parents would ring a bell and the child would be moved around to the care of the brothers or sisters in that community (see Boswell, 1989, for a discussion of this whole phenomenon). Children on the streets of New York were swept into "orphan trains" (Holt, 1994) and taken out to what presumably were healthier environments as farmers or others selected them.

Probably the first well-documented case of child abuse was that of Mary Ellen Wilson in 1874, whose foster parents severely abused her (Figure 24.2). She was removed from her home and her story led to the formation of the New York Society for the Prevention of Cruelty to Children.

Beginning in the early 1900s, increasing attention was drawn to the plight of children who were abused or neglected with a White House conference recommending local foster placement rather than institutional care. By the 1920s states began to regulate this process, and the foster care system, as we know it today, began to emerge.

Only in relatively recent times has child abuse come to be regarded as a medical condition—terms like the *battered child syndrome* and *shaken baby syndrome* came to be used as physicians appreciated the physical findings associated with abuse. Similarly, interest in the response to trauma is also relatively recent (see Chapter 23).

Child abuse and neglect are frequently intertwined. Abuse can be physical, psychological, or sexual in nature. Neglect can also take various forms, ranging from physical or psychological to educational. It is important to note that other problems, like child trafficking or sexual exploitation, are also sometimes included in the broader view of child abuse. Abuse and neglect often co-occur to varying degrees. The term *maltreatment* is used to cover a broader range of problems, including sexual exploitation and trafficking (Kaufman & Hoover, 2018).

It is interesting to note that awareness of physical abuse and its sequelae is a much more recent historical phenomenon. In the 1940s, there was awareness of the unusual presentation of children with subdural hematomas and multiple fractures of unknown etiology. It was only in 1962, with the publication of "The Battered Child Syndrome" by Kempe and colleagues, that there was

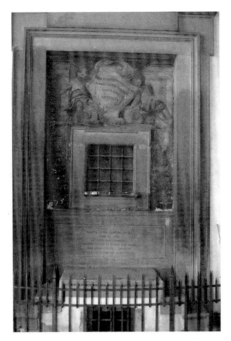

FIGURE 24.1. The Rota or foundling wheel from the Ospedale degli Innocenti, Florence, Italy. (Photo by F. R. Volkmar.)

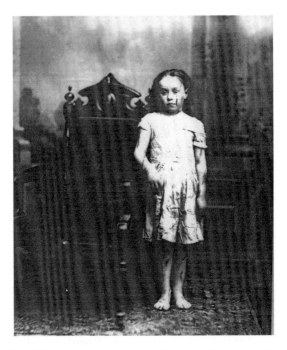

FIGURE 24.2. Mary Ellen Wilson. (Photo courtesy of New York Society for Prevention of Cruelty to Children.)

recognition that these injuries were inflicted by parents. Before this, accounts by parents to (often poorly) explain injuries were simply accepted. After Kempe's paper, pediatricians, radiologists, and others began to pay much more attention to unusual injuries and trauma.

Children and adolescents who are neglected or abused are at increased risk for a range of mental health problems. They may exhibit posttraumatic stress disorder (PTSD), anxiety disorders, mood problems, and aggressive behavior. Severely neglected children may exhibit reactive attachment disorders (RADs). Sexual abuse may have special sequelae in terms of depression, substance abuse, low self-esteem, and dissociative states. Although poverty and low parental education are risk factors, abuse and neglect are observed in families from all social situations and the clinician should be constantly alert to the possibility of abuse or neglect. In some instances, the medical system itself becomes involved in the cycle of abuse— as in the case of the so-called Munchausen by proxy syndrome. Children exposed to trauma within or outside the family are prone to exhibit a range of difficulties, including PTSD (see Chapter 23 and Kaufman & Hoover, 2018).

▌ DEFINITIONS AND CLINICAL FEATURES

Physical abuse entails the intended injury of a child by the caretaker (McCoy & Keene, 2014). For infants, this may take the form of shaking or beating, resulting in the *shaken baby syndrome* (see Box 24.1). Injury may come from inappropriate or excessive punishment. The term *battered child* is often used to refer to victims of physical abuse. In sexual abuse, an adult or older child engages in inappropriate sexual behavior with a child. Psychological abuse takes the form of repeated threats of abandonment or repeated statements to children that they are unwanted, unloved, or damaged. The term *neglect* is generally used to refer to situations where the parent or caretaker does not provide appropriate care (see Kaufman & Hoover, 2018). This can take the form of failure to provide sufficient food, adequate supervision, adequate medical care, or education. Physicians, other health and mental health care providers, teachers, and others are mandated reporters of suspected abuse or neglect. Legal definitions of abuse and neglect vary from state to state; therefore, it is important for health care providers to be

---

| **BOX 24.1** | **Child Abuse** |

Johnny, age 8 months, was brought to the emergency department by ambulance following a frantic call from his mother to 911. His mother had a long history of substance abuse, primarily involving cocaine, and reported that she had left Johnny in the care of her boyfriend only to return and find him left in his crib with the boyfriend nowhere to be found. She reported that Johnny had been a difficult baby "from day one" and she had to have some time away from him. On examination, Johnny was noted to have retinal hemorrhages with one healing and one new fracture. Evaluation was otherwise negative. The mother denied injuring him but did report that he "may" have fallen a few weeks previously. She has few social supports and was on probation for several theft charges. Protective services was called, and Johnny was removed from his mother's care. She subsequently returned to prison for violation of probation and Johnny entered foster care.

Comment: The term *shaken baby syndrome* is often used to refer to a constellation of various injures, ranging from mild to severe, including multiple fractures, retinal hemorrhages, and subdural hematomas. All are warning signs of abuse. In this case, the mother's cocaine habit may have contributed both to some of his early difficulties and to her ability to be an effective parent. Infants are more likely than older children to be abused.

---

aware of the mandates for reporting in their own locations. Unfortunately, the various forms of abuse or neglect frequently co-occur.

Physical abuse should be suspected if a child has injuries that appear to be unexplained or when the history provided does not correspond to the findings. The child who has been abused may look anxious, fearful, depressed, or agitated; older children may be very reticent to reveal the abuse. Marks or bruises, for example, to the face or head, back or buttocks may suggest inappropriate punishment; these are often symmetric (unlike most accidental injuries). Similarly, a belt or rope may leave a characteristic pattern. Burns, for example, from cigarettes, may be noted. The infant or young child may exhibit multiple and spiral fractures. Severe shaking of an infant can lead to the *shaken baby syndrome*, with characteristic retinal hemorrhages. In Munchausen by proxy syndrome (discussed subsequently), there may be a history of repeated emergency department or hospital visits for treatment of unusual problems.

Child neglect may present to the physician with signs of malnutrition and/or with signs of lack of care of the child. Such children may be withdrawn and may be indiscriminate in their affection. These children may exhibit poor hygiene or failure to thrive.

Sexual abuse is often never revealed or comes to light only after a long pattern of abuse (Kaufman & Hoover, 2018). Uncovering the abuse may be difficult. Obvious indicators are unexpected trauma or sexually transmitted diseases. The young child who is sexually abused may display inappropriate sexual knowledge or preoccupation; behavioral manifestations can include mood problems or aggression. The child may be fearful, for example, of men if the perpetrator is himself a male. In interviewing the child with suspected child abuse, the examiner should understand that the child may not always be consistent given understandable anxiety. False allegations of sexual abuse do occur, and in many cases, there is not sufficient evidence to substantiate the claim of sexual abuse. Very young children may have great difficulty providing a coherent verbal account of the abuse. The use of play materials can be helpful, but it is important that the interviewer not inappropriately *lead* the child. Incestuous behavior is most common between older male relatives (fathers, brothers, uncles, stepfathers) and girls. Risk factors include poverty, absent or impaired maternal presence, and substance abuse. Acting out and self-destructive behavior may be a sign of sexual abuse (Wright et al., 2004).

■ EPIDEMIOLOGY AND RISK FACTORS

During fiscal year 2018, the U.S. Department of Health and Human Services reported that over 4 million who work with children had been referred for investigation of possible abuse/neglect. Professionals of all types (teachers, medical personnel, and others) reported about 70% of the abuse, whereas the remaining cases were reported by friends, neighbors, relatives, and other nonprofessionals. There were approximately 678,000 documented cases for a rate of about 9.2 per 1000 children. The youngest children had the highest rates of

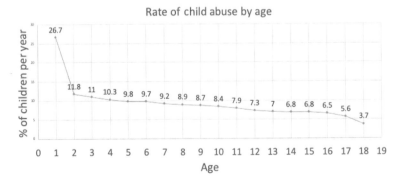

FIGURE 24.3. Rates of child abuse by age (per 1000 children). Data adapted from U.S. Department of Health and Human Services. (2018). *Child maltreatment 2018.* https://www.acf.hhs.gov/cb/report/child-maltreatment-2018

abuse (see Figure 24.3). Girls were more likely (9.6/1000) to face abuse compared with boys (8.57/1000). In terms of ethnicity, Native American families have the highest victimization rates (15.2/1000) followed by African American families (14.0/1000). Whereas most victims suffered from one type of maltreatment, about 15% have faced more than one. Neglect was observed in about three fifths of the cases. It was estimated that 1770 children died because of abuse or neglect. Parents were the perpetrators in most cases (77%). Prenatal substance abuse (drugs or alcohol) results in a substantial number of referrals (McLaughlin et al., 2010; Vanderminden et al., 2019). Risk factors for parents and families include poverty, single-parent household, and parental impairment due to substance abuse (Ben-Arieh, 2010).

Those most likely to die as a result of abuse and neglect are infants and toddlers. These data must be interpreted with some caution, however, because many child fatalities are not correctly reported as abuse (Kaufman & Hoover, 2018). Once a case has been reported, there is increased risk for subsequent referrals. It is typical for the child in protective care to have experienced at least two forms of abuse. Children who suffer from abuse/neglect may exhibit any of several potential risk factors. These include a history of prematurity, physical or cognitive disability, or children who are viewed (rightly or wrongly) as demanding, difficult, or overly active. Girls are at a slightly higher risk than boys.

Although rates remain concerning, it is the efforts at prevention and education, as well as prosecution of offenders, that have had a major effect. Following a peak in 1993, there has been a decline of more than 20%, particularly in the areas of sexual and physical abuse. Sexual abuse in the form of attacks by other children appears, unfortunately, to have increased. Perpetrators often have been abused themselves. Unfortunately, child abuse, spousal abuse, and substance abuse problems tend to co-occur. About 80% of parents who lose their child following investigations for abuse and neglect have histories of substance abuse, and domestic violence is reported in over half of cases involved with child protection services.

COURSE AND PROGNOSIS

Neglect and abuse have varied long-term implications for the mental health and life course of victims, as well as on the developing brain (Bick & Nelson, 2016). Psychiatric problems of children who have experienced abuse/neglect include higher rates of PTSD, depression, attachment problems, dissociative symptoms, substance abuse problems, eating disorders, conduct or oppositional disorder, and borderline personality traits. Other issues may also be present, including problems with peers, low self-esteem, and poor academic performance. In one study, about half of the maltreated children had significant problems in academics, behavior, and social relationships; <5% functioned well in all these domains. In adulthood, these individuals are more likely to be involved in violence with partners and to have problems being parents. Although most parents who are abusive have experienced maltreatment themselves, fortunately overall only about one in three children who are abused go on to become abusing parents. Inappropriate sexual behaviors are possible indicators of sexual abuse but can also be associated with physical abuse, exposure to domestic violence or sexuality, and mental illness (Table 24.1). In the past, it was believed that fecal soiling was an indicator of sexual abuse, but this has not been shown in recent work.

Most children who are sexually abused do not go on to become abusers, but most sexual offenders have experienced maltreatment in some form. Youth who are sexual abusers often have a history of abuse or maltreatment, and most engage in other antisocial activities as well. Fortunately, it appears that many youths who engage in sexual offenses do not do so as adults.

Children removed from parents often enter foster care. The number of children in foster care has increased dramatically over the last several decades. Although many of the over 500,000 children can return home, many of these, between 20% and 40%, will reenter the foster care system. Multiple placements are not at all uncommon, and about 5% of children in care have experienced 10 or more placements. Around 100,000 children live in group homes or institutional settings. Multiple foster placements significantly increase the risk for subsequent antisocial and violent behavior.

TABLE 24.1

Distinctiveness of Sexualized Behaviors in Indicating Abuse History

Moderately Prevalent in Sexually Abused Children, Exceedingly Rare in Psychiatric and Normal Controls	Moderately Prevalent in Sexually Abused Children *and* Psychiatric Controls, Uncommon in Normal Controls	Moderately Prevalent in Sexually Abused Children, Psychiatric Controls, *and* Normal Controls
Puts mouth on sex parts Asks to engage in sexual acts Masturbates with an object Inserts objects in vagina or anus	Stands too close to others Hugs adults they do not know well Talks about sexual acts Wants to watch movies that show nudity Knows more about sex than other children their age	Talks flirtatiously Masturbates with hand Touches sex parts at home Tries to look at nude pictures/undressing people

Reprinted with permission from Martin, A., Bloch, M. H., & Volkmar, F. R., (Eds.). (2018). *Lewis's child and adolescent psychiatry* (5th ed.). Wolters Kluwer.

Important moderating variables in mediating the impact of maltreatment and subsequent difficulties have been identified. Caspi and colleagues identified a genetic risk between child maltreatment and later antisocial behavior—a functional polymorphism of the gene A (monoamine oxidase A, MAOA) involved in neurotransmitter metabolism (Caspi et al., 2002). Children who had been maltreated and who had high levels of MAOA were less likely to develop antisocial problems. This finding has been replicated in other studies. In subsequent work, the same group found that a functional polymorphism in the promoter region of the serotonin transporter (5-HTTLPR) gene was similarly involved in the moderation of maltreatment and life stress or depression.

Other lines of research suggest that support and subsequent positive parenting can modify the effects of child maltreatment. Studies using animal models have shown the potential mitigating effects of support during separation of the young animal from its mother. Similarly, the presence/availability of a supportive caregiver is associated with better outcomes.

■ TREATMENT

In many instances, cases with documented maltreatment referred to child protective services receive no support or services following the investigation. Both children and parents have significant needs that sadly are often not addressed. The failure to provide such services does, of course, increase the likelihood of re-abuse, subsequent placement, and worsened outcome.

Children who have been abused/neglected can present with an unusual range of symptoms and disorders. Compared with children in community samples, those in child protective services are 2–3 times more likely to receive psychotropic medications. Behavioral methods, including treatment specific to PTSD, are underutilized but effective. Given the wide range of potential additional mental health problems, a comprehensive psychiatric assessment is indicated. Work with this population is more than usually complicated, given that not only the child and parent or foster parent but some representative from child protective services will be involved. Given the association of child abuse/neglect with a range of environmental stressors and challenges, various professional services are often needed, for example, to address substance problems in parents, and needs for family supports, academic assistance, and mental health support (Kaufman & Hoover, 2018).

The data on the negative effects of multiple and long foster care placements led Congress to enact the Adoption and Safe Families Act in 1997, which mandates that, in general, permanency in placement should occur for children in out-of-home care for 15 of the last 22 months. Some states require this if children have been in out-of-home care for only 12 months. There are different routes to permanency, including reunification of the family, adoption, or long-term placement with relatives or nonrelatives granted legal guardianship.

Intervention programs often must target parental substance abuse treatment as a priority. This can be accomplished in different ways, including having substance abuse workers in the child welfare program. Various comprehensive programs have been developed. In the next section we review one particular syndrome of abuse/neglect of particular interest to medical professionals, before discussing the problems in attachment and a specific syndrome resulting from neglect through inadequate caretaking and delayed or deviant care.

■ FACTITIOUS DISORDER IN ANOTHER/MUNCHAUSEN SYNDROME BY PROXY

The term *Munchausen syndrome* was used in the 1950s to describe adults who fabricated symptoms of illness. The term referred to the famous Baron Munchausen, a teller of tall tales, and was first described in adults with factitious disorders. It was recognized that the condition also existed relative to children whose parents complained of disorders and put children at risk through their dogged pursuit of diagnostic confirmation. It appears cases of *nonaccidental* poisoning may have represented the first instances of this condition, described by Sneed and Bell in 1976 as the "dauphin of Munchausen" and by Meadow in 1977 as "Munchausen by proxy syndrome."

The condition was listed in an appendix of the *Diagnostic and Statistical Manual (DSM)-IV* as one requiring further study, but now, in *DSM-5*, the condition is recognized and termed *factitious disorder in another*. In *DSM-5*, it now is included with factitious disorder, with the same criteria used for both, that is, falsification of symptoms/signs of illness in another person. The child is presented as impaired or injured, and the deceptive behavior of parents is not better explained by another condition. The parent(s) denies having caused the illness, and there is usually some important psychological gain for the parent/caregiver in assuming, by proxy, the sick role. There is some controversy over the nature of the condition—that is, if this should be categorized as a mental or as another form of child abuse (Meadow, 2002).

Severity can range from mild to severe. There are other circumstances in which symptoms may be falsified, for example, in relation to keeping a child out of school or as part of a custody dispute, and these are not typically considered forms of Munchausen's. Fortunately, the condition is apparently quite rare. In one study in the United Kingdom and Ireland, the rate was 1 per 200,000 in children under 16. A handful of systematic case reviews suggest some commonalities among cases. In addition to the generally expected young age of the children involved (i.e., well before the time they can speak readily for themselves), the perpetrator is usually the mother. The mean age of being reported is between 3 and 4 years, although in one British study, the median age was 20 months. Boys and girls are equally as likely to be affected (Asnes, 2018).

The clinical presentation is highly varied (Asnes, 2018). Usually, the apparent illness seems to be multisystem—at different points in time, the child may appear to have different disorders. In systematic case series reviews the most common clinical presentations were possible seizures, apnea, diarrhea, and fevers, although other presentations are reported as well. Various means are used to produce the symptoms or findings, for example, contamination of intravenous lines or suffocation. The child may be moved from one health care provider or hospital to the next when initial evaluations are negative or as suspicion is aroused.

In some cases, the illness is simulated, for example, by contaminating urine samples, but no damage is done to the child. At other times, the symptom may reflect a dangerous action on the part of the parents (e.g., smothering the child). There may be a history of neglect or of some nonaccidental injury. Siblings may have been the focus of similar reports. In children who present with apnea and where there is a history of sibling death due to apnea, Munchausen by proxy should be included in the differential diagnosis. Other warning signs of factitious disorder in the child include symptoms that are present when a parent is there or other child deaths in the family. At times, the presenting issue may be a complicated, often rare, psychiatric or medical disorder.

Typically the perpetrator has a long history of involvement in the health care system, for example, the mother may herself have had a history of extensive medical evaluations. Typically, the staff report that the mother appears to be a model parent and may develop unusual (and inappropriate) relationships with medical staff, for example, repeatedly bringing gifts and food to the staff. At the same time, there often is a vague sense of uneasiness among the staff. Frequently, the mother will seem to hover over the child and never leave the bedside and be involved to an unusual degree. Once suspected (and with appropriate legal clearance and sometimes court orders), covert videotaping sometimes reveals a rather different pattern when the mother believes she is not being observed. Rather than being distressed in discussing the child's illness, the mother may seem detached or blandly accepting. The perpetrator may fabricate other information about themselves, the child, or family members. Typically, the father seems largely absent and the marital relationship may be poor. In contrast to mothers, fathers who are involved as perpetrators are often demanding and unreasonable (Asnes, 2018).

Risk factors include the mother's own experience of abuse as a child, a pathologic relationship with the child, and an investment in the interaction with the medical care system. Parent perpetrators also contribute their own, sometimes extensive, psychopathology with high rates of somatoform or factitious disorders, along with substance abuse, depression, and personality disorders. The fabrication of illness is often described as "quasi-delusional"; there may be an element of disassociation in their presentation as well (Asnes, 2018). In their review of nearly 800 parent perpetrators, Yates and Bass observed that almost all were female, and a majority married; nearly half had worked in health-related fields. A minority (30%) themselves had a history of maltreatment in childhood and a sizable minority similarly had histories themselves of factitious disorder (Yates & Bass, 2017). Early identification of cases is important but may be challenging (Bass & Glaser, 2014).

Relatively less is written about the psychiatric aspects of the child who is the victim. For older children, it may be the case that the child is involved in the deception. Given the number of intrusive and invasive tests and procedures, children frequently learn to tolerate them rather passively.

Management

These cases present a significant challenge for medical and mental health providers—falling at the intersection of both systems of care. Additional complications for management include the fact that the diagnosis may not be suspected for a long period of time. Once discovered, the diagnosis itself complicates management given the understandable feelings provoked in staff. Often, there is relatively little insight on the part of the mother or motivation to truly engage in psychotherapy (Box 24.2).

Table 24.2 provides a summary of some of the warning signs of Munchausen syndrome by proxy. The child's safety should always be the first priority. The medical care provider should act to involve both a mental health consultant and child protective services. An attempt should be made to disentangle the various complaints, for example, were some things only happening when the mother was present? Can independent sources verify history or observations provided by the mother? How does the mother react to the child's illness and the situations?

Laboratory studies may be helpful, for example, to determine if blood in urine or stool is the child's or the mother's. Although the rationale for continuous observation by staff is clear, this is usually difficult to conduct. Legal guidance should be sought relative to the question of covert video surveillance. Once the diagnosis is clear, the mother should be informed and protective services involved. The father and other family members can be involved as appropriate. The consulting psychiatrist can be helpful in multiple regards.

BOX 24.2   Munchausen's by Proxy

Tammy, a 5-year-old, was seen in consultation. She had been hospitalized for 1 week for observation following her mother's report of possible sleep apnea. At the time of admission, the mother reported that the child had a "variant of Rett's syndrome" and was seeking guidance regarding her school program. Tammy had been born following an uncomplicated pregnancy, labor, and delivery. Her single mother, an LPN, had been worried during the pregnancy about her condition. She was repeatedly reassured by her obstetrician that the pregnancy was progressing normally. Following Tammy's birth, the mother reported that she was slow in both talking and walking (although she was doing both by 18 months). After an episode of asthma, the mother became concerned about Tammy's breathing. She also noted what she believed were staring spells. A pediatric neurologist did an evaluation, including an EEG, which was within normal limits. The mother found a physician who expressed concern that the combination of breathing problems and staring spells raised the question of Rett's disorder. Her head circumference was, however, at the 50th percentile, as were height and weight. Another pediatrician recommended specific testing for Rett's but explained to the mother that the clinical picture did not justify it and that the test was not always positive even in documented cases. On several occasions, the mother had taken the child to the emergency room with complaints of concerns about her breathing. During this hospitalization, two potential apneic episodes had been noted and on both occasions the mother had been alone in the room with the child. The mother appeared quite devoted to the child as well as to the hospital staff who were sympathetic to her situation as the mother explained that she had had to stop working to care for her child. On examination, the child was in the low average range intellectually, with some mild speech articulation difficulties. Neurologic examination was not otherwise unusual. Apart from mild asthma, respiratory functions appeared to be normal. One of the staff became suspicious when she saw the mother apparently engaged in some activity with the apnea monitor just prior to the alarm being sounded. The mother then demanded to remove the child from the hospital and a referral to child protective services was made. Investigation revealed a number of previous evaluations, including two hospitalizations, not reported by the mother. The mother herself had a history of multiple unexplained medical symptoms and problems dating back to her childhood.

Comment: Several aspects of this case are relatively typical for Munchausen by proxy. These include the mother's medical background, the child's age (preschool children are most likely to be involved), multiple medical assessments, a failure to be reassured by the multiple previous assessments, and the over-engagement with staff.

Reprinted from Volkmar, F. R., & Martin, A. (2011). Child abuse, neglect, and the effects of trauma. *Essentials of Lewis's child and adolescent psychiatry* (p. 251). Wolters Kluwer.

The mental health consultant can meet with the mother even before the diagnosis is clear. This can usually readily be justified given the seriousness of the child's illness and allows for a discussion of the mother's history and the assessment of potential risk factors. Comments about the child may provide clues relative to motivation and the interview may also provide information about any overt psychiatric problems in the mother. Being involved with a psychiatrist or other mental health care provider prior to the time she is confronted also gives some potential for building a potentially helpful longer term therapeutic relationship. This person can also work with the medical staff around their feelings and be involved in confronting the mother once the diagnosis is clear. Information provided by the mental health care provider may be extremely helpful to child protection services.

Various factors need to be considered in providing treatment for the mother, for example, the nature of her own psychiatric difficulties, the duration and extent of the abuse, parental

TABLE 24.2

Warning Signals of Munchausen Syndrome by Proxy

Questions to consider when caregiver-fabricated illness in a child is suspected:
1. Are the history, signs, and symptoms of disease credible? 2. Is the child receiving unnecessary and harmful or potentially harmful medical care? 3. If so, who is instigating the evaluations and treatment? Possible indicators of caregiver-fabricated illness: • Diagnosis does not match the objective findings • Signs or symptoms are bizarre • Caregiver or suspected offender does not express relief or pleasure when told that child is improving or that child does not have a particular illness • Inconsistent histories of symptoms from different observers • Caregiver insists on invasive or painful procedures and hospitalizations • Caregiver behavior does not match expressed distress or report of symptoms (e.g., unusually calm) • Signs and symptoms begin only in the presence of one caregiver • Sibling has or had an unusual or unexplained illness or death • Sensitivity to multiple environmental substances or medicines • Failure of the child's illness to respond to its normal treatments or unusual intolerance to those treatments • Caregiver publicly solicits sympathy or donations or benefits because of the child's rare illness • Extensive unusual illness history in the caregiver or caregiver's family; history of somatization disorder in caregiver

Adapted from Asnes, A. G. (2018). Caregiver fabricated illness in a child. In A. Martin, M. Bloch, & F. R. Volkmar (Eds.), *Lewis's child and adolescent psychiatry* (5th ed., p. 670). Wolters Kluwer.

perceptions of the child, and willingness to engage in treatment. There have been reports of parents being able to engage in productive psychotherapy.

Course and Outcome

As might be expected, the outcome is variable. Cases where the condition has been going on for a long period are more challenging, as are cases where severe psychopathology in the mother interferes with treatment. Some activities, for example, simulating sleep apnea by suffocation, are clearly much more dangerous. In Rosenberg's 1987 review, 9% of cases died and 8% of those surviving had some permanent disfigurement or impairment. Suffocation and poisoning are the most frequent causes of death. As noted previously, a family history of mysterious death is a very worrisome sign. Sometimes outplacement is needed given the potential danger to the child's life.

Relatively little is known about the long-term psychiatric effects on the children involved, although a range of difficulties have been described. There is an increased risk for continued fabrication of illness as children become adolescents and adults. More intensive treatment programs may be associated with higher rates of success.

■ REACTIVE ATTACHMENT DISORDERS

Severe neglect and emotional deprivation, either through parental neglect or through institutional rearing, is typically associated with serious negative effects for children's development. Within the child development literature there has long been a focus on processes

TABLE 24.3

Development of Attachment

	0–2 Months	2–7 Months	7–18 Months	18–26 Months
Bowlby's characterization	• Orientation and signals without discrimination	• Orientation and signals directed toward one or more discriminated figures	• Maintenance of proximity to a discriminated figure	• Formation of a reciprocal relationship
Social interaction patterns	• Physical and social attributes attract adults for social interactions • Recognition of maternal face • Olfactory/auditory recognition • Spontaneous smile	• Able to engage adults in reciprocal social interactions • Evidence of differential responses to adults	• Focused attachment • Separation protest • Stranger reactions • Intersubjectivity evident • Social referencing	• Develop negotiating abilities with caregivers ("goal-corrected partnership") • Increased interest in peers; move toward interactive play and exploration
Communication/ methods of cueing adults to needs	• Crying, cooing	• Eye contact • Social smile • Responsive cooing, babbling	• Intentional communication with gestures and then words	• Able to express needs • Rapid vocabulary expansion

Reprinted with permission from Asnes, Z. (2018). Reactive attachment disorder and disinhibited social engagement disorder. In A. Martin, M. H. Bloch, & F. R. Volkmar (Eds.), *Lewis's child and adolescent psychiatry: A comprehensive textbook* (5th ed., p. 659). Wolters Kluwer.

of attachment, building on the work of John Bowlby and his colleague Mary Ainsworth. Bowlby became interested in attachment after he became aware of the effects of maternal separation in a series of children arrested for theft. Mary Ainsworth worked with him and developed a specific procedure for assessing the quality of young children's attachments. In essence, attachment theory proposed that babies come into the world with an inborn predisposition to develop relationships with caregiving adults.

From the moment of birth, typically developing infants have a strong orientation toward people. By 2 months of age, the baby is smiling socially and becoming more discriminating, and by around 8–9 months, the baby becomes extremely attached to parents and anxious around others (stranger anxiety). As babies are able to move, they will maintain physical proximity to parents, and with the onset of language, an entire range of verbal behaviors enhance the attachment process. The development of the concept of attachment is reviewed in Table 24.3.

Definitions and Clinical Features

Although a considerable body of research exists on attachment as a normative process, research on disorders of attachment is much less extensive (see Gleason & Zeanah, 2018). First recognized

Reactive Attachment Disorder (RAD)

Johnny, now 5 years of age (see Box 21.1), was referred for evaluation by his foster parents. Subsequent to removal from his mother's care at 8 months of age, Johnny had been placed in four different foster families. Each had noted difficulties that had appeared to increase over time. Johnny was difficult to console and seemed to have little empathy for others, but was over-affectionate and friendly even with complete strangers. The foster parents complained that, at times, his behavior was disruptive, and they were not sure he could remain with them. He had little evidence of specific attachments to his current foster parents, with whom he had resided for 5 months. There had been no contact from the biological mother for 2 years. On examination, he was superficially friendly but overly familiar with the new adult. He appeared to have some mild learning issues and was referred for additional testing prior to school entry.

Comment: Children in foster care can sometimes be in multiple placements, disrupting the formation of stable attachment relationships with adults. In this case, the child had an unfortunate early history and his vulnerabilities may have contributed to the difficulties he subsequently had with remaining in foster placements.

Reprinted from Volkmar, F. R., & Martin, A. (2011). Child abuse, neglect, and the effects of trauma. *Essentials of Lewis's child and adolescent psychiatry* (p. 254). Wolters Kluwer.

as a diagnostic entity in *DSM-III*, approaches to the diagnosis of the condition have somewhat changed over time. In the *DSM-IV* approach, severe disturbance in social relatedness in the context of grossly negligent care was emphasized, with two subtypes specified: an inhibited and a disinhibited type. The inhibited type was thought to be more typical in children from institutional settings or those who have been severely neglected, who are more passive and disorganized in their approaches to others. The disinhibited type was characterized by many indiscriminate attachments, for example, in situations where care has been provided in group settings or foster care. In *DSM-5* (APA, 2013), two forms of the disorder are still recognized: RAD and disinhibited social engagement disorder. This essentially retains the approach in *DSM-IV*. Some other diagnostic systems have also recognized a mixed type. The condition is not diagnosed in the presence of autism or a similar disorder, although differentiation can occasionally be a problem.

Attachment disorders and PTSD are somewhat unusual in the *DSM*, given that by definition, an etiology is associated with the disorder (Bruce et al., 2019). As Asnes (2018) points out, the two forms of attachment disorder can coexist to some degree, underscoring the complexity of categorical thinking about complex developmental processes.

Clinical presentation varies, depending on the age of the child and developmental level, but invariably the child exhibits severe problems in selective attachment to caregivers and in social interaction (Ellis & Saadabadi, 2019; Gleason & Zeanah, 2018). Infants with the condition may, at times, present with failure to thrive or other growth problems. The child may appear poorly nourished and cared for. Once appropriate care is provided, the child's physical appearance typically improves. As noted previously, the clinical picture may be one of withdrawal and inhibited responding or one in which the child is inappropriately and indiscriminately friendly. The latter group of cases may also exhibit problems with activity and poor attention (Bosmans et al., 2019; Zimmermann & Soares, 2019). As noted, the two forms of the disorder may coexist (Box 24.3).

Epidemiology and Demographics

Solid epidemiologic data are lacking. The problem is frequently observed in clinics serving very young children. Children who have been maltreated/abused are clearly more likely to exhibit the condition. One study found that 40% of foster children assessed within 3 months of placement exhibited the condition. Among children in institutional settings, particularly from a young age, rates of 22% to 56% are reported (see Asnes & Zeanah, 2018 for a detailed discussion).

Etiology

This disorder and the trauma-related conditions are unique in that etiology is specifically included in the definition of the disorder. Put another way, it would be impossible to make a diagnosis of RAD if appropriate care were provided (in such an instance an autism spectrum disorder would presumably be more likely). However, Rutter and colleagues have described a small group of children who suffered severe deprivation and presented with continued features suggestive of autism (Rutter, Sonuga-Barke, & Castle, 2010). The degree of social disturbance appeared to correlate with the duration of institutionalization and symptoms improved with provision of appropriate care. Neglect and patterns of multiple caregivers within a family can also be associated with significant problems in the development of attachment.

Differential Diagnosis and Assessment

Observation of the child in interaction with the caregiver is an important aspect of the assessment. Review of the history and a discussion of the nature and quality of attachment to the caregiver are also indicated. Careful attention should be paid to a history of neglect, repeated changes in caregivers, foster care placement, and so forth. Given the frequent association with a host of other risk factors, including poverty, various other conditions may be seen in this group of cases. There are standard approaches to assessing the quality of attachment using the Ainsworth Strange Situation (Main & Cassidy, 1998), but the responses of the child do not provide a clinical diagnosis and do not substitute for a clinical assessment.

In the typically developing child, selective attachments are usually observed by 9 months of age. Accordingly, care should be taken in making a diagnosis of RAD in a child with severe intellectual deficiency, that is, with a level below about 9 months. Usually, children with intellectual abilities above the 9-month level of cognitive ability will form attachments (children with autism are a notable exception). Occasionally, differentiation from autism and related conditions can be difficult, but usually social, and other gains, will be noted if appropriate care is provided. The most complicated cases are those in which a child may have autism or a related condition *and* a history of some degree of neglect—fortunately, these are not common. Nutritional deficiencies, small size, and growth problems are more typical of the child with RAD. Children with RAD who have experienced severe neglect may show stereotyped movements suggestive of autism or a related disorder.

As with other children who have experienced neglect or abuse, a range of additional conditions may be present. These include disruptive behavior disorders, anxiety disorders, and mood disorders. PTSD can be observed in children who have experienced abuse. As Asnes and Zeanah (2018) emphasize, a broad range of conditions should be considered in the differential diagnosis of attachment disorders. Practice guidelines for diagnosis and assessment are available (AACAP, 2005).

Developmental assessment should be conducted to document current status and monitor change with the provision of a more supportive, nurturing environment. If severe cognitive or other serious developmental delays are noted, a reasonable search for any contributing medical conditions is needed.

Course and Prognosis

When appropriate care is provided, infants usually will rapidly develop new attachments. Longitudinal data, particularly past the school years, are limited.

Treatments

Given the importance of stable child–parent relationships, it is important, whenever possible, to avoid removal of the child from the home, as long as there are provisions for appropriate support to the child and family. However, removal to foster care may be the only choice in some cases, and if the new environment is more facilitating, the child may rapidly improve. Multiple foster placements should be avoided. Often other family members, for example, grandparents, may be the best placement. A child in foster care can be more indiscriminate in their attachments. Children in institutional settings continue to exhibit difficulties. Placement in a supportive family environment is beneficial. For children who are placed in such settings, the inhibited symptoms of attachment disorder are much less persistent than the indiscriminate behaviors. Even when a supportive environment is provided, some difficulties may persist. At times, psychotherapeutic work with the child or parent–child dyad may be indicated. Various models of treatment have been described in the literature. Some of these alternative approaches have little or no substantive empirical basis (see Asnes, 2018).

■ SUMMARY

Children have suffered from the effects of abuse, neglect, and trauma since antiquity. Over the past century, and with an increasingly rapid pace over the last several decades, advances have been made in recognizing abuse and neglect and trauma and their significant sequalae for children's development. There also has been an increased recognition of the importance of several risk factors, including the major role of psychosocial adversity in increasing risk for the child and family. As a result of studies of children who are neglected and deprived, there has been an increasing recognition of the importance of stable parent and child relationships to foster attachment and long-term development. Advances have been made in recognition of the significant effects of trauma on children and ways these effects can be either prevented or lessened and treated when they occur. Several treatment models have been developed. Challenges remain, including the need for better methods of dealing with underlying psychosocial adversity, models that treat perpetrator and victim (often members of the same family), and more integrated adult–child treatment models.

References

American Psychiatric Association. (2013). *Diagnostic and statistical manual (DSM-5)* (5th ed.). Author.

Asnes, A. G. (2018). Caregiver fabricated illness in a child. In A. Martin, M. Bloch, & F. R. Volkmar (Eds.), *Lewis's child and adolescent psychiatry: A comprehensive textbook* (5th ed., pp. 567–572). Wolters Kluwer.

Asnes, A. G. (2018). Caregiver fabricated illness in a child. In A. Martin, M. Bloch, & F. R. Volkmar (Eds.), *Lewis's child and adolescent psychiatry* (5th ed., pp. 667-672). Wolters Kluwer.

Bass, C., & Glaser, D. (2014). Early recognition and management of fabricated or induced illness in children. *Lancet, 383*(9926), 1412–1421. https://doi.org/10.1016/S0140-6736(13)62183-2

Ben-Arieh, A. (2010). Socioeconomic correlates of rates of child maltreatment in small communities. *American Journal of Orthopsychiatry, 80*(1), 109–114. https://doi.org/10.1111/j.1939-0025.2010.01013.x

Bick, J., & Nelson, C. (2016). Early adverse experiences and the developing brain. *Neuropsychopharmacology, 41*, 177–196. https://doi.org/10.1038/npp.2015.252

Boris, N. W., Zeanah, C. H., & AACAP Work Group on Quality Issues. (2005). Practice parameters for the assessment and treatment of reactive attachment disorder in children and adolescents. *Journal of the American Academy of Child & Adolescent Psychiatry, 44*, 1206–1219. https://doi.org/10.1097/01.chi.0000177056.41655.ce

Bosmans, G., Spilt, J., Vervoort, E., & Verschueren, K. (2019). Inhibited symptoms of reactive attachment disorder: Links with working models of significant others and the self. *Attachment & Human Development, 21*(2), 190–204. https://doi.org/10.1080/14616734.2018.1499213

Boswell, J. (1989). *The kindness of strangers*. University of Chicago Press.

Bruce, M., Young, D., Turnbull, S., Rooksby, M., Chadwick, G., Oates, C., Nelson, R., Young-Southward, G., Haig, C., & Minnis, H. (2019). Reactive attachment disorder in maltreated young children in foster care. *Attachment & Human Development, 21*(2), 152–169. https://doi.org/10.1080/14616734.2018.1499211

Caspi, A., McClay, J., Moffitt, T. E., Mill, J., Martin, J., Craig, I. W., Taylor, A., & Poulton, R. (2002). Role of genotype in the cycle of violence in maltreated children. *Science, 297*(5582), 851–854. https://doi.org/10.1126/science.1072290

Ellis, E. E., & Saadabadi, A. (2019). *Reactive attachment disorder.* StatPearls Publishing.

Gleason, M. M., & Zeanah, C. H. (2018). Reactive attachment disorder and disinhibited social engagement disorder. In A. Martin, M. Bloch, & F. R. Volkmar (Eds.), *Lewis's child and adolescent psychiatry: A comprehensive textbook* (5th ed., pp 659–666). Wolters Kluwer.

Holt, M. I. (1994). *The orphan trains: Placing out in America.* University of Nebraska Press.

Kaufman, J., & Hoover, D. (2018). Child abuse and neglect. In A. Martin, M. Bloch, & F. R. Volkmar (Eds.), *Lewis's child and adolescent psychiatry: A comprehensive textbook* (5th ed., pp. 644-651). Wolters Kluwer.

Main, M., & Cassidy, J. (1998). Categories of response to reunion with the parent at age 6: Predictable from infant attachment classifications and stable over a 1-month period. *Developmental Psychopathology, 24*, 1–12. https://doi.org/10.1037/0012-1649.24.3.415

McCoy, M. L., & Keene, S. M. (2014). *Child abuse and neglect.* Psychology Press.

McLaughlin, K. A., Green, J. G., Gruber, M. J., Sampson, N. A., Zaslavsky, A. M., & Kessler, R. C. (2010). Childhood adversities and adult psychiatric disorders in the national comorbidity survey replication II: Associations with persistence of *DSM-IV* disorders. *Archives of General Psychiatry, 67*, 124–132. https://doi.org/10.1001/archgenpsychiatry.2009.187

Meadow, R. (1977). Munchausen syndrome by proxy: The hinterland of child abuse. *Lancet, 2*, 343–345. https://doi.org/10.1016/S0140-6736(77)91497-0

Meadow, R. (2002). Different interpretations of Munchausen syndrome by proxy. *Child Abuse & Neglect, 26*, 501–508. https://doi.org/10.1016/S0145-2134(02)00326-5

Rosenberg, D. A. (1987). Web of deceit: A literature review of Munchausen syndrome by proxy. *Child Abuse & Neglect, 11*(4), 547–563. https://doi.org/10.1016/0145-2134(87)90081-0

Rutter, M., Sonuga-Barke, E. J., & Castle, J. (2010). Investigating the impact of early institutional deprivation on development: Background and research strategy of the English and Romanian Adoptees (ERA) study. *Monographs of the Society for Research in Child Development, 75*(1), 1–20. https://doi.org/10.1111/j.1540-5834.2010.00548.x

Sneed, R. C., & Bell, R. F. (1976). The Dauphin of Munchausen: Factitious passage of renal stones in a child. *Pediatrics, 58*(1), 127–130.

U.S. Department of Health and Human Services. (2018). *Child maltreatment 2018.* Children's Bureau: An Office of the Administration for Children & Families. https://www.acf.hhs.gov/cb/resource/child-maltreatment-2018

Vanderminden, J., Hamby, S., David-Ferdon, C., Kacha-Ochana, A., Merrick, M., Simon, T. R., Finkelhor, D., & Turner, H. (2019). Rates of neglect in a national sample: Child and family characteristics and psychological impact. *Child Abuse & Neglect, 88*, 256–265. https://doi.org/10.1016/j.chiabu.2018.11.014

Wright, J., Friedrich, W., Cinq-Mars, C., Cyr, M., & McDuff, P. (2004). Self-destructive and delinquent behaviors of adolescent female victims of child sexual abuse: Rates and covariates in clinical and nonclinical samples. *Violence & Victims, 19*(6), 627–643. https://doi.org/10.1891/vivi.19.6.627.66343

Yates, G., & Bass, C. (2017). The perpetrators of medical child abuse (Munchausen syndrome by proxy)—A systematic review of 796 cases. *Child Abuse & Neglect, 72*, 45–53. https://doi.org/10.1016/j.chiabu.2017.07.008

Zimmermann, P., & Soares, I. (2019). Recent contributions for understanding inhibited reactive attachment disorder. *Attachment & Human Development, 21*(2), 87–94. https://doi.org/10.1080/14616734.2018.1499207

Suggested Readings

*Indicates Particularly Recommended

Ainsworth, M. D. (1969). Object relations, dependency, and attachment: A theoretical review of the infant-mother relationship. *Child Development, 40*, 969–1025. https://doi.org/10.2307/1127008

Boris, N. W., Zeanah, C. H., & AACAP Work Group on Quality Issues. (2005). Practice parameters for the assessment and treatment of reactive attachment disorder in children and adolescents. *Journal of the American Academy of Child & Adolescent Psychiatry, 44*, 1206–1219. https://doi.org/10.1097/01.chi.0000177056.41655.ce

Bowlby, J. (1962). *Attachment and loss: Attachment*. Basic Books.

*Bretherton, I. (1992). The origins of attachment theory: John Bowlby and Mary Ainsworth. *Developmental Psychology, 28*, 759–775. https://doi.org/10.1037/0012-1649.28.5.759

Burns, B., Phillip, S., Wagner, H., Barth, R., Kolko, D., Campbell, Y., & Landsverk, J. (2004). Mental health need and access to mental health services by youths involved with child welfare: A national survey. *Journal of the American Academy of Child & Adolescent Psychiatry, 43*(8), 960–970. https://doi.org/10.1097/01.chi.0000127590.95585.65

Cicchetti, D., & Toth, S. (1995). A developmental psychopathology perspective on child abuse and neglect. *Journal of the American Academy of Child & Adolescent Psychiatry, 34*(5), 541–565. https://doi.org/10.1097/00004583-199505000-00008

Crosson-Tower, C. (1999). *Understanding child abuse and neglect*. Allyn & Bacon.

Jaghab, K., Skodnek, K. B., & Padder, T. A. (2006). Munchausen's Syndrome and other factitious disorders in children: Case series and literature review. *Psychiatry, 3*(3), 46–55.

Jones, L. M., Finkelhor, D., & Halter, S. (2006). Child maltreatment trends in the 1990s why does neglect differ from sexual and physical abuse? *Child Maltreatment, 11*(2), 107–120. https://doi.org/10.1177/1077559505284375

*Kempe, C. H., Silverman, F. N., Steele, B. F., Droegemueller, W., & Silver, H. K. (1962). The battered child syndrome. *Journal of the American Medical Association, 181*, 17–24. https://doi.org/10.1001/jama.1962.03050270019004

McClure, R. J., Davis, P. M., Meadow, S. R., & Sibert, J. R. (1996). Epidemiology of Münchausen syndrome by proxy, non-accidental poisoning, and non-accidental suffocation. *Archives of Disease in Childhood, 75*, 57–61. https://doi.org/10.1136/adc.75.1.57

*Meadow, R. (1977). Münchausen syndrome by proxy: The hinterland of child abuse. *Lancet, 2*, 343–345. https://doi.org/10.1016/S0140-6736(77)91497-0

Molnar, B. E., Buka, S. L., & Kessler, R. C. (2001). Child sexual abuse and subsequent psychopathology: Results from the National Comorbidity Survey. *American Journal of Public Health, 91*(5), 753–760. https://doi.org/10.2105/AJPH.91.5.753

O'Connor, T. G., & Rutter. M. (2000). Attachment disorder behavior following early severe deprivation: Extension and longitudinal follow-up. *Journal of the American Academy of Child & Adolescent Psychiatry, 9*, 703–712. https://doi.org/10.1097/00004583-200006000-00008

Sheridan, M. S. (2003). The deceit continues: An updated literature review of Münchausen syndrome by proxy. *Child Abuse & Neglect, 27*, 431–451. https://doi.org/10.1016/S0145-2134(03)00030-9

Smyke, A. T., Dumitrescu, A., & Zeanah, C. H. (2002). Disturbances of attachment in young children: I. The continuum of caretaking casualty. *Journal of the American Academy of Child & Adolescent Psychiatry, 41*, 972–982. https://doi.org/10.1097/00004583-200208000-00016

U.S. Department of Health and Human Services. (2018). *Child maltreatment 2018*. Children's Bureau: An Office of the Administration for Children & Families. US Government Printing Office. https://www.acf.hhs.gov/cb/report/child-maltreatment-2018

Zeanah, C. H., Scheeringa, M. S., Boris, N. W., Heller, S. S., Smyke, A. T., & Trapani, J. (2004). Reactive attachment disorder in maltreated toddlers. *Child Abuse & Neglect, 28*(8), 877–888. https://doi.org/10.1016/j.chiabu.2004.01.010

CHAPTER 25 ■ MENTAL HEALTH IN SCHOOLS

■ ISSUES IN SCHOOL CONSULTATION

Since almost all children attend school and since children with mental health problems do not leave their problems at the door when they walk into school, the provision of mental health services presents a unique opportunity for intervention. Mental health services in school are highly varied. Schools have clear mandates to serve the needs of children with disabilities but historically have tended to focus on things like autism and attention-deficit hyperactivity disorder and have generally been less interested in other mental health problems. In one recent national survey (Whitney & Peterson, 2019), 16.5% of children (about 7.7 million) had at least one mental disorder although slightly less than 50% received treatment. Furthermore, marked state-to-state variations were noted both in prevalence and numbers of untreated cases. Unfortunately, the rate of attrition in services outside schools is high (Bostic & Hoover, 2018; Merikangas et al., 2011).

Schools present an obvious place for screening and intervention. At the same time, schools have come under pressure from an increasing range of mandates for meeting education goals and metrics designed to evaluate school performance (Bostic & Hoover, 2018). Consultants must be aware of the potential complexities of the school as an organization, the many different professionals involved, the multiple levels of need, and the potential for sometimes even small gains to have a major impact. Consultation issues to students may change somewhat in dealing with private, parochial, or charter schools. In these settings, some of the pressure from government mandates may not apply although lack of support may be a challenge. It is important for the consultant to have a clear sense of the school and the purpose of the consultation. Visiting the school can provide information on issues as varied as the building, classroom, school personnel, support services, and overall atmosphere (see Bostic & Hoover, 2018 for a detailed discussion), as well as providing opportunities for in-person observation of the child's behavior and that of peers and others including teachers. Students in special education or those with "504" plans because of a learning disability, autism, and so forth present special problems. They may already have some mandated intervention services, but the provision of additional mental health supports in the school can further strengthen their intervention program.

School-based intervention programs stem from various sources. Understanding these various roots of mental health provision in schools helps in understanding the range of models currently available to mental health consultants. Table 25.1 summarizes some of the major events relative to evaluation of school-based consultation services in the United States.

TABLE 25.1

Major Events in Psychiatric Consultation to Schools

Social Event	Mental Health Impact on Schools	Child Psychiatry Response	Lessons Learned
Aftermath of WWII	Displaced orphan students required emotional support to contend with school	Mental health providers worked with educators to manage displaced students	Life events require mindful planning to promote mental health and resiliency in children
Civil rights movement	Equality for all, including those with disabilities, required schools to accept and respond to diverse students	Child psychiatrists identified psychiatric disorders that schools considered as possible educational disabilities	1. Psychiatric disorders did not necessarily "fit" educational disability categories 2. No consensual or empirical school interventions for identified disorders/disabilities existed
Social change and problem behaviors	Problematic behaviors, and their negative impact on schooling, increasingly evident in the classroom	Child psychiatrists provided input on lifestyle variables influencing quality of life	1. Little empirical evidence supported child psychiatry recommendations 2. Efforts to identify the prevalence of substance abuse and other problem behaviors helped illuminate mental health issues
Decrease in psychiatric hospitalization	Students managed in non-school environments returned to schools to receive an education appropriate for them, given complex needs	Child psychiatrists focused on discharge planning to provide outpatient treatment, including in school settings	Psychiatrists and educators partnered, by necessity, to address mental health issues impacting children in daily environments
Impact of mental health on learning	Students with diverse mental health difficulties have similarly diverse struggles at school as well as impact classroom instruction	Embrace broader "Response to Intervention" (RtI) approaches to identify and respond to varying degrees and impacts of psychopathology at school	Proactive efforts to screen, recognize, and respond to students can enhance school achievement

TABLE 25.1

Major Events in Psychiatric Consultation to Schools (*continued*)

Social Event	Mental Health Impact on Schools	Child Psychiatry Response	Lessons Learned
Resilience to traumatic events at schools	Traumatic events at school illuminated the importance of early detection and intervention for all students	Assist in the development of more sophisticated screening and evidence-based interventions for students at risk	Mental health supports can accelerate recovery from traumatic events
Emphasis on social emotional learning	Increased evidence for the positive impact of universal social emotional learning on student psychosocial and academic functioning	Consultation on selection of universal mental health promotion and prevention programming and consideration for how brain science can help inform and evaluate this programming	Psychiatrists' knowledge of brain science and etiology and development of psychopathology can support the shift from treatment-only approaches to promotion/prevention activities, and cultivating social skills

Reprinted with permission from Bostic, J. Q., & Hoover, S. A. (2018). School consultation. In A. Martin, M. H. Bloch, & F. R. Volkmar (Eds.), *Lewis's child and adolescent psychiatry: A comprehensive textbook* (5th ed., p. 958). Wolters Kluwer.

The challenges for providing mental health services include lack of insurance, minority status, and problems in screening and detection of those needing service as well as administrative obstacles to provision of service. Schools sometimes lack sufficient resources, for example, they lack guidance counselors, school psychologists, and social workers who could be expected to address behavioral and emotional issues of students.

There are many potential benefits of school-based mental health centers that provide direct access to services. These can include higher achievement, improved attendance, and lower rates of behavioral problems at schools and at home (Bostic & Hoover, 2018; Oberle et al., 2018; Platt et al., 2020). Benefits can also be observed for teachers and other supporters within the school (Kidger et al., 2016).

There also is the potential for programs to offer expanded services with referrals and links to outside services as needed. Importantly, school-based services provide the opportunity for early intervention and prevention of subsequent mental health and education problems. These models coordinate and integrate family, community, and school services (see Bostic & Hoover, 2018).

Advances in technology and telemedicine (Myers & Roth, 2018) have also impacted provision of consultation services in schools and other settings. Sometimes, these provide services of child psychiatrists to areas or populations with limited access to services. At other times, they help schools plan for intervention for students with special needs. Although offering many potential advantages, other issues including confidentiality and billing can pose obstacles to implementation.

MODELS FOR SCHOOL CONSULTATION

Many models for school-based service provision have now emerged (see Table 25.2). The *mental health consultation* model utilizes the consultant to help clarify how mental health problems may interact with school performance and how interventions might be developed

TABLE 25.2

Contemporary Models of School Consultation

Aspect of the Consultation	Consultation Model		
	Mental Health Consultation	Behavioral Consultation	Organizational Consultation
Initial focus	How mental health impacts student progress	Problematic behaviors exhibited by students/staff	How school contributes to problem
How information is obtained from consultee	Clinical interview with student/parents, review of school data, psychological testing	Direct observation in classroom, counting frequency, length of specified behaviors	Review of school philosophy, curriculum, instructional philosophy, administrative procedures for problem class or group
Objective	Help consultee identify strategies to address mental health problems interfering with school success and strengthen psychological assets	Help consultee measure problem behaviors, alter and shape student responses leading to problem behaviors	Help consultee refine organizational configuration and goals to diminish circumstances
Evaluation of model	Do identified intervention strategies improve student mental health functioning? Does student's school performance improve?	Do specific problem behaviors diminish in frequency/intensity? What does "data collection" reveal?	Does this specific problem illuminate larger problems in policy impacting multiple students? Does the proposed solution benefit everyone?
Example case (17-year-old student who does not attend regularly the year after becoming a teen parent)	Consultee identifies depressive symptoms that occurred post-pregnancy, constructs a plan with the student, teachers, and family to re-engage student in pleasurable activities, teach cognitive coping, and monitor mood	Consultee keeps track of days/times missed, addresses directly with student, and they construct plan for student to be there on time by having others care for child on certain days; they measure success of plan, and revise as needed	Consultee identifies well-intended but misattuned policies for attendance for current school population, and provides alternative schedule for students with children, course credit that can be completed at home, and course credit shifted to allow parenting, study/work to count toward graduation

Reprinted with permission from Bostic, J. Q., & Hoover, S. A. (2018). School consultation. In A. Martin, M. H. Bloch, & F. R. Volkmar (Eds.), *Lewis's child and adolescent psychiatry: A comprehensive textbook* (5th ed., p. 959). Wolters Kluwer.

to optimize student learning and functioning. This model is often an indirect one, that is, information may come to the consultant from parents or school staff and the consultant provides guidance based on this information without necessarily seeing the specific student. In this model, services may be reimbursed either by the school or potentially by insurance or sometimes an outside agency. In this model, the school can decide how best to use (or not use) recommendations made by the consultant.

In the *behavioral consultation model*, the consultant adopts a traditional behavioral psychology approach. Thus, the problem is viewed in the context of its antecedents and consequences; an intervention plan is then developed and refined through further evaluation. The implementation of specific goals and objectives following the behavioral analysis is an important advantage of this model that can engage teachers in implementation and evaluation of the intervention. This model relies heavily on data collection and thoughtful observation. This approach differs from the earlier behavioral models in that it assumes that students often lack appropriate behaviors to employ in dealing with complicated situations and then make use of less adaptive behaviors, for example, aggression or acting out (Putnam et al., 2005; Stephan et al., 2015).

The *organizational consultation model* views schools as systems and uses behavioral principles and the engagement of the range of school staff (i.e., administration staff as well as teachers) to produce organizational change. It seeks to utilize behavioral science concepts and the involvement of multiple system members to evaluate the school in a broader sense. It views difficulties as resulting from discrepancies in expectations and muddled communication leading to inconsistency and ambiguity. This broader systems view may help reveal specific aspects of staff or programs that are associated with student difficulties. In this model, the problems of a single student are viewed more broadly as reflecting system issues, an approach that may clarify how school policies or misunderstanding contribute to mental health and behavioral issues in the student who is confronted by ambiguous or contradictory demands. Models addressing low-achieving schools, such as the Comer School Development Program, precipitated school restructuring and change in school culture and climate, positively impacting student self-esteem, motivation, and achievement (Comer & Woodruff, 1998).

The School Consultation Process

Mental health consultants must be aware of the varied roles of the school staff. Teachers and special educators are the school staff who have the most prolonged and enduring contact with students (Bostic & Hoover, 2018). Other involved staff may include school nurses, social workers, and administrators. Aides may, in actuality, provide the most support to students needing special services during the day; the education requirements of teacher aides are quite varied from state to state. Occupational and physical therapists may be providing services to students with Individualized Education Plans (Bostic & Hoover, 2018). Given the complexity of schools and the marked variations that occur, it is important for a consultant to have a good working relationship and familiarity with schools to which they provide consultations.

The mental health consultant should consider the various aspects of the school environment because they impact students and provision of mental health services. Some of these conditions are summarized in Table 25.3. Box 25.1 provides a framework for the consultant to consider when engaging in a school consultation.

As presented in the table and box, Bostick and Hoover (2018) provide a comprehensive summary of the goals for school consultation. The consultant must be aware of the potential sources of difficulty in this process. Some of the techniques useful in this process are summarized in Box 25.2.

TABLE 25.3

Framework for Evaluating a School

School Component	What to Observe	Potential Questions for Staff
School building	Safety/security: Does the building appear safe? Is the building comfortable (temperature, chairs beyond desks, lighting, noisy)? Does the building value students (student art on the walls, recognition of student achievements, evidence of parent–teacher alliance)? Is this a place a child would want to be in?	How does one enter/exit the building? Where do students go if they are having a hard time? Where are students' classwork or projects kept or displayed? What happens after school is over? Do students stay in the building before or after school?
Classrooms	What do classrooms look like? How big is the room? How many students are in this room, and how many adults? How many learning areas are there, and are they separated so children can be in a quiet place within the classroom? How stimulating (visual, auditory, tactile) is this classroom, and do the students appear over/understimulated?	What is the average number of students in each classroom? How are teachers encouraged to set up their classroom? If a student is having a hard time in the classroom, where do they go? How did you (teacher) decide what to put up in your classroom?
School atmosphere	How is a stranger greeted? Does the school seem organized for students or for staff? Do most students appear engaged with instruction (are students within classrooms, alert, attentive, answering/asking questions?)? How do students and staff interact (smiling, directives, calm, tense)? Do children thrive here?	Whom should I meet when I enter the building? How do students move between classes/to lunch/recess? What do students do when they have finished classroom assignments? What do staff expect from students here? What do staff most worry about here regarding students?
School staff		
Administrators	Are administrators present/accessible? What kind of tone/impression does the administrator convey? Do staff appear comfortable around the administrator? Who does this administrator best serve (students, teachers, parents, other administrators)? What led to this administrator being selected for this building (student needs, up/down move for this administrator)?	What kind of interactions does the administrator have with students (discipline, earned reward time, common interests discussed in halls/lunch)? What is the administrator's priority in this building? What do staff seek from the administrator (support, camaraderie, ideas, discipline, avoidance)?

TABLE 25.3

Framework for Evaluating a School (*continued*)

School Component	What to Observe	Potential Questions for Staff
Teachers	Do teachers want to be in this school (eager to be with students or staff)? Do teachers stay in this building? How do teachers engage students (time to work, demonstrate content, model enthusiasm, surprise students)? How often do teachers alter the instructional approach (every 10 minutes, something different [lecture, student reading, class discussion], or employ different modalities [visual, auditory, tactile]) employed during instruction?	How many teachers left this building last year? Average over the last several (5) years? What is the student to teacher ratio? What is the average length of time teachers have been in this district/building? How many teachers here have advanced (masters, doctoral) degrees? What kind of teachers do best in this school (independent, orderly, collaborative, creative)?
Special staff	Are other school staff present? How do teachers and other school staff interact (take student out, co-teach, friendly/tense)? How do teachers describe other staff (particularly contributions of special educators)?	What kind of special education staff work here? How often are they in this building (always, weekly)? What kind of other teachers are in the classroom (parent aides, "paraprofessionals" aides)? Do they work with particular students, with everyone in the classroom?
Support staff	Are support staff friendly? Do they appear open about discussing the school and students? Do support staff work well with other staff?	What kind of support staff are in this building? How long have most of them been here? How are support staff paired with other staff?

Reprinted with permission from Bostic, J. Q., & Hoover, S. A. (2018). School consultation. In A. Martin, M. H. Bloch, & F. R. Volkmar (Eds.), *Lewis's child and adolescent psychiatry: A comprehensive textbook* (5th ed., pp. 960–961). Wolters Kluwer.

BOX 25.1 **School Consultation Framework**

The psychiatric school consultant should consider how micro problems can lead to macro solutions, that is, how individual student problems can be addressed to improve circumstances for all subsequent students and staff. Five components should be considered in every consultation:

1. Who is the actual consultee, and what are the confidentiality parameters?
2. What is the consultation question, and what is the consultee seeking and wishing will happen?
3. How is the larger system experiencing this problem?
4. What legal or ethical factors should be considered?
5. How does the consultant understand this problem biopsychosocially?

(continued)

BOX 25.1   School Consultation Framework (*continued*)

The Consultee and Confidentiality Parameters

The consultant must establish procedures to clarify who is appropriate to contact or to evaluate. When requested to meet with students, the consultant must obtain parental permission before interviewing any student. If parents refuse evaluation by the consultant of their child, the consultant may still observe, unobtrusively, the student, and consult the staff about their questions on how best to work with this student. Clarification of confidentiality should occur, sometimes recurrently, with staff, students, and parents. Anyone meeting with the consultant should understand how information is shared and whether written clinical information is placed in the student or personnel records.

Clarification of the Consultation Question and Needs/Wishes of the Consultee

Consultants help others define the problem and envision solutions. Although consultees may ask for interventions to assist a student, sometimes they actually wish the consultant will address administrators, or recommend the student be removed from the consultee's classroom. Consultants must "read between the lines" to clarify both the consultee's overt request as well as underlying desires. The success of every consultation depends on the consultant understanding the consultee's concerns and wishes, such that both agree on the problem and on realistic goals for any intervention.

The System Reaction to the Problem

The problem will affect various school staff members differently, and each may have different goals for this consultation. Consultants should clarify who requested a consultation, who knows about the consultation, who has consented to the consultation, and who should be informed about the findings for this consultation. The more that differing goals can be aligned, the higher the probability that participants will invest in a proposed solution.

Legal and Ethical Factors

Special educational laws may provide the student different opportunities, yet families or schools may not see the applicability of such laws in a particular case. Similarly, the case may be confounded by ethical dilemmas, particularly in cases of suspected abuse. If abuse is suspected, the consultant may help staff articulate concerns to the appropriate agency, or assist parents and the school in addressing circumstances or staff perceived as abusive. In acutely dangerous situations such as suicidality or homicidality, the consultant can help consultees facilitate emergency treatment or how to warn others who may be at risk. Potential legal and ethical ramifications should be considered for every proposed intervention.

Biopsychosocial Understanding of the Problem

Child psychiatrists consider people's biologic vulnerabilities to psychopathology, their past experiences, and current family, peer, school, or other social stressors in explaining dysfunctional behaviors. These different influences may provide multiple intervention targets for a particular problem and should take into consideration existing services in the school and community. A student may need interventions biologically, psychologically, and socially, such as a referral for a medication evaluation, a behavioral plan at school and home, and connection to social groups such as sports teams, choir or band, or summer camps.

Reprinted with permission from Bostic, J. Q., & Hoover, S. A. (2018). School consultation. In A. Martin, F. R. Volkmar, & M. Bloch (Eds.), *Lewis's child and adolescent psychiatry: A comprehensive textbook* (5th ed., p. 961). Wolters Kluwer.

BOX 25.2   **School Consulting Techniques**

Ally

1. Validate consultees' perceptions before proposing any solutions. Validating perceptions cultivates consultee trust that the consultant understands their predicament. If in doubt, ask questions or pose solutions as questions ("What would likely happen if we...?").
2. Bind anxiety. Everything the consultant does either increases or decreases anxiety within the system. The more people who share the problem, the less anxious each individual will be. Although consultants may not know the answer to various problems, thinking through how they would find an answer can diminish consultee's anxiety.
3. Create respect for everyone involved. Minimizing splitting of staff, students, and parents decreases the probability that individuals will oppose an intervention. The consultant can attempt to separate personalities from the problem by focusing on terms used, by identifying the common goals between parties, and by identifying the circumstances each party uniquely faces.

Align

4. Find the good intent gone awry. When students or staff act inappropriately, the consultant can back up to the good intention that motivated the person's (mis) behavior so that self-esteem, and thus willingness to attempt different behaviors, is maximized. For example, if a teacher "yells" at students, the consultant can "backtrack" to the diligent efforts by the teacher to get the student's attention and to feel responsible that the student learns the material. Then the consultant is positioned to examine alternatives (visually signal the child, use a very soft voice, etc.), which will seem less critical of the teacher's yelling.
5. Help others to see the child (or staff member) differently. Maladaptive behaviors may be used to solve problems when no other solution is available (e.g., talking in class may be the only way a student "knows" to slow down instruction or to obtain positive attention from others because the student cannot garner positive attention by doing the academic task).
6. Connect others. Look for opportunities to connect others to benefit the staff or student, utilizing existing services in the school and in the larger community.
7. Appeal to shared values by giving people options they cannot argue with. Explore and identify appropriate desires of students and staff so that interventions can be provided to realize those appropriate goals. For example, identifying that a student seeks to attend college, or hold a particular job, provides a "frame" for posed interventions ("You've indicated you want to attend/work at _____, and they require you show up on time; so we have to practice going to sleep at 10 pm so that you can be ready the next morning.").

Mobilize

8. At every opportunity, expand the consultee's skills. Whenever possible, the consultant attempts to assist the consultee in selecting and implementing skills helpful for that situation. The consultant aspires to provide the consultee facility with multiple skills that the consultee can use subsequently independently.
9. Use the consultee's own words to frame interventions. Framing interventions with terms used by the consultee, by staff, and by students, increases each person feeling heard, and improves the probability of each investing in proposed solutions.

(continued)

| **BOX 25.2** | **School Consulting Techniques (*continued*)** |

10. Identify one step up from the current situation. Consultees may need help seeing the steps in a sequence toward appropriate behavior (e.g., Cursing may be "a step up" from physically assaulting others). Even small positive changes generate momentum to achieve greater changes.
11. Move toward anticipating problems rather than reacting to them. Efforts to help consultees see how problems arise, and how they might be prevented in the future can empower consultees to find and face problems early. More importantly, initial reactions may not represent optimal solutions, but instead create additional conflicts or problems.

Reprinted with permission from Bostic, J. Q., & Hoover, S. A. (2018). School consultation. In A. Martin, F. R. Volkmar, & M. Bloch (Eds.), *Lewis's child and adolescent psychiatry: A comprehensive textbook* (5th ed., p. 962). Wolters Kluwer.

ISSUES IN SCHOOL CONSULTATION

A small but growing number of schools have school-based mental health centers that provide direct access to services. Benefits of on-site service include higher achievement, improved attendance, and lower rates of behavioral problems. Some programs now offer expanded services and explicit links and referral arrangements to other agencies. Prevention and early intervention models have been used for high-risk as well as the broader range of children in schools. These models coordinate and integrate family, community, and school services (see Bostic & Hoover, 2018 for a detailed review).

SPECIAL EDUCATION

Students in need of special education service face more than the usual academic challenges and require additional supports. It is important to understand the unique issues that arise for students who have been identified as having these needs. Mental health professionals have several important roles to play in this system: they often take a major role in issues of assessment and identification of eligibility for special services and then in ongoing monitoring and management.

Special education services are designed to use specialized teaching methods that can help students beyond what is presented in the regular education classroom. Students can be identified based on referrals from outside agencies or specialists or within schools because some students are not seen to progress at the same pace as their peers. These services include special instruction from trained special education providers as well as a team of other supporters, including the school psychologist, social workers, occupational therapists, speech-communication therapists, and physical therapists. When students have multiple needs, sometimes including mental health needs, the integration of these services is an important role of the mental health specialist.

Within the United States, several somewhat distinctive sets of entitlements can apply to students with special needs. A growing awareness of the needs of students with learning disability and others for specialized services and a general awareness of the civil rights of all persons in the United States, including the right to an education, led to the passage of the *Education for All Handicapped Children Act* (Public Law [PL] 94-142) by Congress in 1975. This law, subsequently revised several times, required that all public schools receiving any federal support be required to provide a *free and appropriate education* to any child with a physical or mental disability. This marked a sea change from previous policy that allowed schools to decline to serve students if they felt they were not qualified to do so—a practice that led to many children not receiving services at all or ending up in long-stay instructional care. PL 94-142 specifically mentioned a number of handicapping conditions including attention-deficit hyperactivity disorder and autism among others. As noted earlier, the original law has now been amended several times including the Education of the Handicapped Act enacted in 1966 and again in 1975 (see https://sites.ed.gov/idea/ for a history of this act).

These federal mandates for services and education to students with disabilities included provision of an *Individualized Education Plan (IEP)* created by school staff with parental input that includes children with disabilities in the mainstream as much as possible, while also providing them with needed rehabilitative services. The families of children who receive services have access to an entire set of administrative procedures with a right to further judicial review if an agreement cannot be reached. The IEP is designed to have a clear statement of goals and objectives that can be reviewed for progress on a regular basis and then changed as appropriate. The law presumes that children should be educated in the least restrictive environment possible. A number of special provisions for students receiving special services were contained within the original law and its successors, including Part B of the Education of the Handicapped Act. These include protections relative to suspension and expulsion for behavioral problems.

Some children may receive supports in school through the *Americans with Disabilities Act (ADA)*. This act has application in many areas other than in education and essentially prohibits discrimination based on disability. In schools, it provides for accommodations for students with disabilities including such things as extra time on testing, tutoring, and so forth. When requested to do so, schools will provide an assessment and, if needed, a special plan called a "504" plan that outlines the special supports the student needs. The degree and extent of supports provided is usually less extensive than that provided under an IEP. The ADA is more broadly written and can apply to a broader range of students than those needing more specialized and extensive IEP supports. Typical supports under the 504 plans are ones that can be provided within a traditional classroom environment. The assessment process for obtaining a 504 plan is less extensive than that for an IEP. Having an IEP also gives the school more flexibility in modifying the specific educational requirements of the program for the student (something not done in a 504 plan that provides support to help the students meet standard goals). In general, students with needs in multiple areas are more likely to require the more extensive supports of an IEP, for example, those with autism spectrum disorder, whereas a child with a learning disability or attention-deficit hyperactivity disorder might require only a 504 plan. In some cases, existing school district supports may be sufficient. Students with certain specific disabilities like deafness or blindness may have specific rights for services; such students may also have mental health problems (McConachie & Carr, 2008; Swanepoel et al., 2020).

Students with a range of psychiatric disorders may meet criteria for support under these plans. The need of such learning supports for children with developmental disorders like autism spectrum disorder, communication disorders, learning disorders, intellectual disability, and so forth are clear, but students with other problems like anxiety disorders, posttraumatic stress disorder, mood problems, and so forth may also require special supports. Some of the components of these various approaches are summarized in Table 25.4 and some of the classroom and/or programmatic accommodations for students with specific psychiatric difficulties are summarized in Table 25.5.

TABLE 25.4

A. Determining Special Education Eligibility. B. School Service Plans for Students with Psychiatric Disorders

A. Determining Special Education Eligibility

1. Does the child have one or more of the following types of disability (documented by the medical evaluation/diagnosis, educational/ psychological testing, etc.)?
   Autism
   Developmental delay
   Intellectual disability
   Sensory hearing loss, vision, deafness, blindness
   Neurologic
   Emotional
   Communication
   Specific learning
   Other health
2. If one or more of these disabilities is present, is the child making effective progress in school? If the student is being reevaluated to determine if a disability is still impacting the child, would the child continue to make progress in school without the currently provided special education services?
3. Is the lack of progress a result of the child's disability?
4. Does the child require specially designed instruction in order to make effective progress in school or does the child require related services in order to access the general curriculum?

B. School Service Plans for Students with Psychiatric Disorders

	Type of School Service Plan		
	District Service Plan	**504 Plan**	**Individualized Educational Program (IEP)**
Purpose	To respond quickly to mild changes in the student's life that impact learning; focus is on mild and/or brief circumstances that may impact learning	To ensure that all students have equal opportunity to learn, even if they have a disability; focus is student's opportunities as compared to other students in that school	To remediate symptoms of a student's disability; student's unique needs are the focus
Criteria to receive this plan	Student has a symptom or disorder that impacts learning	Student has an impairment that limits a major life activity, but may not require specialized instruction	Student has a disability that interferes with educational progress, and that requires specialized instruction
Who develops this plan	Teacher and administrator, usually with parental input	Teacher, administrator (often the school's designated "504 coordinator"), school counselor, and usually parent, student (if appropriate)	Educational team, including staff certified in special education; may include evaluations by school psychologist, social worker; parent may bring friends, advocates, own evaluators to be part of team
What is usually provided	Changes within classroom to enable student to perform better	Changes within classroom or school building to enable student to complete curriculum expectations	Changes within classroom setting(s) to provide student different instruction, and may substantially alter what is required of student

TABLE 25.4

A. Determining Special Education Eligibility. B. School Service Plans for Students with Psychiatric Disorders (*continued*)

	Type of School Service Plan		
	District Service Plan	**504 Plan**	**Individualized Educational Program (IEP)**
Example of what is provided	Student is allowed to sit closer to teacher during instruction; student is met by familiar staff to decrease anxiety	Student is allowed more time to complete tests; student may be provided device to hear better	Student may leave regular language arts class and receive specialized reading program; student may be exempted from course requirements
Which staff deliver services	Usually regular education staff	Usually regular education staff	Staff with specialized training (special education teachers, speech therapists, occupational therapists, etc.)
Where the student receives services	Regular classroom	Regular classroom with regular peers "to the maximum extent appropriate"	Wide ranging, from regular education classrooms (inclusion) to pullout for special education classrooms, to offsite day-school programs, to 24-hour/day residential schools
Review of the plan	As needed	Plan reviewed at least every year	At least every year plan is reviewed, and every 3 years the student is retested to see if still qualifies
Disciplinary actions	Usually not applicable	If "manifestation hearing" indicates student's impairment or disability caused misbehavior, then student cannot be suspended/expelled; school is not required to provide free, appropriate education for suspended or expelled students	If "manifestation hearing" indicates student's disability caused misbehavior, then student cannot be suspended/expelled; if student is suspended or expelled, school must still provide free, appropriate education
Appeal recourses	None provided	School may alter 504 Plan immediately should circumstances indicate need; "notice" may be provided verbally; family may appeal to the Office for Civil Rights if perceive school is discriminating against child because of a disability	School must provide "prior written notice" before changes in educational plan or placement are made; family may appeal decisions or plan to local, then state departments of education

Reprinted with permission from Bostic, J. Q., & Hoover, S. A. (2018). School consultation. In A. Martin, M. H. Bloch, & F. R. Volkmar (Eds.), *Lewis's child and adolescent psychiatry: A comprehensive textbook* (5th ed., p. 964). Wolters Kluwer.

TABLE 25.5

Components of an Individualized Educational Program (IEP)

Components	Example	Comments
Usual Components		
Present level of functioning	Although in the 5th grade, [student] is currently reading at 3rd grade level.	Both strengths and weaknesses should be described, with current functioning identified for each area of need requiring a goal
Educational goals	In normal classroom discussions, [student] will repeat back accurately instructions for a task, 4/5 times daily.	Goals should include (1) circumstances or setting; (2) observable behavior; and (3) performance measure, as well as staff person responsible for implementing
Educational accommodations and modifications	[Student] will be allowed to take tests verbally or untimed.	Intervention necessary to allow student to access curriculum, or how curriculum will be modified
Special education and related services	[Student] will receive specialized reading instruction 60 minutes/day for 4 days/week in the learning center.	Clarification of staff with special expertise to assist student and how that will occur (teaching, consult to teacher, group instruction, etc.)
Placement and participation specifications	[Student] will receive reading, math, and social group instruction in a pullout resource classroom.	Least restrictive environment for student to receive services
Transition services planning	[Student] will work at _____ 2 days/week starting April 1st.	For all students by age 16, although may start at age 14
Transfer of rights planning	[Student] is aware of right to participate.	Student informed, allowed to participate by age 16, and parental rights transfer when reaches age 18
Additional Components/Related Services		
Adapted physical education	[Student] will be allowed to ride bicycle for physical education (PE) requirement in place of group PE.	Changes in physical education requirements based on disability
Behavioral intervention plan	[Student] will access [staff] and follow de-escalation steps when irritated.	A Functional Assessment of Behavior usually includes (1) antecedents to the negative behaviors, (2) specific negative behavior, and (3) consequences (benefits) of this behavior so that interventions can occur at any of these three points
Counseling services	[Student] will receive 30 minutes of individual counseling per week.	Counseling is usually to help student function better at school; counseling may include parents or family training

TABLE 25.5

Components of an Individualized Educational Program (IEP) (*continued*)

Components	Example	Comments
Extended school year services	[Student] will receive tutoring 2 hour/day for 4 weeks in summer.	Extended-year services are required to "prevent regression" rather than to increase new skills throughout the year
Occupational therapy	[Student] will receive keyboarding training.	Often includes additional training in activities of daily living; may also include special cushions, devices, or techniques to address sensory-motor symptoms
Physical therapy	[Student] will practice writing with special paper and pencil.	Includes development of gross and fine motor skills
School health services	[Student] will have blood pressure checked weekly.	Medication administration, vital sign or other check (blood glucose, etc.), or nutritional services may occur
Speech–language therapy	[Student] will receive speech therapy with another student 30 minutes/week to develop conversation skills.	Includes social-pragmatic training as well as training for dysarthria
Transportation services	[Student] will ride a van with an assistant.	May include special vehicles or configurations based on student's needs

Reprinted with permission from Bostic, J. Q., & Hoover, S. A. (2018). School consultation. In A. Martin, M. H. Bloch, & F. R. Volkmar (Eds.), *Lewis's child and adolescent psychiatry: A comprehensive textbook* (5th ed., p. 965). Wolters Kluwer.

BULLYING

Bullying is a widespread problem in schools, beginning in primary school and particularly prominent in middle school. Using national survey data, the Centers for Disease Control has reported that nearly 20% of children between 14 and 18 years of age report being bullied, with a slightly lower number reporting being victims of cyberbullying (Gladden et al., 2014). There are marked differences in rates of bullying from country to country, with Canada and Norway having the lowest rates and the United States in the middle of the pack (Farrington at al., 2017). Given the amount of time children spend in school and the many unstructured and unsupervised times (e.g., recess, gym, cafeteria), there are many opportunities for bullying.

The term *bullying* is typically used when a child or group of children (or adolescents or adults) use some aspect of dominance/strength to intimidate another. The individual being bullied is typically perceived as weaker and more vulnerable (Juvonen & Graham, 2014) than the perpetrator of the bullying. This inequity of status discriminates bullying from other conflict situations, for example, fighting, in school where status or standing is seen as more equal.

Various types of bullying can occur such as

- verbal bullying—threats, harassment, derogatory comments,
- physical bullying—aggression, physical intimidation,
- emotional bullying—belittling, abusive language
- cyberbullying—use of computer, internet, or online activities to make fun, ostracize, or belittle.

Cyberbullying has some special aspects that differ from other forms of bullying (see Rivara & Le Menestrel, 2016). Other kinds of fighting and aggressive behavior fall outside the scope of bullying. Bullying can occur between individuals or between a group (often with a leader) and an individual target. Because bullying can occur in less supervised contexts, it can go unrecognized. Cyberbullying is particularly complex in this regard (Rivara & Le Menestrel, 2016). There are some gender differences, with boys more likely to use direct methods of bullying and girls indirect ones. Although sometimes an isolated occurrence, bullying often is an ongoing problem.

Risks for bullying have to do with anything that identifies a student as being different, for example, based on a learning difference, gender identification, social standing, social class, ethnicity, physical disability, and so forth (Rivara & Le Menestrel, 2016). Individuals with autism spectrum disorder are at special risk as are LGBTQ youth. Risks for being a bully include the presence of externalizing mental health problems (e.g., problem in conduct and aggression) as well as learning issues, lower degrees of parental involvement, and parental aggression or maltreatment (Shetgiri et al., 2013). Some students who have been bullied go on to be bullies themselves (Rivara & Le Menestrel, 2016).

All involved in bullying are at risk for both short- and long-term problems including issues such as anxiety and depression. A number of school-based interventions have been developed and utilized at multiple levels both of prevention and care once a bullying incident has occurred (Toffoi & Farington, 2011). Mental health problems may be even more common in the group of those who are both victims and bullies themselves. These can include a range of difficulties that persists into adulthood (Rivara & Le Menestrel, 2016).

School attendance and school avoidance can be a problem for the child who is bullied. In addition to school avoidance, other signs of possible bullying include unexplained injuries or bruises, loss of money or electronics, etc. Anxiety and depression can be noted, as well as onset of unexplained physical symptoms and sometimes suicidal ideation (Sansone & Sansone, 2008). Long-term effects of being bullied may cause higher stress levels that, in turn, impact mental and physical health, interpersonal relationships, and work. There may also be an increased risk for later substance abuse (Sanchez et al., 2017).

Understanding the longer term effects of being a bully is somewhat complicated by the fact that bullies often have pre-existing problems with self-esteem, aggression, and conduct. Being a bully may increase risk for a range of difficulties (Schoeler et al., 2018). Sometimes, when bullying is detected, subsequent negative reaction leads to public shaming and social isolation. All 50 U.S. states now have anti-bullying laws, although these vary significantly and the approaches to cyberbullying are particularly varied (Rivara & Le Menestrel, 2016).

A number of effective intervention programs have been developed, and teacher training is now required throughout the United States (Hatzenbuehler et al., 2017). Interventions can be narrow or more broadly focused. Thus, some programs are aimed at the entire school system and aim to decrease bullying through increased awareness and explicit teaching of students/staff on strategies to use to deal with bullying when it occurs. These programs can be effective in reducing rates of bullying in schools (Jimenez-Barbero et al., 2016). Other programs are more specific or selective, targeting groups of students at risk (both for being bullied and for being bullies). These often include training in strategies for coping, anger management, and so forth. These programs do not address broader issues of awareness and tolerance in the family and the broader community as a whole. One meta-analysis has supported the efficacy of such a program for LGBTQ youth (Marx & Kettrey, 2016).

When bullying has occurred, interventions are designed to deal with it and to support both those bullied and those who bully. In their comprehensive review, Ttofi et al. (2011) observed that, overall, there is a significant benefit of programs that aim to reduce bullying, but they did emphasize the need for looking at the broader range of issues involved in bullying. These issues include setting the "no bullying" tone at school, providing more supervision in at-risk settings, and securing parental involvement.

■ SCHOOL-BASED MENTAL HEALTH INTERVENTION PROGRAMS

A number of empirically supported school-based mental health prevention and intervention programs have been developed (see Table 25.6). These all aim to integrate the school with the

TABLE 25.6

Evidence-Based Mental Health Intervention by Tier and Target Outcome

	Trauma	Anxiety	Depression	Conduct Problems/Aggression	Substance Abuse	Social Skills Building/Other
TIER 1 Universal, whole school/classroom strategies for promoting positive mental health in ALL students.	• Psychological first aid: listen, protect, connect, model, and teacher education to identify and address psychological distress (e.g., Kognito) • School-Side Ecologic Strategies—positive, safe school climate	• Friends • Positive action	• Positive action • SOS—Signs of Suicide	• 4 Rs • Al's Pals • Caring School Community • Good Behavior Game (GBG) • High Scope Educational Approach for Preschool • Life Skills Training (LST) • Lion's Quest Skills for Adolescence • Michigan Model for Health • MindUP • Nurturing Parenting Program • Olweus Bully Prevention Program • Open Circle • Peaceworks: Peacemaking Skills for Little Kids • Promoting Alternative Thinking Strategies (PATHS) • PATHS to PAX	• Caring School Community • Life Skills Training (LST) • Lion's Quest Skills for Adolescence • Lion's Quest Skills for Action • Michigan Model for Health • Nurturing Parenting Program • PATHS to PAX • Project ALERT • Project TNT: Toward No Tobacco • Raising Healthy Children • The Too Good for Drugs and Violence Programs	• Competent Kids, Caring Communities Project • SUCCESS • Responsive Classroom (RC) • Teen Outreach Program (TOP) • Tribes Learning Communities

(continued)

TABLE 25.6

Evidence-Based Mental Health Intervention by Tier and Target Outcome (*continued*)

Trauma	Anxiety	Depression	Conduct Problems/ Aggression	Substance Abuse	Social Skills Building/Other
			• Project ACHIEVE • Raising Healthy Children • Resolving Conflict Creatively Program • RULER Approach • Second Step Violence Prevention Program • Social Decision-Making/Problem-Solving Program • Steps to Respect • The Stop and Think Social Skills Program for Schools • Teaching Students to be Peacemakers (Peacemakers) • Tools of the Mind		

TIER 2 Targeted small-group prevention and promotion for at-risk students.	• Bounce Back • Cognitive Behavioral Interventions for Trauma in Schools (CBITS) • Support for Students Exposed to Trauma (SSET)	• CARE (Care, Assess, Respond, Empower) • The C.A.T. Project • Coping Cat	• CARE	• Aggression Replacement Training (ART) • CARE • Coping power • I Can Problem Solve: Raising a Thinking Child (ICPS) • Incredible Years • Nurturing Parenting Program • Strengthening Families Program (SFP)	• CARE • Nurturing Parenting Program • Strengthening Families Program (SFP)	• Girls Circle • Primary Project
TIER 3 More intensive, individualized interventions for students experiencing a mental health challenge	• Trauma-focused cognitive behavioral therapy (TF-CBT)	• The C.A.T. Project • Coping Cat	• Interpersonal Psychotherapy for Depressed Adolescents (IPT-A)	• Multisystemic therapy (MST) • Nurturing Parenting Program	• Nurturing Parenting Program	

Reprinted with permission from Bostic, J. Q., & Hoover, S. A. (2018). School consultation. In A. Martin, M. H. Bloch, & F. R. Volkmar (Eds.), Lewis's child and adolescent psychiatry: A comprehensive textbook (5th ed., p. 972). Wolters Kluwer.

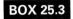

BOX 25.3   School Consultation Websites

www.schoolmentalhealth.org: up-to-date information about national school mental health training, practice, research, and policy

http://www.schoolmentalhealth.org: a repository of useful resources for school clinicians, educators, families, and students on school mental health

http://smhp.psych.ucla.edu: clearinghouse of important mental health, school, and education materials

http://ies.ed.gov/ncee/wwc/: information on broad categories of findings of "what works" in schools including academics and mental health

http://www.ldonline.org: information on classroom changes for students with learning disabilities, including attention-deficit hyperactivity disorder

http://www.wrightslaw.com: information about legal aspects of education, including IDEA 504 Plans

Reprinted with permission from Martin, A., Bloch, M. H., & Volkmar, F. R. (Eds.). (2018). *Lewis's child and adolescent psychiatry* (5th ed., p. 974). Wolters Kluwer.

family and broader community in the coordination and provision of services and help provide school-age youth with increased access to such services. Mental health professionals have an important role in this effort.

Supports in Table 25.6 are grouped by tier level. Tier 1 supports are universal in nature and designed to promote social emotional adjustment and a positive and accepting school environment. These occur throughout the school and within the classroom. They aim to foster positive social emotional functioning and optimal outcome of all students. It appears that about 80% to 85% of students in a school can be successfully addressed through these approaches (Bostick & Hoover, 2018). The Tier 2 approaches focus on the more specific mental health needs of a smaller group (10%–15% of students) at risk for some problem (these are sometimes termed *secondary prevention services*). Finally, Tier 3 supports are those needed for students (perhaps 5%) already exhibiting problems and needing services. As noted previously, telehealth approaches have become increasingly useful and can be integrated into these various programs. Box 25.3 summarizes some of the available school consultation websites. A number of specific interventions may be applicable to youth with a range of developmental and mental health disorders (see Bostic & Hoover, 2018, pp. 967–971).

SUMMARY

An increasing number of schools have partnered with mental health providers and programs to provide school-based services. These can make use of existing community health centers and supports and these programs have assumed increasingly active and prominent roles in recent years. They can be involved at various levels including prevention and intervention, as well as in consultation regarding specific children or youth and/or specific issues and problems like bullying or fostering a positive school climate (Bruns et al., 2004). There has been noteworthy heterogeneity in the number of states and/or local school districts adopting programs that aim to support mental health needs of students. Giving students access on site at school to mental health services is sensible and effective (Benningfield & Stephan, 2015; Fazel et al., 2014) and can readily be integrated into the work of existing community providers (Stephan et al., 2007).

Although many advances have been made, barriers to the provision of effective consultation continue to exist. These include the limited number of mental health providers, tensions between medical (or school) and psychiatric models of care, insurance and time pressures, and difficulties in communication. In some respects, the availability of a consultant who is at least a periodic presence goes a considerable way in dealing with some of these issues. Challenges remain in integrating good mental health principles in pediatric (and educational care), but the range of effective models and solid research has increased dramatically. Mandates for coverage, health care reform, the increased use of technology, and the electronic medical record all have at least the potential for fostering advances in the coming decade.

References

*Indicates Particularly Recommended

Benningfield, M. M., & Stephan, S. H. (2015). Integrating mental health into schools to support student success. *Child and Adolescent Psychiatric Clinics of North America, 24*(2), xv–xvii. https://doi .org/10.1016/j.chc.2014.12.005

*Bostic, J. Q., & Hoover, S. A. (2018). School consultation. In A. Martin, M. H. Bloch, & F. R. Volkmar (Eds.), *Lewis's child and adolescent psychiatry: A comprehensive textbook* (5th ed., pp. 956–974). Wolters Kluwer.

Bruns, E. J., Walrath, C., Glass-Siegel, M., & Weist, M. D. (2004). School-based mental health services in Baltimore: Association with school climate and special education referrals. *Behavior Modification, 28*(4), 491–512. https://doi.org/10.1177/0145445503259524

Comer, J. P., & Woodruff, D. W. (1998). Mental health in schools. *Child & Adolescent Psychiatric Clinics of North America, 7*(3), 499–513, viii. https://doi.org/10.1016/s1056-4993(18)30226-8

*Farrington, D. P., Gaffney, H., Losel, F., & Ttofi, M. M. (2017). Systematic reviews of the effectiveness of developmental prevention programs in reducing delinquency, aggression, and bullying. *Aggression and Violent Behavior, 33*, 91–106. https://doi.org/10.1016/j.avb.2016.11.003

Fazel, M., Hoagwood, K., Stephan, S., & Ford, T. (2014). Mental health interventions in schools in high-income countries. *Lancet Psychiatry, 1*(5), 377–387. https://doi.org/10.1016/ s2215-0366(14)70312-8

Gladden, R. M., Vivolo-Kantor, A. M., Hamburger, M. E., & Lumpkin, C. D. (2014). *Bullying surveillance among youths: Uniform definitions for public health and recommended data elements.* Centers for Disease Control and Prevention, U.S. Department of Education.

Hatzenbuehler, M. L., Flores, J. E., Cavanaugh, J. E., Onwuachi-Willig, A., & Ramirez, M. R. (2017). Anti-bullying policies and disparities in bullying: A state-level analysis. *American Journal of Preventive Medicine, 53*(2), 184–191. https://doi.org/10.1016/j.amepre.2017.02.004

Jimenez-Barbero, J. A., Ruiz-Hernandez, J. A., Llor-Zaragoza, L., Perez-Garcia, M., & Llor-Esteban, B. (2016). Effectiveness of anti-bullying school programs: A meta-analysis. *Children and Youth Services Review, 61*, 165–175. https://doi.org/10.1016/j.childyouth.2015.12.015

Juvonen, J., & Graham, S. (2014). Bullying in schools: The power of bullies and the plight of victims. *Annual Review of Psychology, 65*(1), 159–185. https://doi.org/10.1146/annurev-psych-010213-115030

Kidger, J., Stone, T., Tilling, K., Brockman, R., Campbell, R., Ford, T., Hollingworth, W., King, M., Araya, R., & Gunnell, D. (2016). A pilot cluster randomised controlled trial of a support and training intervention to improve the mental health of secondary school teachers and students—The WISE (Wellbeing in Secondary Education) study. *BMC Public Health, 16*(1), 1060. https://doi.org/10.1186/ s12889-016-3737-y

Marx, R. A., & Kettrey, H. H. (2016). Gay-straight alliances are associated with lower levels of school-based victimization of LGBTQ+ youth: A systematic review and meta-analysis. *Journal of Youth and Adolescence, 45*(7), 1269–1282. https://doi.org/10.1007/s10964-016-0501-7

McConachie, H., & Carr, G. (2008). Mental health in children with specific sensory impairments. In M. Rutter, D. Bishop, D. Pine, S. Scott, J. Stevenson, E. Taylor, & A. Thapar (Eds.), *Rutter's child and adolescent psychiatry* (5th ed., pp. 956–968). Wiley Blackwell. https://doi.org/10.1002/9781444300895 .ch59

Merikangas, K. R., He, J. P., Burstein, M., Swendsen, J., Avenevoli, S., Case, B., Georgiades, K., Heaton, L., Swanson, S., & Olfson, M. (2011). Service utilization for lifetime mental disorders in US adolescents: Results of the National Comorbidity Survey—Adolescent Supplement (NCS-A). *Journal of the American Academy Child and Adolescent Psychiatry, 50*(1), 32–45. https://doi.org/10.1016/j.jaac.2010.10.006

Myers, K., & Roth D. E. (2018). Telepsychiatry with children and adolescents. In A. Martin, M. H. Bloch, & F. R. Volkmar (Eds.), *Lewis's child and adolescent psychiatry: A comprehensive textbook* (5th ed., pp. 885–897). Wolters Kluwer.

*Oberle, E., Guhn, M., Gadermann, A. M., Thomson, K., & Schonert-Reichl, K. A. (2018). Positive mental health and supportive school environments: A population-level longitudinal study of dispositional optimism and school relationships in early adolescence. *Social Science & Medicine, 214*, 154–161. https://doi.org/10.1016/j.socscimed.2018.06.041

Platt, I. A., Kannangara, C., Tytherleigh, M., & Carson, J. (2020). The hummingbird project: A positive psychology intervention for secondary school students. *Frontiers in Psychology, 11*, 2012. https://doi.org/10.3389/fpsyg.2020.02012

Putnam, R. F., Handler, M. W., Rey, J., & McCarty, J. (2005). The development of behaviorally based public school consultation services. *Behavior Modification, 29*(3), 521–538. https://doi.org/10.1177/0145445504273286

Sanchez, F. C., Navarro-Zaragoza, J., Ruiz-Cabello, A. L., Romero, M. F., & Maldonado, A. L. (2017). Association between bullying victimization and substance use among college students in Spain. *Adicciones, 29*(1), 22–32. https://doi.org/10.20882/adicciones.827

Sansone, R. A., & Sansone, L. A. (2008). Bully victims: Psychological and somatic aftermaths. *Psychiatry, 5*(6), 62–64. https://www.ncbi.nlm.nih.gov/pmc/articles/PMC2695751/

Schoeler, T., Duncan, L., Cecil, C. M., Ploubidis, G. B., & Pingault, J.-B. (2018). Quasi-experimental evidence on short-and long-term consequences of bullying victimization: A meta-analysis. *Psychological Bulletin, 144*(12), 1229–1246. https://doi.org/10.1037/bul0000171

Shetgiri, R., Lin, H., & Flores, G. (2013). Trends in risk and protective factors for child bullying perpetration in the United States. *Child Psychiatry and Human Development, 44*(1), 89–104. https://doi.org/10.1007/s10578-012-0312-3

*Stephan, S. H., Sugai, G., Lever, N., & Connors, E. (2015). Strategies for integrating mental health into schools via a multitiered system of support. *Child and Adolescent Psychiatric Clinics of North America, 24*(2), 211–231. https://doi.org/10.1016/j.chc.2014.12.002

Stephan, S. H., Weist, M., Kataoka, S., Adelsheim, S., & Mills, C. (2007). Transformation of children's mental health services: The role of school mental health. *Psychiatric Services, 58*(10), 1330–1338. https://doi.org/10.1176/ps.2007.58.10.1330

Swanepoel, B., Swartz, L., Gericke, R., & Mall, S. (2020). Prevalence and correlates of mental and neurodevelopmental symptoms and disorders among deaf children and adolescents: A systematic review protocol. *BMJ Open, 10*(10), e038431. https://doi.org/10.1136/bmjopen-2020-038431

Ttofi, M. M., Farrington, D. P., Lösel, F., & Loeber, R. (2011). The predictive efficiency of school bullying versus later offending: A systematic/meta-analytic review of longitudinal studies. *Criminal Behaviour and Mental Health, 21*(2), 80–89. https://doi.org/10.1002/cbm.808

Whitney, D. G., & Peterson, M. D. (2019). US national and state-level prevalence of mental health disorders and disparities of mental health care use in children. *JAMA Pediatrics, 173*(4), 389–391. https://doi.org/10.1001/jamapediatrics.2018.5399

Suggested Readings

Benningfield, M. M., & Stephan, S. H. (2015). Integrating mental health into schools to support student success. *Child and Adolescent Psychiatric Clinics of North America, 24*(2), xv–xvii. https://doi.org/10.1016/j.chc.2014.12.005

Christensen, L. L., Fraynt, R. J., Neece, C. L., & Baker, B. L. (2012). Bullying adolescents with intellectual disability. *Journal of Mental Health Research in Intellectual Disabilities, 5*(1), 49–65. https://doi.org/10.1080/19315864.2011.637660

Coady, H. A. (2006). The relationship between learning disabilities, gender and peer victimization. *Dissertation Abstracts International: Section B: The Sciences and Engineering, 67*(1-B), 597.

Committee on the Biological and Psychosocial Effects of Peer Victimization: Lessons for Bullying Prevention; Board on Children, Youth, and Families; Committee on Law and Justice; Division of Behavioral and Social Sciences and Education; Health and Medicine Division; National Academies of Sciences, Engineering, and Medicine. (2016). The National Academies Collection: Reports funded by National Institutes of Health. In F. Rivara & S. Le Menestrel (Eds.), *Preventing bullying through science, policy, and practice*. National Academies Press (US). https://doi.org/10.17226/23482

Didden, R., Scholte, R. H., Korzilius, H., de Moor, J. M., Vermeulen, A., O'Reilly, M., Lang, R., & Lancioni, G. E. (2009). Cyberbullying among students with intellectual and developmental disability in special education settings. *Developmental Neurorehabilitation, 12*(3), 146–151. https://doi.org/10.1080/17518420902971356

Fazel, M., Hoagwood, K., Stephan, S., & Ford, T. (2014). Mental health interventions in schools in high-income countries. *Lancet Psychiatry*, *1*(5), 377–387. https://doi.org/10.1016/s2215-0366(14)70312-8

Greene, R. W., & Ablon, J. S. (2006). *Treating explosive kids: The collaborative problem-solving approach.* Guilford.

Hatton, C., Emerson, E., Robertson, J., & Baines, S. (2018). The mental health of adolescents with and without mild/moderate intellectual disabilities in England: Secondary analysis of a longitudinal cohort study. *Journal of Applied Research in Intellectual Disabilities*, *31*(5), 768–777. https://doi.org/10.1111/jar.12428

Kratochwill, T. R., Albers, C. A., & Shernoff, E. S. (2004). School-based interventions. *Child and Adolescent Psychiatric Clinics of North America*, *13*(4), 885–903. https://doi.org/10.1016/j.chc.2004.05.003

Luciano, S., & Savage, R. S. (2007). Bullying risk in children with learning difficulties in inclusive educational settings. *Canadian Journal of School Psychology*, *22*(1), 14–31. https://doi.org/10.1177/0829573507301039

Maiano, C., Aime, A., Salvas, M.-C., Morin, A. J., & Normand, C. L. (2016). Prevalence and correlates of bullying perpetration and victimization among school-aged youth with intellectual disabilities: A systematic review. *Research in Developmental Disabilities*, *49–50*, 181–195. https://doi.org/10.1016/j.ridd.2015.11.015

McNamara, B. E. (2013). *Bullying and students with disabilities: Strategies and techniques to create a safe learning environment for all.* Corwin Press.

Mishna, F. (2003). Learning disabilities and bullying: Double jeopardy. *Journal of Learning Disabilities*, *36*(4), 336–347. https://doi.org/10.1177/00222194030360040501

Normand, C. L., & Sallafranque-St-Louis, F. (2016). Cybervictimization of young people with an intellectual or developmental disability: Risks specific to sexual solicitation. *Journal of Applied Research in Intellectual Disabilities*, *29*(2), 99–110. https://doi.org/10.1111/jar.12163

Pfeffer, R. D. (2016). Childhood victimization in a national sample of youth with autism spectrum disorders. *Journal of Policy and Practice in Intellectual Disabilities*, *13*(4), 311–319. https://doi.org/10.1111/jppi.12203

Reiter, S., & Lapidot-Lefler, N. (2007). Bullying among special education students with intellectual disabilities: Differences in social adjustment and social skills. *Intellectual and Developmental Disabilities*, *45*(3), 174–181. https://doi.org/10.1352/1934-9556(2007)45[174:basesw]2.0.co;2

Rose, C. A., Espelage, D. L., Monda-Amaya, L. E., Shogren, K. A., & Aragon, S. R. (2015). Bullying and middle school students with and without specific learning disabilities: An examination of social-ecological predictors. *Journal of Learning Disabilities*, *48*(3), 239–254. https://doi.org/10.1177/0022219413496279

Sheard, C., Clegg, J., Standen, P., & Cromby, J. (2001). Bullying and people with severe intellectual disability. *Journal of Intellectual Disability Research*, *45*(5), 407–415. https://doi.org/10.1046/j.1365-2788.2001.00349.x

Spinelli-Casale, S. M. (2009). Bullying of middle school students with and without learning disabilities: Prevalence and relationship to students' social skills. *Dissertation Abstracts International Section A: Humanities and Social Sciences*, *69*(7-A), 2609.

Stephan, S. H., Weist, M., Kataoka, S., Adelsheim, S., & Mills, C. (2007). Transformation of children's mental health services: The role of school mental health. *Psychiatric Services*, *58*(10), 1330–1338. https://doi.org/10.1176/ps.2007.58.10.1330

Zablotsky, B., Bradshaw, C. P., Anderson, C. M., & Law, P. (2014). Risk factors for bullying among children with autism spectrum disorders. *Autism*, *18*(4), 419–427. https://doi.org/10.1177/1362361313477920

Zeedyk, S., Rodriguez, G., Tipton, L., Baker, B., & Blacher, J. (2014). Bullying of youth with autism spectrum disorder, intellectual disability, or typical development: Victim and parent perspectives. *Research in Autism Spectrum Disorders*, *8*(9), 1173–1183. https://doi.org/10.1016/j.rasd.2014.06.001

CHAPTER 26 ■ CHILD MENTAL HEALTH AND THE LEGAL SYSTEM

For mental health professionals as well as other professionals who interact with children and families, there are many situations where work with the legal system may be required (Sharma & Thomas, 2018). These can vary markedly depending on the context. Sometimes mental health or medical professionals will be asked to provide "fact testimony," that is, testifying as to what they observed or know. At other times, the professional may be asked to serve as an "expert witness" and provide expert testimony on a specific issue or situation. In the latter case, the expert will usually be qualified by the court based on their knowledge and expertise. Regardless of whether as a witness of fact or as an expert, the mental health professional may be asked to testify either in court itself or in a deposition before multiple attorneys each of whom will have a chance to ask questions. Legal proceedings can seem very foreign to mental health professionals because the legal system works within a myriad of often significantly differing state and local laws as well as federal laws and guidelines. It can be a source of frustration to clinicians and others that even if the law and case seem straightforward, the legal system may be complex to deal with. Given the nature of the court system, many mental health professionals try, as much as possible, to avoid it—although not always successfully. On the other hand, others may have a practice that includes considerable amounts of forensic work and find this rewarding. Sometimes, mental health or health care professionals find it quite rewarding to help a child or youth deal with what can seem a "Dickensian" situation, that is, as in his novel *Bleak House* where endless legal proceedings overshadow the needs of those involved.

Adding to this complexity is the nature of the justice system in the United States with dual federal and state legal systems, each with its own processes for appeal. In the federal system, all cases are heard in District Court by a District Judge appointed by the President or a federal magistrate. State Court systems have various specialized courts, for example, the juvenile courts, and often specialized courts like probate courts that often seek testimony from mental health experts. This has become increasingly true over the past decade as the emphasis with the juvenile justice system has shifted away from an emphasis on rehabilitation. Table 26.1 provides a summary of some of the definitions of terms that are frequently used but may be foreign to those not involved in the legal system. For mental health professionals working for a state or private organization, notification should be immediately given to the relevant legal representative or to the private practitioner's attorney if the professional is served with a subpoena. Sometimes an expert is asked to assist the court and provide an independent assessment—this has its own set of special rules (Sharma & Thomas, 2018).

TABLE 26.1

Definitions of Legal Terms

Confidentiality: Secrecy; the state of having the dissemination of certain information restricted.
Cross-examination: The questioning of a witness at a trial or hearing by the party opposed to the party who called the witness to testify. The purpose of cross-examination is to discredit a witness before the fact finder in any of several ways, as by bringing out contradictions and improbabilities in earlier testimony, by suggesting doubts to the witness, and by trapping the witness into admissions that weaken the testimony. The cross-examiner is allowed to ask leading questions but is traditionally limited to matters covered on direct examination and to credibility issues.
Defendant: A person sued in a civil proceeding or accused in a criminal proceeding.
Deposition: A witness's out-of-court testimony that is reduced to writing (usually by a court reporter) for later use in court for discovery purposes.
Direct examination: The first questioning of a witness in a trial or other proceedings conducted by the party who called the witness to testify.
Expert witness: A witness qualified by knowledge, skill, experience, training, or education to provide a scientific, technical, or other specialized opinion about the evidence or a fact issue.
Fact witness: A witness who may testify only to information that is based on firsthand knowledge.
Guardian ad litem: A caretaker, usually a lawyer, appointed by the court to appear in a lawsuit on behalf of an incompetent or minor party.
Plaintiff: The party who brings a civil suit in a court of law.
Preponderance of evidence: The greater weight of the evidence; superior evidentiary weight that, though not sufficient to free the mind wholly from all reasonable doubt, is still sufficient to incline a fair and impartial mind to one side of the issue rather than the other. It is also referred to as preponderance of proof or balance of probability.
Privilege: A special legal right, exemption, or immunity granted to a person or class of persons; an exception to a duty.
Reasonable doubt: The doubt that prevents one from being firmly convinced of a defendant's guilt, or the belief that there is a real possibility that a defendant is not guilty.
Redirect examination: A second examination, after cross-examination, the scope ordinarily being limited to matters covered during cross-examination.
Subpoena: A writ commanding a person to appear before a court or other tribunal, subject to a penalty for failing to comply.
Subpoena duces tecum: A subpoena ordering the witness to appear and to bring specified documents or records.
Voir dire: A preliminary examination to determine the qualifications of a prospective witness or evidence.

Reprinted from Sharma, S., & Thomas, C. R. (2018). The child and adolescent psychiatric in court. In A. Martin, M. Bloch, & F. R. Volkmar (Eds.), *Lewis's child and adolescent psychiatry: A comprehensive textbook* (Table 7.4.1.1, p. 975). Wolters Kluwer.

PARTICIPATION IN THE JUDICIAL PROCESS

It is very important that the mental health provider understands the rules of confidentiality and privacy since some health-related information can remain protected and confidential (Sharma & Thomas, 2018). In such situations, the patient may be willing to grant a release of the information or the court may order it, but there are some situations, for example, if there are claims of malpractice, when special rules may apply. These issues are especially complex in situations where clinical care is ongoing, for example, when a child is being seen for treatment and parents are divorcing (Sharma & Thomas, 2018), and when issues of juvenile competence arise (Soulier, 2012).

A response to requests for medical records may differ for individuals in private practice and those working for organizations where a central repository of such records exist. In some situations, the patient or parents may be requesting that the child's therapist be involved although it is important that the professional clearly understands the nature of the request, for example, relative to providing facts or serving as an expert witness.

The mental health or health care professional should have some basic familiarity with the court and court procedures. Unfortunately, what seems exciting and dramatic on television can be vastly different when you spend long periods of time waiting to testify and then do not enjoy the adversarial nature of the process once it starts! Depending on the nature of the proceeding, an appearance in court may be involved and this might be open or closed or the request may involve a deposition (sworn testimony taken in an attorney's office in advance). Professional dress and demeanor should be appropriate for a court appearance. Even though a specific time may be arranged, it is frequently the case that court proceedings run late or that changes in schedule occur. A court reporter will typically transcribe or audio record testimony that becomes part of the official court record. Often the testimony will begin with a request for the professional to list past training and other qualifications. Where the professional is serving as a fact witness, there is no reimbursement except where permitted for travel costs by local court rules, nor can an insurance company be asked to reimburse. On the other hand, time spent as an expert witness is, however, typically reimbursed.

It is important for the mental health or health professional to realize that both (and sometimes even more) sides will have an opportunity to ask questions. The order of questioning may vary depending on the context. Typically, after the "direct" testimony (questions from the first lawyer), there will be cross-examination by the other attorney (or attorneys) and then a chance for additional ("redirect") questions from the original attorney followed by another round from the opposing attorney. At the end of the testimony, the judge will indicate that the witness is excused. In some situations, for example, in a family or juvenile court or in probate court, the judge may take a more active role in the questioning process. It is important to remain calm and professional and give responsive answers to questions.

In providing testimony, the mental health professional should think carefully about the question before giving a direct and straightforward response. It is best if this is as straightforward as possible (sadly this is not always possible). It is often the tendency of mental health and other professionals to give overly elaborate answers. Put another way, be short and to the point and speak to the facts/situation as you know it. It is best to firmly give a simple and responsive answer. If something is complex, one can try to explain that this is the case but keep in mind that attorneys (on all sides) will be thinking about potential implications of literally everything that is said. Anything the professional brings with them by way of notes or records or materials may itself be subpoenaed on the spot; so, as a general rule, only bring with you what you are prepared to have entered into evidence. It is important to realize that the attorney usually will be careful to ask questions where they think they already know the answer. If the question is unclear, ask for it to be rephrased so that you are not answering the wrong question. If you cannot answer the question, then say so. If the question is one that can be addressed based on medical records, it is perfectly appropriate to ask to see the record (or other documentation). It is also possible to indicate uncertainty in an answer or to indicate no relevant knowledge of the answer. If called to testify on certain facts, that is, as a fact-based witness, it is important that the psychiatrist NOT stray into becoming an expert witness; this is particularly complex when the patient remains in ongoing treatment.

At times, the various attorneys will raise objections—these are of various types but from the point of view of the witness, it is important to stop speaking and wait for the judge to sort things out and make a decision and give direction to the witness either to answer the question or not. Often, questions will be asked in very specific ways. Again, if the meaning is unclear, the witness should ask for clarification. The lawyer may ask if a question can be answered within a reasonable degree of "medical certainty:" for example, "Did X cause Y?" Be sure you understand what this means: usually it means more likely than not, but different standards arise in different situations. It can be a source of confusion for those who constantly cope with uncertainty as they revise diagnoses and treatment plans.

By its very nature, the legal system is divisive, and lawyers may employ a number of tactics in questioning in the hope of helping bolster their case. For example, the lawyer may offer up a summary of earlier testimony; often, this will be cast in a certain way and the witness is well advised to carefully listen and correct any errors or misrepresentations. Similarly, witnesses should be careful about rather vague and general questions that may precede a much more specific and loaded one. When being asked about earlier testimony, it is always possible to ask to have a previous answer repeated. Similarly, when asked about medical records, it is also quite reasonable to ask to review the specific material in question. Being thoughtful and deliberate in answering is important and so is not being ruffled when proceedings are prolonged or attorneys poorly prepared.

Depositions are an important aspect or seemingly hostile of the legal system. They are conducted as part of what the attorneys call the *discovery* phase and help the attorneys involved plan their strategy for trial. They also provide the attorneys (on all sides) a chance to observe a witness. The deposition is a legal proceeding and the testimony obtained becomes part of the court record and can be reviewed or presented at the time of a trial. Depositions are usually done in a lawyer's office or even sometimes in the mental health professional's office. A court reporter is present to make a record and to swear in the witness. Sometimes, depositions are videotaped. During a deposition, a judge is not present. Attorneys make objections but the witness will still be asked to answer the question (the judge can later decide on the objection). The witness will be given a copy of the deposition to review. Sharma & Thomas (2018) provides a very helpful summary for the mental health professional going to court.

■ CHILD CUSTODY

Legal conceptualizations of children and childhood have evolved significantly over time (Mroczkowski, 2018). This evolution has reflected many factors. Historically, children were viewed within the legal system as "chattels" (property) and, like women, had few specific rights. Fathers typically were assumed to "rule" the family and make major decisions for family members. These notions began to change as women began to demand, and receive, additional rights and as child development research began to emphasize the important role of parent–child (including mother–child) relationships for healthy development. Courts began to recognize the principle of "best interests of the child" (Goldstein, Freud, & Solnit, 1973) in decision making regarding child custody. Often, particularly for young children, mothers began to be considered the more natural custodial parents, but over time this notion has changed with fathers assuming an increasingly important role in child rearing.

The increasing frequency, and acceptance, of divorce has raised other issues with current trends suggesting that about 50% of marriages will end in divorce. Other issues arise given the frequency of single-parent households, particularly for children growing up in poverty (Herman, 1997; Mroczkowski, 2018). Parental separation and divorce increase the risk for children and adolescents to have various mental health problems–probably doubling this risk relative to intact families. Children can be the focus of prolonged, bitter, and protracted fights for custody. These long-term disputes may also have an even more negative impact on the child.

It is important to understand that the issue of child custody (the ability to make a range of decisions for the child) is not the same thing as parental rights, for example, on issues like visitation. Increasingly, there is a focus on joint legal custody, so that both parents participate in major decisions. This situation, although obviously theoretically fair and ideal, may, in reality, have quite a difficult result for the child if it results in continued battles in which the child moves into the role of pawn rather than a central concern. The advent of same-sex marriage has added a further wrinkle to this complex legal landscape. Yet another set of challenges has arisen with the advent of new technologies from obstetrics with procedures like in vitro fertilization and surrogacy presenting new opportunities for legal contest.

There are many potential areas of mental health impact of separation and divorce for children and youth (Mroczkowski, 2018). Following the separation, children may exhibit a range of reactions including anxiety and distress, anger, and sorrow. This can happen even when the separation is amicable; it can become much more toxic if the process is less than amicable. Problems vary with age and developmental level. The younger child may experience an upsurge of anxiety, sleeping problems, and so on. For the older children, problems with anxiety, mood, and school-related issues may emerge. These issues may be particularly challenging in adolescence—itself a time when most teens gradually distance and separate from parents.

Increasingly, courts have encouraged continued involvement of both parents viewing this as in the best interest of the child (Goldstein, Freud, & Solnit, 1973). Depending on the specifics of the situation, the mental health professional may be engaged (ideally by the court) to make recommendations after doing an assessment. Laws vary considerably from state to state and it is always the case that judges have considerable discretion.

Mental health professionals may be engaged either by court or lawyers for the child (children) to make recommendations relative to the best interest of the child (children). Sometimes, parents will seek mental health testimony in their favor (or against their former partner). Issues can be complex, as facts may be unclear when children are very young and thus less able to speak for themselves. The consultant can make any number of potential recommendations to the courts regarding custody and visitation. Special issues arise when there are concerns about the child's safety, allegations of abuse, serious psychopathology, or other problems relative to one or another parent. To be effective, the clinician will have to be skilled in understanding aspects of child development, family functioning, and mental health issues and problems. The consultant must also be aware of the specific applicable law. In some states, specific additional, or ongoing, training, is required for work in this area.

It is essential that the consultant maintain ethical and professional boundaries and not be drawn into ongoing disputes. This is sometimes easier said than done. In providing an independent opinion for the court, the consultant should carefully explain their role and the special nature of the professional contact; for example, usual confidentiality rules do not apply in the sense that anything that is said may appear in a written report or be noted in testimony to the court. Referrals should usually come from the court with the agreement of the various attorneys involved and a clear description of the nature of the question(s) to be addressed by the consultant. Sometimes, the child is represented by their own attorney (a guardian ad litem) who will be involved in this process as well.

Sometimes, discussion is required to refine the initial question into one that the consultant feels that they may be able to address. Data may be provided, or requested, from various sources and a series of clinical interviews will usually be conducted typically with each of the parents and the child or children. Depending on the situation, interviews might be done in the home. Information collected will usually include a review of the history of the child and family, the factors leading to divorce, the psychosocial history of the parents, vulnerabilities in them and the child, areas of strength, and so forth. In some situations, additional consultations, for example, psychological testing, may be requested.

The interview of the child should be appropriate to the developmental level of the child with careful attention to evidence of attachments and relationships with the parents. Exploration of the parents' views of the child, of the home environment, and observation of the parent–child interaction are all relevant. Collateral sources of information, for example, from pediatricians, schools, and so forth, may also inform the process. A final written summary typically includes a review of the background of the consultation including the specific questions of interest to the court and a summary of the sources of information used by the evaluator. Usually, the next section of the report provides a narrative description of the process of the assessment and summaries of interviews and observations, and the final section includes recommendations and conclusions. Once the report is submitted, conferences with the various parties or a deposition may be requested.

A host of special issues/situations may arise in custody cases, for example, the rights of grandparents or stepparents to visitation, issues of reunification of children with parents who have been abusive or neglectful, and so forth. Issues increasingly arise from new approaches to reproductive technologies, for example, the woman carrying the child to term may not be the biological mother. Courts frequently turn to mental health consultants in these situations. Often, the preference of courts is to honor biological relationships, but clear evidence of the child's best interest may outweigh such considerations. Visitation of grandparents has been an area of active legislation, and litigation, in recent years. Most states now give some form of visitation rights to grandparents, but the U.S. Supreme Court has placed some limitations on such rights.

Increasingly, fathers seek custody and the past presumption that mothers should automatically be custodial parents, particularly of younger children, has given way to a more balanced view that seeks to encourage continued relationships among all involved. Usually, sustained contact with frequent visitation and joint custody are preferred, but some situations may make this less than ideal, for example, if a parent has seriously harmed a spouse, the child, or a sibling. When the divorce process has become bitter, the joint custody arrangement may present a culmination and complex continuation of this long struggle. This is not in the best interest of the children involved. For some parents, desperation following adverse legal decisions leads to parental kidnapping. These situations are fraught with risks for the child and consultants should be familiar with relevant state and federal laws in the area.

Sometimes, allegations of parental physical or other abuse occur as part of the custody dispute and must be carefully evaluated even though they can be, at times, very difficult to sort out. For parents who have substance abuse or mental health problems, the existence of a problem is less important than what any impact this might have on caring for a child. These can easily involve health care professionals who are mandated to report suspected or reported abuse.

Given the highly mobile U.S. society, there is potential for multiple jurisdictions to be involved. In most states, there is recognition of the need for stability and coordination of care for the child. Increasingly, divorced parents live at some distance from each other. In most states, there is recognition that parents may need to move although specific issues may arise that lead to a revisitation of custodial or visitation issues. There can be highly specialized and complex issues, for example, when a parent is a member of a recognized Native American tribe where the tribe's own rules and laws may apply.

Often in an attempt to avoid the time and expense of protracted legal proceedings, there may be attempts at alternative disputes resolutions, for example, through mediation. It is important in such situations to realize that what seems a simple and fair solution to the adults may not be so to the child or children involved. Even in such proceedings, the interests of the child or children should be considered in the process. Mroczkowski (2018) provides an excellent summary of the role of mental health professionals in custody cases (Box 26.1).

ADOPTION

Adoption represents a specialized custody issue, albeit one not always involving mental health professionals (Brown, 2018). Adoption has been practiced since ancient times, often including adults and children if, for example, an heir was needed. In the United States, informal adoption preceded the first laws on the topic, for example, as orphan children were taken care of by family members, friends, or neighbors. Adoption arose in the context of parents taking care of orphaned babies, in apprenticeship of children, and in the practice of sending homeless children from large cities to work on farms. Legal formalization of adoption is a much more recent historic phenomenon in this country with statutes now present both at the state and federal levels. In the past, a major source of adoptees came from unmarried mothers; with birth control, this population has dwindled and foreign adoptions and adoptions of children from foster care has increased, particularly with the emphasis on longer term permanency planning (Brown, 2018). Over the last two decades, there has been a noteworthy upsurge in adoption of children from other countries.

BOX 26.1	Case Illustration—Subpoena for Custody Case

Dr. Jones has worked with a family for approximately 1 year. The 6-year-old daughter, Anna, has been treated for an anxiety disorder while Dr. Jones also worked with the parents for some behavioral problems. Mrs. Smith was the parent that usually brought Anna to her appointments and Mr. Smith came for the initial evaluation and for two other sessions. The parents during this period have had a breakdown in their marriage and the mother has told Dr. Jones about numerous family problems that are affecting Anna, which were discussed in the course of treatment. Dr. Jones has not seen the family for several months and then receives a phone call from Mrs. Smith stating that the parents have decided to divorce, and she asks Dr. Jones to write a letter to the court in support of her having full custody of Anna. She feels that Dr. Jones knows the problems in the family well and would be the best person to explain to the court why she would be the better primary parent for their daughter. Dr. Jones tries to explain that he does not feel comfortable complying with the request and feels that it would be unethical of him to do so. The mother then asks Dr. Jones if she can bring Anna in for a custody evaluation to allow Dr. Jones to feel comfortable writing the letter. Dr. Jones explains that it would be inappropriate for him to change roles from treating psychiatrist to forensic evaluator. Shortly thereafter, Dr. Jones is issued a subpoena duces tecum from Mrs. Smith's lawyer because he feels Dr. Jones's testimony will be helpful to her case. There is also a release of information included from both parents that will allow Dr. Jones to discuss protected health information. Dr. Jones reviews and discusses this request with his attorney. He then blocks his entire clinic day, gathers his case materials, and is in court on the scheduled date and time. During direct examination, the mother's attorney asks Dr. Jones if he thinks the father is emotionally capable of taking care of Anna alone if the parents divorce, and what custody arrangement would be in the child's "best interests" in terms of visitations. Dr. Jones is later asked regarding the child's specific medical treatment rendered and what the long-term prognosis and plan would be for the patient. Dr. Jones has a release to discuss any specifics of the evaluation and treatment of Anna and is required to answer those questions to the best of his ability. However, regarding the earlier questions about the father's capability to raise Anna alone or what type of custody arrangement should be undertaken, Dr. Jones did not perform a custody evaluation and therefore does not have an opinion on those topics relating to Anna and informs the court of this through his answers.

Reprinted with permission from Thomas, C. (2018). The child and adolescent psychiatrist in court. In A. Martin, M. Bloch, & F. R. Volkmar (Eds.), *Lewis's child and adolescent psychiatry: A comprehensive textbook* (5th ed., pp. 974–990). Wolters Kluwer.

Around 135,000 children a year are adopted in this country and another 428,000 are in foster care (see https://adoptionnetwork.com/adoption-statistics). In some situations, the birth parents, usually mothers, maintain ongoing contact with the child and adoptive family (this is termed *open adoption*). There are some special challenges for foreign adoptions depending, particularly, on the age of the child and whether or not the child has been cared for in an institutional setting, the latter significantly increasing the risk for a range of potential problems (Brown, 2018; Rutter, 1998). One of other risks for adoption relates to the medical history of birth mothers, for example, the use of things like alcohol during pregnancy. For children adopted internationally, there may be little or no information on biological parents, their caretaking history before adoptions, and so forth.

Fortunately, most of the time, children and their adoptive families do well. The usual practice now is to encourage parents to be open about adoption to discourage the problem of family secrets that were observed in the past. Sometimes children, as they become older, become more interested in their birth parents or birth countries. As is true for children in a divorce, the child may feel personally responsible in some way for their adoption. There may be fantasies about why the child was unwanted. Sometimes, the wish of the child to protect their adoptive parents from these concerns complicates discussion. Adolescence, in particular, may present some special challenges given that the normative developmental task is individuation from parents and leaving adoptive parents may be particularly difficult. Sometimes, adoptees will search for information on biological parents. This can be the source of distress and sadness for the adoptive parents, because it may be experienced as rejection even when this is not in fact intended.

Adoptive parents face some unique challenges including anxiety and/or concerns relative to delay in the actual adoption process sometimes undertaken when parents have trouble conceiving. Adoption is of relatively low risk, although, as a group, there are somewhat higher rates of externalizing problems—particularly in adolescent boys. There is also some suggestion of increased risk for mood and anxiety problems. As compared to multiple foster placements, the stability of adoption is a benefit and one usually associated with a much better outcome.

Adoption of children within the child welfare system has been an important and controversial topic for many years. In the past, overtly expressed policy favored reunification of child and parent(s) but this has now shifted to encourage early foster placement to insure stability. Unfortunately, it is clear that adoptive children are more likely to have problems if they have been placed at an older age. Mental health clinicians will, of course, tend to have contact only with situations where the adoptive child is not doing well. Occasionally, clinicians see situations where the adoption is not completed.

GUARDIANSHIP

When some adolescents with significant developmental, or sometimes mental health–emotional issues, turn 18, parents may be motivated to seek some degree of guardianship (also called "conservatorship" in some places). Essentially, this entails a legal process (differing in the various states) and ensuring the rights of the individual to legal protection. This often arises for children with more significant levels of intellectual disability, sometimes for those with autism, severe psychosis, and so forth. Guardianship issues sometimes arise as children become legal-aged adults. There may be a question about the person's ability to make realistic decisions for themselves as a result of mental health, developmental, or other difficulties. Various levels of guardianship exist. Guardianship might be full and complete so that the guardian controls where the individual lives, how they spend their time, and money. Or it may be more limited, for example, limited only to money. This might, for example, happen when the person is the recipient of a large gift or settlement or otherwise holds significant assets.

The mental health professional may be asked to provide an opinion about the capacities of the person to care for themselves and make independent life decisions. It is important to realize that the presence of any specific diagnosis does not always mean that a person needs a guardian. The court may need help in understanding any assessment done and the person's abilities to make informed life choices. For the psychologist, this may involve tests of intelligence and adaptive behavior. For other mental health professionals, issues may have to do with specifics of the diagnosis. Typically, a parent, sibling, friend, relative, or some other concerned person will be asked to be the guardian.

THE INTERFACE OF EDUCATIONAL SYSTEMS AND THE LAW

In the past several decades, the role of mental health professionals in the identification of children who present to schools with special educational needs has expanded (Bostic & Hoover,

TABLE 26.2

Educational Law: Key Concepts and Terms

IDEA	The Individuals with Disabilities Education Act—an act of Congress giving specific rights to children with disabilities for educational services.
PL 94-142	The original (1975) law passed by Congress mandating school services to children with disabilities.
FAPE	Free and appropriate public education
IEP	Individualized education plan
LRE	Least restrictive environment
ADA	Americans with Disabilities Act
504 Plan	A plan developed to accommodate the special needs of a child with a handicap.
IFSP	Individualized family service plan—a plan similar to the IEP but for younger children (under age 3).

Rights and Safeguards Under IDEA

Notice requirements: The school must give written notice to parents of proposed changes (e.g., in placement or program) and of the parents' rights (e.g., to voice complaints or contest a planned change).

Consent of parents: Parents must give consent for an evaluation to be done or if reevaluation is done; schools have the right to seek such an evaluation if parents do not consent but must go through due process procedures or mediation to do so.

Mediation: Rather than go through due process, parents and schools can use the more informal mediation process to resolve disputes.

Due process: Parents or the school can initiate a due process hearing to resolve disputes at any stage in the process (from evaluation, planning and placement, and review). Parents must be informed of their rights and the possibilities for free or low-cost legal representation. The due process hearing is similar to a regular court hearing (but less formal) and parents and/or school may be represented by attorneys. An entire appeals process is also available.

Stay put: The stay put provision means that if a child is in a program and there is a dispute about moving the child to another program, this cannot be done until a placement decision is reached, that is, the school cannot unilaterally remove a child from a program (parents, of course, can). Practically, this usually means that when a dispute is under way, the child stays where they are until the dispute is resolved.

From Volkmar, F. R., & Wiesner, L. A. (2009). *A practical guide to autism.* John Wiley & Sons, Inc. Reprinted by permission of John Wiley & Sons, Inc.

2018). In addition, they may be asked to provide consultation and/or recommendations relative to disorders/disabilities that may affect the child's ability to profit from their educational program. These accommodations can range from very small to much larger, for example, modifications in homework or test taking with extra time for support from other members of the school staff regarding speech-communication intervention, social skills training, special classes, and so on. There are a number of important concepts and terms like *Free and Appropriate Education, least restrictive environment,* and so forth (see Table 26.2) that refer to children's rights to education in the United States.

To complicate matters, several different laws can be relevant. The *Americans with Disabilities Act* (ADA) applies to children as well as adolescents and adults. It specifically forbids denial of educational services to students who exhibit disabilities and also prohibits discrimination against such students. Parents can request an evaluation to document the presence of a disability and identify the accommodations that can be made to help the student. Under the law, if a child needs some (although not many) accommodations, there is a "504" plan (504 refers to the section of the law). 504 services can be used for individuals with a wide range of difficulties and usually accommodations are carried out while maintaining the student in the regular educational setting. Regardless of the specific diagnostic label, it is important to understand that the intention is the identification of problems/disabilities that interfere with the student's ability to learn.

For students who need more extensive services, a different law usually applies. Originally passed in 1975 and now modified several times, Public Law 94-142 marked a very major shift in services provided within school settings. Before it was passed, only a small number of children with severe disabilities received services within public school settings. Children would be turned away from school and parents were told they needed residential or institutional placements. The passage of Public Law 94-142 mandated school services for all children. This law has been most recently revised as the *Individual with Disabilities Education Act*. Schools are now required to provide free and appropriate public education to students whose difficulties require special instruction and services. A number of different disorders are specifically mentioned in the law. Students must need specialized instruction (i.e., if a child has a condition but does not need such instruction, they will not qualify). The most common way to establish that special instruction is needed is the child's failure to progress effectively in school; for some children, early intervention services would have established special needs. An Individualized Educational Plan (IEP) will be developed; components of the IEP are summarized in Table 26.2.

The process of establishing eligibility under IDEA is more involved than that for a 504 plan. The IEP does allow for important modifications of the program that do not necessarily require the student to meet the same academic requirements as other students in the classroom. The IEP development process typically includes an assessment conducted by a multidisciplinary team of professionals and often includes an evaluation of cognition, language-communication, academics, social-emotional skill, health status overall, and screening for sensory and motor difficulties (see Bostic & Hoover, 2018 for a detailed review). In cases where eligibility has once been established, reevaluation may be used to document whether the disability continues to affect the child and whether special services are still needed. Parents must be involved in this process; if they are not in agreement with the results, they can request an independent assessment (although the school is NOT required to necessarily agree with it).

Any number of relevant modifications can be considered in putting the IEP together, including educational/academic goals along with accommodations and modifications, participation in special educational or other programs or in the mainstream (sometimes with support), behavioral interventions and accommodations, extended school services, transition planning, modifications of the curriculum, special services (occupational, speech language, or physical therapy and/or counseling) along with school health services and even transportation. Specific interventions can be made relative to specific psychiatric symptoms (Table 25.4B). The law provides for special services up to age 21 years and gives states incentives via funding to insure participation.

For older individuals, for example, those in college or in technical school after age 21, IDEA does not apply but other laws, such as the Americans with Disability Act, may do so. The age of the child is also relevant for younger children because requirements for early intervention (before age 3) differ from those of public schools.

A number of special situations can arise, for example, if a student is dangerous or threatening or is involved in substance abuse at school, where an emergency IEP meeting can be held, and alternative placement implemented. Special rules relate to student suspension with provision for rapid response to emergent situations as well as continued provision of due process protections. Protections also extend to children where a disability is suspected but an evaluation process has not yet been completed.

The IDEA provides relatively extensive procedural protections to parents of children with disabilities, including "the right to participate in the development of the IEP, the right to independent evaluations, the right to inspect educational records" and "the opportunity to present complaints with respect to any matter relating to the identification, evaluation, or educational placement of the child, or the provision of a free appropriate public education to such child." Such a proceeding, referred to as a *due process hearing*, requires a neutral adjudicator, a right to counsel at the parent's expense, and the right to present evidence and cross-examine witnesses. If dissatisfied, either party has a right to judicial review in the appropriate state or federal court. With a growing number of students doing well in more mainstream settings, more students with some developmental and/or psychiatric vulnerability are entering school and college programs. It is important for them, and their parents, to realize that mandates for service under IDEA do NOT apply to college settings whereas ADA mandates still do. Several excellent resources with detailed information on educational advocacy, rights, and entitlements are provided in the suggested reading list.

THE JUVENILE JUSTICE SYSTEM

Historically (see Chapter 1), one of the origins of the child mental health system was the desire to rehabilitate rather than simply punish juvenile offenders. Although, at least in theory, this remains the guiding principle of the juvenile justice system, important challenges have emerged (Underwood & Washington, 2016). For example, during the 1990s, many states developed ways to prosecute juveniles, particularly those committing violent crimes, within the adult judicial and penal system.

During 2019, there were almost 700,000 juveniles arrested—most of these (https://www .ojjdp.gov/ojstatbb/crime/qa05101.asp) being youth 16 years and older. From an economic point of view (Greenwood, 2008), it clearly would make much more sense to work to prevent juvenile crimes; it is clear that community-based alternatives to detention have been shown to lower rates of re-offending. Unfortunately, there has been an increased tendency to resort to the youth correctional system to deal with youth with mental illness (Underwood & Washington, 2016).

Unfortunately, the juvenile justice systems are not well equipped to deal with child-adolescent mental health problems (Trupin & Boesky, 1999), with services often either totally unavailable or inadequate. Clearly, better coordination of the various systems of care (educational, social service/child protection, mental health, and juvenile justice) would be ideal in preventing problems and minimizing needs for incarceration (Underwood & Washington, 2016). This would also be very consistent with the notion that the problems of these youth are complex and interrelated.

Not surprisingly, rates of mental health and developmental disorders are higher for those involved in the juvenile justice system with an estimated two thirds of males and three fourths of females having at least one disorder, and many also having associated substance abuse problems (Wasserman et al., 2002). Given the importance of aggression in prompting incarceration, it is not surprising that disorders that involve aggression and impulse control increase risk for incarceration. Accordingly, conduct problems and attention deficit disorder are frequent among the externalizing disorder; for the internalizing disorder, anxiety and mood problems including depression and psychosis are more common. Mood problems can lead to irritability and acting out and also increase risk for self-injury. About two thirds of juvenile offenders exhibit at least two mental health disorders (Abram et al., 2003).

Treatment needs in juvenile justice systems are varied (Underwood & Washington, 2016). Several different treatment models have been shown to be effective. Of these, *cognitive behavioral therapy* and the *multisystemic therapy* approaches have been among the most frequently studied and well validated. Mental health consultants have an important role in management and treatment. This may include participation both in activities aimed to prevent incarceration as well as for youth who are incarcerated (Kraus & Thomas, 2011).

MALPRACTICE, LIABILITY, AND CONFIDENTIALITY

Both state and, to some extent, federal laws regulate medical practice. Allegations of misconduct can be raised at the level of the state medical licensing board or through litigation on allegations of malpractice (see Ash & Nurcomb, 2018 for a review). The current system is somewhat arbitrary and haphazard in nature given the lack of national licensure programs. However, relative to many other specialties, mental health specialists are rather less likely to be investigated or sued, although when such investigations occur they are sources of great anxiety and distress to those involved. The available data suggest that when mental health professionals are sued, only a small minority of claims result in any payment. However, an investigation by medical or other licensing boards can be highly intrusive and problematic.

Usually, to show malpractice, it must be shown that a physician or other professional had a duty of reasonable care of a patient but that this care was lacking in some important way. Usually, the standard of care is that typically provided in the community. Although this seems straightforward, there are some gray areas. For example, does giving free advice maybe mean a professional relationship exists? Accordingly, it is very important in this age of the internet to carefully consider implied relationships and to have an explicit statement of individuals and parents to obtain their care from practitioners familiar with them.

These issues get complicated particularly around things like psychopharmacology. These issues can arise when a psychiatrist, other physician, or nurse practitioner is responsible for medication management but some other professional, for example, a social worker or psychologist, is the person actually engaged in psychotherapy with the individual.

Treatment termination also can present some problems. Usually, over the long term the practitioner owes the patient continued confidentiality and an obligation to share medical records when these are requested (this can be an issue for the 30-year-old who requests a copy of his evaluation at age 3). It is important that the therapist be aware of any potential appearance of having abandoned a patient or client. Accordingly, the child and their family should have reasonable notice if treatment is to be terminated and the practitioner should assist in arrangements for subsequent care if this is needed. If there are specific complexities around termination, for example, patient noncompliance, it may be important to document these in the record (Ash & Nurcomb, 2018).

Inadequate or improper diagnostic assessments can also lead to liability, for example, failure to detect psychosis or suicidality, although lawsuits of this type are relatively uncommon. Similarly, inappropriate treatment can be alleged although may be difficult to prove except in certain circumstances, for example, sexual exploitation of the patient. Liability issues can also arise around medication use and problems in any of several different ways. In one case, for example, a patient who had been treated for a period of time with psychotherapy sued after being transferred to a different setting and being treated, successfully, with medications. Errors can also arise when a medication is given based on an incorrect diagnosis, when a contraindication to administration was present but missed, or when medications are used inappropriately.

Other issues can arise, for example, relative to supervision of trainees or employees. Consultations and second opinions represent another area of potential liability. The rise of telehealth and even a message board or email suggestion has some risk. This is an area of some complexity.

In instances of malpractice, the issue is often not so much whether an error was made but whether the error was below the standard of care, that is, in general clinicians are on safe ground if they exercise reasonable judgment and a reasonable standard of care. This means, for example, that physicians cannot be held liable for a bad outcome as long as they adhered to a reasonable standard of care in treatment; the latter can, of course, be the topic of much debate particularly in some areas in mental health where a clear consensus has not always developed. There have been some attempts at the national level to develop such standards including practice guidelines and parameters that should guide clinical management.

Malpractice claims can arise based on negligence or some wrong conduct on the part of the professional giving service. Clinicians should realize that for minors, the statute of limitations relative to malpractice suits usually does not begin until the child has reached legal adulthood. A series of relevant legal issues and principles applies in this area (see Ash & Nurcomb, 2018). There also can be important variations in the law from state to state. Among the many complexities are the young age of the patients who often cannot consent to treatment without the parents' involvement. Parents are themselves often involved in treatment raising further complications. Table 26.3 summarizes some of the areas where malpractice is more frequently alleged.

Issues of professional liability often arise around the potential for children or youth to engage in self-harm, violence, or dangerous behavior. This is an area of potential malpractice liability for all mental health professionals. A series of legal decisions have led to major exceptions in usual confidentiality laws because these apply to threats and assessment of dangerousness. In malpractice cases arising in these contexts, major issues have to do with whether the danger could reasonably be foreseen and if the clinician took appropriate steps to protect the patient or a potential victim. Similarly, the high rates of suicidal thoughts in adolescents present major challenges for clinicians (see Chapter 14). Accordingly, the documentation of a careful as well as of a thoughtful assessment and reasonable standard of care is important in these cases. This should include documentation of consideration of risk and protective factors. There is a higher standard for this care in inpatient settings. Family involvement is important in considering precautions relative to youth suicide. Discussion with parents can be used to help them monitor the child's condition or need for hospitalization. The child or youth should know about, and potentially be involved in, these discussions.

The Tarasoff decision in 1974 radically changed the standard of care relative to warning of potential violence against third parties. In this case, the California Supreme Court found that the "duty to warn" was indicated when a patient confided a plan to harm a third party.

TABLE 26.3

Common Issues in Malpractice Litigation

Area of Practice	Example Plaintiff Allegation
Dangerousness	
Suicide	Weak suicide assessment documentation
Homicide	No violence risk assessment in chart
Failure to protect from danger	Inpatient sexually assaulted by another inpatient
Failure to protect third parties	Dangerous patient escapes from hospital and family not notified
Protecting and releasing information	Confidential information released without authorization
Treatment	
Failure to obtain informed consent	Possible side effects not discussed
Psychotherapy	Implanted memories of sexual abuse
Sex with patient	Therapist had sex with patient
Medication	Girl with bipolar disorder treated with sodium divalproex for 8 months gives birth to baby with birth defects and there is no documentation of pregnancy status when medication is started
Ending treatment	
Negligent discharge	Patient discharged while still suicidal
Abandonment	Therapist terminated treatment without referral when patient failed to pay bill

Reprinted with permission from Ash, P., & Nurcombe, B. (2018). Malpractice and professional liability. In A. Martin, M. Bloch, & F. R. Volkmar (Eds.), *Lewis's child and adolescent psychiatry* (5th ed., Table 7.4.4.1, p. 999). Wolters Kluwer.

Because of serious concerns about potential for reducing confidentiality, the court revised this in a subsequent decision clarifying that there was duty to protect (i.e., rather than warn) if a serious danger of violence existed for a foreseeable potential victim. The issue of what constituted reasonable care in this regard was left unresolved. Following this decision, both state lawmakers and courts have struggled with the myriad of complex issues created by the Tarasoff decision. Requirements vary from state to state with many states agreeing there is a duty to warn, others do not require warning, and in a few the issue remains ambiguous. Fortunately, this issue is a relatively uncommon problem in dealing with children and youth. In situations where there is a serious threat to self or others, the mental health professional needs to take appropriate action. Table 26.4 summarizes some basic risk management principles.

Concerns around issues of confidentiality have always been a major concern in psychiatry and become even more complex in child psychiatry since consultation/collaboration with parents and, often, others are frequent and since the advent of the electronic medical record. Good clinical judgment is needed to weigh issues of the child's desire for privacy relative to parental rights to know (and release) information relative to their child's care. Some variation exists between states in terms of what information can or cannot be withheld from parents/guardians. For example, parents clearly should be informed if their child is engaging in potentially dangerous behavior. In most cases, a discussion of confidentiality issues should be held very early in treatment to clarify exactly what information is shared and in what circumstances. Privilege, for example, from having to testify, has been established by law or court decision in many states. The U.S. Supreme Court has held that a mental health privilege, that is, relative to confidentiality, applies in the federal court system.

Even if the clinician receives a subpoena, they may not necessarily be compelled to testify about confidential information unless authorization from the patient is provided or if, for example, the judge orders the clinician to do so. The latter might occur in a situation where the mental health issues are relevant to a lawsuit or criminal action. The passage of the Health Insurance Portability and Accountability Act of 1996 (HIPAA) resulted in a new set of regulations that became effective in 2003. This sets a federal standard relative to protected health information (states can provide for even higher levels of protection). The implications of these regulations are complex and important aspects remain to be resolved. However, it is clear that violations can result in prosecution. Patients (or parents) must be given a Notice of Privacy Practices during their first appointment. In addition, HIPAA specifically gives patients rights to see their records (with rare exceptions). HIPAA also restricts third parties (e.g., insurance companies) access to information that is the "minimum necessary." Within psychiatry, the latter will usually include identifying information, a treatment plan, diagnosis, and dates when services were provided but does not allow more extensive access to material. As part of the process, a new form of medical record, *the psychotherapy note*, has been established and can be kept apart and might even be destroyed by the clinician (except under certain circumstances). These notes are only released when the patient consents; for example, concerns about HIPAA can also arise relative to unprotected email communications.

Confidentiality issues also can arise regarding reporting of potential child abuse or neglect. All states mandate reporting if a reasonable suspicion is present. The laws that mandate reporting also provide legal protections for clinicians who, in good faith, report potential abusive activities. Gray areas and ambiguities can arise, for example, around allegations made in custody cases and consultation with legal counsel may be helpful. Clearly, a referral to Child Protective Services may endanger ongoing work with a child or family but may be appropriate if circumstances warrant it.

Failures to provide proper treatment can arise in many ways. These may include failures to obtain informed consent or to provide information sufficient for that process. Consent cannot always be obtained in emergency situations, although even here attempts should be made if possible, for example, to obtain consent from parents or others. In many states, it is possible for adolescents to give consent, for example, emancipated minors, for evaluation of certain problems, for example, sexually transmitted disease. Given variations from state to state, clinicians must be aware of the current law in their own jurisdiction. Inappropriate admission to a mental health hospital, for example, without adequate evaluation or monitoring, can also result in liability for the mental health care provider involved.

Liability issues can also arise when patients are "abandoned," for example, when treatment is terminated abruptly and unilaterally without appropriate arrangements for transfer of care or when appropriate coverage and accessibility is not provided. Termination can be done unilaterally in some circumstances, although usually only with adequate notice, provision of alterative treaters, and a follow-up (certified) letter to document the discussion and the reasons why treatment is being terminated. Liability is also potentially the result of inappropriate disclosure of confidential information, for example, in presentations or research reports.

■ SERVING AS AN EXPERT WITNESS

Mental health professionals sometimes serve as expert witnesses, for example, in cases within the juvenile justice system, custody cases, medical malpractice, and sometimes in suits related to educational services. In this role, the court expects the professional to offer specific information relevant to the case based on their knowledge and experience as it applies to the case at hand. In the role of expert, the professional is given somewhat more leeway than is usually the case. Sometimes, the psychiatrist is appointed by the court and issues a report to the judge or the child's attorney rather than to a specific attorney (although the other attorneys, if any, will typically have access to it). Standards of proof differ in civil versus criminal proceedings. In juvenile court, the standard of proof is like that in an adult criminal court, that is, beyond a reasonable doubt, whereas in the civil or family court the standard is a preponderance of the evidence. In serving as an expert witness, it is critical to avoid conflicts of interest, for example, serving both as an expert witness and treating physician raises issues. The specific requirements for what constitute an expert medical witness vary from one state to another as, to some extent, do other court procedures.

In dealing with requests to serve as an expert witness, it is important that the mental health professional have a clear understanding of what is being asked. Often this is reasonable, but sometimes it is not. A clear understanding and agreement on what question(s) is being asked will help clarify some aspects of what is involved, for example, record review, examination of a child or adolescent, or an evaluation in relation to a custody dispute typically. The latter will involve meetings with parents and child (separately and together) and, if relevant, other people important to the child's life. In taking a case (and there is no obligation that one is required to do so), the potential expert witness should be clear that the issues involved fall within their areas of expertise (of course, sometimes, other issues will emerge). The initial discussion should also be done so as to reveal any potential conflicts of interest that might exist and will also give a chance for the expert to provide a fee schedule, typically an hourly rate, and have an initial review of the basic aspects of the case with the attorney. Given the nature of these assessments and the considerable time they often require, it can be perfectly reasonable to decline an invitation to serve as an expert witness. In some cases, the expert and attorney or judge may agree on an initial record review before a decision is made regarding additional work.

A forensic evaluation has similarities and some important differences from routine clinical evaluations. The issues may have less to do with current diagnosis and treatment than with past status, for example, mental disorders present at the time a crime was committed. Similarly, in a custody assessment, issues will have to do not only with the child but also with the child's relationship to the parents and parental capacities to parent. It is particularly important in forensic evaluations that all those involved be clear about the purpose and nature of the evaluation, for example, a parent should understand that anything they say might end up in a report to the court or might be repeated if the psychiatrist testifies in court. Depending on the context, ancillary sources of information, for example, school records, may be helpful.

It is not the job of the expert to ferret out records or materials; rather the court or attorneys involved should request relevant records and be informed if it becomes clear that some records have not been provided. Depending on the context, the expert may ask that other

TABLE 26.4

Risk Management Principles

General Principle	Special Consideration in Child and Adolescent Work	Example of Potential Problem
Open communication	Clear understanding of minor's confidentiality and exceptions	Parents have right to see chart. Parents need to be told of dangerous situations.
Clarity of role definition	Whether the child or the whole family is the patient	In family work, there may be a doctor–patient relationship with each person in the family.
Need to obtain informed consent	Assent from minor is useful; consent from parents is usually required	In nontraditional family or post-divorce situations, need to be sure which parent(s) has authority to consent
Appropriate medication use	Much use is off label	Insufficient explanation of possible side effects
Compliance and cooperation with treatment	May be reduced by immaturity or minor's lack of agreement	Jury may see immature child as less responsible than an adult and so attribute more responsibility for safety to the clinician
Documentation of treatment	Documentation of communications with collateral sources (parents, school) is important	Failure to document telling parents that their child had some suicidal symptoms
Careful risk assessment	Risk factors less researched and less predictive than with adults Ratio of suicidal ideation to completed suicide is much higher than with adults	Unforeseen impulsive suicide

Reprinted with permission from Ash, P., & Nurcombe, B. (2018). Malpractice and professional liability. In A. Martin, M. Bloch, & F. R. Volkmar (Eds.), *Lewis's child and adolescent psychiatry* (5th ed., Table 7.4.4.1, p. 1008). Wolters Kluwer.

consultations be arranged, for example, psychological testing might be requested to evaluate psychotic thinking or intellectual functioning.

Before writing the report, it is often helpful to discuss preliminary findings with the retaining attorney or the judge even before a final report is submitted. This gives them the opportunities to clarify any questions that have not been answered. Such conversations should not, of course, change the report (unless new facts come to light based on these discussions). Composition of the report should parallel, in many ways, the approach to providing testimony as a witness. The report should be clear, easy to read, and free, as much as possible, of jargon. Usually, it includes a discussion of the background of the case and the questions the expert is asked to address. A list of interviews conducted, any special procedures or testing, and results of record review should precede a summary of opinions. Direct quotations can be helpful and those interviewed should always be reminded at the outset that this might be the case. The report should be professional in its tone and not inflammatory or pejorative. The rationale for any specific recommendations should be clear and the expert should be prepared to defend their recommendations in court. The court procedures and advice presented in the section on treatment or fact witness apply to expert testimony as well. Attorneys retaining expert witnesses most likely want to go over the material that will be presented and the questions likely to come up in court. Depositions are frequently used, and the experts will receive a transcript of the deposition for authentication and correction, for example, of any medical terms. If followed by later courtroom testimony, statements made in the deposition may be used to challenge the consistency of expert opinion by answers that the expert has made in court.

The process and the advice for handling of direct, cross, redirect, and recross examinations in expert testimony are essentially the same as with fact witnesses. In addition to the qualifications of expertise, the testimony of a child and adolescent psychiatrist is expected to meet the general acceptance rule or Frye Test, named after the case of *Frye v. United States* (1923), which holds that a medical test, procedure, or disorder has been generally accepted in the scientific community. For example, describing a person as suffering from a particular syndrome is unlikely to be considered unless it is included in the *Diagnostic and Statistical Manual of the American Psychiatric Association*. A new standard for scientific opinion in federal cases was set by the U.S. Supreme Court's ruling in *Daubert v. Merrill Dow Pharmaceuticals, Inc.* (1993), which determined that the judge is the one to determine if the offered evidence is scientifically valid and it will assist the court in understanding or determining facts relevant to the case. In addition, this assessment by the judge of expert opinion must be made prior to it being presented in court before a jury. Sometimes, opposing attorneys will object to expert testimony as "hearsay," as evidence based on the statements or experience of those other than the expert witness. Such evidence is permitted for expert witnesses, because the use of others' statements and experience gathered as part of clinical evaluation is a recognized practice in formulating psychiatric opinions. Opposing attorneys may also ask if the child and adolescent specialist accepts or recognizes another professional as an expert in the field or a particular study, paper, or book as authoritative. This is usually in order to present information that may conflict or appear to contradict the evidence presented by the expert witness. It is important to maintain objectivity throughout testimony and avoid the appearance of personal bias. The expert is not a patient advocate in such situations but presents psychiatric opinion and the data on which it is based (Box 26.2).

BOX 26.2   **Case Illustration—Disposition Hearing for Juvenile Case**

Dr. Smith is contacted by the local juvenile court with a request to conduct a transfer evaluation of Jim, a 16-year-old boy, currently held in juvenile detention following his arrest for armed robbery. A court hearing has been scheduled but the district attorney and judge agree to reschedule in order to allow time for the completion of the forensic evaluation. Dr. Smith agrees and arrangements are made for billing the court. A copy of the court order, arrest reports, probation record, and psychological testing are sent to Dr. Smith. She contacts the juvenile detention center and arranges times to interview both Jim and his mother, his legal guardian.

Dr. Smith reviews the records and learns that Jim was on probation for possession of a controlled substance (marijuana) when he was arrested for allegedly robbing a pizza delivery boy at gunpoint. No one was injured and apparently the gun was not loaded. He has one other recorded arrest for shoplifting (beer at a convenience store) when he was 13. Psychological testing reveals no current psychiatric complaints other than symptoms associated with his drug use. In addition, it notes that he would be considered competent to stand trial as an adult, although the psychologist expresses the opinion that Jim's needs would be better met by the juvenile court system.

On interview with Jim, Dr. Smith explains that she is preparing a report for the court as it considers sending his case for trial in adult criminal court. Jim understands and agrees to the interview. Jim describes feeling sad since his incarceration but does not have sufficient symptoms for a diagnosis of major depression. He admits to using alcohol and marijuana on almost a daily basis, having begun drinking at age 11 and smoking at age 12. He has drunk until he passed out, but denies blackouts or other symptoms associated with alcohol use. He has had hallucinations associated with marijuana use. He has experimented with cocaine by snorting it on two occasions and has tried Ecstasy several times but denies using or trying any other drugs. He also does not think that the marijuana that he uses is laced with other drugs but is not sure. He admits to arrests listed in his criminal record and to having stolen some money from his mother in order to pay for marijuana but denies other antisocial behavior, including physical fights, fire setting, vandalism, cruelty to animals, rape, and involvement with a gang. He states that he had been using both alcohol and marijuana with friends at the time that the pizza delivery boy arrived.

He also remembers taking his friend's gun and threatening the delivery boy as a joke, although now he thinks what he did was stupid. His probation officer had made plans to refer him for drug treatment, but that had not taken place at the time of the incident. He also was noncompliant with his probation visits because he did not want to be found in violation with a positive drug screen. He was a student in ninth grade at the time of his arrest, having been held back for failing due to truancy and poor academic performance. He expresses a desire to get his GED and enter a trade school.

His mother also understands the purpose of the interview and agrees to answer Dr. Smith's questions. She reports that she and Jim's father were never married and that they amicably separated when Jim was 3 years old. His father has stayed involved with Jim, taking him every other weekend. She admits that both she and Jim's father have problems with drinking. She currently works evenings cleaning offices and says that it has been hard to supervise Jim. She corroborates Jim's description of his behavior and previous troubles with the law.

Dr. Smith considers that while Jim is mature, his offense was serious and previous probation has not contained his behavior, he does not have a pattern of violent offense, and that there has never been a serious effort made to deal with drug use that is central to his antisocial behavior. She calls the district attorney to learn why the request for a transfer hearing was made. The district attorney points out the history of arrests, the appearance of threatening and potentially violent behavior, and that Jim will soon be 17 and beyond the scope of juvenile probation. Dr. Smith asks if the court has the option of deferred or concurrent sentencing, where Jim would be sent for drug treatment by court order and his progress reviewed at age 17, when he would either be released or sentenced as an adult. The district attorney said that was possible but did not know of treatment facilities that would take Jim. Dr. Smith then prepares a report for the court outlining her findings and opinion that Jim should not be transferred because there was no prior rehabilitation for his drug use and the lack of previous violent offenses. She recommends a facility that would accept Jim for drug treatment on court order. The court and district attorney accept Dr. Smith's report and recommendation at the hearing and she does not have to testify.

■ SUMMARY

Mental health professionals who work with children and adolescents have an increasing role in various legal proceedings. Involvement may range from serving as a "fact" witness to serving as an expert witness or consultant to the court, in helping mediate a custody dispute or providing an opinion about needed accommodations to address a developmental or psychiatric problem in school. It is vital that professionals remain aware of changes in the law and are aware of new laws and decisions that may impact their care of children and families. Having some awareness of the judicial process and procedures facilitates this effort.

Changes in practices of custody and custody dispute resolution have been an active area for involvement of mental health professionals over the last several decades. Considerable progress has been made in considering the child's needs (rather than only those of the adults) in this process, and advances have been made in terms of facilitating, as much as possible, the continued involvement of both parents in the child's life. As with other aspects of forensics, it is important that the professional remains current with laws and practices in their jurisdiction.

Adoption touches many lives. Many adults joyfully become parents through adoption and for most children, adoption has a positive outcome, contributes to positive psychological adjustment, and is clearly protective; for a minority, adoption may be associated with emotional and behavioral problems and psychiatric disorders. Children at particular risk include those adopted later in life, after early adverse experiences, as well as those at particular risk, for example, through toxic exposure prenatally. Clinicians working with adopted children and their families should be aware of the complexity and variability of the circumstances in which adoption takes place, as well as the meaning of the process for all the individuals involved.

Mental health consultants have had an increasing role both within the juvenile justice system and the complex areas of care that aim to prevent incarceration. Rates of mental disorders, often comorbid mental health conditions, are high and sometimes the goal of rehabilitation rather than punishment is lost. Fortunately, a number of effective treatment models are available.

Lawsuits of mental health professionals who work with children and adolescents are not common. They can be very stressful when they occur. These can arise in several ways, for example, through patient abandonment, poor clinical management, and failure to observe proper (community-based) standards of care. One of the complexities of work with children and adolescents has to do with issues of confidentiality, particularly when, as is frequent, parents are also understandably involved in some way in the treatment.

In summary, although work in the forensic area can be challenging, it can also be rewarding. Some practitioners choose either to specialize in this area or maintain some part of their practice devoted to it. Recent Supreme Court decisions have had an important impact on the juvenile justice system (see Sharma & Thomas, 2018). On the other side, advances in neuroscience may have important implications for the legal system (Pope, Luna, & Thomas, 2012).

References

Abram, K., Teplin, L., McClelland, G., & Dulcan, M. (2003). Comorbid psychiatric disorders in youth in juvenile detention. *Archives of General Psychiatry*, 60(11), 1097–1108. https://doi.org/10.1001/archpsyc.60.11.1097

Ash, P., & Nurcomb, B. (2018). Malpractice and professional liability. In A. Martin, M. Bloch, & F. R. Volkmar (Eds.), *Lewis's child and adolescent psychiatry: A comprehensive textbook* (5th ed., pp. 999–1010). Wolters Kluwer.

Bostic, J. F., & Hoover, S. A. (2018). School consultation. In A. Martin, M. Bloch, & F. R. Volkmar (Eds.), *Lewis's child and adolescent psychiatry: A comprehensive textbook* (5th ed., pp. 956–974). Wolters Kluwer.

Brown, R. M. A. (2018). Adoption. In A. Martin, M. Bloch, F. R. Volkmar, (Eds.), *Lewis's child and adolescent psychiatry: A comprehensive textbook* (5th ed., pp. 991–995). Wolters Kluwer.

Daubert v. Merrell Dow Pharmaceuticals, Inc., 113 S.Ct. 2786, 1993.

Frye v. United States 293 F. 1013–1014 D.C. Cir., 1923.

Goldstein, J., Freud, A. & Solnit, A. J. (1973). *Beyond the best interests of the child.* Macmillan.

Greenwood, P. (2008). Prevention and intervention programs for juvenile offenders. *The Future of Children*, 18(2), 185–210. https://doi.org/10.1353/foc.0.0018

Herman, S. P. (1997). Practice parameters for child custody evaluation. American Academy of Child and Adolescent Psychiatry. *Journal of the American Academy of Child and Adolescent Psychiatry*, 36, 57S–68S. https://doi.org/10.1097/00004583-199710001-00005

Mroczkowski, M. D. (2018). Divorce and child custody. In A. Martin, M. Bloch, & F. R. Volkmar, (Eds.), *Lewis's child and adolescent psychiatry: A comprehensive textbook* (5th ed., pp. 982–990). Wolters Kluwer.

Pope, K., Luna, B., & Thomas, C. R. (2012). Developmental neuroscience and the courts: How science is influencing the disposition of juvenile offenders. *Journal of the American Academy of Child & Adolescent Psychiatry, 51*(4), 341–342. https://doi.org/10.1016/j.jaac.2012.01.003

Rutter, M. (1998). Developmental catch-up, and deficit, following adoption after severe global early privation. *Journal of Child Psychology and Psychiatry, 39*(4), 465–476. https://doi.org/10.1111/1469-7610.00343

Soulier, M. (2012). Juvenile offenders: Competence to stand trial. *Psychiatric Clinics of North America, 35*(4), 837–854. https://doi.org/10.1016/j.psc.2012.08.005

Thomas, C. (2018). The child and adolescent psychiatrist in court. In A. Martin, M. Bloch, & F. R. Volkmar (Eds.), *Lewis's child and adolescent psychiatry: A comprehensive textbook* (5th ed., pp. 974–990). Wolters Kluwer.

Trupin E., & Boesky L. (1999). Working together for change: Co-Occurring mental health and substance use disorders among youth involved in the juvenile justice system: Cross training, juvenile justice, mental health, substance abuse. Delmar, NY: The National GAINS Center.

Underwood, L. A., & Washington, A. (2016). Mental illness and juvenile offenders. *International Journal of Environmental Research and Public Health, 13*(2), 228. https://doi.org/10.3390/ijerph13020228

Wasserman, G. A., McReynolds, L. S., Lucas, C. P., Fisher, P., & Santos, L. (2002). The voice DISC-IV with incarcerated male youths: Prevalence of disorder. *Journal of the American Academy of Child & Adolescent Psychiatry, 41*(3), 314–321. https://doi.org/10.1097/00004583-200203000-00011

Suggested Readings

American Academy of Child and Adolescent Psychiatry. (1997). Practice parameters for child custody evaluations. *Journal of the American Academy of Child and Adolescent Psychiatry, 36*, 57S–67S. https://doi.org/10.1097/00004583-199710001-00005

Ash, P., & Nurcombe, B. (2018). Malpractice and professional liability. In A. Martin, M. Bloch, & F. R. Volkmar (Eds.), *Lewis's child and adolescent psychiatry: A comprehensive textbook* (5th ed., pp. 996–1010). Wolters Kluwer.

Barkley, R. (1996). Attention-deficit/hyperactivity disorder. In E. Mash & R. Barkley (Eds.), *Child psychopathology* (pp. 63–112). Guilford Press.

Bernet, W. (1998). The child and adolescent psychiatrist and the law. In J. D. Noshpitz (Ed.), *Handbook of child and adolescent psychiatry* (pp. 438–468). John Wiley and Sons, Inc.

Billick, S. B., & Ciric, S. J. (2003). Role of the psychiatric evaluator in child custody disputes. In *Principles and practice of forensic psychiatry* (2nd ed., pp. 331–347). CRC Press.

Borland, M., O'Hara, G., & Triseliotis, J. (1991). Placement outcomes for children with special needs. *Adoption and Fostering, 15*, 18–28. https://doi.org/10.1177/030857599101500205

Borum, R., Fein, R., Vossekuil, B., & Berglund, J. (1999). Threat assessment: Defining an approach for evaluating risk of targeted violence. *Behavioral Science Law, 17*, 323–337. https://doi.org/10.1002/(SICI)1099-0798(199907/09)17:3<323::AID-BSL349>3.0.CO;2-G

Bostic, J. Q., Stein, B., & Scwab-Stone, M. (2005). Schools. In A. Martin & F. R. Volkmar (Eds.), *Lewis's essentials of child and adolescent psychiatry: A comprehensive textbook* (5th ed.). Wolters Kluwer.

Brown, J. M. A. (2018). Adoption. In A. Martin, M. Bloch, & F. R. Volkmar (Eds.), *Lewis's child and adolescent psychiatry: A comprehensive textbook* (5th ed., pp. 991–995). Wolters Kluwer.

Cederblad, M., Hook, B., Irhammar, M., & Mercke, A. M. (1999). Mental health in international adoptees as teenagers and young adults: An epidemiological study. *Journal of Child Psychology and Psychiatry, 40*, 1239–1248. https://doi.org/10.1111/1469-7610.00540

Charney, D., Deutch, A., Krystal, J., Southwick, S., & Davis, M. (1993). Psychobiologic mechanisms of posttraumatic stress disorder. *Archives of General Psychiatry, 50*(4), 294–305. https://doi.org/10.1001/archpsyc.1993.01820160064008

Goldstein, J., Solnit, A. J., Goldstein, S., & Freud, A. (1996). *In the best interest of the child.* Free Press.

Grisso, T. (2008). Adolescent offenders with mental disorders. *The Future of Children, 18*(2), 143–164. https://doi.org/10.1353/foc.0.0016

Hannibal, M. E. (2002). *Good parenting through your divorce.* Marlow and Co.

Hetherington, M. E., & Kelly, J. (2002). *For better or for worse.* W. W. Norton & Co.

Hodges, J., & Tizard, B. (1989). Social and family relationships of ex-institutional adolescents. *Journal of Child Psychology & Psychiatry, 30*, 77–97. https://doi.org/10.1111/j.1469-7610.1989.tb00770.x

Howe, D. (1997). Parent reported problems in 211 adopted children: Some risk and protective factors. *Journal of Child Psychology & Psychiatry, 38*, 401–411. https://doi.org/10.1111/j.1469-7610.1997.tb01525.x

Huizinga, D., Loeber, R., Thornberry, T., & Cothern, L. (2000). *Co-occurrence of delinquency and other problem behaviors.* Office of Juvenile Justice and Delinquency Prevention.

Juffer, F., & van Ijzendoorn, M. H. (2007). Adoptees do not lack self-esteem: A meta-analysis of studies on self-esteem of transracial, international, and domestic adoptees. *Psychological Bulletin, 133*(6), 1067–1083. https://doi.org/10.1037/0033-2909.133.6.1067

Kelly, J. B., & Emery, R. (2003). Children's adjustment following divorce: Risk and resilience perspectives. *Family Relations, 52*, 352–262. https://doi.org/10.1111/j.1741-3729.2003.00352.x

Keyes, M. A., Sharma, A., Elkins, I. J., Iacono, W. G., & McGue, M. (2008). The mental health of US adolescents adopted in infancy. *Archives of Pediatrics & Adolescent Medicine, 162*(5), 419–425. https://doi.org/10.1001/archpedi.162.5.419

Kraus, L. J., Thomas, C. R., Bukstein, O. G., Walter, H. J., Benson, R. S., Chrisman, A., Farchione, T. R., Hamilton, J., Keable, H., Kinlan, J., Schoettle, U., Siegel, M., Stock, S., Ptakowski, K. K., & Medicus, J. (2011). Practice parameter for child and adolescent forensic evaluations. *Journal of the American Academy of Child and Adolescent Psychiatry, 50*(12), 1299–1312. https://doi.org/10.1016/j.jaac.2011.09.020

Kuo, A. D., & Sikorski, J. B. (2005). Divorce and child custody. In A. Martin & F. R. Volkmar (Eds.), *Lewis's essentials of child and adolescent psychiatry: A comprehensive textbook.* Wolters Kluwer.

Martin, A., Krieg, H., Esposito, F., Stubbe, D., & Cardona, L. (2009). Reduction of restraint and seclusion through collaborative problem solving: A five-year prospective inpatient study. *Psychiatric Services, 60*(3), 406. https://doi.org/10.1176/ps.2008.59.12.1406

Ash, P., & Nurcombe, B. (2007). Malpractice and and professional liability. In A. Martin & F. R. Volkmar (Eds.), *Lewis's child and adolescent psychiatry: A comprehensive textbook* (4th ed.). Wolters Kluwer.

Maughan, B., & Pickles, A. (1990). Adopted and illegitimate children grown up. In L. Robins & M. Rutter (Eds.), *Straight and devious pathways from childhood to adulthood.* Cambridge University Press.

Mossman, D., & Kapp, M. B. (1998). "Courtroom whores?"—Or why do attorneys call us? Findings from a survey on attorneys' use of mental health experts. *The Journal of the American Academy of Psychiatry and the Law, 26*, 27–36.

Mroczkowski, M. M. (2018). Divorce and child custory. In A. Martin, M. Bloch, & F. R. Volkmar (Eds.), *Lewis's child and adolescent psychiatry: A comprehensive textbook* (5th ed., pp. 982–999). Wolters Kluwer.

O'Connor, S. (2004). *Orphan trains: The story of Charles Loring brace and the children he saved and failed.* University of Chicago Press.

Recupero, P. R. (2005). E-mail and the psychiatrist-patient relationship. *Journal of the American Academy of Psychiatry Law, 33*, 465–475. https://doi.org/10.1521/jaap.2005.33.3.465

Reed, J. (2004). Cybermedicine: Defying and redefining patient standards of care. *Indiana Law Review, 37*, 845–877.

Rutter, M. (1998). Developmental catch-up, and deficit, following adoption after severe global early privation. *Journal of Child Psychology & Psychiatry, 39*, 465–476. https://doi.org/10.1017/S0021963098002236

Schetky, D. (2002). History of child and adolescent forensic psychiatry. In D. H. Schetky & E. P. Benedek (Eds.), *Principles and practice of child and adolescent forensic psychiatry* (pp. 3–14). American Psychiatric Publishing, Inc.

Schetky, D. H., & Guyer, M. J. (1990). Civil litigation and the child psychiatrist. *Journal of the American Academy of Child & Adolescent Psychiatry, 29*, 963–968. https://doi.org/10.1097/00004583-199011000-00023

Sharma, S., & Thomas, C. R. (2018). The child and adolescent psychiatrist in court. In A. Martin, M. Bloch, & F. R. Volkmar (Eds.), *Lewis's child and adolescent psychiatry: A comprehensive textbook* (5th ed., pp. 974–982). Wolters Kluwer.

Simon, R. I. (2004). *Assessing and managing suicide risk: guidelines for clinically based risk management.* American Psychiatric Publications.

Skolnick, A. (1998). Solomon's children: The new biologism, psychological parenthood, attachment theory, and the best interests standard. In S. D. Sugarman (Ed.), *All our families.* Oxford University Press.

Skowyra, K., & Cocozza, J. (2007). *A blueprint for change: improving the system response to youth with mental health needs involved with the juvenile justice system.* National Center for Mental Health and Juvenile Justice.

Stepanyan, S. T., Sidhu, S. S., & Bath, E. (2016). Juvenile competency to stand trial. *Child and Adolescent Psychiatric Clinics of North America, 25*(1), 49–59. https://doi.org/10.1016/j.chc.2015.08.008

Stoddard-Dare, P., Mallett, C., & Boitel, C. (2011). Association between mental health disorders and juveniles' detention for a personal crime. *Child and Adolescent Mental Health, 16*(4), 208–213. https://doi.org/10.1111/j.1475-3588.2011.00599.x

Teplin, L. A., Abram, K. M., McClelland, G. M., Dulcan, M. K., & Mericle, A. A. (2002). Psychiatric disorders in youth in juvenile detention. *Archives of General Psychiatry, 59*(12), 1133–1143. https://doi.org/10.1001/archpsyc.59.12.1133

Teplin, L., Abram, K., McClelland, G., Mericle, A., Dulcan, M., & Washburn, D. (2006). *Psychiatric disorders of youth in detention*. Office of Juvenile Justice and Delinquency Prevention.

Tesler, P. (2001). *Collaborative law: Achieving effective resolution in divorce without litigation*. American Bar Association.

Tizard, B. (1991). Intercountry adoption: A review of the evidence. *Journal of Child Psychology & Psychiatry, 32*, 743–756. https://doi.org/10.1111/j.1469-7610.1991.tb01899.x

Volkmar, F. R., & Wiesner, L. A. (2009). *A practical guide to autism: what every parent, family member, and teacher needs to know*. John Wiley & Sons, Inc.

Wallerstein, J. S., Lewis, J. M., & Blakeslee, S. (2000). *The unexpected legacy of divorce*. Hyperion.

Zajac, K., Sheidow, A. J., & Davis, M. (2015). Juvenile justice, mental health, and the transition to adulthood: A review of service system involvement and unmet needs in the U.S. *Children and Youth Services Review, 56*, 139–148. https://doi.org/10.1016/j.childyouth.2015.07.014

Zeanah, C. H., Larrieu, J. A., Heller, S. S., Valliere, J., Hinshaw-Fuselier, S., Aoki, Y., & Drilling, M. (2001). Evaluation of a preventive intervention for maltreated infants and toddlers in foster care. *Journal of the American Academy of Child and Adolescent Psychiatry, 40*, 214–221. https://doi.org/10.1097/00004583-200102000-00016

CHAPTER 27 ■ THE INTERFACE OF MENTAL HEALTH AND MEDICINE

In this chapter, we consider some aspects of mental health care in pediatrics and the medical care/hospital system. We begin with a short discussion of the role of primary care providers before turning to emergency care. As we discuss emergency mental health, referrals are of many types and some special issues, for example, suicidality and its assessment, as well as evaluation of aggressive behavior are of special importance. We also discuss when to consider hospitalization. In the final section of this chapter, we discuss the role of the mental health consultant within inpatient pediatric consultations. This includes consideration of the role of the consultant, the process of the consultation, and special areas of mental health services including conditions like pediatric oncology, delirium, pediatric transplants, epilepsy, and palliative care. Mental health consultation is an area of great and growing interest to many disciplines including not only psychiatry and child psychiatry but also psychology, social work, nursing, and child life support staff within larger hospital settings. As we note, the dearth of providers creates significant challenges in many settings.

■ MENTAL HEALTH ISSUES IN PRIMARY CARE

The integration of mental health resources and treatments into primary pediatric care settings presents many opportunities and challenges (Pumariega & Winters, 2018). Most children in the United States have at least one visit with the primary care provider each year. The primary care provider may be required to interact with other systems, for example, school, child welfare, legal, as well as mental health. Although provision of medical care (including mental health care) has improved, mental health services remain lacking for many youth (Asarnow et al., 2005; Pumariega & Winters, 2018).

Typically, the primary care provider serves as a resource and potentially a gatekeeper in facilitating access to mental health services. The need for mental health providers is underscored by epidemiologic studies suggesting high rates of mental health problems in children, with probably one in five children having a significant problem (Pumariega & Winters, 2018). These problems take a significant toll on school success and may impact peer and family relationships. The public health significance of these problems is underscored by work suggesting that about half of all mental health disorders have their onset by age 14 years and 75% by age 24 years.

Unfortunately, the historic divisions between medical and psychiatric service systems have tended to fragment service delivery and complicate provision of effective, integrated care. This unfortunate dichotomy is now greatly compounded by issues of insurance reimbursement and the organization (or lack thereof) of health care. These issues become further complicated for some disorders specifically covered within the mandates of schools for providing services. There are a few model programs, for example, that of Massachusetts, that aim to integrate care (Sarvet et al., 2010).

Mental health conditions frequently present with physical problems, and patients with physical problems have associated psychiatric disabilities. Psychiatric conditions also have important associated medical risks, for example, for accidents and injuries, suicide, violence, substance abuse, and teen pregnancy, among others. Most chronic physical illnesses increase the risk for subsequent mental health problems. Conversely, the association of depression with a chronic condition like diabetes may be associated with significant risk for problems. It is important to be aware of medical conditions that increase the risk for mental health disturbances in the child (see Table 27.1).

Sadly, despite the awareness of the effective mental health interventions, most children and adolescents do not receive treatments they need and even those who do do not necessarily receive treatments considered best practice, evidence-based interventions. Primary care providers can offer clinical management for most psychosocial problems and account for the majority of prescriptions of psychoactive medications. This is true for various conditions ranging from depression, anxiety, and mood problems to attention-deficit disorder (see Havens et al., 2018). Fortunately, there have now been some attempts on the part of the American Academy of Pediatrics to produce guidelines for management of mental health care issues in primary pediatric care. The field of Developmental-Behavioral Pediatrics arose from concerns about the need for more sustained and effective training of pediatricians in behavioral health. This approach has focused on common behavioral and developmental problems, and the subspecialty has been officially recognized and now includes a period of fellowship training. The medical home model (Sheldrick & Perrin, 2010) has now been used with good results in a range of conditions, for example, autism, to provide better integrated care.

Primary care providers may feel more comfortable in the management of some disorders, like ADHD, but not others, for example, depression (Asarnow et al., 2005; Schonfeld & Campo, 2018). There are many obstacles to providing mental health services including lack of

TABLE 27.1

Common Medical Causes of Psychiatric Disturbance in Children and Adolescents

Fever
Nonconvulsive status epilepticus
Temporal lobe seizures
Absence seizure
Encephalitis
Cerebral systemic lupus erythematosus
Childhood confusional migraine
Head trauma or post-concussive syndrome
Porphyria
Sickle cell disease
Substance intoxication
Withdrawal from illicit substances
Anticholinergic delirium
Steroid psychosis or steroid-induced mania
Central nervous system neoplasm or other occult malignancy
Medication adverse effects such as akathisia from risperidone or irritability from levetiracetam

Reprinted with permission from J. F. Havens, R. S. Gerson, and M. March. (2018). Designing emergency psychiatry services for children and adolescents. In A. Martin, M. Bloch, & F. R. Volkmar (Eds.), *Lewis's child and adolescent psychiatry,* (5th ed., p. 349). Wolters Kluwer.

access, social stigma, the shortage of child and adolescent psychiatrists, reimbursement, and administrative issues. Clearly, priorities in this area include better training, new models of care like the medical home, and new methods of service delivery, for example, school-based clinics. Communities in rural and impoverished areas may have the least access to good models of care, and telemedicine has some important potential advantages in these situations.

Although they can occur at any age, child mental health emergencies become more common as children enter school and high school. The urgency of the situation depends on the nature of the psychiatric symptoms, available supports, and issues of safety for the child and others. Unfortunately, as with other aspects of medical care, psychiatric emergency services are frequently, but inappropriately, used to deal with problems more appropriate to less urgent settings, but, given an absence of community resources, such problems may present on an emergent basis or directly in the emergency department. Sometimes, issues have been simmering for a long time and something finally tips the situation over the edge (Havens et al., 2018). At other times, there may be rapid emergence of difficulties. Referrals may come from many sources including parents and family, schools, juvenile justice, community agencies, and so forth. Referrals from junior high and high schools are frequent except in the summer. Heightened sensitivities to violence have often led schools to adopt a policy of zero tolerance; these policies may require some sort of psychiatric assessment before the child returns to the school.

Mental health emergency referral of all kinds has become more common in recent years. Kalb and colleagues (2019) reported a nearly 30% overall increase with a 2.5-fold increase in visits related to suicidal thoughts/actions. Sadly, only about 16% of youth were actually evaluated in the emergency department (ED) by a mental health professional. The reasons for the increased number of referrals remain unclear but include higher rates of suicidal thinking and increased rates of violent behavior. Dwindling options for community-based care force more children and adolescents to emergency settings when crises occur. Many mental health professionals in private practice are willing to see patients on an urgent basis but if issues of hospitalization or suicidality or violence arise, they typically will refer the patient and their family to the ED. Insurance coverage pressures have also forced shorter lengths of stay when mental health hospitalization is indicated. Finally, of course, the ED remains the place of last resort for the many uninsured children and adolescents who need acute mental health care.

■ CONSULTATION IN THE EMERGENCY DEPARTMENT

Child psychiatric emergencies are characteristically times of great stress for all concerned. The sense of urgency is often complicated by anxiety about the outcome and/or the ongoing issues or conflicts. Typically, many different factors are involved in precipitating the trip to the ED and often a relevant place to begin is with the question "why now" (Havens et al., 2018).

Clarifying the relationships of the various individuals centrally involved is another important priority. Children function in several different contexts: home and family, school, and community. A crisis can occur with any number of changes to these overlapping systems—for example, school failure, parental discord, violence, bullying, and victimization. Sometimes a sudden upsurge in the level of severity of an ongoing problem can precipitate the crisis. Often clarifying the questions of why now and who is involved become the first steps in thinking about a resolution of the crisis.

In understanding the nature of the emergency, the evaluator typically has several important goals:

- understanding the factor(s) that led to the referral (including interviewing all the relevant participants),
- developing a shared or working alliance with the child and family about goals for evaluation,
- obtaining a history of the child's current difficulties as well as long-standing issues and problems and relevant support systems, and
- conducting a mental status examination focused not only on issues of differential diagnosis and treatment but also with attention to the presence of suicidal or homicidal ideation, symptoms of psychosis or delirium, and so forth.

It is important to develop an emergency treatment plan and arrive at a disposition, with due consideration for the safety of the child (and others) with follow-up and collaboration with other clinicians involved in the child's care, including the primary care provider.

Given the intense pressures on a busy hospital ED, it is not surprising that often the focus in an emergency is the question of dangerousness and potential needs for hospitalization. This approach misses the potential therapeutic value, that is, using a crisis to stimulate change, of the ED visit and the opportunity it presents for significant benefit. In contrast to the somewhat more leisurely pace of typical assessments, the urgency of the ED situation typically leads to rapid clinical decisions and treatment formulation. This process can be severely hampered, for example, by the absence of key adults who can provide information or by limited community resources for treatment after discharge from the ED. The latter can be even more of a problem when, as is often the case, the evaluation is conducted at night or on the weekend rather than during regular business hours. Given the pressures involved, the clinician must be efficient and well organized. With experience, clinicians rapidly develop a clear sense of the priority of problems and often begin to formulate their ideas about diagnosis and treatment planning as soon as the evaluation has begun.

The typical ED is a busy place with little privacy and many distractions. Depending on the situation, it can be very helpful if the clinician can locate a quieter and less stimulating area to use for interviewing the child and others. This area must, however, be safe and the clinician should feel that help is at hand should the need arise. Typically, an adult, rather than the child, will have been the source of the referral to the ED. Similar to other situations that require mental health evaluation (see Chapter 4), assessment often requires eliciting information from multiple sources, but in contrast to the usual outpatient situation, the adult bringing the child may not necessarily be the parent but a police officer, social service worker, or a teacher who might be involved in the crisis. A lack of relevant information and/or conflicting sources of information can complicate the task of assessment. Practically speaking, the examiner often ends up collecting information in a piecemeal fashion but with an overall understanding of the most critically important issues to address. Whoever is present becomes a legitimate source of information, that is, the child and whoever has transported them, for example, police or schoolteachers and resource officer or parents. It may be important to touch base with all concerned; in emergency situations, the clinician has considerable leeway in gathering information but parental contact is indicated as quickly as possible if parents do not come with the child. In many states, adolescents may be able to give consent when parents are not available and the clinician should be aware of applicable state laws and guidelines to mental health emergencies, consent issues, and involuntary hospitalization.

The chief complaint may vary, sometimes markedly, depending on who serves as the informant. These discrepant views (also termed *informant variance*) simultaneously complicate the task of the clinician but also provide helpful information about the factors that led to the emergency evaluation. They also can serve as a starting point for intervention because they reflect major areas of discrepancy between the views of the child and important adults. Other variations arise depending on the setting or context within which the child or adolescent is observed and levels of demands/expectations placed on them. The complaint, for example, that "Becky needs medication because of her behavior on the bus" suggests an important initial area of inquiry ("Only on the bus?") that can tremendously streamline subsequent discussion! Benarous and colleagues (2019) examined data on ED use by children. Overall, there was a 3.85 times increase in the annual number of ED visits, with a sharp rise in primary complaints of anxiety or depression rising from 5% in 1981 to 34% in 2017.

A simple way to view mental health emergencies is to realize that children and adolescents can be disturbed or disturbing or both. It is the child who is disturbing or exhibiting "externalizing" problems who frequently is the focus of parental or school concern and complaint. On the other hand, the child who is disturbed (anxious, depressed, or quietly suicidal—that is, exhibiting "internalizing" problems) but does NOT exhibit high levels of behavior problems may be less likely to present for emergent evaluation. Parents may have a selective bias in their recognition of family or personal factors contributing to difficulties in the child, for example, marital conflict or violence in the home. The examiner should be alert to the child who is vague or minimizes problems because often this results from an attempt on the child's part to protect the parent(s) and/or to maintain some family secret within the family, for example, parental violence, illegal behavior, mental illness, substance abuse, or physical or sexual abuse. Evaluation in these cases is particularly difficult.

The Interview of the Child or Adolescent

The child interview in emergency situations requires considerable focus. Given the nature of the setting, the examiner must cope (and help the patient cope) with intrinsic distress associated with the ED setting. Although not easy to do, every effort should be made to help the child feel as comfortable as possible. Unfortunately, by the time the child psychiatrist or the social worker has arrived to conduct an evaluation, the child often has been sufficiently stressed that they are angry, withdrawn, or overtly oppositional and antagonistic. In situations like this, the clinician can invoke the "constructive use of ignorance": for example, "I don't know much about why you are here. Can you help me out?" and thus invite the child to provide a view of the events leading to the current situation (Havens et al., 2018).

The attitudes of the child and their parents and their ability to work with each other provide important information relative to the safety of potential discharge home with follow-up in outpatient settings. The child or adolescent's ability to reflect on their contributions to the current situation and the events leading up to the ED visit also become important in terms of disposition planning. Difficulties arise when children refuse to acknowledge their contributions to problems or when parents attempt to minimize "the problem" and attribute it to external sources and unreasonable expectations. On the other hand, the child/family who acknowledge the realities of the difficulties and seem motivated to change have a much greater likelihood to use outpatient treatment successfully. The next sections of this chapter will review three of the more important topics: aggressive behavior, suicidal thoughts and behavior, and the decision on whether to hospitalize.

Aggressive Behavior as a Mental Health Emergency

Aggressive and/or uncooperative patients present special problems for assessment in the ED. Aggressive outbursts are a frequent cause of ED referrals and the patient may be transported to the ED by law enforcement or emergency medical services. The child or adolescent, sometimes in physical restraints, may be agitated, belligerent, and prone to act out. The child's threats and yelling may understandably disturb other patients and staff. Despite the pressure for a rapid solution/resolution, the clinician should approach the aggressive child/adolescent patient in a thoughtful, calm, and deliberate fashion. Both in terms of doing an adequate assessment and contributing to the resolution of the crisis, the clinician should try, as much as possible, not to be caught up in the maelstrom but ally themselves with whatever capacity the child or adolescent has to remain in control. Unfortunately, the stressors of being in the ED environment can contribute to irritability, anger, aggression, or defiant behaviors.

The clinician should be aware of the many causes of aggressive behavior and its association with different psychiatric conditions. To complicate the situation further, frequently oppositional defiant and more overtly aggressive/violent behaviors have multiple origins and determinants and often a long history antedating a specific event. In evaluating such behavior and developing a differential diagnosis, the clinician should be aware of the many factors that may contribute. Impulsive behavior and poor impulse control are frequent in various conditions including attention-deficit disorders, hypomania, autism, and conduct disorder. Learning difficulties, cognitive delays, and associated coping difficulties may also contribute to such behaviors. Exposure through observation or direct experience of aggression in violent families is another risk factor. Substance use/abuse can impair judgment, increase irritability, and contribute to disinhibited, impulsive behaviors. Psychotic conditions of various types can similarly present with overt aggression, for example, as the child or adolescent responds to a state of considerable confusion with paranoia or auditory (command) hallucinations. Aggression and apparent psychosis may also be seen as a feature of various medical conditions including delirium, encephalitis, seizure disorder, post-concussive states as discussed later in the chapter. Careful medical history is important, and the clinician should be particularly alert to the presence of such conditions (Havens et al. 2018). Treatments vary with associated conditions (see Table 27.2).

The history should focus both on recent and on past aggressive behavior: for example, is this a new problem or one that emerges in the context of years of increasing difficulty? A thorough history of the events leading up to the present problem is critical, with attention to the precipitants of the aggressive outburst. The perspective of the patients and the various relevant adults often provides important information on these issues. In situations where the child is involved as a victim, the child's account, the setting of the event, and broader context should be identified. Often, problems will have come about as an adult attempted to set a limit. In such cases, the context may clarify issues/factors that contributed to the child's response. Areas to be assessed are summarized in Table 27.3.

The safety of the child and others (including the clinician) is the first consideration in management. The clinician should feel comfortable in the setting with adequate support. In the absence of this, the clinician cannot be nearly as effective or helpful. Several steps can be taken to ensure that the patient is in sufficient control for a thorough assessment to be conducted. In approaching the patient and family, the clinician should be professional and respectful and avoid becoming angry or irritable even when dealing with the most challenging patients. The clinician should not place themselves in a situation of danger where backup is not available, and sensible precautions, for example, sitting between the patient and the door, should occur as a matter of course. As in other areas of mental health, one's own inner sense will provide important clues, for example, if a patient makes the clinician very anxious, there probably is a good reason. The waiting area and examination room should be one free of safety hazards and objects that might be used in an aggressive outburst; as much as is reasonable, it should provide minimal stimulation (certainly as compared to other parts of the ED) and have some privacy. At the same time, it should also be an area close enough to have help at hand and there should be some potential for visual contact with other staff, with use

TABLE 27.2

Psychiatric Disorders and Treatment of Acute Aggression

Illness/Symptom	Treatment Focus
ADHD	Address impulsivity
ODD	Set clear limits, reinforce positive behaviors
Psychosis	Treat command hallucinations/paranoia that are triggering aggression
Mania	Stabilize mania to address impulsivity/irritability
Anxiety or OCD	Identify and address triggers (such as being blocked from completing compulsions)
PTSD	Identify trauma reminders, promote safe coping behaviors
Autism	Promote verbal problem solving and other coping behaviors
Conduct disorder	Set clear consequences for antisocial behaviors and reinforce positive behaviors
Substance use	Increase supervision, motivation enhancement techniques to reduce use

Reprinted with permission from J. F. Havens, R. S. Gerson, and M. March. (2018). Designing emergency psychiatry services for children and adolescents. In A. Martin, M. Bloch, & F. R. Volkmar (Eds.), *Lewis's child and adolescent psychiatry* (5th ed., p. 849). Wolters Kluwer.

TABLE 27.3

Components of a Comprehensive Assessment

Identifying information
Chief complaint
History of present illness
Past psychiatric history
Current medications and medication history
Past medical history
Substance use history
Trauma history
Social history including trauma and child welfare involvement
Developmental and educational history
Family history
Legal history
Mental status examination including cognitive examination when indicated
Medical clearance including physical examination if indicated

Reprinted with permission from J. F. Havens, R. S. Gerson, and M. March. (2018). Designing emergency psychiatry services for children and adolescents. In A. Martin, M. Bloch, & F. R. Volkmar (Eds.), *Lewis's child and adolescent psychiatry* (5th ed., p. 850). Wolters Kluwer.

of appropriate codes/procedures for alerting staff if necessary. The possibility of seclusion and/or restraining should also be available if needed.

Clear expectations and firm but nonconfrontational limit setting may help de-escalate violent or potentially violent behavior. Communication of rules and expectations can be done to clarify what behavior is and is not considered acceptable. This should be provided both to the patient and family. Agitation and aggression related to confusion and disorganization make it particularly important that patients be monitored carefully. For such patients, avoiding an overstimulating, disorganizing environment is important as is the presence of another person, for example, a family member, who can provide reassurance and orientating/organizing information. Although there is often a temptation to proceed directly to medication and sedation, it is important to have a clear sense of the nature of the difficulty, for example, observing the patient for signs of other medical conditions, changes in levels of consciousness, and so forth (see next section).

Pharmacologic intervention may be needed if behavioral approaches are not successful; in such situations, consideration of sedation should involve an awareness of the severity of the symptoms, potential underlying causes of the behavioral difficulties as well as the patient's medical status, history, and goals of the sedation. Careful medical monitoring is indicated. Various agents, but particularly the neuroleptics and/or benzodiazepines, are frequently used. The shorter acting benzodiazepines can be used for both sedative and anxiolytic properties. Unfortunately, at times, the benzodiazepines can also result in a seemingly paradoxical disinhibition; this seems particularly likely in children and adolescents. Sometimes, higher potency neuroleptics are used for more aggressive and agitated patients (but only after careful assessment). For younger children, the antihistamine diphenhydramine (Benadryl®) can be given. If medications are used, understanding their potential side effects and any interactions with medications the individual is receiving is important.

The use of physical restraints is regulated by several sets of standards and should be reserved for situations in which there is immediate danger to self or others. Restraints should be used only in such situations and only for as long as they are needed. Institutional policies for seclusion and restraint should be in place. These typically clarify indications for use, the role of key personnel, and guidance on monitoring (e.g., to be sure vital signs are stable, that the airway is not restricted, and so forth) and on periodic reassessment and removal. Such policies provide guidance on the ways orders can be written and the child monitored.

Suicidal Behavior in Children and Adolescents

Along with aggressive behavior, one of the most frequent reasons for ED referral is suicidal ideation and behavior. Prevention of suicide in children and adolescents has been increasingly recognized as an important public health problem in the United States and internationally (Pfeffer, 2018).

This awareness has been fostered by a number of highly publicized cases as well as recognition of the problem at the national level, for example, the Surgeon General's Report (www.hhs.gov/surgeongeneral/reports-and-publications/suicide-prevention/index. html). The sensitivity of parents, teachers, and primary care providers to this important topic has been substantially increased as a result. This work has encompassed a range of topics including suicidal behaviors (including suicidal thoughts and acts) and important psychiatric and psychosocial correlates, for example, with depression and general psychopathology. Researchers have identified a continuum of behaviors ranging in severity from nonsuicidal behavior to suicidal ideas, attempts, and actual suicide (Pfeffer, 2018). As in other areas of child psychiatry, age and developmental factors are relevant and sometimes complicating considerations. Historically, the publication of Goethe's *The Sorrows of Young Werther* precipitated a wave of youth suicide. The topic was the focus of much interest, including to the Vienna Psychoanalytic Society in the first decade of the 20th century when Freud emphasized the importance of conflict with significant others in suicide. Starting in the late 1960s and peaking in 1977, rapid increase in rates of suicide in teenage and young adult men drew increased attention to the issue as did reports of "cluster cases." As a result, there has been an increased demand for new and better approaches to suicide prevention. This effort stimulated further research as well as important attempts to achieve a consensus on the need for more consistent approaches to definition, database development, research approaches, and work on education, treatment, and prevention of suicidal behavior.

Since 2006, suicide has been a leading cause of death for adolescents and young adults. Data from the National Institute of Mental Health suggest rates of suicide ranging from a rate of 11.8 (per 100,000) in adolescents (15-19 years of age) and 2.5/100,000 in children aged 10-14 years with rates rising over the last decade. Historically, suicide risk has been highest in white men of all ages followed by nonwhite men, white women, and nonwhite women. Over time, rates of suicide among black youths have increased, possibly related to greater degrees of assimilation into U.S. society. Native Americans have particularly high rates of suicide; loss of traditional cultural values, unemployment, and alcohol problems likely contribute to this risk. Men tend to use more lethal means, accounting for the discrepancy between higher rates of suicidal ideation in girls but higher completed rates in boys. Clinicians should carefully consider the potential suicidality of any self-injurious act in the child or adolescent, that is, both the seriousness of the act *and* the seriousness of the intent.

Approaches to Suicidal Children and Youth

Various factors contribute to suicidal ideation and attempts and should be considered in the assessment of any child/adolescent. These include the presence of comorbid psychiatric problems (particularly depression but not *only* depression), stressful life events, and sociocultural factors. A strong role of family genetic factors has also increasingly been recognized. Accordingly, attention to the multiple factors potentially contributing is important. This includes the presence of significant psychiatric or developmental disorders, biologic and environmental factors, and social adaptation and coping.

Information derived from psychological autopsy studies has given us new perspectives on youth suicide. In the majority of cases (about 90%), the child or adolescent has some psychiatric disorder. Although the relative risk varies from study to study, it is clear that clinicians should be alert to the presence of possible suicidal thoughts in all youth who are evaluated. A prior suicide attempt substantially increases the risk for another suicide attempt, suggesting that the clinician should inquire about such attempts and, in their presence, be particularly alert to the risk for suicide.

Many youths who complete suicide have a mood disorder or bipolar disorder (Pfeffer, 2018). Substance abuse conditions are the next most frequent problem and usually are seen in the presence of mood disorder as well. This risk factor is a stronger one among older adolescents (16 years of age or older). Other disorders, including anxiety disorders, eating disorders, and schizophrenia, are less frequently associated with suicide, although even in these conditions there is some risk. The nature of gender differences has also been clarified by results of psychological autopsy studies; one study noted greater risk for men with prior suicide attempts while greater risk for women was observed in those with current major depressive disorder.

For youth who commit suicide but without apparent psychiatric disorders, history of previous attempts or suicidal ideation, access to firearms, and conduct problems have been observed. Studies of youth who attempt but do not complete suicide suggest rather a similar pattern of associations with psychiatric conditions and behavior and substance abuse problems. In community samples, suicidal ideation is relatively common, with about 4% of men and nearly 9% of women reporting at least moderate levels (Pfeffer, 2018). There is some suggestion that seriousness and severity of the attempt can be related to the degree of associated mood problems and alcohol/substance abuse. For men, sexual orientation also contributes to increased risk.

Studies of neurobiological risk factors in children and adolescents have been less common than in adults where there is evidence of dysregulation in the serotonergic neurotransmitter system. Some suggestion of similar findings in adolescents has also been noted with lowered levels of serotonin-related compounds in the CSF of adolescents who had attempted suicide. This suggests an important potential focus for suicide prevention research. Other lines of neurobiological work have focused on the hypothalamic–pituitary–adrenal axis and the stress response system. Other work has focused on sleep dysregulation, particularly in adolescents with major depressive disorder who attempt suicide.

Family factors can increase suicide risk. These include high levels of stress at home, parents who have significant emotional problems, are abusive, or have a history of suicide attempts themselves. The latter increases risk among men about 5-fold and in women about 3-fold. Family histories of substance abuse also increase risk. There is some suggestion that problems at birth may increase risk as do chronic medical problems like diabetes.

Exposure to models of suicide, for example, through the media, may result in clusters of cases. This seems to be particularly true when reports are exaggerated and romanticized. An important implication is that suicide prevention strategies should be considered in a community when a child or adolescent commits suicide.

As part of assessing suicidal potential, the clinician should evaluate the extent of social and environmental support. The presence of a sympathetic adult, of supportive peers, and a supportive environment will assist the child or adolescent in coping adaptively; conversely, a poorly supportive social network will only compound the isolation, despair, and hopelessness of the youth. In this regard, it is of interest that having dropped out of school increases suicide risk. Other factors that contribute to risk include poor coping ability with few resources for dealing with negative feelings as do less adaptive defense mechanisms, for example, of denial or reaction formation. The latter may contribute to risk-taking behavior. Cultural issues also can be important in terms of issues of support, cultural affiliation, and so on.

Assessment of Suicide Risk

The assessment of suicide risk should include an interview of the youth as well as caregivers and a systematic review of present (and past) suicidal acts or ideation as well as the presence of other risk factors, environmental and social stress and supports, history of impulsive behavior, family history, and so forth. The presence of significant concern should prompt a plan for repeated assessment and if the child or adolescent appears to be a danger to self, psychiatric hospitalization is recommended.

Several different rating scales for assessment of suicidal risk are available and readily administered. Other approaches can be used, for example, human figure drawings may be helpful with younger children. These instruments supplement but do not replace a careful clinical assessment (see Pfeffer, 2018). The assessment should take into account the degree of intended self-harm and the relative risk. For younger children (and sometimes even older ones), exploration of the child's understanding of death may also be important, for example, the child may believe that it is reversible or have the fantasy that they will be "around" to observe the suffering of a significant other who has rejected them. Suicidal thought in a child with psychotic symptoms is also a great concern as is access to highly lethal means (guns, poisons, drugs).

The ED evaluation can be helpful in beginning the treatment process. One part of the assessment should include consideration of the motivations underlying the suicidal ideas, for example, breakup of a close relationship, anger at a parent, or overwhelming emotions. Treatment typically is multimodal. Various approaches have been developed, but, unfortunately, controlled studies of their effectiveness are uncommon. Family involvement and support and improved communication can be helpful as can be thoughtful involvement of nonfamily supports, for example, school personnel.

One study, the Treatment of Adolescent Depression Study (TADS), addressed the medication (fluoxetine) alone, against placebo, combined with cognitive-behavioral therapy (CBT), and against CBT alone in a study of adolescents with major depression but without high risk for suicide (the latter were excluded) (March et al., 2007). The most effective treatment was the combined drug–CBT (71% improved) over medication alone (61%), over CBT alone (43%), and placebo (35%). In this study, those receiving the SSRI had a noteworthy increase in suicidal thinking and acts. The FDA mandated black box warnings for antidepressant medications given to children and adolescents and also recommended increased clinical monitoring of adverse effects. Special consideration also arises when giving medications that may lead to disinhibition (e.g., benzodiazepines) or impulsivity.

The Decision to Hospitalize

One of the most challenging tasks for the clinician in the ED is the assessment of potential risk, for example, if the child returns home and the decision to hospitalize. Various guidelines have been developed but considerable clinical judgment is required. In some situations, this decision is straightforward, for example, the presence of a serious medical problem such as delirium, intoxication, a florid psychosis, high suicidal risk, or dangerous behavior. More typically, the decision about disposition is more complicated. The history (from child and adults) along with the interview and mental status examination of the child should help guide such decisions. Important considerations also include the factor(s) leading to the referral and the resources that the child or adolescent may be able to draw upon outside the ED setting.

Hospitalization offers important advantages of providing a structured, contained environment with staff immediately available. Although not to be undertaken lightly, hospitalization is indicated in the presence of significant suicidal ideation. In cases where risk is lower and when a more supportive family and psychosocial environment are available, other alternatives can include partial hospitalization and outpatient services.

A child or adolescent who has suicidal ideas should not be discharged from the ED without a clear and explicit discussion with them and family regarding their condition and agreement for participation in a treatment plan. This discussion can also include limiting access to lethal materials.

When considering these issues, it is important to examine and document what will be different following the clinical contact. This might include arrangements for clinical follow-up, the child's positive attempts at coping with crisis intervention management, arrangements for supports to be in place at home, and so forth. On the other hand, if the risk of danger to self or others is high and when the clinician has a strong sense of the lack of adequate supports, inpatient hospitalization may be needed. Similarly, a deteriorating course, often with an acute decompensation in ED, is a strong argument for inpatient assessment as are escalating levels of dangerous behaviors—regardless of whether suicidal intent is present, for example, the individual with a severe eating disorder. In assessing risk, it is important to be aware that the child's behavior in other settings (home or school) may be more informative of risk than the child's behavior in the ED setting. Conversely, some children who initially present as aggressive or violent may be discharged to supportive settings with a clear and practical follow-up plan in place.

Effective management and crisis intervention in the ED may result in at least a temporary solution for the child and family. Unfortunately, when hospitalization is indicated, considerable time and energy may be spent both in acquiring insurance approval and finding an often scarce, inpatient bed. The clinician should be aware of all relevant laws and regulations, for example, relative to confidentiality issues, seclusion/restraint, involuntary hospitalization, HIPAA, and so forth. Laws vary from state to state, so it is important to be aware of the existing laws in your specific location.

CONSULTATION LIAISON AND THE INTERFACE WITH PEDIATRICS

General Principles and Models of Consultation

The recognition of child mental health difficulties in medical settings can be traced back to the 1930s with the work of Leo Kanner at Johns Hopkins. Over time, there has been a sustained increase in the need for both individual and program consultation by specialists in mental health. This includes individuals from various backgrounds including child psychiatrists, pediatric psychologists, and social workers as well as educators, speech and communication specialists, occupation and physical therapists, and others. It is clear that chronic illness increases risk for psychiatric conditions in children and adolescents. Concomitant medical illness may color the presentation of behavioral difficulties and can be compounded by associated stress and concern in parents and family members. Consultation issues can arise in different contexts, for example, outpatient or emergency settings, but most typically arise in the context of pediatric inpatient hospitalization.

An initial mental health consultation in pediatrics can often be obtained quickly, although developing a treatment plan for mental health intervention may be a longer term process. An appreciation of the nature of the underlying medical conditions and their impact on behavior and mental health may be highly relevant; for example, are symptoms a feature of the underlying disorder or might they be a manifestation of treatment?

Medical procedures may be painful and stressful and are often associated with behavioral and emotional difficulties. Similarly, acute and chronic medical problems can represent different challenges for children and family members. The reactions and behaviors of parents may also be important factors in relation to levels of distress in the child. Peer relationships may also be important, for example, management of type I diabetes where availability of more supportive peers resulted in better control. The age and cognitive level of the child also has an influence on children's understanding of and responses to illness and medical procedures. An awareness of developmental principles including Piaget's approach to understanding children's thinking (see Chapter 1) helps inform how we understand the child's understanding of what is taking place. Children in the phase of concrete operations (roughly early primary school) may see their illness as a punishment and may benefit from an age-appropriate explanation. In contrast, adolescents have a more adult understanding of pathophysiology although in adolescents a sense of invulnerability may complicate compliance with medical treatments.

Mental health professionals must be aware of the context in which they are asked to consult and be familiar with the range of problems frequently encountered along with their potential treatments. For the mental health consultant, a familiarity with issues of differential diagnosis, potential behavioral and psychiatric symptoms, and complications associated with specific illnesses and treatments is important. In addition to working around a specific case, consultants are, ideally, involved on a longer term basis as they provide suggestions for programmatic approaches designed to minimize stress, maximize coping, and facilitate outcomes.

Mental Health Consultation in Pediatric Inpatient Settings

Mental health professionals can draw on a number of treatments, both more narrowly and more broadly focused. Intervention strategies from the CBT model are frequently used to help deal with pain and anxiety and they have been adapted for medical procedure–related pain and anxiety. These behavioral and cognitive-behavioral methods may also help ensure adherence to medical treatments for children as they leave the hospital setting (see Table 27.4).

Consultation may be requested to help in management issues of depression and suicidal ideation as well as management of anxiety or other psychiatric symptoms and lack of adherence to treatment. The latter may come about as adolescents strive to deny the reality of chronic illness. Referral rates vary widely and also may vary in nature depending on the level of services provided in the hospital, for example, for treatment of cancer, sickle cell disease, and so on. Patients who are expected to have long lengths of stay may need special supports.

Typically, in doing a consultation, the consultant first tries to understand the specific question around which the consultation centers (see Cardona, 2018). Then the consultant reviews the record and talks with the staff before actually interviewing the patient and/or parents. Following this, there may be suggestions for additional tests or assessments and perhaps coordination with other agencies or providers (schools or mental health service providers). The consultant should be continuously aware of potential issues of coordination and communication (or lack thereof), as these impact the patient. There is usually a feedback with specific recommendations. Depending on the context, various services may be provided and the consultant usually wishes to follow up.

TABLE 27.4

Principles From the AACAP Practice Parameter for the Psychiatric Assessment and Management of Physically Ill Children and Adolescents (2009)

1. Mental health clinicians should understand how to collaborate effectively with medical professionals to facilitate the health care of physically ill children.
2. The reason for and purpose of the mental health referral should be understood.
3. The assessment should integrate the impact of the child's physical illness into a developmentally informed biopsychosocial formulation.
4. General medical conditions and/or their treatments should be considered in the etiology of a child's psychological and behavioral symptoms.
5. Psychopharmacologic management should consider a child's physical illness and its treatment.
6. Psychotherapeutic management should consider multiple treatment modalities.
7. The family context should be understood and addressed.
8. Adherence to the medical treatment regimen should be evaluated and optimized.
9. The use of complementary and alternative medicine should be explored.
10. Religious and cultural influences should be understood and considered.
11. Family contact with community-based agencies should be considered and facilitated where indicated.
12. Legal issues specific to physically ill children should be understood and considered.
13. The influence of the health care system on the care of a physically ill child should be considered.

Reprinted from L. Cardona. (2018). Pediatric consultation-liason. In A. Martin, M. Bloch, & F. R. Volkmar (Eds.), *Lewis's child and adolescent psychiatry* (5th ed., p. 908). Wolters Kluwer.

The interview with the child typically includes a comprehensive mental status examination appropriate to the child's age and level of functioning. Observation of the child in the hospital setting can provide important information. At times, specific self-report inventories might be administered. If there are questions of potential neurologic dysfunction, repeated interviews are essential to document baseline function and changes, and specific psychological and/or neurologic assessments may be needed. Even before the encounter is documented in the medical record, the consultant usually provides a verbal report to the patient and family.

Behavioral management approaches can be also used to target issues of treatment noncompliance within a family context. Although some interventions can be instituted within a hospital setting, others may require helping families access community and school-based services.

Providing effective mental health consultation services in general and in pediatric hospital settings can be complicated by a number of barriers. These include a shortage of potential consultants, limited insurance reimbursement, and differences in models of service delivery in the pediatric and mental health systems. The pace of pediatric care moves much more quickly than that of mental health work and an adequate psychiatric consultation can take several hours. Other issues have to do with resistance, on the part of families and medical professionals, to use of mental health services. The complex issues of confidentiality (see Chapter 26) can also be an issue. At the most basic level of course, the child or adolescent shares something with the consultant that they do not want revealed to parents or medical staff, for example, being sexually active, using drugs. Sometimes, these become nonissues (e.g., as toxicology screen or pregnancy tests are positive). In some instances where danger to the child is involved, the consultant has to explain the requirements about breaking confidentiality (this should have been told to the child originally). The consultant should attempt to keep the assessment and recommendations understandable, action oriented, and concise. On larger inpatient services, the presence of the consultant can reduce barriers to communication and facilitate improved service delivery. This is most practical in teaching hospital settings.

Special Consultation Areas

Pediatric Oncology

About 1 in 285 youth will have a cancer diagnosis before age 20 (Walsh and Zubrick, 2018). Advances in treatment have increased long-term survival and, in many cases, recovery. With increased survival rates, intervention programs have shifted focus to include both acute and longer term issues with greater attention to foster coping and dealing with stress-related symptoms and disorders (Walsh and Zebrack, 2018). There is growing recognition of the importance of family and family factors for positive outcome. Even with positive outcomes, the child and family may continue to need support, for example, around fears of recurrence.

Supports are needed at the time of initial diagnosis as well as during and after treatment. Supports should be provided to family members as well. Children and adolescents are frequently amenable to straightforward discussion of relevant issues with mental health professionals and others. Their ability to participate in discussion with medical staff also may help lessen their anxiety. As with other chronic diseases, lack of adherence to treatments is frequent. Cultural differences in understanding illness may also complicate compliance. In some hospitals, the availability of a teacher may help the child maintain at least some continuity with schoolwork.

Delirium

There has been a growing recognition of the identification of delirium, confused thinking, and reduced awareness of surroundings in children and adolescents in hospital settings. Delirium can result from a range of difficulties and manifest in myriad ways. By definition, it is usually transient and typically reversible and can have an acute or more subacute pattern

BOX 27.1	**Features of Delirium**

- Psychosis: hallucinations (often visual), loose association, delusions—paranoid and often poorly formed
- Language problems: aphasia-like symptoms, word-finding problems, altered language problems
- Affective issues: labile, altered affect with lability, congruent affect to context, irritability
- Sleep–wake cycle problems: altered sleep cycle, wakefulness, fragmented sleep
- Temporal course/onset: usually acute onset, fluctuating, reversible, subclinical presentation before/after episode is common
- Reactivity alterations: hypo-, hyper-mixed reactivity
- Diffuse cognitive deficits: problems in memory, executive functioning, orientation

Adapted from Table 5.11.1 in William, D. T. (2018). Delirium and catatonia. In A. Martin, M. Bloch, & & F. R. Volkmar (Eds.), *Lewis's child and adolescent psychiatry* (5th ed., p. 605). Wolters Kluwer.

of onset. Alternations in thinking, perception, mood disturbance, and various psychomotor features may be observed. However, given the potential for delirium to sometimes progress, identification of delirium in children and adolescents presenting with apparent psychiatric problems is critical. Features of delirium are summarized in Box 27.1.

Various factors can predispose individuals to delirium and children seem at higher risk presumably due to continued CNS development. Delirium can result from many different etiologies, and in children and adolescents, the pattern of etiology is often somewhat different from that in adults, for example, illicit drug use, hypoxia, head trauma, various medical conditions, and postsurgery are frequent causes (William, 2018). Other predisposing factors in children include history of prior episodes, cognitive difficulties, the presence of a neurologic or sensory disorder, or conditions that result in greater blood–brain barrier permeability. Indeed, hospitalization often provides a striking confluence of various factors that can result in delirium. Anticholinergic drugs like atropine are particularly known to be associated with delirium. Careful monitoring is needed for children at risk, particularly in hospital settings, because the impression of regression, for example, with hospitalization, on the part of staff may prevent early identification and treatment of delirium. Interestingly, some procedures known to be associated with delirium in adults, for example, post-cardiotomy, are less common in children. When possible, planned admission with preoperative interventions to help the child become familiar with the setting and cope more adaptively reduces perioperative management difficulties in children. In emergency situations, this is not of course always possible and high levels of stress increase the likelihood of a delirium developing. Some of the difficulties associated at times with hospitalization such as sensory overload and sleep deprivation contribute to risk. Medical factors including metabolic and nutritional abnormalities and drug interactions can contribute to increased risk. As William (2018) has noted, the many and varied etiologies for delirium make it more reasonable to think of delirium as a final common pathway leading to various, often fluctuating, symptoms. Delirium can be associated with significant morbidity and mortality. In their review of a large case series, Turkel and Tavare (2003) reported a mortality rate of 20%. Abrupt changes in mental status or in cognition or attention should prompt thorough evaluation.

Pediatric Transplantation

There have been major advances in pediatric transplantation over the last decades with successful solid organ and bone marrow/stem cell transplant procedures, now frequent. There are similarities and a few differences from adults. At present, transplant specialists have become more interested in obtaining appropriate mental health supports before transplantation to prevent subsequent problems and to enhance compliance with treatment after.

Complexities include understanding that in some cases there has to be a lifetime commitment to antirejection medications and their various side effects—some of these may include agitation, mood problems, paranoid thinking, and cognitive changes. Preexisting psychiatric problems may worsen. The mental health consultant has an important role in assessing potential side effects, both in terms of risk and as these emerge. Helping children and youth comply with treatment protocols may be an issue.

Pediatric Epilepsy

Recurrent seizures (epilepsy) place children at significantly increased risk for a range of mental health problems. A seizure arises from abnormal electrical activity in the brain and can have behavioral or sensory aspects (or both). Various factors may predispose children to seizures, for example, high fever, brain infection, tumor, and so forth. Between the seizures (the interictal period), the brain problems associated with the seizures can continue and thus have associated behavioral and psychological impact. Common causes of seizures are listed in Table 27.5.

The association of epilepsy with mental health problems like depression has been noted since ancient times; indeed, Hippocrates first observed the association with depression. For some children and their families, the psychiatric difficulties that co-occur with epilepsy are often even more problematic than the seizures. Developmental skills in children with seizure disorders can be impacted, including cognitive, language, and adaptive skills, leading to problems in learning and worsening of self-esteem. Mental health workers can have an important role in treating, and hopefully minimizing, the repercussions of epilepsy. These issues are reviewed in detail by Munhi and colleagues (2018).

Sometimes, differentiation of epileptic and nonepileptic events can be difficult. Video and EEG monitoring often is helpful. Absence seizures can sometimes present as attentional problems. Sometimes, somatoform disorders, particularly conversion disorder (see Chapter 18),

TABLE 27.5

Common Causes of Seizures

High fever[a]
Systemic or CNS infection (meningitis, encephalitis, etc.)
Hyperthermia (exogenous)
Congenital disorders of brain development[a]
Perinatal hypoxic/ischemic injury[a]
Tuberous sclerosis
Phenylketonuria
Head trauma[a]
Intracranial hemorrhage
Neoplasm
Metabolic derangements (hypoglycemia, hyponatremia, etc.)
Anoxia
Cardiac disorders
Intoxication (medications, recreational drugs, environmental toxins)
Autoimmune disorders
Lupus, CNS vasculitis, etc.

[a]Most common in children.
Reprinted with permission from Muchi, Brownstein, Rottenberg, et al. (2018). Epilepsy. In A. Martin, M. Bloch, & F. R. Volkmar (Eds.), *Lewis's child and adolescent psychiatry* (5th ed., p. 923). Wolters Kluwer.

can present as an apparent seizure. Sometimes, an individual child exhibits seizures along with other paroxysmal behaviors making differentiation difficult. The choice of a drug treatment must take into account the type of seizure, potential side effects, and potential for drug interaction. Sometimes, more than one drug is needed.

Treatment of psychiatric disorder in children with epilepsy should include a broad view of the various areas of the child's life and functioning. Educational interventions and psychotherapeutic interventions for child and/or family should be used as appropriate. In considering drug treatment for comorbid psychiatric difficulties, the potential risks and benefits should be carefully considered.

Palliative Care and Bereavement

In the past, childhood death was relatively common but, over the last century and a half, advances in public health, immunization, and the development of antibiotics led to a dramatic decrease in childhood mortality. As a result, there has been an increased recognition of the need to support children and families facing end-of-life issues; the latter include pain, anxiety, depression, and other problems. The modern hospice movement has achieved greater prominence in end-of-life care for adults although only more recently for children.

Pediatric palliative care encompasses a range of issues including pain management, other medical issues, psychosocial issues, spiritual issues, planning for care needs, and practical matters such as where and how services are best delivered. Care for the family following the loss of the child is also part of this process. Life-limiting illness represents a growing phenomenon, with advances in care prolonging lives in illnesses that were previously terminal in childhood or adolescence, for example, cystic fibrosis. Advances in chemotherapy, transplantation, and other areas are significantly extending life for many children and adolescents. The child's own understanding of the meaning of death is important and reflects their age and developmental level.

SUMMARY

Although many advances have been made, barriers to the provision of effective mental health care in primary care, emergency, and hospital settings still exist. These include the limited number of child psychologists, social workers, and other mental health providers, the tensions between medical, mental health, and educational care as well as insurance and time pressures. There can be difficulties in communication. In some respects, the availability of a consultant who is at least a periodic presence goes a considerable way in dealing with some of these issues. Challenges remain in integrating good mental health principles in pediatric and educational care but the range of effective models and solid research has increased dramatically. Mandates for coverage, health care reform, the increased use of technology, and the electronic medical record all have at least the potential for fostering advances in the coming decade.

References

*Indicates Particularly Recommended

Asarnow, J. R., Jaycox, L. H., Duan, N., LaBorde, A. P., Rea, M. M., Tang, L., Anderson, M., Murray, P., Landon, C., Tang, B., Huizar, D. P., & Wells, K. B. (2005). Depression and role impairment among adolescents in primary care clinics. *Journal of Adolescent Health, 37,* 477–483. https://doi.org/10.1016/j.jadohealth.2004.11.123

Benarous, X., Milhiet, V., Oppetit, A., Viaux, S., El Kamel, N. M., Guinchat, V., Guilé, J. M., & Cohen, D. (2019). Changes in the use of emergency care for the youth with mental health problems over decades: A repeated cross sectional study. *Frontiers in Psychiatry, 10,* 26. https://doi.org/10.3389/fpsyt.2019.00026

*Cardona, L. (2018). Pediatric consultation liaison. In A. Martin, M. Bloch, & F. R. Volkmar (Eds.), *Lewis's child and adolescent psychiatry: A comprehensive textbook* (5th ed., pp. 906–911). Wolters Kluwer.

*Havens, J. F., Gerson, R. S., & Marr, M. (2018). Designing emergency psychiatric services for children and adolescent. In A. Martin, M. Bloch, & F. R. Volkmar (Eds.), *Lewis's child and adolescent psychiatry: A comprehensive textbook* (5th ed., pp. 844–855). Wolters Kluwer.

Kalb, L. G., Stapp, E. K., Ballard, E. D., Holingue, C., Keffer, A., & Riley, A. (2019). Trends in psychiatric emergency department visits among youth and young adults in the U.S. *Pediatrics, 143*(4), e20182192. https://doi.org/10.1542/peds.2018-2192.

March, J. S., Silva, S., Petrycki, S., Curry, J., Wells, K., Fairbank, J., Burns, B., Domino, M., McNulty, S., Vitiello, B., & Severe, J. (2007). The treatment for adolescents with depression study (TADS): Long-term effectiveness and safety outcomes. *Archives of General Psychiatry, 64*(10), 1132–1143. https://doi.org/10.1001/archpsyc.64.10.1132

Munhi, K., Browstein, C., Rotternberg, A., Rao, G. K., Poncin, Y. B., & Gonzales-Heydrich, J. (2018). Epilepsy. In A. Martin, M. Bloch, & F. R. Volkmar (Eds.), *Lewis's child and adolescent psychiatry: A comprehensive textbook* (5th ed., pp. 932–945). Wolters Kluwer.

Pfeffer, C. (2018). Child and adolescent suicidal behavior. In A. Martin, M. Bloch, & F. R. Volkmar (Eds.), *Lewis's child and adolescent psychiatry: A comprehensive textbook* (5th ed., pp. 500–508). Wolters Kluwer.

Pumariega, A. L., & Winters, N. C. (2018). Community based treatments and services. In A. Martin, M. Bloch, & F. R. Volkmar (Eds.), *Lewis's child and adolescent psychiatry: A comprehensive textbook* (5th ed., pp. 873–884). Wolters Kluwer.

Sarvet, B., Gold, J., Bostic, J., Masek, B. J., Prince, J. B., Jeffers-Terry, M., Moore, C. F., Molbert, B., & Straus, J. H. (2010). Improving access to mental health care for children: The Massachusetts child psychiatry access project. *Pediatrics, 126,* 1191–1200. https://doi.org/10.1542/peds.2009-1340

Schonfeld, D., & Campo, J. V. (2018). Integrating behavioral services for pediatric care settings: Principles and models. In A. Martin, M. Bloch, & F. R. Volkmar (Eds.), *Lewis's child and adolescent psychiatry: A comprehensive textbook* (5th ed., pp. 898–905). Wolters Kluwer.

Sheldrick, R. C., & Perrin, E. C. (2010). Medical home services for children with behavioral health conditions. *Journal of Developmental and Behavioral Pediatrics: JDBP, 31*(2), 92–99. https://doi.org/10.1097/DBP.0b013e3181cdabda

Turkel, S. B., & Tavaré, C. J. (2003). Delirium in children and adolescents. *The Journal of Neuropsychiatry and Clinical Neurosciences, 15*(4), 431–435. https://doi.org/10.1176/jnp.15.4.431

Walsh, C., & Zebrack, B. (2018). Cancer. In A. Martin, M. Bloch, & F. R. Volkmar (Eds.), *Lewis's child and adolescent psychiatry* (5th ed., pp. 912–918). Wolters Kluwer.

William, D. T. (2018). Delirium and catatonia. In A. Martin, M. Bloch, & F. R. Volkmar (Eds.), *Lewis's child and adolescent psychiatry: A comprehensive textbook* (5th ed., pp. 604–642). Wolters Kluwer.

Suggested Readings

American Academy of Pediatrics, Committee on Quality Improvement. (2001). Clinical practice guidelines: Treatment of the school-aged child with attention-deficit/hyperactivity disorder. *Pediatrics, 108,* 1033–1044. https://doi.org/10.1542/peds.108.4.1033

Berg, A. T., Shinnar, S., Levy, S. R., Testa, F. M., Smith-Rapaport, S., & Beckerman, B. (2001). Early development of intractable epilepsy in children: A prospective study. *Neurology, 56*(11), 1445–1452. https://doi.org/10.1212/WNL.56.11.1445

Bosic, J., Stein, B., & Schwab-Stone, J. (2005). Schools. In A. Martin & F. R. Volkmar (Eds.), *Lewis's child and adolescent psychiatry: A comprehensive textbook* (pp. 981–998). Wolters Kluwer/Lippincott Williams & Wilkins.

Brophy, P., & Kazak, A. E. (1994). Schooling. In F. L. Johnson & E. L. O'Donnell (Eds.), *The candlelighters guide to bone marrow transplants in children* (pp. 68–73). Candlelighters Childhood Cancer Foundation.

Brunquell, P., McKeever, M., & Russman, B. S. (1990). Differentiation of epileptic from nonepileptic head drops in children. *Epilepsia, 31*(4), 401–405. https://doi.org/10.1111/j.1528-1157.1990.tb05495.x

Campbell, J. M., & Cardona, L. (2005). The consultation and liaison process to pediatrics. In A. Martin & F. R. Volkmar (Eds.), *Lewis's child and adolescent psychiatry: A comprehensive textbook* (pp. 912–920). Wolters Kluwer/Lippincott Williams & Wilkins.

*Cardona, L. (1994). Behavioral approaches to pain and anxiety in the pediatric patient. *Child and Adolescent Psychiatric Clinics of North America, 3,* 449–464. https://doi.org/10.1016/S1056-4993(18)30481-4

Carison, A., Babl, F. E., Hill, A., & O'Donnell, S. M. (2020). Children and adolescents with severe acute behavioural disturbance in the emergency department. *Emergency Medicine Australasia, 32*(5). https://doi.org/10.1111/1742-6723.13515

Carter, B. D., Kronenberger, W. G., Baker, J., Grimes, L. M., Crabtree, V. M., Smith, C., & McGraw, K. (2003). Inpatient pediatric consultation-liaison: A case-controlled study. *Journal of Pediatric Psychology, 28,* 423–432. https://doi.org/10.1093/jpepsy/jsg032

Cavusoglu, H. (2001). Depression in children with cancer. *International Pediatric Nursing, 16*(5), 380–385. https://doi.org/10.1053/jpdn.2001.0000

Christ, G., Bonanno, G., Malkinson, R., & Rubin, S. (2003). Bereavement experiences after the death of a child. In M. Field & R. Behrman (Eds.), *When children die: Improving palliative and end-of-life care for children and their families* (pp. 553–579). National Academies Press.

Comer, J. P., & Woodruff, D. W. (1998). Mental health in schools. *Child Adolescent Psychiatry Clinics of North America, 7*(3), 499–513, viii. https://doi.org/10.1016/S1056-4993(18)30226-8

Costello, E. J., Burns, B. J., Costello, A. J., Edelbrock, C., Dulcan, M., & Brent, D. (1988). Service utilization and psychiatric diagnosis in pediatric primary care: The role of the gatekeeper. *Pediatrics, 82,* 435–441.

Erchul, W. P., & Martens, B. K. (1997). *School consultation: Conceptual and empirical bases of practice.* Plenum.

Glazer, J. P., Pao, M., & Schoenfeld, D. S. (2018). Life-threatening illness, palliative care, and bereavement. In A. Martin, M. Bloch, & F. R. Volkmar (Eds.), *Lewis's child and adolescent psychiatry: A comprehensive textbook* (5th ed., pp. 946–955). Wolters Kluwer.

Gothelf, D., Rubinstein, M., Shemesh, E., Miller, O., Farbstein, I., Klein, A., Weizman, A., Apter, A., & Yaniv, I. (2005). Pilot study: Fluvoxamine treatment for depression and anxiety in children and adolescents with cancer. *Journal of the American Academy of Child and Adolescent Psychiatry, 44,* 1258–1262. https://doi.org/10.1097/01.chi.0000181042.29208.eb

Greene, R. W., & Ablonm, J. S. (2006). *Treating explosive kids: The collaborative problem-solving approach.* Guilford Press.

Guerrero, A. P. S., Lee, P. C., & Skokauskas, N. (Eds.). (2018). *Pediatric consultation-liaison psychiatry: A global, healthcare systems-focused, and problem-based approach* (1st ed.). Springer.

Hesdorffer, D. C., Ludvigsson, P., Olafsson, E., Gudmundsson, G., Kjartansson, O., & Hauser, W. A. (2004). ADHD as a risk factor for incident unprovoked seizures and epilepsy in children. *Archives of General Psychiatry, 61*(7), 731–736. https://doi.org/10.1001/archpsyc.61.7.731

Himelstein, M. D., Bruce, P., Hilden, M. D., Joanne, M., Morstad-Boldt, M. S., & Weissman, A. (2004). David: Pediatric palliative care. *The New England Journal of Medicine, 350,* 1752–1762. https://doi.org/10.1056/NEJMra030334

Jennings, J., Pearson, G., & Harris, M. (2000). Implementing and maintaining school-based mental health services in a large, urban school district. *Journal of School Health, 70*(5), 201–205. https://doi.org/10.1111/j.1746-1561.2000.tb06473.x

Kanner, A. M. (2003). Depression in epilepsy: Prevalence, clinical semiology, pathogenic mechanisms, and treatment. *Biological Psychiatry, 54*(3), 388–398. https://doi.org/10.1016/S0006-3223(03)00469-4

Kelleher, K. J., McInerny, T. K., Gardner, W. P., Childs, G. E., & Wasserman, R. C. (2000). Increasing identification of psychosocial problems: 1979–1996. *Pediatrics, 105*(6), 1313–1321. https://doi.org/10.1542/peds.105.6.1313

Kessler, R. C., Berglund, P., Demler, O., Jin, R., & Walters, E. (2005). Lifetime prevalence and age-of onset distributions of *DSM-IV* disorders in the National Comorbidity Survey Replication. *Archives of General Psychiatry, 62,* 593–602. https://doi.org/10.1001/archpsyc.62.6.593

Kestenbaum, C. J. (2000). How shall we treat the children in the 21st century? *Journal of the American Academy of Child and Adolescent Psychiatry, 39*(1), 1–10. https://doi.org/10.1097/00004583-200001000-00001

Kriechman, A., Salvador, M., & Adelsheim, S. (2010). Expanding the vision: The strengths-based, community-oriented child and adolescent psychiatrist working in schools. *Child & Adolescent Psychiatric Clinics of North America, 19*(1), 149–162. https://doi.org/10.1016/j.chc.2009.08.005

Lauria, M. M. (2001). Common issues and challenges for families dealing with childhood cancer. In M. M. Lauria, E. J. Clark, J. F. Hermann, & N. M. Stearns (Eds.), *Social work in oncology: Supporting survivors, families, and caregivers* (pp. 117–142). American Cancer Society.

Levinson, J. L., & Olbrisch, M. E. (2000). Psychosocial screening and selections of candidates for organ transplantation. In P. T. Trepacz & A. F. DiMartini (Eds.), *The transplant patient* (pp. 27–28). Cambridge University Press.

Lewis, M. (2002). The consultation process in child and adolescent psychiatric consultation-liaison in pediatrics. In M. Lewis (Ed.), *Child and adolescent psychiatry: A comprehensive textbook* (3rd ed., pp. 1111–1115). Lippincott Williams & Wilkins.

Li, J., Precht, D., Mortensen, P., & Olsen, J. (2003). Mortality in parents after death of a child in Denmark: A nationwide follow-up study. *Lancet, 361,* 363–367. https://doi.org/10.1016/S0140-6736(03)12387-2

McLaren, J., & Bryson, S. E. (1987). Review of recent epidemiological studies of mental retardation: Prevalence, associated disorders, and etiology. *American Journal of Mental Retardation, 92*(3), 243–254.

McGrath, P. J., Dick, B., Unruh, A. M. (2003). Psychologic and behavioral treatment of pain in children and adolescents. In N. L. Schechter, C. B. Berde, & M. Yaster (Eds.), *Pain in infants, children and adolescents* (pp. 303–316). Lippincott Williams & Wilkins.

Mintzer, L. L., Stuber, M. L., Seacord, D., Castaneda, M., Mesrkhani, V., & Glover, D. (2005). Traumatic stress symptoms in adolescent organ transplant recipients. *Pediatrics, 115*(6), 1640–1644. https://doi.org/10.1542/peds.2004-0118

Olson, A. L., Kelleher, K. J., Kemper, K. J., Zuckerman, B. S., Hammond, C. S., & Dietrich, A. J. (2001). Primary care pediatricians' roles and perceived responsibilities in the identification and management of depression in children and adolescents. *Ambulatory Pediatrics, 2*, 91–98. https://doi.org/10.1367/1539-4409(2001)001<0091:PCPRAP>2.0.CO;2

Pendley, J. S., Kasmen, L. J., Miller, D. L. Donze, J., Swenson, C., & Reeves, G. (2002). Peer and family support in children and adolescents with type I diabetes. *Journal of Pediatric Psychology, 27*, 429–438. https://doi.org/10.1093/jpepsy/27.5.429

Piña-Garza, J. E., & James, K. C. (Eds.) (2019). *Fenichel's clinical pediatric neurology: A signs and symptoms approach* (8th ed.). Elsevier.

Rando, T. (1993). *Treatment of complicated mourning*. Research Press.

Rao, J., Poncin, Y. B., & Gonzales-Heydrich, J. (2005). *Epilepsy*. In A. Martin & F. R. Volkmar (Eds.), *Lewis's child and adolescent psychiatry: A comprehensive textbook* (pp. 958–970). Wolters Kluwer/Lippincott Williams & Wilkins.

Ringeisen, H., Oliver, K. A., & Menvielle, E. (2002). Recognition and treatment of mental disorders in children. *Pediatric Drugs, 4*, 697–703. https://doi.org/10.2165/00128072-200204110-00001

Rushton, J., Bruckman, D., & Kelleher, K. J. (2002). Primary care referral of children with psychosocial problems. *Archives of Pediatric and Adolescent Medicine, 156*, 592–598. https://doi.org/10.1001/archpedi.156.6.592

Sarvet, B. D., & Wegner, L. (2010). Developing effective child psychiatry collaboration with primary care: Leadership and management strategies. *Child & Adolescent Psychiatric Clinics of North America, 19*(1), 139–148. https://doi.org/10.1016/j.chc.2009.08.004

Sawyer, M., Antoniou, G., Rice, M., & Baghurst, P. (2000). Childhood cancer: A 4-year prospective study of the psychological adjustment of children and parents. *Journal of Pediatric Hematology/Oncology, 22*(3), 214–220. https://doi.org/10.1097/00043426-200005000-00006

Schechter, N. L., Berde, C. B., & Yaster, M. (2003). Pain in infants, children, and adolescents an overview. In N. L. Schechter, C. B. Berde, & M. Yaster (Eds.), *Pain in infants, children and adolescents* (pp. 3–18). Lippincott Williams & Wilkins.

Schlozman, S. C., & Prager, L. (2005). The role of the child and adolescent psychiatrist on the pediatric transplant service. In A. Martin & F. R. Volkmar (Eds.), *Lewis's child and adolescent psychiatry: A comprehensive textbook* (pp. 939–945). Wolters Kluwer/Lippincott Williams & Wilkins.

Shaw, R. J., & Demaso, D. R. (2020). *Clinical manual of pediatric consultation-liaison psychiatry* (2nd ed.). American Psychiatry.

Smilansky, S. (1987). *On death: Helping children understand and cope*. Peter Lang.

Speece, M., & Brent, S. (1984). Children's understanding of death: A review of three components of a death concept. *Child Development, 55*, 1671–1686. https://doi.org/10.2307/1129915

Stuber, M. L., Kazack, A. E., Meeske, K., Barakat, L., Guthrie, D., Garnier, H., Pynoos, R., & Meadows, A. (1997). Predictors of posttraumatic stress symptoms in childhood cancer survivors. *Pediatrics, 100*, 958–964. https://doi.org/10.1542/peds.100.6.958

Swick, S. D., & Rauch, P. K. (2006). Children facing the death of a parent: The experiences of a parent guidance program at the Massachusetts General Hospital Cancer Center. *Child and Adolescent Psychiatric Clinics of North America, 15*(3), 779–794. https://doi.org/10.1016/j.chc.2006.02.007

U.S. Department of Health and Human Services; U.S. Department of Education; U.S. Department of Justice. (2000). *Report of the Surgeon General's conference on children's mental health: A national action agenda*. Department of Health and Human Services.

Weigers, M. E., Chesler, M. A., Zebrack, B. J., & Goldman, S. (1998). Self-reported worries among long-term survivors of childhood cancer and their peers. *Journal of Psychosocial Oncology, 16*(2), 1–23. https://doi.org/10.1300/J077V16N02_01

SECTION IV ■ TREATMENTS

CHAPTER 28 ■ PSYCHOTHERAPY

INTRODUCTION

The origins of psychotherapy can be traced to diverse sources (see Chapter 5 for a brief overview of psychotherapies and their roots). Freud attempted to understand the horse phobia of a child (Little Hans) in light of his own theories of development and the unconscious. Early behaviorists noted the important role of learning in fear and fear conditions, for example, the case described by Mary Jones in 1923. Over time, the field of psychotherapy as it applies to children and adolescents has expanded dramatically. The predominant mode of scientific inquiry has now shifted from a focus on single clinical case studies to research methods using groups of children in clinical trials. Modern approaches pay considerable attention to issues of study method and design, use of standard measures, manualization to ensure replicability, and so forth (see Weersing & Dirks, 2007).

EFFICACY OF PSYCHOTHERAPY

An important, and immediate, issue is the question of whether psychotherapy works. The first review of psychotherapy, now six decades old, raised important questions about the effectiveness of psychotherapy, that is, over rates of improvement noted in children and adolescents. This result corresponded, in many ways, to an influential review questioning the efficacy of psychotherapy in adults. Both sets of findings were the source of much debate. Thoughtful consideration of these early efforts identified several important limitations of then available research. These included nonrandom assignment to treatment, lack of attention to independent evaluations, need for careful control and comparison groups, and so forth. Recognition of these limitations led to the development of more rigorous clinical trial research.

A large and substantive body of research is now available and it has become possible to conduct meta-analytic reviews in which the results of carefully selected studies can be pooled and analyzed. Results can then be summarized in terms of overall effect size (see Chapter 3). Typically, a statistic like the one proposed by Cohen's d quickly conveys how different a treatment group is from a comparison group in terms of units of standard deviation. For example, a d of 0.2 would usually be termed a small effect size whereas a d of 0.8 would be viewed as large.

In the first review of this kind in psychotherapy for children, Casey and Berman (1985) noted a reasonably good effect size (0.71). Subsequent work has generally confirmed that medium to large effect sizes are frequently observed—similar to those reported in adults. Subsequent research has also addressed issues that may moderate treatment outcome, for example, variables in child, family, environment. Interestingly, the nature of the child or adolescent's difficulties does not appear to straightforwardly relate to degree of improvement. Children and adolescents with internalizing type problems (depression, anxiety) are as likely to profit from intervention as are those with externalizing difficulties (conduct disorder, attentional problems).

The movement toward evidence-based treatments has factored heavily in attempts to evaluate psychotherapies. To qualify as evidence based, a treatment must have been shown to work in two independent, carefully designed, controlled studies with random assignment to treatment and comparison to either a placebo or comparison treatment group. The term *probably efficacious* has been used when study design is less stringent, for example, through comparison of treated cases to a wait list control. Even when the efficacy of a specific treatment model has been established, typically in a highly research oriented setting, important questions surrounding the effectiveness of the treatment in real-world settings must also be addressed. The typical university setting for clinical trials offers many advantages in terms of access, for example, extensive logistical support, the potential for careful training and monitoring treatment methods over time, and so forth. If conducted as part of a research project, participation may be free or participants may even be paid for being involved. Unfortunately, only much smaller number of studies have actually addressed the issue of treatment effectiveness in more usual treatment settings, and findings have not been nearly as promising as those from clinical trials conducted in university settings. Thus, there is a major gap between what can be done in research settings and what actually happens in the community.

Attempts have been made, particularly in the areas of depression and anxiety disorders, to address these issues with some encouraging results. Studies have also examined combined treatments, for example, medication and cognitive behavioral therapy (CBT), suggesting a modest benefit from adding CBT to drug treatment. Other efforts have focused on the effectiveness of work with parents, notably in the area of parent management training, where studies evaluating both clinical use and cost-effectiveness of this approach have produced promising results, for example, in reducing the number of arrests. Given the public health and social policy significance of youth conduct problems, these results are particularly encouraging and the approach has been adapted for other populations including for substance abuse.

Psychotherapy clearly can work for children and adolescents. The question of how it works remains an important topic for research and active area of debate. The question is a difficult one to answer for many reasons. Even a highly structured treatment will usually include multiple components, any of which, or any combination of which, may be most relevant to particular problems and patients. For example, in work on anxiety using CBT, is it the targeting of maladaptive cognitions that is most important or is it the exposure to the anxiety-provoking situation, or the combination of both? Further problems arise given our limited understanding of the pathophysiology of mental conditions. It will be important for future work in this area to develop more relevant measures, for example, beyond the typical child/parent report and observation scales to more direct measures, for example, of behavior or physiology.

PSYCHODYNAMIC PSYCHOTHERAPY

Insight-oriented or psychodynamic psychotherapy is the oldest of the psychotherapies and has its origins in the attempt, beginning in the 19th century, to understand mental activity, the interplay of mind and brain, and symptoms/conditions that could be related to these processes. Sigmund Freud's contribution remains substantial and modern methods owe a considerable intellectual debt to him, for example, for the conscious and unconscious mind and the importance of developmental issues in understanding symptoms. Freud's case of

"Little Hans" provides one of the first reports of attempts to engage in psychotherapy with children. Because of Freud's emphasis on the importance of early experience in the analysis of adults, he and his students had a strong developmental orientation. Several of his early trainees, including his daughter Anna, began direct work with children. From early on, this work noted the importance of an awareness of development, of the role of parents, and the special complexities of work with children, for example, the role of education, the place of play activities, and so forth. In England, Melanie Klein developed the notion of play analysis as the analog of free association in adult psychoanalysis and emphasized interpretation with a focus on core issues. In contrast, Anna Freud, who moved to England with her family shortly before World War II and who had been trained as a teacher, emphasized the "educative" functions of child therapy as well as interpretation. The war in Europe and increased interest in mental health issues after the war contributed to an influx of European-trained psychiatrists and analysts to the United States. Their ideas influenced a generation of therapists and also impacted the approaches to treatment used in child guidance clinics, congregate care programs, and similar settings.

Goals of psychodynamic psychotherapy often involve changing patterns of thought, feeling, or behavior that are partly, or even fully, not in the individual's consciousness. This process relies on the importance of the relationship with the therapist attempting to help the patient. The notion of *transference* arises in this regard and refers to the tendency of patients to project onto their therapist feelings stemming from earlier relationships with meaningful figures in their lives. In addition, there is a significant "real" relationship with the therapist that also may further the psychotherapeutic process; this is particularly the case in work with children. Usually, the therapist attempts to understand the patient's difficulties in light of early history and experience as well as in the context of the direct observations and interaction with the patient. (See Ritvo & Shapiro, 2018 for a discussion.)

Freud elaborated a complex theory of psychological functioning, and, at different points in his professional life, emphasized different features, but his theory was always strongly developmental. He highlighted the interplay of biologic factors and psychological ones in both normal development and psychopathology. He emphasized the importance of sexual development and believed that the surface (conscious behaviors, thoughts, and feelings reported by people) could be studied scientifically, were multiply determined, and that aspects of unconscious or not fully conscious issues could be inferred based on observation and discussion with the patient. His theory also emphasized the importance of conflict (external or internal) in the formation of difficulties and of various "drives" (sexual or aggressive) that the individual must cope with. As a practical matter, his therapy took the form of talking, or with children, playing, to clarify the nature of conflicts, developmental arrests, and distortions. One of the goals was to make conscious patterns that would otherwise remain unconscious and continue to be acted out/acted upon in some way. Freud also viewed the tendency of the patient to relive past relationships within the therapy (transference) as important and also noted that the therapist could similarly have feelings about the patient (counter transference) that also provide useful clinical information.

Freud's theory evolved over time but had a tremendous influence on the development of models of the mind and mental illness in the 20th century. Many aspects of Freud's views have been incorporated into other aspects of psychology and many of his concepts have influenced educational practices and childcare. Over time, a myriad of other models and approaches have appeared. For example, one group, the ego psychologists, developed a strong interest in understanding the working of the ego. Many members of this group were interested in children's development and child psychotherapy. Another group developed in response to some of Freud's notions about female development and female sexuality. Another school of psychoanalytic thought, object relations theory, emphasizes the centrality of internal representations both of the self and others in typical development and psychopathology. This school has been very much concerned theoretically with the earliest development of the mind and clinically with some of the more challenging patients, for example, those with borderline personality disorders, and emphasizes issues like early modulation of aggression and ability to tolerate affect and develop relationships with parents and others.

Regardless of the specific theoretical orientation of the therapist, psychodynamic psychotherapy is centrally concerned with the therapist–patient relationship both as a lens for viewing the past and understanding how this past colors the present. The therapist looks as well for patterns in the patients' relationships and daily life to clarify these issues. In addition, the patient has, to some degree, a "real relationship" with the therapist. For therapists working with children, this real relationship is often very much present and provides, at least in theory, a greater potential for learning from new experiences. Accordingly, there is great emphasis on how the therapist conducts themselves with the child (or adult) patient. The therapist also models a reflective and thoughtful stance encouraging examination, introspection, and insight. This attitude of respect and concern also has the benefit of encouraging the treatment alliance—the commitment of the patient to seek greater self-understanding even in the face of anxiety or unpleasant feelings.

Goals of individual psychodynamic therapy include developing an understanding of the various influences in the life of the child or adolescent and how past experience and patterns of adaptation continue to be expressed in the present, for example, as symptoms or problem behaviors. Because such therapy is typically time consuming, it often is not undertaken if a less intensive approach is available. In this regard, however, it is important to note that in contrast to other forms of psychotherapy the goals of intensive psychodynamic psychotherapy are not limited solely to symptom reduction or elimination. Rather, the goals have to do with helping the individual child or adolescent assume a more normative developmental path with increased capacities for self-regulation, improved relations with others, and an enhanced ability to take appropriate pleasure in school or work activities.

The opening phase of psychodynamic therapy usually is concerned both with fostering the treatment and engagement of the child as well as clarifying aspects of diagnosis and interpersonal dynamics. For younger children, initial visits with the parents can provide important historic information and allow the parents to establish a sense of trust in the therapist that can then be conveyed to the child. For adolescents, issues of autonomy, confidentiality, and trust may have special importance. Meeting with the parents early on also helps clarify some aspects of the therapeutic relationship with them, that is, in general, the therapist strives to maintain confidentiality for the child and typically refrains from conveying information from sessions to the parents (with certain very specific exceptions related, for example, to thoughts of suicide or aggression). Children, and particularly younger children, may choose to make use of play materials, toys, games, and other activities. For some adolescents, the use of such activities, for example, cards or chess, may also provide a structure within which the patient can be more comfortable talking "on the side" with the therapist. Negotiating the complexities of working with the child and meeting periodically with the parents can be challenging. It is important for the therapist to be aware of these complexities and cope as effectively as possible.

The initial or opening phase of treatment focuses on obtaining important information on the child/adolescent and their difficulties as well as modeling a new approach for the child in attempting to understand these difficulties. This comes about through both implicit processes (modeling, empathizing) and more explicit ones, for example, interpretation. Interpretation consists of helping the child or adolescent understand, with the therapist's help, a new way to understand thoughts, feelings, or impulses. For younger children, the integrative process begins through ongoing commentary of the therapist on the child's play or about the child's behavior or language. The therapist may draw the child or adolescent's attention to something by wondering about or questioning something with the overarching goal of helping the child become more consciously aware of defense patterns, impulses, or maladaptive ways of coping. The opening phase of treatment typically lasts for weeks to several months.

Once a treatment alliance has been established, the middle phase of the treatment will concentrate on helping the child develop a new "defense" and give up old ones. This period, usually the longest phase of treatment, can last from months to even years. By this time, the child or adolescent is actively engaged in treatment as reflected in their ability to make use of the therapist's consistency and nonjudgmental approach. Play during this time becomes richer, and, with older children and adolescents, some activity may alternate with or gradually be replaced by talking. Difficulties in the treatment take the form of resistance, for example, the child may actively resist coming to sessions or be silent and "bored" during session, or, in some cases, the child may be overly compliant but relatively unengaged and passively resistant. The expected moments of resistance or difficulty in therapy, expressed by a sudden shift in topic, feeling, behavior, or withdrawal, can be important clues for the therapist regarding the child's inner experience. It is during the middle phase of treatment that the transference relationship develops most vividly. Thus, the patient will tend to experience the therapist in very specific and unique ways reflecting previous experiences, particularly with the parents. Important differences from the adult transference relationship exist, because the child continues to live with the parents, has a child–adult relationship with the therapist, and the therapist also exists as a new and real person to the child. As a result, the transference relationship in the child patient may be less deep and complex than that observed in adult patients.

During the middle phase of treatment, the work with parents includes understanding the parents' fears and beliefs about treatment, their hopes for the child in the future, and their fantasies and unrealistic expectations, for example, that the child will be "rescued." In some situations, the parents can see the therapist as a rival or see them as the authority figure. As much as possible, the therapist should attempt to form an alliance supporting the parents' positive striving for their child.

The termination phase of treatment involves both the decision to terminate and the process during which treatment is ended. The decision to end treatment can come from the child, therapist, or parents. Ideally, all agree on the appropriateness of setting an end date. Sometimes, a decision will be made unilaterally because of external factors, for example, a family move. At other times, it may stem from a unilateral decision, for example, by a parent who feels threatened or ambivalent about the treatment. The final phase of treatment provides an opportunity for a review and reworking of many of the themes/issues raised earlier in the treatment. The child or adolescent's fantasies and expectations about termination become important. The therapist will consider various factors in considering termination including the gains made and the child or adolescent's ability to maintain these gains and the degree to which developmental process have been facilitated. Termination awakens issues of separation and loss for both patient and therapist alike. In this context regression may occur and symptoms not seen for some time may reemerge. Such situations provide the child or adolescent with an opportunity to face and discuss these issues and consolidate the insight and self-awareness that hopefully have emerged over treatment. The child or adolescent's ability to internalize some of the therapist's "observing ego" functions is a hallmark of a successful treatment and facilitates longer term development. As much as possible, the child/adolescent patient should be actively involved in the process of termination. Depending on the situation, a follow-up plan may be put into place; in any event, the door should be left open for the patient to return if the need arises.

In contrast to other treatments, notably CBT (see next section), the quality and quantity of research is limited and in many respects psychoanalysis and related psychodynamic psychotherapies face major challenges for the future given the absence of this research. Challenges for research include the diversity of theoretical approaches, the continued reliance on case reports rather than controlled trials, and the scarcity of rigorous research studies. Fortunately, some work has appeared based on meta-analyses suggesting important gains associated with treatment with reasonably good effect sizes for general psychiatric difficulties, specific targeted problems, and overall functioning at follow-up.

COGNITIVE BEHAVIORAL THERAPY

CBT is the most frequently used evidence-based treatment (see Boettcher et al., 2018). The term refers to a number of interventions designed to address both cognitive and behavioral issues that impact mental health problems. This set of techniques has its origin in learning principles and has had a very strong research basis. As a method, it has grown considerably over the past decades. In addition to being strongly data based, these techniques are readily learned, useful for focused, short-term treatment, and are both patient and clinician friendly.

CBT has been used in a wide range of disorders including anxiety disorders, eating disorders, habit and tic disorders, posttraumatic stress disorder (PTSD), conduct disorders, depression, and attention-deficit hyperactivity disorder. It has also been used in targeting social skills and maladaptive behaviors (including anxiety and depression) in individuals with autism and related disorders.

The behavioral foundations of CBT rest strongly in learning theory. This work emphasizes the central role of changing behavior with the latter being examined within a broad context, including both antecedences and consequences. This perspective helps clarify what elicits and maintains the behavior and allows for intervention aimed to disrupt some aspect of this process. It is important to understand those factors that maintain the behavior and not just those that initially seem to cause it. This approach draws on aspects of both classical and operant conditioning. The work in the 1920s by Mary Cover Jones in demonstrating the learning of fear responses in children was widely applied in the understanding of phobias in general. In phobias, continued avoidance behavior helps to maintain the phobia by preventing exposure to the fear-inducing situation and thus prevents extinction of the fear response. Aspects of classic conditioning can also be used to understand emotional reactions other than fear as well as other mental health problems including substance abuse, depression, and some psychosomatic disorders. As might be expected, treatments based on this model aim to encourage extinction of the learned maladaptive behaviors. Other techniques, for example, exposure can be used as well. Operant conditioning is similarly based on analysis of antecedents and consequences. In contrast to classic conditioning, operant conditioning can explain acquisition of new behaviors. This work, based on the work of learning theorists like Skinner, understands acquisition of new behaviors through reinforcement, for example, an association of a behavior with a positive outcome. Removal of the reinforcement would, over time, result in a decrease in the behavior. Within this model, rewards or punishments will increase or decrease the frequency of the target behavior. Aspects of operant conditioning have been well studied and widely used, for example, in the treatment of children with autism in applied behavior analysis along with parent management training for children with behavior/conduct problems as well as for many other conditions. Extinction occurs when reinforcement is no longer provided and the behavior ceases. This process may be, initially, associated with higher levels of the behavior of interest (the so-called extinction burst) before rates of the behavior decrease. Some of the common techniques derived from operant condition principles are listed in Table 28.1.

CBT also focuses more broadly on aspects of thinking, feeling, and behavior that may be relevant to the genesis or maintenance of a problem. For example, rather than an overt event, it may be a thought or feeling that serves as an important antecedent event, for example, thinking about a fear-inducing stimulus may elicit anxiety even in the absence of the stimulus itself. Thus, CBT is concerned with both behavioral and cognitive techniques in an effort to put emotional difficulties in a broader context. Much of the work of CBT focuses on understanding why some unpleasant experiences or thoughts persist rather than disappear over time. The individual who spends considerable time avoiding a fear-inducing event might, for example, be inadvertently perpetuating and compounding their anxiety because there is no opportunity for exposure to the event. For example, the child with obsessive-compulsive disorder who, having engaged in a number of ritualistic actions, discovers that their parents' health, which they obsessively worry about, remains fine may believe that their good health is because of the child's own compulsive rituals. Attentional issues have importance in the CBT model. An adolescent who is, for example, anxious and depressed, may overly attend to cues that support continued feelings of anxiety or depression. Similarly, thoughts or images may be associated with specific reactions: for example, the child with OCD who is concerned that angry thoughts about their father increase the probability that the father will be hurt. Aspects of memory also play an important role; for example, the person with an anxiety problem may frequently be reminded of past situations in which they were anxious or the child with PTSD may recall the traumatic event in response to some relatively minor stimulus and become highly anxious. An over focus on past mistakes and failings may similarly perpetuate feelings of depression or poor self-esteem. Preoccupation with past negative events may also make it seem more likely that such events will recur.

TABLE 28.1

Common Therapy Techniques Associated with Principles of Operant Conditioning

Type and Technique	Description
Reinforcement to increase behaviors	
Token economy	Reinforcing target behavior with "tokens" (e.g., stickers, points, poker chips) that can then be traded in for reinforcers once multiple tokens have been earned
Differential reinforcement of other behavior (DRO)	Reinforcing specific appropriate behaviors while ignoring inappropriate behaviors that serve the same function
Shaping	Reinforcing gradual approximations of a behavior
Punishment to decrease behaviors	
Overcorrection	Applied consequence that involves engaging in a series of retribution steps that are related to the inappropriate behavior (e.g., washing soiled clothes after toileting accident)
Response cost	Removal of previously earned reinforcers as consequence of negative behavior; used especially in conjunction with token economy when "tokens" are removed.
Time out	Removing all sources of reinforcement for allotted period of time; typically involves placing the individual in a location where access to reinforcing activities, including social attention, is not available
Decreasing behavior with extinction	Removing previously available reinforcement from an inappropriate behavior to decrease the probability that the behavior will occur in the future

Reprinted with permission from Boettcher, M. A., & Piancentini, J. (2007). Cognitive and behavioral therapies. In A. Martin & F. R. Volkmar (Eds.), *Lewis's child and adolescent psychiatry: A comprehensive textbook* (4th ed., p. 798). Lippincott Williams & Wilkins.

Cognitive Behavioral Therapy in Children and Adolescents

The approach to the patient in CBT is a collaborative one where the therapist works with the patient to better understand and monitor behaviors and thoughts, formulate hypotheses about them, and develop alternate ways of coping, behaving, and thinking. Children present some challenges in that they may have difficulty in self-monitoring. In addition, parental and family influences may also have a major impact on the child. Thus, it is essential that the therapist work within a developmental framework to tailor the treatment to the child's level of understanding and functioning. Issues of autonomy and degree of support must be carefully balanced. The impact of family members or other systemic issues may be an important factor to consider as well, because, often unwittingly, schools or parents may help maintain problems. Accordingly, work with parents or other adults significant in the child's life may be indicated. Difficulties that children, and sometimes adolescents, have with abstract thinking can require adaption of technique, for example, explanations may need to be made more concrete or the child can be encouraged to adopt a role, such as a detective, in gathering information and testing hypotheses. Modeling/role playing, for example, with puppets, can be used both to insure the child's attention and illustrate concepts/issues. For children with higher language and cognitive levels, more traditional cognitive techniques can be used. Issues of frequency/intensity and duration of treatment are determined considering the child's developmental level.

Family factors are an important issue in child CBT. Having parents, and others, focus on antecedents and consequences of behavior can help them notice accommodations that support and even encourage maladaptive behaviors. Similarly, helping parents change routines and disciplinary practices is often an essential aspect of helping the child change. This is particularly true with younger children who often need adult support in treatment, for example, in maintaining a focus on treatment goals and homework. Conversely, with older children, parents may need support in allowing the child or adolescent to have greater responsibility for the treatment.

CBT is concerned with generalization of treatment effects in several ways: across settings, and between domains of functioning (behavior and thinking). There is also a concern with generalization over time (maintenance). Techniques and methods should be applied across settings, in various contexts, and over time, that is, not only in the setting of therapy.

Regardless of the individual's age, CBT approaches share some basic features such as active involvement of the patient in developing new strategies, use of homework, use of data to monitor treatment, an explicit focus on symptoms and daily functioning, a focus on generalization, and time-limited treatment. The initial phase of treatment will usually focus on assessment of the presenting problem, developing a working relationship, and preparation of the child for the active phase of treatment. The assessments should address detailed information about the symptoms and identification of maintaining factors. Normalization of the patient's problems can be an important therapeutic aspect of the assessment phase, which may lead to immediate symptomatic relief. The goal of this phase should be to develop a cognitive behavioral model of the presenting problem to guide treatment. Thus, the assessment phase will gather data on when symptoms occur and their context (location, antecedents, and consequences), the cognitions, behaviors, and emotions associated with the symptoms, and the factors that relieve symptoms, make them worse, or help to maintain them. In addition, there is a focus on relevant historic information, for example, previous treatment history, factors associated with the onset of the symptoms, as well as on the cognitions, beliefs, and other experiences that contribute to them.

As symptomatic difficulties and other relevant variables are identified, a treatment plan is developed that usually starts with a focus on educating about symptoms and how these can be understood and treated. The active (middle) phase of treatment focuses on implementing and mastering new cognitive behavioral treatment strategies; this is done with a combination of regular treatment sessions and assigned homework. This phase includes systematic monitoring with the possibility of adjustment as needed. Psychoeducation is an important element of CBT, given the explicit focus on helping the patient understand and change symptoms, feelings, and behaviors. This can include a focus on understanding physiologic symptoms and their cognitive components: for example, the child with PTSD may be helped to understand that intrusive thoughts are common following a traumatic experience. This effort may also itself relieve some anxiety, for example, about the potential medical seriousness of some symptoms. Helping the child make connections between thoughts and events can help the child question prior assumptions: for example, for the child with OCD that thinking a bad thought is not the same thing as engaging in a bad behavior.

As symptoms become less problematic, the final phase of treatment focuses on generalization and maintenance of techniques and preventing relapse. Usually, visits are less frequent and the child has greater responsibility for ongoing maintenance. Sometimes "booster sessions" may be needed even after treatment has been completed to facilitate maintenance. Treatment frequency can vary somewhat between inpatient and outpatient treatment settings. It is important that the child have some time between sessions to practice and complete homework. Therapy typically lasts for between 3 and 6 months.

Cognitive Behavioral Therapy Techniques

A number of different techniques are employed in CBT (see Boettcher & Piacentini, 2005 for a detailed discussion). These include **cognitive restructuring** that focuses on understanding the role of cognitive distortions in symptoms and replacing them with more accurate and adaptive ones and **identifying automatic thoughts,** those spontaneous thoughts or responses to situations that contribute to symptoms (Table 28.2). The method of **Socratic Questioning/**

TABLE 28.2

Common Cognitive Errors Found in Cognitive Restructuring

Cognitive Error	Description	Example
Catastrophizing	Placing unrealistic importance on thoughts and events and assuming terrible negative outcomes will occur as a result	"I got a C on my report card, so I will never get into college and I will fail in life."
Magnifying/ Minimizing	Placing an inaccurate amount of importance on thoughts, feelings, events, and so forth (either too much or too little)	Believing getting caught doing drugs is not important because the implications of having a drug problem are too anxiety provoking (minimizing).
Absolutism (black and white thinking)	All events and experiences are thought of in extreme categories, rather than moderately.	"I will **never** lose any weight because I just ate a cookie."
Personalization	Attributing responsibility for external events to the self with no basis for the attribution	"It is my fault that my parents are getting divorced."
Selective abstraction	Taking information out of context and ignoring relevant details	"My soccer coach hates me" when they did not play the child in spite of the fact that they have started the last three games
Arbitrary inference	Making arbitrary conclusions contrary to or without evidence	Believing homework is too hard when, in fact, the child completed the same work that day in class
Ignoring evidence	Leaving out important information when forming thoughts about events	Believing that werewolves are a danger at night in spite of the fact that multiple adults have told the child they do not exist, and all the doors in the house are locked
Overgeneralization	Believing the outcome of one situation applies in many situations, when it may not	"All my teachers hate me" when one teacher yelled at the child at school
Attending to negative features of events	Placing greater cognitive importance on negative features of events and ignoring positive features	Focusing on one poor grade when all others are good

Reprinted with permission from Boettcher, M. A., & Piacentini, J. (2007). Cognitive and behavioral therapies. In A. Martin & F. R. Volkmar (Eds.), *Lewis's child and adolescent psychiatry: A comprehensive textbook* (4th ed., p. 803). Lippincott Williams & Wilkins.

Examining the Evidence is used as an important part of cognitive restructuring and involves questioning the patient to help elicit automatic thoughts and then raising issues regarding their validity. This is particularly important for children who may not understand that thoughts, worries, and so forth are not intrinsically true. This method also helps to **correct misinterpretations,** which may cause individuals, for example, with depression, to consistently misinterpret events, their own experience, and the behavior of others. **Behavioral experiments** are used, particularly as part of psychoeducation, to help clarify the importance of cognitive distortions; for example, the patient may be asked not to think about a particular topic during a short period of time to illustrate how attempts at thought suppression actually result in an overfocus on the avoided topic or idea. Particularly for patients with anxiety, **modification of imagery** may be used to help patients cope with an anxiety-provoking event, for example, in imagining a positive outcome or learning that their images of an event have specific cognitive distortions that result in exaggerated or misplaced anxiety. Certain core beliefs or cognitive schema underlying maladaptive thoughts/symptoms may be identified during treatment; for example, the fundamental core belief that "I am stupid" may result in various compensatory behaviors that are never totally successful. A range of **physiologic techniques** can also be useful, particularly when anxiety leads to significant physical symptoms and bodily sensations. These methods are less dependent on higher levels of cognition and thus more readily used in children. They can take the form of **regulated breathing,** where breathing exercises help reduce physical tension and the tendency to hyperventilation and have the additional benefit of helping patients be more comfortable coping with bodily experiences and sensations. Similarly, **progressive muscle relaxation** (tensing and relaxing of muscle groups) can help with anxiety and anger management. **Exposure techniques** are based on the idea that the child's anxious and unwarranted avoidance only exacerbates their response to feared situations. Typically, the child is given a series of gradual, progressive exercises to create or recreate situations associated with anxiety, for example, this might include thinking about fearful situations or actual graded exposure.

Self-monitoring can be used in various ways including for work on habit disorders, modification of eating and exercise in eating disorders, and tracking use of behavioral techniques and relaxation in anxiety disorders. **Self-management procedures** include responsibility for implementation of a specific behavioral plan and similarly can be used in a range of conditions both in terms of improving desired skills and decreasing undesired behaviors. Another approach, **activity scheduling,** is frequently used in the treatment of depression to help increase the individual's involvement in daily activities and break the negative cycles of depressed mood, thoughts, and behavior that result in lack of participation in previously pleasurable activities, further contributing to depressed mood. **Behavior modification and applied behavior analysis** techniques are helpful in increasing desired behaviors and decreasing undesirable ones. **Counter conditioning** pairs a maladaptive behavior with an incompatible behavior in order to reduce and eliminate the maladaptive behavior. **Habit reversal** training procedures are most frequently used in the treatment of habit disorders (trichotillomania and skin-picking) and in Tourette syndrome and tic disorders. This approach involves awareness training combined with training in an incompatible competing response.

■ INTERPERSONAL PSYCHOTHERAPY

Interpersonal therapy (IPT) was originally developed as a brief treatment for adults with nonpsychotic depression (see Mufson & Young, 2018). It assumes that social relationships are important mitigating and protective factors in depression. The goals of IPT include education about connections between depression and interpersonal relationships with an aim to improve the latter as an important aspect of treatment. This model has its origins in the work of Adolf Meyer and Harry Stack Sullivan as well as the work of John Bowlby on attachment. The approach is concerned with helping clients cope with conflicts and losses. The two major goals of this approach have to do with improving social functioning and diminishing/mitigating depressive symptomatology. A series of specific strategies involve identification of problem

TABLE 28.3

Interpersonal Psychotherapy: Primary Components of Treatment

Education	Affect Identification	Interpersonal Skills Building
Psychoeducation	Labeling emotions	Modeling
Limited sick role	Clarification of emotions	Use of therapeutic relationship as sample of interpersonal interaction
Treatment contract	Facilitating expression of emotions Monitoring emotions	Communication analysis Perspective taking Interpersonal problem-solving Role playing

Reprinted with permission from Mufson, L., & Young, J. F. (2007). Interpersonal psychotherapy. In A. Martin & F. R. Volkmar (Eds.), *Lewis's child and adolescent psychiatry: A comprehensive textbook* (4th ed., p. 821). Lippincott Williams & Wilkins.

area(s), effective approaches to problem-solving, and communication and practice on use of these approaches. The IPT approach has been used for depressed adolescents as an active and structured treatment approach that involves a significant psychoeducational aspect. The goal, as treatment progresses, is to help the teenager develop more effective, action-oriented approaches to coping. This model is particularly relevant to adolescents who have the task of becoming increasingly independent and autonomous. Parents are typically involved to some degree in the treatment. At a minimum, this includes some involvement in the opening phase of treatment when much of the focus is on education. Parents may be involved again as treatment works on specific strategies, and, at the end, as part of the process of reviewing treatment progress and future needs. Various other modifications are made for adolescents to help concretize the process and to focus on more basic aspects of social skills and negotiation of parent issues. Other modifications can be made in special circumstances, for example, around issues of abuse, school refusal, suicidality, and so forth. Table 28.3 summarizes some of the components of IPT.

GROUP PSYCHOTHERAPY

Group therapy has many potential advantages in the treatment of children and adolescents (Moss et al., 2018). Peers can be powerful mediators of change, bring different perspectives than those of parents and adult therapists, and may more readily provide useful feedback and information. Group treatments originated in part with the use of congregate care facilities for children in the juvenile justice system at the end of the 19th century. Over time, groups focused on specific activities/issues have also been developed, for example, groups for teaching social skills to children with difficulties on the autism spectrum or to support children exposed to trauma. As with other psychotherapies, there has been a movement toward increased standardization and development of specific curricula. Depending on its focus and leadership, a therapy group will typically move through several phases.

Groups can be time limited or ongoing. The role of the group leaders will vary depending on the purposes and nature of the group; for example, in highly focused short-term groups, the leader may have an active role throughout the group's duration. In open-ended groups, the leader's role may be more important in early stages, in helping ensure effective group functioning and in helping new group members enter as others leave. The interventions of the group leader will vary depending on the nature of the group and its stage of existence.

Various theoretical perspectives have been used in the organization of group treatment programs. Having a specific theoretical orientation can help group leaders in management of the group. An overall theoretical perspective may also be important strategically, for example, in guiding decisions of when to, and when not to, intervene.

Groups for children and adolescents must cope with several important tasks. Depending on the age and developmental level of participants, play or verbalization may be a major mode of communication. Some groups will have a more traditional insight-oriented, psychodynamic orientation whereas others will be briefer and more highly focused. Some groups, like social skills groups, may aim to increase skill levels. Such groups can include typically developing children as well as those with social vulnerabilities or may be limited only to children with vulnerabilities. Support groups may be primarily concerned with helping the child or adolescent deal with a very specific problem, for example, substance abuse, loss, or trauma. Groups can be more or less didactic. Members of the group should have a clear sense of the purpose of the group. Activities of the group will vary depending on the nature, focus, and developmental levels of participants but typically are divided, to varying degrees, around processes that help the group focus on its specific areas of activity/interest as well as those activities that are essential in maintain the group. Issues that group leaders, and sometimes the group itself, will have to consider including recruiting members into the group, the specific composition of the group, for example, around a focus on a specific problem or around a specific diagnostic category. Issues of composition encompass issues of diversity (age, gender, and so forth) and sensitivity to group composition is important because a person who is, or becomes, a solitary member representing some specific group or issue can feel isolated. In some groups, there may be a deliberate attempt to include typically developing peers both as role models and to serve, to some degree, as potential allies of the leaders, for example, in social skills groups. Both the developmental level and chronologic ages of the child or adolescent are relevant.

Typically, each group encounter will last for a specific length of time (e.g., from 60 to 90 minutes), although in public school settings shorter lengths of time are frequent. Depending on the context, the group may be time limited (meeting for x number of sessions or during the school year); in other cases, the group is ongoing. In the latter case, issues of departure of "graduating" members and of entry of new members will arise. Typically, the leaders will provide a structure for the group that is conveyed initially and then reasonably adhered to throughout the life of the group. Depending on the nature of the group, for children this usually will include some period of time for talking, for an activity (games, play, or projects), snack time, and wrap-up. The group leader(s) has an important role in monitoring the group and providing reminders of continuity from one meeting to the next. Sometimes, a journal can be used to summarize the overall focus of a group meeting or can be used to document group rules and history. Periods of time can be adapted for various purposes; for example, telling jokes at a snack period in social skills groups provides important opportunities for feedback from peers (and adults). Group leaders will pay attention to potentially informative and communicative aspects of all undesired behaviors while simultaneously helping such behaviors not disrupt the group. Various techniques can be used to cope with behavioral difficulties including changes in group activities or structure, verbal interpretation, limit setting, and so forth. Sometimes an individual will not be able to tolerate the demands of being in a group, and in such cases removal of a group member should provide an opportunity for explanation as well as discussion.

The degree to which parents are involved can vary dramatically. For outpatient groups, parents may be physically present (having transported their child or several children). Sometimes, parents can have their own group that meets at the same time.

In addition to providing a safe environment, the group leaders provide models for interpersonal relationships and for open and honest communication. Groups typically are led by two leaders and this gives the working dyad a chance to develop their own approaches to effectively process the wealth of clinical information and make myriad process decisions encountered in the group. The leaders can and should disagree with each other at times and model a process by which such events are handled. By providing a degree of predictability and reliability, the leaders also set a tone for the group's activity.

In weighing the potential benefits of group therapy, several issues should be considered including the nature of the individual's difficulties, the degree to which a group experience may counter a tendency toward isolation and/or self-blame, or the degree to which group therapy may be more tolerable than individual or family therapy. In some cases, the nature of the clinical situation may suggest that individual treatment is more appropriate. As with other aspects of psychotherapy, research documenting the efficacy of group therapy has become more rigorous in recent years. A series of studies has now demonstrated its benefits in a range of populations.

SUMMARY

Psychotherapy for treatment of behavioral and emotional disorders in children and adolescents has a long history. A large body of work has now confirmed that psychotherapy can be effective. Challenges remain in generalizing highly structured, research-based methods into more typical clinical treatment settings. The evidence for "treatment as usual" is not, unfortunately, particularly strong but a growing body of work has established the effectiveness of several different structured treatment approaches.

ACKNOWLEDGMENT

Large portions of this chapter previously appeared as Chapter 22 in Volkmar, F. R., & Martin, A. (2011). *Essentials of Lewis's child and adolescent psychiatry*. Lippincott Williams & Wilkins, with permission.

References

Boettcher, M. A., Montague, R. A., Fox, E. A., & Piancentini, J. (2018). Cognitive and behavioral therapies. In A. Martin, M. Bloch, & F. R. Volkmar (Eds.), *Lewis's child and adolescent psychiatry: A comprehensive textbook* (5th ed., pp. 757–787). Wolters Kluwer.

Moss, N. E., Racusin, G. R., & Moss-Racusin, C. (2018). Group therapy. In A. Martin, M. Bloch, & F. R. Volkmar (Eds.), *Lewis's child and adolescent psychiatry: A comprehensive textbook* (5th ed., pp. 822–833). Wolters Kluwer.

Mufson, L., & Young, J. F. (2018). Interpersonal psychotherapy. In A. Martin, M. Bloch, & F. R. Volkmar (Eds.), *Lewis's child and adolescent psychiatry: A comprehensive textbook* (5th ed., pp. 788–779). Wolters Kluwer.

Ritvo, R. Z., & Shapiro, M. (2018). Psychodynamic principles in practice. In A. Martin, M. Blochkh, & F. R. Volkmar (Eds.), *Lewis's child and adolescent psychiatry: A comprehensive textbook* (5th ed., pp. 788–792) Wolters Kluwer.

Weersing, V. R., & Dirks, M. A. (2007). Psychotherapy for children and adolescents: A critical review. In A. Martin & F. R. Volkmar (Eds.), *Lewis's child and adolescent psychiatry: A comprehensive textbook* (pp. 789–796). Wolters Kluwer.

Suggested Readings

Bion, W. R. (1961). *Experiences in groups and other papers*. Basic Books.

Brent, D. A., Holder, D., Kolko, D., Birmaher, B., Baugher, M., Roth, C., Iyengar, S., & Johnson, B. A. (1997). A clinical psychotherapy trial for adolescent depression comparing cognitive, family, and supportive therapy. *Archives of General Psychiatry, 54*, 877–885. https://doi.org/10.1001/archpsyc.1997.01830210125017

Burlingame, G. M., Fuhriman, A. J., & Johnson, J. (2004). Current status and future directions of group therapy research. In J. L. De-Lucia-Waack, D. A. Gerrity, C. R. Kalodner, & M. T. Riva (Eds.), *Handbook of group counseling and psychotherapy* (pp. 651–660). Sage Publishing.

Casey, R. J., & Berman, J. S. (1985). The outcome of psychotherapy with children. *Psychological Bulletin, 98*, 388–400. https://doi.org/10.1037/0033-2909.98.2.388

Chambless, D. L., & Hollon, S. D. (1998). Defining empirically supported therapies. *Journal of Consulting and Clinical Psychology, 66*(1), 7–18. https://doi.org/10.1037/0022-006X.66.1.7

Chambless, D. L., & Ollendick, T. H. (2001). Empirically supported psychological interventions: Controversies and evidence. *Annual Review of Psychology*, *52*, 685–716. https://doi.org/10.1146/annurev.psych.52.1.685

Chorpita, B. F. (2003). The frontier of evidence based practice. In A. E. Kazdin & J. R. Weisz (Eds.), *Evidence based psychotherapies for children and adolescents* (pp. 42–59). Guilford Press.

Clarke, G. N., Debar, L., Lynch, F., Powell, J., Gale, J., O'Connor, E., Ludman, E., Bush, T., Lin, E. H., Von Korff, M., & Hertert, S. (2005). A randomized effectiveness trial of brief cognitive-behavioral therapy for depressed adolescents receiving antidepressant medication. *Journal of the American Academy of Child Psychiatry*, *44*(9), 888–898. https://doi.org/10.1016/S0890-8567(09)62194-8

Cohen, J. (1992). A power primer. *Psychological Bulletin*, *112*, 155–159. https://doi.org/10.1037/0033-2909.112.1.155

Curtis, N. M., Ronan, K. R., & Borduin, C. M. (2004). Multisystemic treatment: A meta-analysis of outcome studies. *Journal of Family Psychology*, *18*, 411–419. https://doi.org/10.1037/0893-3200.18.3.411

Fonagy, P., Target, M., Cottrell, D., Phillips, J., & Kurtz, Z. (2005). *What works for whom? A critical review of treatments for children and adolescents*. Guilford Press.

Freud, A. (1946). *The psycho-analytical treatment of children*. Imago Publishing.

Freud, S. (1955). Analysis of phobia in a five-year-old boy. In *Standard editions of the complete psychological works of Sigmund Freud* (Vol. 10, pp. 3–149). Hogarth.

Haley, J. (1963). *Strategies of psychotherapy*. Grune & Stratton.

Henggeler, S. W., & Lee, T. (2003). Multisystemic treatment of serious clinical problems. In A. E. Kazdin & J. R. Weisz (Eds.), *Evidence-based psychotherapies for children and adolescents*. Guilford Press.

Henggeler, S. W., Rowland, M. D., Pickrel, S. G., Henggeler, S. W., Rowland, M. D., Pickrel, S. G., Miller, S. L., Cunningham, P. B., Santos, A. B., Schoenwald, S. K., Randall, J., & Edwards, J. E. (1997). Investigating family-based alternatives to institution-based mental health services for youth: Lessons learned from the pilot study of a randomized field trial. *Journal of Clinical Child Psychology*, *26*, 226–233. https://doi.org/10.1207/s15374424jccp2603_1

Henggeler, S. W., Schoenwald, S. K., Borduin, C. M., Rowland, M. D., & Cunningham, P. B. (1998). *Multisystemic treatment of antisocial behavior in children and adolescents*. Guilford Press.

Hinshaw, S. P., Owens, E. B., Wells, K. C., Kraemer, H. C., Abikoff, H. B., Arnold, L. E., Conners, C. K., Elliott, G., Greenhill, L. L., Hechtman, L., Hoza, B., Jensen, P. S., March, J. S., Newcorn, J. H., Pelham, W. E., Swanson, J. M., Vitiello, B., & Wigal, T. (2000). Family processes and treatment outcomes in the MTA: Negative/ineffective parenting practices in relation to multimodal treatment. *Abnormal Child Psychology*, *28*, 555–568. https://doi.org/10.1023/A:1005183115230

Jones, M. C. (1924). A laboratory study of fear: The case of Peter. *Pedagogy Seminar*, *31*, 308–315. https://doi.org/10.1080/08856559.1924.9944851

Kazdin, A. E. (2000). Developing a research agenda for child and adolescent psychotherapy. *Archives of General Psychiatry*, *57*, 829–835. https://doi.org/10.1001/archpsyc.57.9.829

Kazdin, A. E., Siegel, T. C., & Bass, D. (1992). Cognitive problem-solving skills training and parent management training in the treatment of antisocial behavior in children. *Journal of Consultative Clinical Psychology*, *60*, 733–747. https://doi.org/10.1037/0022-006X.60.5.733

Kazdin, A. E., & Weisz, J. R. (2003). *Evidence-based psychotherapies for children and adolescents*. Guilford Press.

Klein, M. (1932). *The psychoanalysis of children*. Hogarth Press.

Krasny, L., Williams, B. J., Provencal, S., & Ozonoff, S. (2003). Social skills interventions for the autism spectrum: Essential ingredients and a model curriculum. *Child and Adolescent Psychiatric Clinics of North America*, *12*, 107–122. https://doi.org/10.1016/s1056-4993(02)00051-2

Minuchin, S. (1974). *Families and family therapy*. Harvard University Press.

Mufson, L., Dorta, K. P., Moreau, D., & Weisman, M. M. (2004). *Interpersonal psychotherapy for depressed adolescents* (2nd ed.). Guilford Press.

Muratori, F., Picchi, L., Bruni, G., Patarnello, M., & Romagnoli, G. (2003). A two-year follow-up of psychodynamic psychotherapy for internalizing disorders in children. *Journal of the American Academy of Child and Adolescent Psychiatry*, *42*(3), 331–339. https://doi.org/10.1097/00004583-200303000-00014

Patterson, G. R. (1982). *A social learning approach to family interventions: III. Coercive family process*. Castalia.

Reiss, D., Neiderhiser, J. M., Hetherington, E. M., & Plomin, R. (2000). *The relationship code, deciphering genetic and social Influences on adolescent development*. Harvard University Press.

Schectman, Z. (2004). Group counseling and psychotherapy with children and adolescents. In J. L. De-Lucia-Waack, D. A. Gerrity, C. R. Kalodner, & M. T. Riva (Eds.), *Handbook of group counseling and psychotherapy* (pp. 429–444). Sage Publishing.

Sholevar, G. P. (2007). Family therapy. In A. Martin & F. R. Volkmar (Eds.), *Lewis's child and adolescent psychiatry: A comprehensive textbook* (pp. 854–864). Wolters Kluwer.

Weersing, V. R., & Weisz, J. R. (2002). Mechanisms of action in youth psychotherapy. *Journal of Child Psychology and Psychiatry, 43*, 3–29. https://doi.org/10.1111/1469-7610.00002

Weisz, J. R., Donenberg, G. R., Han, S. S., & Weiss, B. (1995). Bridging the gap between laboratory and clinic in child and adolescent psychotherapy. *Journal of Consulting Clinical Psychiatry, 63*, 688–701. https://doi.org/10.1037/0022-006X.63.5.688

Weisz, J. R., Doss, A. J., & Hawley, K. M. (2005). Youth psychotherapy outcome research: A review and critique of the evidence base. *Annual Review of Psychology, 56*, 337–363. https://doi.org/10.1146/annurev.psych.55.090902.141449

Weisz, J. R., Weiss, B., & Donenberg, G. R. (1992). The lab versus the clinic: Effects of child and adolescent psychotherapy. *American Psychological Association, 47*, 1578–1585. https://doi.org/10.1037/0003-066X.47.12.1578

Weisz, J. R., Weiss, B., Han, S. S., Granger, D. A., & Morton, T. (1995). Effects of psychotherapy with children and adolescents revisited: A meta-analysis of treatment outcome studies. *Psychological Bulletin, 117*, 450–468. https://doi.org/10.1037/0033-2909.117.3.450

Wells, K. B., Sherbourne, C., Schoenbaum, M., Duan, N., Meredith, L., Unutzer, J., Miranda, J., Carney, M. F., & Rubenstein, L. V. (2000). Impact of disseminating quality improvement programs for depression in managed primary care: A randomized controlled trial. *Journal of the American Medical Association, 283*, 212–220. https://doi.org/10.1001/jama.283.2.212

CHAPTER 29 ■ PSYCHOPHARMACOLOGY

■ GENERAL ISSUES AND PRINCIPLES

In considering medications for behavioral and emotional problems, it is important to keep in mind the entire range of treatment options—not just pharmacologic ones. Child and adolescent psychiatrists, the medical specialists with the greatest expertise in this area, are the ones least frequently likely to use them, especially as first interventions. Additional information is provided in other chapters as it relates to specific conditions. An understanding of more basic issues of neurochemistry and drug metabolism is important, but is beyond the scope of this introductory chapter (see Anderson & Martin, 2018 for a comprehensive review). Keep in mind that knowledge changes, and always check on current best practices! In this chapter, we will review some of the issues and principles in pharmacologic treatments and the major drug classes commonly used. Given the nature of the topic, for example, the stimulants, we focus almost entirely in their use in attention-deficit hyperactivity disorder (ADHD). For the other classes of medications, we will discuss specific disorders in relation to the medication class.

That certain drugs derived from plants, for example, opium, have psychoactive effects has of course been known for millennia (Braslow & Marder, 2019). Modern interest in the scientific study of psychoactive medications on children and adolescents began with the clinical trial conducted by Charles Bradley (1937) who examined the effects of Benzedrine (a mix of levo- and dextroamphetamine) in an open trial of children with behavioral emotional problems and observed that the children became more manageable. About the same time, a placebo-controlled study of Benzedrine was done in a large group of delinquent boys who then showed improved learning and memory (Molitch & Eccles, 1937) These studies mark the beginning of psychopharmacology in children an area of research that now includes many placebo-controlled studies showing the efficacy of stimulants in the treatment of ADHD (Bloch, Beyers, Scahill, et al., 2018b; Multimodal Treatment Study of Children with ADHD [MTA] Group, 1999, 2004). In other areas like autism, important studies like those done by the Research Units on Pediatric Psychopharmacology (RUPP) group (McDougle et al., 2000) on risperidone and on stimulants in autism have been done and are helpful but are few and far between, and the core social dysfunction of autism has, to date, been resistant to drug treatment. Similarly, despite their demonstrated safety, efficacy, and widespread use in adults, the use of selective serotonin reuptake inhibitors (SSRIs) in children and adolescent rests on a much less extensive database, although research with adolescents has notably increased.

Pharmacologic agents are routinely prescribed in primary care practice for disorders like ADHD and anxiety (Chen et al., 2016). Often these practitioners are well able to manage cases that are uncomplicated. However, as cases increase in complexity, for example, due to side effects, associated comorbid conditions, and unusual clinical presentations, specialists tend to get involved. Finding good ways to support primary care providers in their use of these agents remains an important area of work (Meyers & Roth, 2018)

Although research in pediatric psychopharmacology has lagged behind that in adults (for a number of reasons), there have been some noteworthy and important initiatives that we will discuss subsequently. Recent congressional and governmental initiatives have also encouraged drug companies to study the use of agents in children and adolescents as well as adults (Oesterheld et al., 2018).

As Martin et al. (2004) have observed, there are some important considerations in prescribing psychoactive medications for children. They note seven major principles that guide work in this area (see Box 29.1).

BOX 29.1   Guiding Principles in Medication Management

1. Developmental differences in metabolism and elimination often result in shorter drug half-life in children.
2. Realization that comorbidity is common and that childhood disorders are complex and heterogenous. These issues may be relevant in deciding which issues are most important to target and what the impact of drug treatments may be on other conditions/problems that are present.
3. Identification of specific target symptoms (and their measurement) and the ability to integrate information from multiple informants (child, parents, teachers) is important. This creates some important practical problems in ongoing monitoring and dose adjustment.
4. Monitoring risks and benefits is important. Various methods can be used but is always important to weigh potential risks and benefits and to be sure all involved are aware of potential side effects and drug interactions.
5. Parents/caregivers must be engaged in treatment. As with all medications the most usual reason they don't work is that they are not taken (or not taken correctly). It is important to engage with children and youth as well as parents to ensure that drugs are taken appropriately and that all concerned are engaged in the treatment process. Discussion of the onset of benefit as well as of potential side effects is important; some drugs will have a more or less immediate effect, whereas others will take some time to be effective. Discussion of the meaning of the medicine to the child is important. Consideration can be given to use of longer acting agents to prevent children from feeling stigmatized by being called off to the nurses' office for mid-day mediations!
6. Usually medications are combined with other intervention methods. These may be as simple as ongoing special education or special services or more complex like participation in special psychotherapies or other treatments. It is important to be cognizant of these treatments. More information, particularly from practice parameters and guidelines, is now available as are guide clinicians for use in combination treatments. There are now good data on several combination treatment approaches.

(continued)

| **BOX 29.1** | **Guiding Principles in Medication Management (*continued*)** |

7. Treatment should be evidence based and guided by the available data. The treatment plan is clearly individualized for the particular child or youth but should be based in a realization of the levels of strength of evidence for the treatments proposed taking into account the myriad individual family, cultural, and other factors that impact the given child.

Adapted from Martin, A., Oesterhed, J. R., Bloch, M. H., et al. General principle and clincal practice. In A. Martin, M. Bloch, & F. R. Volkmar (Eds.), *Lewis's child and adolescent psychiatry: A comprehensive textbook* (5th ed., pp. 715–716). Wolters Kluwer.

In considering the use of medications, it is important to understand if there are alternatives to medication and whether these have been given an adequate trial. As part of considering medication, the prescriber will want to understand whether any medical conditions or life changes have contributed to the difficulties. Other considerations include problem severity, the degree to which it impacts across settings (e.g., both school and home) or is more limited, and the history of the problem and its impact on the child or adolescent's life functioning. The potential risks of pharmacologic intervention must be weighed against possible benefits. Sometimes problems are of recent onset and at other times issues arise in the context of long-standing issues and concerns. Often a careful behavioral assessment is helpful. Medications can be used with behavioral interventions, but once multiple interventions occur simultaneously, it gets more difficult to understand why things change; so a careful and thoughtful approach is needed trying, if at all possible, to change just one thing at a time.

There are important developmental changes that impact the use and efficacy of medications in children. These include changes both in drug absorption, metabolism, and excretion as well as in specific mechanisms of action (see Anderson & Martin, 2018). The term "pharmacokinetics" describes how the body deals with a drug, whereas pharmacodynamics refers to the effect of a drug on the body (see Figure 29.1).

There can be important differences in the effect of medication at different ages as brain regions develop at different rates. This can impact both the hoped-for treatment response as well as side effects. These issues are reflected, for example, in different side-effect profiles of the neuroleptic medications, developmental differences in responses to agents like antidepressants and SSRIs and so forth (Oesterheld et al., 2018). An understanding of pharmacokinetics as well as pharmacodynamic factors is important and may be relevant in issues of choice of specific agent within a drug class.

Several different issues are involved in pharmacokinetic effects. These include absorption and distribution that impact onset of effects, whereas metabolism and excretion help determine duration of drug effects (Oesterheld et al., 2018). Some drugs follow a linear pattern of drug kinetics so there is essentially a linear relationship between dose and plasma concentration. For drugs with this pattern, dose–response relationships are often easiest to interpret. In other situations nonlinear (also called zero-order) kinetics occur when a given amount of the agent is metabolized per unit time (i.e., without respect to plasma level). In drugs with this pattern, dose–response relationships are more complicated to interpret (see Oesterheld et al., 2018). A range of factors impact the *bioavailability* of any drug including its absorption, its initial clearance (first-pass effects) by gastrointestinal and liver metabolism, and conjugation. For some agents, for example, lithium, urinary excretion is the major path for elimination of the drug, whereas for others metabolism in the liver occurs. Drugs vary in the efficiency with which this first-pass mechanism impacts bioavailability, with some very efficiently metabolized and others much less so. Although oral administration of a drug is most common, it is also less predictive in terms of bioavailability. Many psychoactive agents are absorbed just after they pass through the stomach. Our understanding of drug absorption and distribution in the body has greatly advanced over the last decades (Oesterheld et al., 2018).

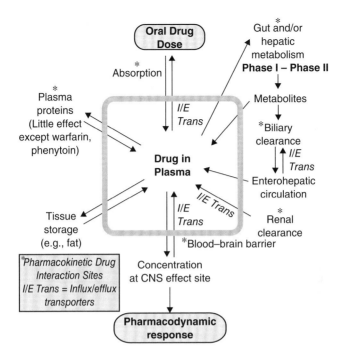

FIGURE 29.1. Pharmacokinetics and pharmacodynamics of a central nervous system (CNS) drug. Reprinted with permission from Oesterheld, J., Shader, R., & Martin, A. (2018). Clinical and developmental aspects of pharmacokinetics and drug interactions. In A. Martin, F. R. Volkmar, & M. Bloch (Eds.), *Lewis's child and adolescent psychiatry: A comprehensive textbook* (5th ed., p. 703). Wolters Kluwer.

STIMULANTS AND OTHER MEDICATIONS FOR ADHD

As noted earlier, the stimulants were some of the first medications used in the treatment of behavioral and emotional difficulties and now have become the first-line treatments for ADHD. These medications (methylphenidate and various forms of amphetamine) have been shown to be generally effective and exist both in short and longer acting forms. As discussed in Chapter 10, ADHD is one of the most common child mental health problems in school-age children, primarily boys. Longitudinal studies have shown the persistence of the condition into adolescence and adulthood in many cases (Spetie & Arnold, 2018). Although the effectiveness of these (and other) medications is clear, it is also clear that many children do not receive treatment (Scahill et al., 1999).

Stimulant Medications

Methylphenidate- and dextroamphetamine-related agents and mixed preparation of dextro- and levo-amphetamine are most frequently used. Table 29.1 summarizes many of the features of these medications that have now been shown to be effective in literally hundreds of studies going back many decades. More recent and technologically sophisticated work has clarified important issues of dose–response as well as potential differences in these agents and their potential side effects. One study (Rapport & Denney, 1997) of dose–response found that all

TABLE 29.1

Stimulant Medications for Attention-Deficit Hyperactivity Disorder

Drug Name (Brand)	Active Ingredient	Onset of Action	Duration of Effect	Required Number of Doses/Day	Suggested Dosing and Titration
Short Acting					
Ritalin® Methylin® Focalin® Metadate®	Methylphenidate	20–60 minutes peak effect: 2 hours	3–6 hours	2–3 doses; occasionally 4 doses	Start with one 5-mg tablet (2.5 for Focalin®) 2–3× a day. Increase by 5 mg (or 2.5 mg for Focalin®) until target behavior controlled, maximum dose is 60 mg per day
Dexedrine® Dextrostat®	D-amphetamine	20–60 minutes peak effect: 1–2 hours	4–6 hours	2–3 doses	Start with one 5-mg tablet 2–3× per day[a]
Adderall®	D,L-amphetamine	30–60 minutes peak effect: 1–2 hours	4–6 hours	2–3 doses	Start with one 5-mg tablet 2–3× per day[a]
First Generation: Long Acting					
Ritalin SR® Metadate ER® Methylin ER®	Methylphenidate	60–90 minutes peak effect: 8 hours	5–8 hours	1–2 doses	Start with one 10-mg tablet 1–2× per day[a]
Dexedrine Spansules®	D-amphetamine	60–90 minutes peak effect: 8 hours	6–8 hours	1–2 doses	Start with one 5-mg capsule 1–2× per day[a]
Second Generation: Long Acting					
Concerta®	Methylphenidate	30 minutes–2 hours	12 hours	1 tablet	Start with one 18-mg tablet once per day[a]
Metadate CD® Ritalin LA®	Methylphenidate	30 minutes–2 hours	6–8 hours	1–2 capsules	Start with one 10-mg capsule once per day[a]
Daytrana®	Methylphenidate	20–60 minutes peak effect: 10 hours after single application, 8 hours after repeat applications	8–12 hours	1 patch	Start with 10-mg patch worn 9 hours daily. Maximum dose: 30 mg patch worn 9 hours daily
Focalin XR®	Dexmethylphenidate	1–4 hours	8–12 hours	1 capsule	Start with one 5-mg capsule once per day[a]

TABLE 29.1

Stimulant Medications for Attention-Deficit Hyperactivity Disorder (*continued*)

Quillivant XR®	Methylpheni-date	30 minutes peak effect: 5 hours	8–12 hours	1 liquid dose	Start with 20 mg liquid suspension once per day[a]
Adderall XR®	D,L-amphetamine	1–2 hours	10–12 hours	1 capsule	Start with one 5- or 10-mg capsule once per day[a]
Vyvanse®	L-lysine-dextroam-phetamine	2 hours peak effect: 3–4 hours	10–12 hours	1 capsule	Start with one 30-mg capsule once daily[a]

[a]Titrate upward until target behavior controlled.
Reprinted with permission from Bloch, M., Beyer, C., & Martin, A. (2018). ADHD: Stimulant and nonstimulant agents. In A. Martin, M. H. Bloch, & F. R. Volkmar (Eds.), *Lewis's child and adolescent psychiatry: A comprehensive textbook* (5th ed., p. 719). Wolters Kluwer.

levels of medication were better than placebo. Similarly, meta-analyses have shown that the most common side effects include (given the nature of stimulants) problems with insomnia, appetite, and sometimes obsessive thinking and behavior, among others (see Bloch, Beyer, Martin, et al., 2018a).

The two stimulant agents appear to be about equally as effective (Elia, 1991). One of the major problems with methylphenidate has been the short duration of action so that the advent of extended-release forms has been welcome (Pelham et al., 2001). It is important to note that only a handful of studies have addressed long-term use, although data available suggest fewer overall side effects of methylphenidate (Greenhill et al., 1996). The large Multimodal Treatment Study (MTA) of ADHD in children provided powerful evidence of the superiority of this agent (sometimes in combination with other treatments) over behavioral treatment alone and to a community care group (the latter generally providing less frequent doses of the agent; see MTA, 1999 for details). Issues in the community care group were noted to include discontinuation of the medication, possibly reflecting undertreatment. The two research groups (medication alone and medication with behavioral intervention) had more frequent visits and intensive follow-up, including teacher reports. Overall, this study suggested that in the community, medication may be underdosed and not followed sufficiently closely. It is the case that individual differences are noted, and some children and youth do respond better to one over the other agents.

The mechanism of action of the stimulants remains the focus of some debate (Solanto, 1998). It is clear that methylphenidate and amphetamine work, in slightly different ways, to impact the dopamine system in the brain (and some other systems as well). Within the brain these effects are centered in the striatum and, to some degree, in the prefrontal cortex. Both kinds of agents also impact the norepinephrine (NE) system (Biederman & Spencer, 1999) via the locus coeruleus. It is interesting that the drugs like guanfacine (see next section) are more selective in their action but with smaller clinical impact.

The immediate-release forms of these agents (see Table 29.1) are readily absorbed and generally have behavioral effects within 30–60 minutes and reach peak levels within 90–150 minutes. The clinical benefit lasts several hours. Both drugs are metabolized in the liver, although through different pathways (see Oesterheld et al., 2018). The mixed amphetamine preparations have a somewhat longer period of action (Swanson, Wigal, Greenhill, et al., 1998). The sustained release (SR) forms provide the option of once-daily dosing and more flexibility and convenience.

There has been some disagreement about best approaches to dosing, for example, by weight or fixed dose; in one well-designed study, a linear dose–response relationship was noted (Rapport & Denney, 1997). Dosing of methylphenidate is usually done multiple times during the day to achieve optimal benefit without side effects, for example, on appetite or sleep (see Bloch, Beyer, Martin, et al., 2018a, for additional dosing information). The input of parents and teachers on effectiveness is important. Information from both sources is helpful to clinicians in management.

With D-amphetamine and D,L-amphetamine, the approach is similar. Usually, only twice-daily dosing is needed: in the morning and then again at noon to achieve maximum benefit at school. The extended-release preparations are also effective with similar side-effect profiles but with the advantage of less frequent administration. They may improve compliance and avoid some of the problems of rebound effects seen in shorter acting forms. A patch form is also now available to provide extended release for children who have difficulties with oral medications.

There has been concern, given their effect on appetite suppression, that growth retardation may be an adverse effect. The data on this issue are mixed (see Bloch, Beyer, Martin, et al., 2018a). One approach is to give stimulant medications with food or just after eating and monitor weight and height on a regular basis. By their very nature stimulants have the potential to cause sleep disturbance (one of the common reasons they are abused by college students attempting to "pull all-nighters"). Changes in mood, tics, headaches, and other problems can also occur. Taking a careful sleep history prior to use of these agents is important, and use of extended-release forms may avoid rebound phenomena and minimize some side effects. When methylphenidate is used, it is frequently the case that the end-of-day dose, if needed at all, is lower than other doses. The association of tics and stimulant administration has been controversial. One complexity is that many children with tics also have ADHD and the latter responds to stimulants (Bloch et al., 2009). A major meta-analytic study failed to suggest increased rates of tics with stimulants (Cohen et al., 2015).

Nonstimulants for ADHD

Given the concerns regarding possible side effects of stimulants, a number of other agents have been developed for use in treatment of ADHD. Table 29.2 provides a summary of these agents. The drug atomoxetine (Strattera) was approved by the Food and Drug Administration (FDA) as a treatment for ADHD (and comorbid oppositional defiant disorder following placebo-controlled trials, e.g., Michelson et al., 2002; Newcorn et al., 2005). Both once- and twice-daily dosing have been used (Michelson et al., 2002). Although better than placebo, the degree of improvement is less than that of the more traditional stimulants (Wigal et al., 2005). Some of the side effects include gastrointestinal (GI) problems, fatigue, mood swings, and dizziness. There is a black box warning relative to liver problems, higher levels of aggression/hostility, as well as suicidal thinking.

The drug bupropion (Wellbutrin) has been approved for the treatment of depression and smoking cessation in adults. Its exact mechanism of action is unclear, but it does seem to have both dopaminergic and noradrenergic effects. In one large placebo-controlled trial, it was effective for ADHD, although again the magnitude of the effect was less than that for stimulants (Conners et al., 1996). Side effects can include GI problems and agitation and a reduced seizure threshold. A SR preparation is available.

The shorter acting adrenergic agents—clonidine (Catapres, Kapvay) and guanfacine (Tenex)—have been used for many years in the treatment of tics and ADHD, although they were only FDA approved for hypertension. More recently, the extended-release forms of both clonidine (Kapvay) and guanfacine (Intuniv) have been approved for ADHD as have the shorter acting forms. A meta-analysis of the efficacy of alpha-2 agonists for ADHD (Hirota et al., 2014) has shown reduction in overall ADHD as well as specific individual symptoms generally, with a moderate effect size for the major symptoms of hyperactivity,

TABLE 29.2

Nonstimulant Medications for Attention-Deficit Hyperactivity Disorder

Medication	Drug Name	Frequency	Daily Dose Range
Atomoxetine	Strattera®	Daily or twice daily	0.5–1.2 mg/kg/day (<70 kg) 40–80 mg/day (≥70 kg)
Clonidine	Clonidine IR®	Twice daily to 4× per day	0.05–0.4 mg/day
	Clonidine ER (Kapvay®)	Daily	0.1–0.4 mg/day
Guanfacine	Guanfacine IR®	Twice daily to 4× per day	0.5–0.4 mg/day
	Guanfacine ER (Intuniv®)	Daily	1–4 mg/day
Desipramine	Norpramin®	Twice daily to 3× per day	2–5 mg/kg/day
Bupropion	Wellbutrin®	Twice daily	50–150 mg

Reprinted with permission from Bloch, M., Beyer, C., & Martin, A. (2018). ADHD: Stimulant and nonstimulant agents. In A. Martin, M. H. Bloch, & F. R. Volkmar (Eds.), *Lewis's child and adolescent psychiatry: A comprehensive textbook* (5th ed., p. 722). Wolters Kluwer.

impulsivity, and inattention. These agents may be particularly useful for children with both tics and ADHD (Weisman et al., 2013). The presumed mechanism of actions relate to central noradrenergic activity. Starting doses are small and gradually increased, patch and extended-release forms are available. Side effects of both clonidine and guanfacine are rather similar and include sedation, irritability, sleep problems. At doses usually given to children and adolescents, hypotension is not a problem although blood pressure should be monitored. Rapid withdrawal may be associated with rebound hypertension.

THE ANTIDEPRESSANT MEDICATIONS

The various antidepressant medications are a rather diverse set of drugs, all of which have been shown to be effective in the treatment of depression in adults as well as for some other conditions, notably obsessive compulsive disorder, various anxiety disorders, autism, and posttraumatic stress disorder, among others (see Chapters 12, 13, and 23). These agents have somewhat different chemical structures and mechanisms of action. Some are SSRIs, whereas others are selective norepinephrine reuptake inhibitors (SNRIs), or inhibitors of monoamine oxidase inhibitors. There are some newer agents with different mechanisms of action as well (Bloch, Beyer, Martin, et al., 2018b). Of all of these, the SSRIs are the most extensively used and studied. This group of agents strongly inhibit reuptake of the neurotransmitter into presynaptic neurons. This is in contrast to other agents like the older tricyclics, which inhibit reuptake both of NE and serotonin. The group of SSRIs have been FDA approved for the treatment of obsessive compulsive disorder (OCD) in adults and, except for fluvoxamine, are all approved for use in adult depression as well. Table 29.3 summarizes features of these agents.

Research has been much more extensive in adults than in children, although these medications are frequently used with children. When these agents were first introduced they had a major impact on pediatric drug treatments because they were easier to use than the older tricyclic antidepressants (TCAs), did not have the same cardiac side effects of the TCAs,

TABLE 29.3

Clinical Guidance for Antidepressant Medications Utilized in Pediatric Practice

	Pediatric		Adult		
	Starting Dose (mg/day)	Typical Dose Range (mg/day)	Starting Dose (mg/day)	Typical Dose Range (mg/day)	Half-Life
Selective Serotonin Reuptake Inhibitors					
Citalopram	10	20–40	20	40	20 hours
Escitalopram	5	10–40	10	20–40	27–32 hours
Fluoxetine	10–20	20–80	20	20–80	4–6 days
Fluvoxamine	25–50	5–0	100–300	100–300	16 hours
Paroxetine	10	20–60	10–20	40–60	21 hours
Sertraline	25–50	100–200	50	150–250	26 hours
Serotonin Norepinephrine Reuptake Inhibitors					
Venlafaxine	37.5	150–225	37.5–75	75–375	10 hours
Duloxetine	40	40–60	20–60	20–80	12.5 hours
Desvenlafaxine	10	10–100	50	50–400	11 hours
Atypical Antidepressants					
Bupropion	100	150–300	100–150	150–300	21 hours
Mirtazapine	7.5	15–45	15	15–45	20–40 hours
Vilazodone	Not studied		10	10–40	25 hours
Vortioxetine	Not studied		10	10–80	66 hours
Trazodone	25–50	100–150	150	150–300	3–9 hours
Tricyclic Antidepressants					
Clomipramine	25	50–200	25	100–250	32 hours
Desipramine	25	50–200	100–200	150–300	12–27 hours
Nortriptyline	30–50	30–150	100	75–150	18–44 hours

Reprinted with permission from Bloch, M., Beyer, C., & Martin, A. (2018). Antidepressants. In A. Martin, M. H. Bloch, & F. R. Volkmar (Eds.), *Lewis's child and adolescent psychiatry: A comprehensive textbook* (5th ed., p. 727). Wolters Kluwer.

generally were well tolerated, and, in a series of studies, proved superior to the TCAs for the treatment of depression as well as OCD (Riddle et al., 2001).

Obsessive Compulsive Disorder

Several different SSRIs have now been approved for the treatment of OCD. These agents, sertraline, fluvoxamine, fluoxetine, and paroxetine, have proven benefit in well-controlled placebo-controlled studies (Geller et al., 2001, 2012; March et al., 1998; Riddle et al., 2001). Some children with OCD may have only some benefit (March et al., 1998). The combination of SSRI and cognitive behavioral therapy (CBT) has been shown to be superior to either alone (Bloch et al., 2006).

Autism Spectrum Disorder

Some children and youth with autism spectrum disorder (ASD) also have features of OCD, and there has been interest in the use of SSRIs in this group. One of the difficulties, of course, is that the repetitive behaviors so common (indeed frequently seen as a defining features of ASD) may differ from OCD in important ways, but clearly some children with ASD do have intrusive thoughts and recurrent behaviors suggestive of OCD. Unfortunately, evidence for the efficacy of SSRIs in this group of patients is mixed. King et al. (2009) in a large well-designed study found no benefit after 12 weeks of treatment with citalopram. Recent meta-analyses (Carrasco et al., 2012; Williams et al., 2013) found a small effect that might be attributed to publication bias (i.e., for positive reports only to be published).

Depressive Disorders

Various SSRIs including fluoxetine, sertraline, paroxetine, and citalopram have been used in the treatment of depression in children and youth. The study by Emslie et al. (1997) was the first to show superiority of fluoxetine over placebo. Subsequent work has confirmed this finding and extended these results to other agents in this group (Bloch, Beyer, Martin, et al., 2018b). Although studies observe some variability of response to the various agents, meta-analytic studies have failed to show significant differences although fluoxetine has seemed to have the best risk–benefit profile (Bloch, Beyer, Martin, et al., 2018b; Cipriani et al., 2016).

In the Treatment for Adolescents with Depression Study (TADS) (March et al., 2004), fluoxetine alone was compared to pill placebo, CBT alone, and the combination of CBT with active agent. The greatest treatment response was noted for the combined drug CBT group after 12 weeks of therapy. Both CBT by itself and fluoxetine by itself were superior to placebo. However, concern over the potential for increased suicidal ideation led to a FDA-mandated black box warning (see Rey & Martin, 2006). As Bloch, Beyer, Martin et al. (2018b) summarize, this is a complicated topic and there are reasons to question the black box warning. The recommendations for increased monitoring during early phases of treatment may be difficult to implement and hesitancy to use may contribute to increased suicide rates in children and adolescents. For example, practitioners may hesitate to use these agents if they are unable to provide the intensive monitoring recommended. This has become especially problematic in underserved areas, where nonspecialists may be reluctant to prescribe antidepressants to this population.

Anxiety Disorders

Sertraline has been shown to be effective (particularly if combined with CBT) in the treatment of social phobia and generalized anxiety disorder (Walkup et al., 2008) and has received FDA approval for these two conditions. The SSRI fluvoxamine has shown efficacy in the treatment of generalized anxiety disorder, social phobia, and separation anxiety, although it has not yet received FDA approval for these indications in children and adolescents (see Bloch, Beyer, Martin, et al., 2018b).

Mechanisms of Action and Pharmacokinetics

The specifics of clinical management and dosing recommendations are discussed extensively in Bloch, Beyer, Martin, et al. (2018b). Generally, these agents are well tolerated, although there is some potential for serious side effects but not in the usual dosage range. These agents can interact with other drugs. They sometimes cause activation, for example, restlessness, insomnia, disinhibition, agitation, and so forth (King et al., 1991). As noted earlier, despite the FDA black box warning, the apparent risk for increased suicidal thinking is actually probably low (Jane Garland et al., 2016). In adults, sexual dysfunction has been noted, but this has not frequently been reported in adolescents. Sometimes, a flu-like condition is noted following acute discontinuation of some of the shorter acting SSRIs; so a slow withdrawal is typically recommended. If effective, SSRIs can be continued longer term with periodic reassessments.

Partly reflecting their effectiveness, ease of use, and favorable side-effect profiles, the SSRIs have become very popular in the treatment of children and adolescents. All medical providers should be aware of medication status and potentials for drug interactions in this group of medications as well as recommendations for monitoring.

Tricyclic Antidepressants

The TCAs have been used over the years for a range of childhood disorders. Evidence in their favor is limited and somewhat mixed. There may be some potential use for ADHD and enuresis although not as first-line treatments (Spetie & Arnold, 2018). These drugs inhibit reuptake of NE and serotonin presynaptically, and it is thought that this enhances noradrenergic neurotransmission. There are significant concerns regarding potential cardiac toxicities and adverse effects of these agents, which should be used cautiously by experienced clinicians. Clomipramine is unusual in this group in that it has more of an effect on inhibition of serotonin reuptake, possibly accounting for its better effectiveness in the treatment of OCD. As a general rule, at present the TCAs are not used as first-line interventions. When they are used, electrocardiogram (ECG), pulse, and blood pressure at baseline and then monitoring treatment are important.

Given the better side-effect profile and safety of the SSRIs, the TCAs have become much less frequently used in children and adolescents. Many of their side effects relate to the anticholinergic effects of the agents including dry mouth, sedation, weight gain, agitation, tremor, and dizziness, among others. Cardiac conduction side effects can be dose related to prolonged QTc on the ECG. The TCAs also lower seizure thresholds. Drug interactions should be carefully monitored. Other antidepressant medications are available but are not well studied in children.

■ THE NEUROLEPTIC (ANTIPSYCHOTIC) MEDICATIONS

These medications have long been used in the treatment of a diverse group of disorders. These include psychosis and bipolar disorder as well as for tics, Tourette syndrome, and irritability in ASD (Bloch, Beyer, Scahill, et al., 2018a). These agents became available in the 1950s for the treatment of adults with psychotic conditions and provided one of the first truly effective drug treatments for psychosis. They quickly became studied in children. They can be grouped in various ways, for example, by chemical family and relative potency in dopamine blockage (their main mechanism of action). The more recent introduction of new types of these agents (the second- and third-generation neuroleptics or atypical neuroleptics) began with the use of clozapine and continued with drugs like risperidone and aripiprazole. Tables 29.4 and 29.5 give details on dosing, indication, and side effects. It is important to understand that the FDA approvals of these medications vary with the age of the child (see Bloch, Beyer, Scahill, et al., 2018a).

Treatment of psychosis has, overall, been the major use of these medications. Originally, studies were conducted in adults and adolescents and more recently in children. However, given concerns about the use of placebo in this serious condition, data in children are sparse. The available data (Bloch, Beyer, Scahill, et al., 2018a) do suggest their effectiveness in childhood psychosis. Differences between the agents in terms of their efficacy are minimal (Kumar et al., 2013), although the second-generation drugs are associated with greater weight gain (Sikich et al., 2008) but otherwise have some advantages in terms of side-effect profile.

These medications have also been studied for the treatment of bipolar disorder and shown to be effective. One large multisite study showed risperidone more effective in the treatment of manic symptoms in pediatric bipolar disorder (Geller et al., 2012). In tic disorders, several meta-analyses of randomized controlled trials (RCTs) have shown these agents safe and effective (Bloch, Beyer, Scahill, et al., 2018a; Ching & Pringsheim, 2012).

TABLE 29.4

Clinical Guidance for Antipsychotic Medications Utilized in Pediatric Practice

	Pediatric			Adult		
	Starting Dose (mg/day)	Typical Dose Range (mg/day)	Number of Daily Doses	Starting Dose (mg/day)	Typical Dose Range (mg/day)	Number of Daily Doses
Second-Generation (Atypical) Antipsychotics						
Risperidone	0.5–2	1–6	1–2	2	2–6	1–2
Aripiprazole	2–5	5–30	1	5–15	10–30	1
Quetiapine	25–50	100–800	2–3	50–100	150–800	2–3
Olanzapine	2.5–5	5–20	1	5–10	5–20	1
Ziprasidone	5–20	40–160	2	40–80	80–160	2
Clozapine	12.5–50	300–900	2	25–50	300–900	1–2
Paliperidone	3	3–12	1	3–6	3–12	1
Lurasidone	20	20–160	1	20–40	20–160	1
Asenapine	5	5–20	2	10–20	10–20	2
First-Generation (Typical) Antipsychotics						
Haloperidol	1–10	2–30	2–3	2–15	2–50	2–3
Molindone	25–75	50–225	3–4	50–75	50–225	3–4
Pimozide	0.5–2	1–6	1–2	1–2	2–10	1–2
Chlorpromazine	30–75	50–200	4	30–75	200–400	3–4
Perphenazine	6–12	12–32	2–4	12–24	16–32	2–4
Fluphenazine	1–10	2.5–20	3–4	2–10	10–40	3–4
Thioridazine	25–50	25–200	2–4	150–300	200–800	2–4

Reprinted with permission from Bloch, M., Beyer, C., & Scahill, L. (2018). Antipsychotics. In A. Martin, M. H. Bloch, & F. R. Volkmar (Eds.), *Lewis's child and adolescent psychiatry: A comprehensive textbook* (5th ed., p. 734). Wolters Kluwer.

Several RCTs of the atypical antipsychotics have shown significant improvement in irritability and aggression in children both with and without ASD (Ching & Pringsheim, 2012; Loy et al., 2012). For irritability in ASD, risperidone and aripiprazole have been the agents most frequently used and are effective.

Although well-controlled studies have not yet been done in severe and treatment-refractory OCD the augmentation of SSRI treatment has been suggested (Bloch et al., 2006). These medications typically are only used after a realistic treatment trial of an SSRI and should be discontinued if improvement is not observed after 6–12 weeks of treatment (Bloch & Storch, 2015). In treatment-refractory depression, antipsychotic augmentation has also proven useful (Nelson & Papakostas, 2009).

Information on dosing is provided in Table 29.4. The use of these agents is discussed in greater detail in Bloch, Beyer, Scahill, et al. (2018a). Probably the greatest interest has centered on the use of the new agents like risperidone (Risperdal), which has, in adults, been shown to be effective with a lower risk of side effects as compared to the older traditional agents like

TABLE 29.5

Side-Effect Profile of Commonly Prescribed Antipsychotic Medications

	Extrapy-ramidal	Sedation	Weight Gain	Hypergly-cemia	Anticho-linergic	Ortho-static Hyperten-sion
Second-Generation (Atypical) Antipsychotics						
Risperidone	+ +	+ +	+ +	+ +	−	+ +
Aripiprazole	+	+	+	−	−	+
Quetiapine	+	+ + +	+ +	+ + +	+ +	+ +
Olanzapine	+	+ + +	+ + +	+ + +	+ + +	+
Ziprasidone	+	+ +	+	+	+	+ +
Clozapine	+	+ + +	+ + +	+ + +	+ + +	+ +
Paliperidone	+	+	+	−	−	+
Lurasidone	+ + +	+ + +	−	−	−	−
Asenapine	+	+	+	+	−	+
First-Generation (Typical) Antipsychotics						
Haloperidol	+ + +	+	+ +	+ +	+	+
Molindone	+ +	−	−	−	+	+
Pimozide	+ + +	+ +	Not reported		+ +	+
Chlorpromazine	+ +	+ + +	+ + +	+ + +	+ + +	+ + +
Perphenazine	+ +	+ +	Not reported		+	+
Fluphenazine	+ + +	+	+	+	+	+
Thioridazine	+	+ +	+	+	+ +	+ +

Key: + + + ≥20% incidence; + + 10–20% incidence; + 1–10% incidence; −minimal evidence of effect.
Reprinted with permission from Bloch, M., Beyer, C., & Scahill, L. (2018). Antipsychotics. In A. Martin, M. H. Bloch, & F. R. Volkmar (Eds.), *Lewis's child and adolescent psychiatry: A comprehensive textbook* (5th ed., p. 735). Wolters Kluwer.

haloperidol. Several studies have now demonstrated its safety and efficacy in children for the treatment of schizophrenia, mania, and irritability in autism (McCracken et al., 2002). The major side effect of this agent has been weight gain.

Aripiprazole (Abilify) is a third-generation antipsychotic that functions as a partial dopamine agonist as well as having serotonin blocking properties. Like risperidone it has been shown to be effective in the treatment of adolescents with schizophrenia, mania, tic disorders, and irritability in children with ASD (Owen et al., 2009). This agent and risperidone are the only FDA-approved medications for the treatment of irritability in ASD.

Other agents sometimes used include quetiapine (Seroquel), a second-generation antipsychotic that is increasingly studied in the pediatric population. It has been used in the treatment of both schizophrenia and the manic phase of bipolar mania (Pathak et al., 2013). The drug ziprasidone (Geodon) is another antipsychotic medication useful in the treatment of adults with schizophrenia and used in at least one study of Tourette Syndrome. The neuroleptic olanzapine (Zyprexa) (Owen et al., 2009) has atypical features in lower dose ranges in adults and has been approved for the treatment of bipolar I depression in children and adolescents. There has been concern about significant weight gain with this agent (McClellan et al., 2007).

Various other drugs in this category are available (Bloch, Beyer, Scahill, et al., 2018a). The mechanisms of these agents relate to blockage of postsynaptic dopaminergic D2 receptors with differences in effect related to the regional specificity of this action and impact on other neurotransmitter systems. The newer atypical antipsychotics have their action through blockage of both serotonin and dopamine and serotonin postsynaptic receptors. This addition of serotoninergic blockage may account for the lower rates of neurologic side effects. All these agents also have effects related to their anticholinergic, antihistamine, and adrenergic-blocking properties; these differences account for many of the differences in side effects observed (see Bloch, Beyer, Scahill, et al., 2018a). Neurologic side effects like dystonic reactions, akathisia, and rigidity and stiffness are clearly more frequent with the higher potency antipsychotics. The first-generation agents also have an association with weight gain, increased risk of diabetes, and increased prolactin (gynecomastia in boys and galactorrhea or amenorrhea with girls; Bloch, Beyer, Scahill, et al., 2018a). The anticholinergic side effects can include dry mouth, constipation, and blurry vision. Some of these agents also can prolong cardiac conduction times (Blair et al., 2004). Careful monitoring is needed (see Bloch, Beyer, Scahill, et al., 2018a). Given their much better side-effect profiles, the atypical antipsychotics have come into more frequent use but also have side effects. The drug clozapine is associated with serious side effects and is typically used only for treatment-resistant schizophrenia. Weight gain has been noted with clozapine, olanzapine, quetiapine, and risperidone particularly in the first months of treatment (Ratzoni et al., 2002).

Tardive dyskinesia is one of the most serious adverse reactions to antipsychotic medications (Riddle et al., 1987). Accordingly careful follow-up and monitoring for abnormal movement is needed. At times withdrawal dyskinesia can be difficult to distinguish from tardive dyskinesia (Wagner et al., 2002). Unfortunately data on best practice approaches to discontinuing these agents are limited. Usually this should be done on a gradual, thoughtful basis with consideration of discontinuation on an annual basis. The goal is to have the lowest effective dose.

The rare adverse side effect of neuroleptic malignant syndrome (NMS) is characterized by high fever, autonomic instability, and muscle breakdown and is a serious medical emergency with a significant mortality rate in children (nearly 10%) (Silva et al., 1999). Parents and caregivers and all medical care professionals involved should be aware of this potentially life-threatening side effect. Typically, discontinuation of the medication is all that is needed but at times intravenous (IV) hydration and hospitalization may be needed.

Some of the side effects of these agents can be prevented or treated with the use of anticholinergic agents. The motor side effects are particularly common with the higher potency medications, and although these are less common with the newer atypical medications they still can be noted particularly at higher dose levels. Anticholinergic/antihistaminic drugs can reverse many of these neurologic side effects, but care needs to be taken given the potential for the side effects of these agents to further complicate treatment. Usually diphenhydramine (Benadryl) is the initial treatment followed by longer term treatment with benztropine (Cogentin). Diphenhydramine is typically available both at home as well as in the emergency room but its longer term use is associated with sedation. Benztropine is usually preferred as a longer term treatment given the absence of the sedative effect. These agents should be avoided in very young children due to their side effects.

MOOD STABILIZERS

Lithium was discovered to be an effective mood stabilizer over 50 years ago and quickly became the standard treatment for bipolar illness. It remains one of two agents approved by the FDA for youth (over 12 years) with acute mania and maintenance therapy for bipolar disorder in youth. A number of other mood stabilizers are available and approved for use in adults. Mood stabilizers have frequently been used for the treatment of lability and aggression in children, although the supporting scientific data are, at best, modest. Table 29.6 summarizes the information on these agents in pediatric populations.

In addition to the mood stabilizers, several atypical antipsychotics have been found to be effective and are also approved for the treatment of acute mania and mixed episodes as well as chronic treatment of bipolar disorder in the pediatric age group (Bloch, Beyer, Scahill, et al., 2018b). One well-designed RCT found risperidone more effective than lithium or valproic in mania (Geller et al., 2012). A second study with younger children compared risperidone to valproic acid and found similar results (Kowatch et al., 2015). Accordingly now mood stabilizers in bipolar disorder usually are used in conjunction with an atypical antipsychotic.

As Bloch, Beyer, Scahill, et al. (2018b) point out, a major complication for this literature has been continued controversies and inconsistencies in diagnosis. Recent work in the pediatric age group suggests two somewhat distinctive disorders—one the more classic bipolar and the other disruptive mood dysregulation disorder (DMDD) (Regier et al., 2013). Clarification of this issue remains an important challenge for the field.

Lithium (Lithobid, Eskalith)

A solid body of research demonstrates the efficacy of lithium both for the acute manic phase as well as maintenance phase of children and youth with the more classical forms of bipolar disorder (Bloch, Beyer, Scahill, et al., 2018b). Given the results discussed earlier of the efficacy of risperidone, it is now more frequent to use lithium in conjunction with the atypical neuroleptic (Kafantaris et al., 2001). There are some limited data on the use of lithium in the acute depression phase of bipolar 1 disorder (Delbello et al., 2006). Lithium has also been found to be superior to placebo in the treatment of aggression in conduct disorders (Rifkin et al., 1997). A Cochrane meta-analysis found lithium was effective in reducing suicide risk in individuals with mood disorder. This may reflect its impact on issues of aggression and impulsive behavior (Bloch, Beyer, Scahill, et al., 2018b). Lithium does impact a number of neurotransmitter systems, but its main effect appears to relate to intracellular signaling processes (Manji & Lenox, 1998).

Typically peak levels of lithium are achieved 1–4 hours after ingestion. Both a liquid form and extended-release forms are available. The drug is excreted directly by the kidney and the half-life in children (18 hours) is slightly shorter than that in adults. One implication of this shorter half-life in children is the more rapid achievement of reliable blood levels (typically after about 4 days).

Drugs that impact kidney functioning may interact with lithium excretion in the kidney. These include anti-inflammatory drugs, tetracyclines, and certain diuretics. Before a lithium trial is done, a medical evaluation should include assessment of thyroid and kidney functioning and complete blood count and electrolytes. A very handy guide for dosing has been developed by Weller et al. (1986); doses vary with age and size. Usually, once a response is achieved at maintenance levels, it is important that lithium levels be closely monitored and maintained in the range of 0.6–1.1 mEq/L to find the lowest effective dose (see Bloch, Beyer, Scahill, et al., 2018b). Usually effects are seen in a few days but can take as long as several weeks (Kowatch et al., 2000). Regular medical follow-up is needed.

Generally lithium is well tolerated. Some of the more common side effects can include tremor, ataxia, GI problems, fatigue, and cognitive dulling. Kidney disease is a contraindication to use given the central role of the kidneys in excretion. Lithium toxicity can appear even at relatively low levels and can include weakness and cognitive impairment. Dehydration is a frequent source of toxicity and other side effects have been noted (Bloch, Beyer, Scahill, et al., 2018b).

TABLE 29.6

Clinical Guidance on Mood Stabilizers Used in Pediatric Practice

Drug	Mechanism of Action	Main Indications and Clinical Uses	Dosage	Schedule	Adverse Effects	Comments
Lithium	Inhibition of phosphatidylinositol and protein kinase C signaling pathways; enhancement of serotonergic transmission	Bipolar disorder, manic; prophylaxis of bipolar disorder; MDD aggressive behavior/conduct disorder; adjunct treatment in refractory MDD	10–30 mg/kg/day, dose adjusted to serum levels in the range of 0.6–1.1 mEq/L	bid/tid	Polyuria, polydipsia, tremor, ataxia, nausea, diarrhea, weight gain, drowsiness, acne, hair loss; possible effects on thyroid and renal functioning with long-term administration; children prone to dehydration are at higher risk for acute lithium toxicity; lithium levels>2 mEq/L can be life threatening	Therapy requires monitoring of lithium levels, thyroid and renal function
Divalproex	Inhibition of catabolic enzymes of GABA and of protein kinase C signaling	Bipolar disorder; aggressive behavior; conduct disorder; seizure disorders	15–60 mg/kg/day, dose adjusted to serum levels in the range of 50–125 mcg/L	bid/tid	Sedation, nausea, liver toxicity (requires baseline and close monitoring), thrombocytopenia, pancreatitis	Polycystic ovarian disorder has been reported during long-term use for seizure control

(continued)

TABLE 29.6

Clinical Guidance on Mood Stabilizers Used in Pediatric Practice (*continued*)

Drug	Mechanism of Action	Main Indications and Clinical Uses	Dosage	Schedule	Adverse Effects	Comments
Carbamazepine	Inhibition of glial steroidogenesis; inhibition of alpha 2 receptors; blocks sodium	Bipolar disorder; complex partial seizures	10–20 mg/kg/day, dose adjusted to serum levels in the range of 4–14 mcg/L	bid	Bone marrow suppression (requires baseline and close monitoring of blood counts); dizziness, drowsiness, rashes, nausea, liver toxicity, especially under 10 years of age	Potent inductor of CYP3A4, leading to auto-induction requiring periodic dose adjustment
Oxcarbazepine	Channels block glial calcium influx	Seizure disorders	Maintenance dose of 18.5–48 mg/kg/day, not to exceed 2100 mg/day		No reports of bone marrow suppression, more benign drug interaction profile compared to carbamazepine; no blood level monitoring necessary	No empirical data available for children and adolescents
Lamotrigine	Weak 5HT3 inhibition; release of aspartate and glutamate	Bipolar depression and maintenance therapy; seizure disorders	75–300 mg/day	qd	Potentially life-threatening rash; Stevens–Johnson syndrome (dose-[direct] and age-[inverse] related event rates)	Slow dose titration (12.5 mg qo wk) may reduce risk of skin reactions

GABA, gamma aminobutyric acid; MDD, major depressive disorder.
Reprinted with permission from Bloch, M., Beyer, C., & Scahill, L. (2018). Mood stabilizers. In A. Martin, M. H. Bloch, & F. R. Volkmar (Eds.), *Lewis's child and adolescent psychiatry: A comprehensive textbook* (5th ed., p. 743). Wolters Kluwer.

Valproate (Depakote, Depakene)

The anticonvulsant Valproate has been effective in adults as a mood stabilizer. However, studies in the pediatric population are rather limited. It appears to have multiple mechanisms of action (Czapiński et al., 2005). Several forms are available (Bloch, Beyer, Scahill, et al., 2018b). A physical examination and laboratory studies should be obtained before treatment and the agent regularly monitored. Side effects include GI difficulties, liver toxicity, and occasional hair loss. Most important there is significant risk for fetal malformation in teenage females who become pregnant so education and use of birth control is very strongly advised. There are a number of other risks (Alsdorf & Wyszynski, 2005).

Carbamazepine (Tegretol)

This anticonvulsant was first approved by the FDA in 2004 for the treatment of acute mania and mixed bipolar disorder in adults. There have been some open-label and case series studies in children. One study of conduct disordered children did not find it better than placebo (Cueva et al., 1996). Another open-label study (Joshi et al., 2010) of bipolar disorder in children found a modest benefit. One well-designed study using extended-release forms of the agent did find it effective for acute manic or mixed episodes (Joshi et al., 2010).

The mechanisms of action are poorly understand. There are both immediate-release forms as well as SR preparations available. The agent is absorbed relatively slowly with a peak level in 2–8 hours. A lower initial dose is gradually increased in divided daily doses. Adjustments are often needed early in treatment, and prior to treatment a physical examination and liver, complete blood count (CBC), and kidney function studies are obtained. There is some evidence of fetal toxicity.

Other Agents

The anticonvulsant Lamotrigine (Lamictal) has been effective in adults for the treatment of bipolar 1 depression as well as in mood stabilization and prophylaxis in rapid cycling and bipolar 2 patients (Gao & Calabrese, 2005). One recent well-designed multicenter and placebo-controlled trial did not show significant benefit on the primary outcome measure, but some secondary benefits were noted (Fung et al., 2004). The agent frequently causes skin rashes usually mild and early in treatment, but it can be associated with Stevens–Johnson Syndrome (a potentially fatal condition associated with widespread skin sloughing) so careful follow-up and patient education are needed (see Bloch, Beyer, Scahill, et al., 2018b).

▰ SUMMARY

In this chapter, we have summarized much of the available literature on pediatric psychopharmacology. Yet other agents that we have not discussed in this chapter, for example, drug treatments for enuresis, are discussed in other chapters in this book. Clearly this is an area where knowledge has increased dramatically. Still as compared to work with adults, much remains to be done in terms of understanding not only the practical uses of medications but also their basic mechanisms of actions and potential risks and benefits. Recent mandates for study registration will help us understand more about drugs (and studies) that don't work. For the student who is interested in more detailed reading, the chapters from *Lewis's Child and Adolescent Psychiatry, 5th ed.*, (2018) provide important and more detailed reading and a number of specialized texts are available.

References

Alsdorf, R., & Wyszynski, D. F. (2005). Teratogenicity of sodium valproate. *Expert Opinion on Drug Safety*, 4(2), 345–353. https://doi.org/10.1517/14740338.4.2.345

Anderson, G. M., & Martin, A. (2018). Neurochemsitry pharmacodynamics, and biological psychiatry. In A. Martin, M. Bloch, & F. R. Volkmar (Eds.), *Lewis's child and adolescent psychiatry* (pp. 688–702). Wolters Kluwer.

Biederman, J., & Spencer, T. (1999). Attention-deficit/hyperactivity disorder (ADHD) as a noradrenergic disorder. *Biological Psychiatry*, 46(9), 1234–1242. https://doi.org/10.1016/s0006-3223(99)00192-4

Blair, J., Taggart, B., & Martin, A. (2004). Electrocardiographic safety profile and monitoring guidelines in pediatric psychopharmacology. *Journal of Neural Transmission*, 111(7), 791–815. https://doi .org/10.1007/s00702-004-0153-8

Bloch, M., Beyer, C., Martin, A., & Scahill, L. (2018a). ADHD: Stimulants and nonstimulant agents. In A. Martin, M. Bloch, & F. R. Volkmar (Eds.), *Lewis's child and adolescent psychiatry* (5th ed., pp. 718–724). Wolters Kluwer.

Bloch, M., Beyer, C., Martin, A., & Scahill, L. (2018b). Antidepressants. In A. Martin, M. Bloch, & F. R. Volkmar (Eds.), *Lewis's child and adolescent psychiatry* (pp. 724–732). Wolters Kluwer.

Bloch, M., Beyer, C., Scahill, L., & Martin, A. (2018a). Anti-psychotics. In A. Martin, M. Bloch, & F. R. Volkmar (Eds.), *Lewis's child and adolescent psychiatry* (5th ed., pp. 733–741). Wolters Kluwer.

Bloch, M., Beyer, C., Scahill, L., & Martin, A. (2018b). Mood stabilizers. In A. Martin, M. Bloch, & F. R. Volkmar (Eds.), *Lewis's child and adolescent psychiatry* (5th ed., pp. 742–749). Wolters Kluwer.

Bloch, M. H., Landeros-Weisenberger, A., Kelmendi, B., Coric, V., Bracken, M. B., & Leckman, J. F. (2006). A systematic review: Antipsychotic augmentation with treatment refractory obsessive-compulsive disorder. *Molecular Psychiatry*, 11(7), 622–632. https://doi.org/10.1038/sj.mp.4001823

Bloch, M. H., Panza, K. E., Landeros-Weisenberger, A., & Leckman, J. F. (2009). Meta-analysis: Treatment of attention-deficit/hyperactivity disorder in children with comorbid tic disorders. *Journal of the American Academy of Child & Adolescent Psychiatry*, 48(9), 884–893. https://doi.org/10.1097/ CHI.0b013e3181b26e9f

Bloch, M. H., & Storch, E. A. (2015). Assessment and management of treatment-refractory obsessive-compulsive disorder in children. *Journal of the American Academy of Child & Adolescent Psychiatry*, 54(4), 251–262. https://doi.org/10.1016/j.jaac.2015.01.011

Bradley, C. (1937). The behavior of children receiving benzedrine. *American Journal of Psychiatry*, 94(3), 577–585. https://doi.org/10.1176/ajp.94.3.577

Braslow, J. T., & Marder, S. R. (2019). History of psychopharmacology. *Annual Review of Clinical Psychology*, 15, 25–50. https://doi.org/10.1146/annurev-clinpsy-050718-095514

Carrasco, M., Volkmar, F. R., & Bloch, M. H. (2012). Pharmacologic treatment of repetitive behaviors in autism spectrum disorders: Evidence of publication bias. *Pediatrics*, 129(5), e1301–e1310. https://doi .org/10.1542/peds.2011-3285

Chen, L. Y., Crum, R. M., Strain, E. C., Alexander, G. C., Kaufmann, C., & Mojtabai, R. (2016). Prescriptions, nonmedical use, and emergency department visits involving prescription stimulants. *The Journal of Clinical Psychiatry*, 77(3), e297–e304. https://doi.org/10.4088/JCP.14m09291

Ching, H., & Pringsheim, T. (2012). Aripiprazole for autism spectrum disorders (ASD). *Cochrane Database of Systematic Reviews*, 5, CD009043, https://doi.org/10.1002/14651858.CD009043.pub2

Cipriani, A., Zhou, X., Del Giovane, C., Hetrick, S. E., Qin, B., Whittington, C., Coghill, D., Zhang, Y., Hazell, P., Leucht, S., Cuijpers, P., Pu, J., Cohen, D., Ravindran, A. V., Liu, Y., Michael, K. D., Yang, L., Liu, L., & Xie, P. (2016). Comparative efficacy and tolerability of antidepressants for major depressive disorder in children and adolescents: A network meta-analysis. *Lancet*, 388(10047), 881–890. https:// doi.org/10.1016/S0140-6736(16)30385-3

Cohen, S. C., Mulqueen, J. M., Ferracioli-Oda, E., Stuckelman, Z. D., Coughlin, C. G., Leckman, J. F., & Bloch, M. H. (2015). Meta-analysis: Risk of tics associated with psychostimulant use in randomized, placebo-controlled trials. *Journal of the American Academy of Child & Adolescent Psychiatry*, 54(9), 728–736. https://doi.org/10.1016/j.jaac.2015.06.011

Conners, C. K., Casat, C. D., Gualtieri, C. T., Weller, E., Reader, M., Reiss, A., Weller, R. A., Khayrallah, M., & Ascher, J. (1996). Bupropion hydrochloride in attention deficit disorder with hyperactivity. *Journal of the American Academy of Child & Adolescent Psychiatry*, 35(10), 1314–1321. https://doi .org/10.1097/00004583-199610000-00018

Cueva, J. E., Overall, J. E., Small, A. M., Armenteros, J. L., Perry, R., & Campbell, M. (1996). Carbamazepine in aggressive children with conduct disorder: A double-blind and placebo-controlled study. *Journal of the American Academy of Child & Adolescent Psychiatry*, 35(4), 480–490. https://doi .org/10.1097/00004583-199604000-00014

Czapiński, P., Blaszczyk, B., & Czuczwar, S. J. (2005). Mechanisms of action of antiepileptic drugs. *Current Topics in Medicinal Chemistry*, 5(1), 3–14. https://doi.org/10.2174/1568026053386962

Delbello, M. P., Kowatch, R. A., Adler, C. M., Stanford, K. E., Welge, J. A., Barzman, D. H., Nelson, E., & Strakowski, S. M. (2006). A double-blind randomized pilot study comparing quetiapine and divalproex for adolescent mania. *Journal of the American Academy of Child & Adolescent Psychiatry*, 45(3), 305–313. https://doi.org/10.1097/01.chi.0000194567.63289.97 PMID: 16540815.

Elia, J. (1991). Stimulants and antidepressant pharmacokinetics in hyperactive children. *Psychopharmacology Bulletin*, 27(4), 411–415.

Emslie, G. J., Rush, A. J., Weinberg, W. A., Kowatch, R. A., Hughes, C. W., Carmody, T., & Rintelmann, J. (1997). A double-blind, randomized, placebo-controlled trial of fluoxetine in children and adolescents with depression. *Archives of General Psychiatry*, 54(11), 1031–1037. https://doi.org/10.1001/archpsyc.1997.01830230069010

Fung, J., Mok, H., & Yatham, L. N. (2004). Lamotrigine for bipolar disorder: Translating research into clinical practice. *Expert Review of Neurotherapeutics*, 4(3), 363–370. https://doi.org/10.1586/14737175.4.3.363

Gao, K., & Calabrese, J. R. (2005). Newer treatment studies for bipolar depression. *Bipolar Disorder*, 7(5, Suppl.), 13–23. https://doi.org/10.1111/j.1399-5618.2005.00250.x

Geller, B., Luby, J. L., Joshi, P., Wagner, K. D., Emslie, G., Walkup, J. T., Axelson, D.A., Bolhofner, K., Robb, A., Wolf, D. V., Riddle, M. A., Birmaher, B., Nusrat, N., Yan, N. D., Vitiello, B., Tillman, R., & Lavori, P. (2012). A randomized controlled trial of risperidone, lithium, or divalproex sodium for initial treatment of bipolar I disorder, manic or mixed phase, in children and adolescents. *Archives of General Psychiatry*, 69(5), 515–528. https://doi.org/10.1001/archgenpsychiatry.2011.1508

Geller, D. A., Hoog, S. L., Heiligenstein, J. H., Ricardi, R. K., Tamura, R., Kluszynski, S., Jacobson, J. G., & Fluoxetine Pediatric OCD Study Team. (2001). Fluoxetine treatment for obsessive-compulsive disorder in children and adolescents: A placebo-controlled clinical trial. *Journal of the American Academy of Child & Adolescent Psychiatry*, 40(7), 773–779. https://doi.org/10.1097/00004583-200107000-00011

Greenhill, L. L., Abikoff, H. B., Arnold, L. E., Cantwell, D. P., Conners, C. K., Elliott, G., Hechtman, L., Hinshaw, S. P., Hoza, B., Jensen, P. S., March, J. S., Newcorn, J., Pelham, W. E., Severe, J. B., Swanson, J. M., Vitiello, B., & Wells, K. (1996). Medication treatment strategies in the MTA Study: Relevance to clinicians and researchers. *Journal of the American Academy of Child & Adolescent Psychiatry*, 35(10), 1304–1313. https://doi.org/10.1097/00004583-199610000-00017

Hirota, T., Schwartz, S., & Correll, C. U. (2014). Alpha-2 agonists for attention-deficit/hyperactivity disorder in youth: A systematic review and meta-analysis of monotherapy and add-on trials to stimulant therapy. *Journal of the American Academy of Child & Adolescent Psychiatry*, 53(2), 153–173. https://doi.org/10.1016/j.jaac.2013.11.009

Jane Garland, E., Kutcher, S., Virani, A., & Elbe, D. (2016). Update on the use of SSRIs and SNRIs with children and adolescents in clinical practice. *Journal of the Canadian Academy of Child and Adolescent Psychiatry*, 25(1), 4–10.

Joshi, G., Wozniak, J., Mick, E., Doyle, R., Hammerness, P., Georgiopoulos, A., Kotarski, M., Aleardi, M., Williams, C., Walls, S., & Biederman, J. (2010). A prospective open-label trial of extended-release carbamazepine monotherapy in children with bipolar disorder. *Journal of Child and Adolescent Psychopharmacology*, 20(1), 7–14. https://doi.org/10.1089/cap.2008.0162

Kafantaris, V., Coletti, D. J., Dicker, R., Padula, G., & Kane, J. M. (2001). Adjunctive antipsychotic treatment of adolescents with bipolar psychosis. *Journal of the American Academy of Child & Adolescent Psychiatry*, 40(12), 1448–1456. https://doi.org/10.1097/00004583-200112000-00016

King, B. H., Hollander, E., Sikich, L., McCracken, J. T., Scahill, L., Bregman, J. D., Donnelly, C. L., Anagnostou, E., Dukes, K., Sullivan, L., Hirtz, D., Wagner, A., Ritz, L., & STAART Psychopharmacology Network. (2009). Lack of efficacy of citalopram in children with autism spectrum disorders and high levels of repetitive behavior: Citalopram ineffective in children with autism. *Archives of General Psychiatry*, 66(6), 583–590. https://doi.org/10.1001/archgenpsychiatry.2009.30

King, R. A., Riddle, M. A., Chappell, P. B., Hardin, M. T., Anderson, G. M., Lombroso, P., & Scahill, L. (1991). Emergence of self-destructive phenomena in children and adolescents during fluoxetine treatment. *Journal of the American Academy of Child & Adolescent Psychiatry*, 30(2), 179–186. https://doi.org/10.1097/00004583-199103000-00003

Kowatch, R. A., Scheffer, R. E., Monroe, E., Delgado, S., Altaye, M., & Lagory, D. (2015). Placebo-controlled trial of valproic acid versus risperidone in children 3–7 years of age with bipolar I disorder. *Journal of Child and Adolescent Psychopharmacology*, 25(4), 306–313. https://doi.org/10.1089/cap.2014.0166

Kowatch, R. A., Suppes, T., Carmody, T. J., Bucci, J. P., Hume, J. H., Kromelis, M., Emslie, G. J., Weinberg, W. A., & Rush, A. J. (2000). Effect size of lithium, divalproex sodium, and carbamazepine in children and adolescents with bipolar disorder. *Journal of the American Academy of Child & Adolescent Psychiatry*, 39(6), 713–720. https://doi.org/10.1097/00004583-200006000-00009

Kumar, A., Datta, S. S., Wright, S. D., Furtado, V. A., & Russell, P. S. (2013). Atypical antipsychotics for psychosis in adolescents. *Cochrane Database of Systematic Reviews, 10,* CD009582. https://doi .org/10.1002/14651858.CD009582.pub2

Loy, J. H., Merry, S. N., Hetrick, S. E., & Stasiak, K. (2012). Atypical antipsychotics for disruptive behaviour disorders in children and youths. *Cochrane Database of Systematic Reviews, 9,* CD008559. https://doi.org/10.1002/14651858.CD008559.pub2

Manji, H. K., & Lenox, R. H. (1998). Lithium: A molecular transducer of mood-stabilization in the treatment of bipolar disorder. *Neuropsychopharmacology, 19*(3), 161–166. https://doi.org/10.1016/ S0893-133X(98)00021-9

March, J., Silva, S., Petrycki, S., Curry, J., Wells, K., Fairbank, J., Burns, B., Domino, M., McNulty, S., Vitiello, B., Severe, J., & Treatment for Adolescents with Depression Study (TADS) Team. (2004). Fluoxetine, cognitive-behavioral therapy, and their combination for adolescents with depression: Treatment for Adolescents with Depression Study (TADS) randomized controlled trial. *JAMA, 292*(7), 807–820. https://doi.org/10.1001/jama.292.7.807

March, J. S., Biederman, J., Wolkow, R., Safferman, A., Mardekian, J., Cook, E. H., Cutler, N. R., Dominguez, R., Ferguson, J., Muller, B., Riesenberg, R., Rosenthal, M., Sallee, F. R., Wagner, K. D., & Steiner, H. (1998). Sertraline in children and adolescents with obsessive-compulsive disorder: A multicenter randomized controlled trial. *JAMA, 280*(20), 1752–1756. https://doi.org/10.1001/ jama.280.20.1752

Martin, A., Scahill, L., Anderson, G. M., Aman, M., Arnold, L. E., McCracken, J., McDougle, C. J., Tierney, E., Chuang, S., & Vitiello, B. (2004). Weight and leptin changes among risperidone-treated youths with autism: 6-month prospective data. *American Journal of Psychiatry, 161*(6), 1125–1127. https://doi.org/10.1176/appi.ajp.161.6.1125

McClellan, J., Sikich, L., Findling, R. L., Frazier, J. A., Vitiello, B., Hlastala, S. A., Williams, E., Ambler, D., Hunt-Harrison, T., Maloney, A. E., Ritz, L., Anderson, R, Hamer, R. M., & Lieberman, J. A. (2007). Treatment of early-onset schizophrenia spectrum disorders (TEOSS): Rationale, design, and methods. *Journal of the American Academy of Child & Adolescent Psychiatry, 46*(8), 969–978. https://doi .org/10.1097/CHI.0b013e3180691779

McCracken, J. T., McGough, J., Shah, B., Cronin, P., Hong, D., Aman, M. G., Arnold, L. E., Lindsay, R., Nash, P., Hollway, J., McDougle, C. J., Posey, D., Swiezy, N., Kohn, A., Scahill, L., Martin, A., Koenig, K., Volkmar, F. R., Carroll, D.,... McMahon, D. (2002). Research units on pediatric psychopharmacology autism network. Risperidone in children with autism and serious behavioral problems. *New England Journal of Medicine, 347*(5), 314–321. https://doi.org/10.1056/ NEJMoa013171

McDougle, C. J., Scahill, L., McCracken, J. T., Aman, M. G., Tierney, E., Arnold, L. E., Freeman, B. J., Martin, A., McGough, J. J., Cronin, P., Posey, D. J., Riddle, M. A., Ritz, L., Swiezy, N. B., Vitiello, B., Volkmar, F. R., Votolato, N. A., & Walson, P. (2000). Research Units on Pediatric Psychopharmacology (RUPP) Autism Network. Background and rationale for an initial controlled study of risperidone. *Child and Adolescent Psychiatric Clinics of North America, 9*(1), 201–224.

Meyers, K. and Roth, D. E. (2018). Telepsychiatry with children and adolescents. In A. Martin, M. Bloch, & F. R. Volkmar (Eds.), *Lewis's child and adolescent psychiatry* (6.3.5, pp. 885–897). Wolters Kluwer.

Michelson, D., Allen, A. J., Busner, J., Casat, C., Dunn, D., Kratochvil, C., Newcorn, J., Sallee, F. R., Sangal, R. B., Saylor, K., West, S., Kelsey, D., Wernicke, J., Trapp, N. J., & Harder, D. (2002). Once-daily atomoxetine treatment for children and adolescents with attention deficit hyperactivity disorder: A randomized, placebo-controlled study. *American Journal of Psychiatry, 159*(11), 1896–1901. https:// doi.org/10.1176/appi.ajp.159.11.1896

Molitch, M., & Eccles, A. K. (1937). The effect of benzedrine sulfate on the intelligence scores of children. *American Journal of Psychology, 94*(3), 587–590. https://doi.org/10.1176/ajp.94.3.587

Multimodal Treatment Study of Children with ADHD Cooperative Group. (1999). A 14-month randomized clinical trial of treatment strategies for attention-deficit/hyperactivity disorder. *Archives of General Psychiatry, 56*(12), 1073–1086. https://doi.org/10.1001/archpsyc.56.12.1073

Multimodal Treatment Study of Children with ADHD Cooperative Group. (2004). National Institute of Mental Health Multimodal Treatment Study of ADHD follow-up: Changes in effectiveness and growth after the end of treatment. *Pediatrics, 113*(4), 762–769. https://doi.org/10.1542/peds.113.4.762

Nelson, J. C., & Papakostas, G. I. (2009). Atypical antipsychotic augmentation in major depressive disorder: A meta-analysis of placebo-controlled randomized trials. *The American Journal of Psychiatry, 166*(9), 980–991. https://doi.org/10.1176/appi.ajp.2009.09030312

Newcorn, J. H., Spencer, T. J., Biederman, J., Milton, D. R., & Michelson, D. (2005). Atomoxetine treatment in children and adolescents with attention-deficit/hyperactivity disorder and comorbid oppositional defiant disorder. *Journal of the American Academy of Child & Adolescent Psychiatry, 44*(3), 240–248. https://doi.org/10.1097/00004583-200503000-00008

Oesterheld, O. J. R., Shader, R. J., & Martin A. (2018). Clinical and developmental aspects of pharmocokinetics and drug interactions. In A. Martin, M. Bloch, & F. R. Volkmar (Eds.), *Lewis's child and adolescent psychiatry* (pp. 703–714). Wolters Kluwer.

Owen, R., Sikich, L., Marcus, R. N., Corey-Lisle, P., Manos, G., McQuade, R. D., Carson, W. H., & Findling, R. L. (2009). Aripiprazole in the treatment of irritability in children and adolescents with autistic disorder. *Pediatrics, 124*(6), 1533–1540. https://doi.org/10.1542/peds.2008-3782

Pathak, S., Findling, R. L., Earley, W. R., Acevedo, L. D., Stankowski, J., & Delbello, M. P. (2013). Efficacy and safety of quetiapine in children and adolescents with mania associated with bipolar I disorder: A 3-week, double-blind, placebo-controlled trial. *Journal of Clinical Psychiatry, 74*(1), e100–e109. https://doi.org/10.4088/JCP.11m07424

Pelham, W. E., Gnagy, E. M., Burrows-Maclean, L., Williams, A., Fabiano, G. A., Morrisey, S. M., Chronis, A. M., Forehand, G. L., Nguyen, C. A., Hoffman, M. T., Lock, T. M., Fielbelkorn, K., Coles, E. K., Panahon, C. J., Steiner, R. L., Meichenbaum, D. L., Onyango, A. N., & Morse, G. D. (2001). Once-a-day concerta methylphenidate versus three-times-daily methylphenidate in laboratory and natural settings. *Pediatrics, 107*(6), E105. https://doi.org/10.1542/peds.107.6.e105

Rapport, M. D., & Denney, C. (1997). Titrating methylphenidate in children with attention-deficit/hyperactivity disorder: Is body mass predictive of clinical response? *Journal of the American Academy of Child & Adolescent Psychiatry, 36*(4), 523–530. https://doi.org/10.1097/00004583-199704000-00015

Ratzoni, G., Gothelf, D., Brand-Gothelf, A., Reidman, J., Kikinzon, L., Gal, G., Phillip, M., Apter, A., & Weizman, R. (2002). Weight gain associated with olanzapine and risperidone in adolescent patients: A comparative prospective study. *Journal of the American Academy of Child & Adolescent Psychiatry, 41*(3), 337–343. https://doi.org/10.1097/00004583-200203000-00014

Regier, D. A., Kuhl, E. A., & Kupfer, D. J. (2013). The DSM-5: Classification and criteria changes. *World Psychiatry: Official Journal of the World Psychiatric Association (WPA), 12*(2), 92–98. https://doi.org/10.1002/wps.20050

Rey, J. M., & Martin, A. (2006). Selective serotonin reuptake inhibitors and suicidality in juveniles: Review of the evidence and implications for clinical practice. *Child and Adolescent Psychiatric Clinics of North America, 15*(1), 221–237. https://doi.org/10.1016/j.chc.2005.08.012

Riddle, M. A., Hardin, M. T., Towbin, K. E., Leckman, J. F., & Cohen, D. J. (1987). Tardive dyskinesia following haloperidol treatment in Tourette's syndrome. *Archives of General Psychiatry, 44*(1), 98–99. https://doi.org/10.1001/archpsyc.1987.01800130110023

Riddle, M. A., Reeve, E. A., Yaryura-Tobias, J. A., Yang, H. M., Claghorn, J. L., Gaffney, G., Greist, J. H., Holland, D., McConville, B. J., Pigott, T., & Walkup, J. T. (2001). Fluvoxamine for children and adolescents with obsessive-compulsive disorder: A randomized, controlled, multicenter trial. *Journal of the American Academy of Child & Adolescent Psychiatry, 40*(2), 222–229. https://doi.org/10.1097/00004583-200102000-00017

Rifkin, A., Karajgi, B., Dicker, R., Perl, E., Boppana, V., Hasan, N., & Pollack, S. (1997). Lithium treatment of conduct disorders in adolescents. *American Journal of Psychiatry, 154*(4), 554–555. https://doi.org/10.1176/ajp.154.4.554

Scahill, L., Schwab-Stone, M., Merikangas, K. R., Leckman, J. F., Zhang, H., & Kasl, S. (1999). Psychosocial and clinical correlates of ADHD in a community sample of school-age children. *Journal of the American Academy of Child & Adolescent Psychiatry, 38*(8), 976–984. https://doi.org/10.1097/00004583-199908000-00013

Sikich, L., Frazier, J. A., McClellan, J., Findling, R. L., Vitiello, B., Ritz, L., Ambler, D., Puglia, M., Maloney, A. E., Michael, E., De Jong, S., Slifka, K., Noyes, N., Hlastala, S., Pierson, L., McNamara, N. K., Delporto-Bedoya, D., Anderson, R., Hamer, R. M., & Lieberman, J. A. (2008). Double-blind comparison of first-and second-generation antipsychotics in early-onset schizophrenia and schizo-affective disorder: Findings from the treatment of early-onset schizophrenia spectrum disorders (TEOSS) study. *American Journal of Psychiatry, 165*(11), 1420–1431. https://doi.org/10.1176/appi.ajp.2008.08050756

Silva, R. R., Munoz, D. M., Alpert, M., Perlmutter, I. R., & Diaz, J. (1999). Neuroleptic malignant syndrome in children and adolescents. *Journal of the American Academy of Child & Adolescent Psychiatry, 38*(2), 187–194. https://doi.org/10.1097/00004583-199902000-00018

Solanto, M. V. (1998). Neuropsychopharmacological mechanisms of stimulant drug action in attention-deficit hyperactivity disorder: A review and integration. *Behavioural Brain Research, 94*(1), 127–152. https://doi.org/10.1016/s0166-4328(97)00175-7

Spetie, L., & Arnold, B. E. L. (2018). Attention deficit hyperactivity disorder. In A. Martin, M. Bloch, & F. R. Volkmar (Eds.), *Lewis's child and adoelscnet psychairy* (pp. 364–285.) Wolters Kluwer.

Wagner, K. D., Weller, E. B., Carlson, G. A., Sachs, G., Biederman, J., Frazier, J. A., Wozniak, P., Tracy, K., Weller, R. A., & Bowden, C. (2002). An open-label trial of divalproex in children and adolescents with bipolar disorder. *Journal of the American Academy of Child & Adolescent Psychiatry, 41*(10), 1224–1230. https://doi.org/10.1097/00004583-200210000-00012

Swanson, J. M., Wigal, S., Greenhill, L. L., Browne, R., Waslik, B., Lerner, M., Williams, L., Flynn, D., Agler, D., Crowley, K., Fineberg, E., Baren, M., & Cantwell, D. P. (1998). Analog classroom assessment of Adderall in children with ADHD. *Journal of the American Academy of Child and Adolescent Psychiatry, 37*(5), 519–526.

Walkup, J. T., Albano, A. M., Piacentini, J., Birmaher, B., Compton, S. N., Sherrill, J. T., Ginsburg, G. S., Rynn, M. A., McCracken, J., Waslick, B., Iyengar, S., March, J. S., & Kendall, P. C. (2008). Cognitive behavioral therapy, sertraline, or a combination in childhood anxiety. *New England Journal of Medicine, 359*(26), 2753–2766. https://doi.org/10.1056/NEJMoa0804633

Weisman, H., Qureshi, I. A., Leckman, J. F., Scahill, L., & Bloch, M. H. (2013). Systematic review: Pharmacological treatment of tic disorders—Efficacy of antipsychotic and alpha-2 adrenergic agonist agents. *Neuroscience & Biobehavioral Reviews, 37*(6), 1162–1171. https://doi.org/10.1016/j.neubiorev.2012.09.008

Weller, E. B., Weller, R. A., & Fristad, M. A. (1986). Lithium dosage guide for prepubertal children: A preliminary report. *Journal of the American Academy of Child Psychiatry, 25*(1), 92–95. https://doi.org/10.1016/s0002-7138(09)60603-8

Wigal, S. B., McGough, J. J., McCracken, J. T., Biederman, J., Spencer, T. J., Posner, K. L., Wigal, T. L., Kollins, S. H., Clark, T. M., Mays, D. A., Zhang, Y., & Tulloch, S. J. (2005). A laboratory school comparison of mixed amphetamine salts extended release (Adderall XR) and atomoxetine (Strattera) in school-aged children with attention deficit/hyperactivity disorder. *Journal of Attention Disorders, 9*(1), 275–289. https://doi.org/10.1177/1087054705281121

Williams, K., Brignell, A., Randall, M., Silove, N., & Hazell, P. (2013). Selective serotonin reuptake inhibitors (SSRIs) for autism spectrum disorders (ASD). *Cochrane Database of Systematic Reviews, 8*, CD004677. https://doi.org/10.1002/14651858.CD004677.pub3

Suggested Readings

American Psychiatric Association. (2013). *Diagnostic and statistical manual of mental disorders* (5th ed.). American Psychiatric Publishing.

Angold, A., Costello, E. J., & Erkanli, A. (1999). Comorbidity. *Journal of Child Psychology and Psychiatry and Allied Disciplines, 40*(1), 57–87. https://doi.org/10.1111/1469-7610.00424

Aparasu, R. R., & Bhatara, V. (2007). Patterns and determinants of antipsychotic prescribing in children and adolescents, 2003–2004. *Current Medical Research and Opinion, 23*(1), 49–56. https://doi.org/10.1185/030079906X158075

Arnsten, A. F. (1997). Catecholamine regulation of the prefrontal cortex. *Journal of Psychopharmacology (Oxford, England), 11*(2), 151–162. https://doi.org/10.1177/026988119701100208

Avery, R. A., Franowicz, J. S., Studholme, C., van Dyck, C. H., & Arnsten, A. F. (2000). The alpha-2A-adrenoceptor agonist, guanfacine, increases regional cerebral blood flow in dorsolateral prefrontal cortex of monkeys performing a spatial working memory task. *Neuropsychopharmacology, 23*(3), 240–249. https://doi.org/10.1016/S0893-133X(00)00111-1

Barrickman, L. L., Perry, P. J., Allen, A. J., Kuperman, S., Arndt, S. V., Herrmann, K. J., & Schumacher, E. (1995). Bupropion versus methylphenidate in the treatment of attention-deficit hyperactivity disorder. *Journal of the American Academy of Child & Adolescent Psychiatry, 34*(5), 649–657. https://doi.org/10.1097/00004583-199505000-00017

Biederman, J., Faraone, S., Milberger, S., Curtis, S., Chen, L., Marrs, A., Ouellette, C., Moore, P., & Spencer, T. (1996). Predictors of persistence and remission of ADHD into adolescence: Results from a four-year prospective follow-up study. *Journal of the American Academy of Child & Adolescent Psychiatry, 35*(3), 343–351. https://doi.org/10.1097/00004583-199603000-00016

Biederman, J., Newcorn, J., & Sprich, S. (1991). Comorbidity of attention deficit hyperactivity disorder with conduct, depressive, anxiety, and other disorders. *American Journal of Psychiatry, 148*(5), 564–577. https://doi.org/10.1176/ajp.148.5.564

Bowers, R., Jackson, J., & Weston, C. (2018). *Green's child and adolescnet clinical psychopharmacology* (6th ed.). Wolters Kluwer.

Cipriani, A., Hawton, K., Stockton, S., & Geddes, J. R. (2013). Lithium in the prevention of suicide in mood disorders: Updated systematic review and meta-analysis. *BMJ, 346*, f3646. https://doi.org/10.1136/bmj.f3646

Detke, H. C., DelBello, M. P., Landry, J., & Usher, R. W. (2015). Olanzapine/fluoxetine combination in children and adolescents with bipolar I depression: A randomized, double-blind, placebo-controlled trial. *Journal of the American Academy of Child & Adolescent Psychiatry, 54*(3), 217–224. https://doi.org/10.1016/j.jaac.2014.12.012

Findling, R. L., Cavuş, I., Pappadopulos, E., Vanderburg, D. G., Schwartz, J. H., Gundapaneni, B. K., & DelBello, M. P. (2013). Ziprasidone in adolescents with schizophrenia: Results from a placebo-controlled efficacy and long-term open-extension study. *Journal of Child and Adolescent Psychopharmacology*, 23(8), 531–544. https://doi.org/10.1089/cap.2012.0068

Findling, R. L., McKenna, K., Earley, W. R., Stankowski, J., & Pathak, S. (2012). Efficacy and safety of quetiapine in adolescents with schizophrenia investigated in a 6-week, double-blind, placebo-controlled trial. *Journal of Child and Adolescent Psychopharmacology*, 22(5), 327–342. https://doi.org/10.1089/cap.2011.0092

Geller, B., & Luby, J. (1997). Child and adolescent bipolar disorder: A review of the past 10 years. *Journal of the American Academy of Child & Adolescent Psychiatry*, 36(9), 1168–1176. https://doi.org/10.1097/00004583-199709000-00008

Geller, B., Warner, K., Williams, M., & Zimerman, B. (1998). Prepubertal and young adolescent bipolarity versus ADHD: Assessment and validity using the WASH-U-KSADS, CBCL and TRF. *Journal of Affective Disorders*, 51(2), 93–100. https://doi.org/10.1016/s0165-0327(98)00176-1

Gray, J. (1997). *Evidence-based healthcare: How to make health policy and management decisions.* Churchill-Livingstone.

Hamilton, B. E., Miniño, A. M., Martin, J. A., Kochanek, K. D., Strobino, D. M., & Guyer, B. (2007). Annual summary of vital statistics: 2005. *Pediatrics*, 119(2), 345–360. https://doi.org/10.1542/peds.2006-3226

Heiligenstein, J. H., Hoog, S. L., Wagner, K. D., Findling, R. L., Galil, N., Kaplan, S., Busner, J., Nilsson, M. E., Brown, E. B., & Jacobson, J. G. (2006). Fluoxetine 40–60 mg versus fluoxetine 20 mg in the treatment of children and adolescents with a less-than-complete response to nine-week treatment with fluoxetine 10–20 mg: A pilot study. *Journal of Child and Adolescent Psychopharmacology*, 16(1–2), 207–217. https://doi.org/10.1089/cap.2006.16.207

Hetrick, S. E., McKenzie, J. E., Cox, G. R., Simmons, M. B., & Merry, S. N. (2012). Newer generation antidepressants for depressive disorders in children and adolescents. *Cochrane Database of Systematic Reviews*, 11, CD004851. https://doi.org/10.1002/14651858.CD004851.pub3

Keller, M. B., Ryan, N. D., Strober, M., Klein, R. G., Kutcher, S. P., Birmaher, B., Hagino, O. R., Koplewicz, H., Carlson, G. A., Clarke, G. N., Emslie, G. J., Feinberg, D., Geller, B., Kusumakar, V., Papatheodorou, G., Sack, W. H., Sweeney, M., Wagner, K. D., Weller, E. B.,... McCafferty, J. P. (2001). Efficacy of paroxetine in the treatment of adolescent major depression: A randomized, controlled trial. *Journal of the American Academy of Child & Adolescent Psychiatry*, 40(7), 762–772. https://doi.org/10.1097/00004583-200107000-00010

Ketter, T. A., Wang, P. W., Chandler, R. A., Alarcon, A. M., Becker, O. V., Nowakowska, C., O'Keeffe, C. M., & Schumacher, M. R. (2005). Dermatology precautions and slower titration yield low incidence of lamotrigine treatment-emergent rash. *Journal of Clinical Psychiatry*, 66(5), 642–645. https://doi.org/10.4088/jcp.v66n0516

Leckman, J. F., Ort, S., Caruso, K. A., Anderson, G. M., Riddle, M. A., & Cohen, D. J. (1986). Rebound phenomena in Tourette's syndrome after abrupt withdrawal of clonidine. Behavioral, cardiovascular, and neurochemical effects. *Archives of General Psychiatry*, 43(12), 1168–1176. https://doi.org/10.1001/archpsyc.1986.01800120054011

Marcus, R. N., Owen, R., Kamen, L., Manos, G., McQuade, R. D., Carson, W. H., & Aman, M. G. (2009). A placebo-controlled, fixed-dose study of aripiprazole in children and adolescents with irritability associated with autistic disorder. *Journal of the American Academy of Child & Adolescent Psychiatry*, 48(11), 1110–1119. https://doi.org/10.1097/CHI.0b013e3181b76658

Mooney, L., Fosdick, C., & Erickson, C. A. (2019). Psychopharmacology of autism spectrum disorders. In F. R. Volkmar (Ed.), *Autism and the pervasive developmental disorders* (3rd ed., pp. 158–175). Cambridge University Press.

Norn, S., Kruse, P. R., & Kruse, E. (2005). Opiumsvalmuen og morfin gennem tiderne [History of opium poppy and morphine]. *Dansk medicinhistorisk arbog*, 33, 171–184.

Riddle, M. A. (2019). *Pediatric psychopharmacology for primary care* (2nd ed.). American Academy of Pediatrics.

Riddle, M. A., Scahill, L., King, R. A., Hardin, M. T., Anderson, G. M., Ort, S. I., Smith, J. C., Leckman, J. F., & Cohen, D. J. (1992). Double-blind, crossover trial of fluoxetine and placebo in children and adolescents with obsessive-compulsive disorder. *Journal of the American Academy of Child & Adolescent Psychiatry*, 31(6), 1062–1069. https://doi.org/10.1097/00004583-199211000-00011

Robb, A. S. (2017). Practical pediatric psychopharmacology for pediatricians and non-child psychiatrists [conference abstract]. *Journal of the American Academy of Child & Adolescent Psychiatry*, 56(10), S150. https://doi.org/10.1016/j.jaac.2017.07.567

Sallee, F. R., Kurlan, R., Goetz, C. G., Singer, H., Scahill, L., Law, G., Dittman, V. M., & Chappell, P. B. (2000). Ziprasidone treatment of children and adolescents with Tourette's syndrome: A pilot study. *Journal of the American Academy of Child & Adolescent Psychiatry, 39*(3), 292–299. https://doi .org/10.1097/00004583-200003000-00010

Smith, A. (2017). Commentary: Pediatric psychopharmacology for the primary care clinician [comment]. *Current Problems in Pediatric and Adolescent Health Care, 47*(1), 25–26. https://doi.org/10.1016/j .cppeds.2016.12.003

Smith, A. (2018). Commentary: Recent advances in pediatric psychopharmacology [note]. *Current Problems in Pediatric and Adolescent Health Care, 48*(2), 63–64. https://doi.org/10.1016/j.cppeds.2017.12.004

Sprague, R. L., & Sleator, E. K. (1977). Methylphenidate in hyperkinetic children: Differences in dose effects on learning and social behavior. *Science, 198*(4323), 1274–1276. https://doi.org/10.1126/ science.337493

Sultan, R. S., Correll, C. U., Zohar, J., Zalsman, G., & Veenstra-VanderWeele, J. (2018). What's in a name? Moving to neuroscience-based nomenclature in pediatric psychopharmacology [editorial]. *Journal of the American Academy of Child & Adolescent Psychiatry, 57*(10), 719–721. https://doi.org/10.1016/j .jaac.2018.05.024

Varigonda, A. L., Jakubovski, E., Taylor, M. J., Freemantle, N., Coughlin, C., & Bloch, M. H. (2015). Systematic review and meta-analysis: Early treatment responses of selective serotonin reuptake inhibitors in pediatric major depressive disorder. *Journal of the American Academy of Child & Adolescent Psychiatry, 54*(7), 557–564. https://doi.org/10.1016/j.jaac.2015.05.004

Vitiello, B. (2015). Principles in using psychotropic medication in children and adolescents. In J. M. Rey (Ed.), *IACAPAP e-textbook of child and adolescent mental health.* International Association for Child and Adolescent Psychiatry and Allied Professions.

Vitiello, B., Behar, D., Malone, R., Delaney, M. A., Ryan, P. J., & Simpson, G. M. (1988). Pharmacokinetics of lithium carbonate in children. *Journal of Clinical Psychopharmacology, 8*(5), 355–359.

Vitiello, B., & Jensen, P. S. (1995). Developmental perspectives in pediatric psychopharmacology. *Psychopharmacology Bulletin, 31*(1), 75–81.

Wagner, K. D., Ambrosini, P., Rynn, M., Wohlberg, C., Yang, R., Greenbaum, M. S., Childress, A., Donnelly, C., Deas, D., & Sertraline Pediatric Depression Study Group. (2003). Efficacy of sertraline in the treatment of children and adolescents with major depressive disorder: Two randomized controlled trials. *JAMA, 290*(8), 1033–1041. https://doi.org/10.1001/jama.290.8.1033

CHAPTER 30 ■ FAMILY-BASED THERAPY

Family therapy is a broad "umbrella concept" that encompasses a great many specific clinical interventions that share certain characteristics but that differ significantly in their underlying theoretical principles and orientation, their techniques and implementation, and the specific problems and disorders they aim to ameliorate. Within this broad category can be found psychodynamic approaches, cognitive and behavioral approaches, strategic approaches, and others. Since its early development, around the middle of the 20th century, family therapy has evolved considerably. The strict divide between the field of family therapy and the fields of psychiatry and psychology has been gradually (and partially) bridged, and family therapy has gained a place of prominence and respect in the overall landscape of mental health services. This chapter reviews key parts of the history of family therapy and discusses several of the theoretical models and applied implementations, as they relate to the treatment of children and adolescents.

■ BACKGROUND AND HISTORY

The roots of family therapy are often traced to the decade following World War II, and to the challenges and problems caused by the large-scale reunification of families who sought mental health counseling to address them. Roles that had been traditionally filled by the broader community, including extended family, schools, and religious organizations, became the purview of clinical providers. These providers began to turn their attention increasingly to the family system as an integrated unit, where previously the focus had been almost exclusively on the individual and the problems of the "patient."

An important early influence on the development of family therapy as a theoretical field was the work of Gregory Bateson (Bateson et al., 1956). Bateson, a linguist and anthropologist, applied concepts from communications and cybernetics to human communication, including within family systems. Most notably, in collaboration with other researchers, Bateson developed the double-bind theory as a proposal for understanding the etiology and symptoms of schizophrenia. The double-bind refers to situations in which a person receives contradictory messages or injunctions through different forms of communication. For example, a parent whose words convey love for a child but whose actions express disdain or detachment. When the contradictory injunctions demand a response from the child, who is unable to satisfy both and perceives a threat of punishment for not doing so, the double-bind can trigger anxiety, stress, and confusion. Ultimately, over repeated such instances the child may become suspicious of all communication and may respond to the confusing messages with equally disjointed communication of their own. This was suggested to be the onset of the schizophrenic illness. Although researchers today no longer attribute the etiology of schizophrenia to parental behaviors or specific forms of maladaptive parenting, the influence of the theory lies in its departure from individual models that emphasize only the inner psyche, in favor of an emphasis on relationships and interpersonal systems.

Another proposal for the etiology of schizophrenia that exerted an early influence on the field of family therapy was the work of Frieda Fromm-Reichmann on the so-called schizophrenogenic mother (Fromm-Reichmann, 1948). The theory posited that distant and aloof, but possessive and manipulative mothers, in combination with passive and ineffective fathers, cause children to feel inadequate and bewildered and ultimately to develop schizophrenia. Like the double-bind, the schizophrenogenic mother theory is no longer viewed as an empirically sound theory for the etiology of schizophrenia, but it remains important for its impact on family therapy and contribution to the shift toward a systemic family-based view of psychopathology.

Other early contributors to the field include Theodore Lidz who emphasized the importance of maladaptive fathering and disrupted marital relationships, Murray Bowen who emphasized multigenerational transmission of unhealthy relationships, Nathan Ackerman who published the first paper addressing treatment with an entire family in 1937 (Ackerman, 1937), John Bell who was among the first to regularly meet with families in a clinical setting, Carl Whitaker who began working with families during the 1940s and organized early family therapy conferences that included interviewing families behind a one-way mirror, and many others.

By the 1960s, family therapy had gained a respected place in the field of mental health, although it remained dominated, at least in practice, by social workers rather than psychologists or psychiatrists who continued to focus on the individual patient and on intrapsychic processes rather than interpersonal systems. A journal, *Family Process,* was established and remains highly influential to this day, although numerous other journals that emphasize family-based approaches have since come into existence. And despite the early focus on adults with mental illness (and in particular schizophrenia), applications of family therapy to the problems of children and adolescents also emerged.

The work of Salvador Minuchin is particularly influential in this regard. Minuchin developed *structural family therapy*, a theory-driven approach to family therapy grounded in empirical research and inspired by his work with youth in underprivileged communities (Minuchin & Nichols, 1998). Structural family therapy aims to map relationships between family members and to dislodge unhealthy patterns of intra-family transactions, allowing the emergence and stabilization of healthier and more adaptive patterns.

Although much of the work in the field of family therapy occurred in the United States, important centers also emerged in other locations. Notably, Mara Selvini-Palazzoli founded the Institute for Family Studies in Milan, a group that became highly influential in the field for a long time.

The 1980s are the decade many consider to be the heyday of family therapy. Journals dedicated to the field proliferated, national and international professional associations sprung up with many active members, the American Psychological Association established a division dedicated to family psychology, and professionals could become board certified in family therapy. This surge in focus on family therapy also led to certain criticisms, including that the field was placing excessive focus on pragmatic solutions, at the expense of deep and full understanding of the family system in which the problems are emerging, and that treatments were being advanced without enough empirical evidence to support their efficacy. In recent decades, family therapy has broadened its scope and has placed increased emphasis on establishing competency benchmarks for clinicians and on establishing evidence-based practices for the field.

MODELS OF FAMILY THERAPY

Psychodynamic Family Therapy

Psychodynamic therapy originates with the work of Freud and places special emphasis on drives and processes that occur outside of conscious awareness. In psychodynamic therapy, the role of the analyst involves understanding these processes through (among other things) interpretation of transference and countertransference and of resistance on the part of the patient (see Chapter 5 for a brief overview of psychodynamic therapy). Ackerman published early research describing the entire family as a single psychosocial unit and was the first to apply the concepts of psychodynamic theory and practice to family therapy (Ackerman, 1958). His work with families emphasized the unconscious processes that occur between family members and he sought to tackle defensiveness in family members by encouraging open and frank discussion of any topic. However, Ackerman did not delineate a specific theoretical model underlying his work.

An example of a more clearly laid out theory of psychodynamic family therapy is the work of David Scharff and Jill Savege Scharff (a married couple) (Scharff, 1989). This work built on objects relations theory, a development of psychoanalysis that emphasizes the relationship between infant and caregiver as the foundation for adult identity and personality. In object relations family therapy, the therapist elicits unconscious material from dreams and fantasies to help patients gain insight into how past experiences are impacting their current relationships. Transference, rather than being viewed as something that happens exclusively between patient and therapist, is thus understood to occur between family members and between the family and the therapist and can be interpreted by the therapist to advance the therapeutic process. Observing the family and how family members interact with each other provides the therapist with information about each member's object relations and can enable increased understanding, and ultimately a stabilization of the family system.

Other forms of psychodynamic therapy have also been translated to the family therapy domain, including Kohut's self-psychology and, more recently, relational psychoanalysis.

Transgenerational Family Therapy

Transgenerational models of family therapy posit that current problems experienced by family members have their roots in the passed-on issues of previous generations. Essentially, when problems are not successfully resolved in one generation, they echo onward through future generations, sometimes growing in severity and leading to symptoms of psychopathology. Particularly notable in this context is the work of Murray Bowen (Bowen, 1966). Bowen emphasized the conflicting drives within families for both cohesive togetherness and for separation and autonomy. He posited this conflict as a central issue impacting all people. Bowen suggested that over-entanglement between children and parents, through the process of enmeshment, could lead to triangulation within families—involving everyone in the family and not only the mother-child dyad (Bowen, 1972). He articulated a theory comprising several key concepts relating to both the current family and to the transgenerational impact of previous generations.

Believing that all human beings must contend with anxiety, Bowen suggested that the transgenerational transmission of anxiety can lead the current family to an imbalanced resolution of the conflicting drives for togetherness and autonomy. This in turn causes enmeshment and triangulation, and even more anxiety. Bowen's *Family Systems Therapy* aimed to "detriangulate" families and to increase family members' individuation, thus reducing the level of anxiety experienced by the family members and by the family as a whole. Family systems therapy includes a set of strategies and techniques to foster communication and insight, including the use of genograms to chart family history over generations.

Of note, in the context of children and adolescents, Bowen's approach centered on work with couples, even when the identified patient was a child. The belief that the marital relationship, influenced by each spouse's generational history, is at the root of children's difficulties led to this focus, which differs from most forms of family therapy that involve the entire family unit in the therapeutic process.

Structural Family Therapy

In *Structural Family Therapy,* the underlying structure and organization of the family system is carefully mapped out. This refers to the complex set of rules, norms, and demands that determine how family members interact with each other within the family system.

Salvador Minuchin, the developer of structural family therapy, proposed that this self-perpetuating structure and its degree of flexibility are critical to a family's ability to contend with the changing challenges of life (Minuchin, 1974; Minuchin & Fishman, 1981; Minuchin & Nichols, 1998). A family that is open to change in its underlying structure will be better able to cope adaptively with transitions and novel demands. Conversely, a family that is rigidly clinging to a firmly fixed structure will struggle with periods of change and become less functional. Thus, the structural family therapist will help families by enabling changes in the structure of dysfunctional families, paving the way for more adaptive patterns to emerge.

The concepts of family boundaries and family subsystems (e.g., parents vs. children; males vs. females) are central to mapping the family organization in structural family therapy. Overly diffuse boundaries between family members prevent healthy individuation in children, causing them to take on roles such as family protector, leading to overwhelming stress in the child, and the emergence of psychopathological symptoms. These symptoms can act as a stress reliever, helping the family to focus on the symptoms while still maintaining the unhealthy organization and structure. In other cases, overly rigid boundaries can lead to disengagement and alienation, with little sense of belonging and cohesiveness, poor communication, and scant family support.

Key to helping families understand, and gradually improve, their family structure is the technique of "family mapping." The procedure involves creating a visual map of the complex interactional patterns within the family. The map denotes the boundaries between family members and the various subsystems, with a notation system for indicating the style of boundary (e.g., clear, diffuse, rigid, etc.). Once the structure has been mapped, it is continually monitored, and the therapist can implement active interventions to challenge and modify it in more adaptive ways.

Strategic Family Therapy

Strategic family therapy originates with the work of the Mental Research Institute in Palo Alto and was developed and refined by such people as Jay Haley and Milton Erickson, and, in a somewhat different direction, Mara Selvini-Palazzoli (Haley, 1963; Selvini-Palazzoli & Viaro, 1989).

Strategic family therapy emphasizes solution-based approaches focused on addressing the symptoms most important to the family at the present moment, rather than on understanding or modifying the overall family system or structure. Strategic therapists are usually highly directive, offering prescriptive instructions to families and not being content with only striving for increased insight through observation, reflection, and interpretation. Perhaps as a result, strategic family therapy is also highly tailored and specific to each case, with the family setting the priorities for the treatment and the therapist selecting the active intervention components most relevant to addressing them. Among the interventions best known for their role in strategic family therapy are those referred to as *paradoxical interventions.* The term refers to the deliberately provocative nature of these interventions aimed at eliciting resistance or even defiance in the family member or members (West & Zarski, 1983). These are particularly useful when the family is exhibiting resistance to change or to the process of therapy and offer a means of engaging the family and overcoming the resistance. Examples of paradoxical interventions include the relabeling of symptoms in a positive light, explicitly "prescribing" that family members engage in some symptomatic behavior that they express the desire to stop, or recommending that the family change nothing at all in their behavior for some set period of time. In one typical example, a mother who is highly controlling of her children might be instructed to maintain complete control over them and their behavior for the coming week, and to meticulously monitor her exercise of control in every instance. In this case, if the mother follows the instruction, she is actually relinquishing some control by following the instructions of the therapist. If, on the other hand, she defies the instruction and is less controlling, then the problem has been alleviated and the relationship with the children may improve. Thus, the therapist gains a degree of control over the family dynamic, even when the family initially was resistant to allowing the therapist to intervene. The Milan school of Selvini-Palazzoli also made use of paradoxical intervention, often recommending that families refrain from premature change early in the treatment process and reframing symptoms as positive or well-intentioned as they contribute to stability and predictability within the system.

Behavioral and Cognitive Behavioral Family Therapy

Behavioral family therapy has its roots in the 1950s although it took almost two decades for it to enter the mainstream of family therapy, and it has been gaining prominence ever since. Behaviorism views behavior, including maladaptive behaviors and symptoms, as learned phenomena shaped by the influence of contingencies such as punishments and rewards. Theories of learning, including classical conditioning, operant conditioning, social learning theory, and social exchange theory all contributed to the conceptualization of strategies for modifying problematic behavior patterns (Liberman, 1972; Stuart, 1969).

In the context of treatment for children, family members, in particular parents, are generally understood to provide many of the contingencies likely to exert a shaping influence on the child's behavior. Accordingly, intervention with the family rather than with the child alone has significant appeal. Important pioneers in this domain included such figures as Richard Stuart, Gerald Patterson, and Richard Liberman. They emphasized a focus on observable behaviors rather than inferred, but not directly observable, processes and on the extinction of maladaptive behaviors through the systematic and strategic use of reinforcements.

The integration of cognitive approaches, and the emergence of cognitive behavioral therapy, occurred during the 1970s, with the recognition that cognitive processes such as thoughts and attributions also influence behavior. Cognitive therapy was originally developed by Aaron Beck and Albert Ellis (Beck, 1970; Ellis, 1969) and posits that how individuals process information plays critical roles in determining function. Essentially, the underlying premise is that thoughts and behaviors influence each other in reciprocal manners and, thus, attending only to behavior limits the ability to effectively intervene.

More recently, a third wave in cognitive behavioral therapy has emerged, with reduced emphasis on eliminating problematic thoughts, feelings or behaviors, and instead emphasizing acceptance of one's self and of the other (Jacobson et al., 2000; West, 2013). Acceptance building strategies such as empathetic joining and tolerance building are typical of these approaches, which may be particularly useful when attempts to directly reduce or eliminate a behavioral or cognitive pattern have not been successful.

Cognitive behavioral therapy has long emphasized the importance of establishing sound empirical foundations for evidence-based treatments. Indeed, cognitive behavioral family therapy has been extensively researched and studied in clinical trials, more so than other family-based approaches.

Parent-Based Treatments

Although most family therapy aims to involve the entire family unit in the therapeutic process, there are also parent-based treatment approaches for a variety of childhood and adolescent problems. In some disorders, such as oppositional defiant disorder, parent-based treatment is the most commonly used, and the most researched, treatment modality (Michelson et al., 2013). Parent management training (PMT) stands out for the number of clinical studies supporting its efficacy in the treatment externalizing problems (Reyno & McGrath, 2006). PMT teaches parents skills to interact positively and productively with children, through reinforcement of desirable behaviors and the removal of inadvertent rewards for undesirable ones. Parents learn to correctly label their children's behaviors, to provide reinforcement consistently, and to respond effectively to noncompliance in the child by controlling their own attention and through tools such as time-outs.

Parent training has also been applied to attention-deficit hyperactivity disorder (Daley et al., 2018). In this context, parents learn to enhance their child's capacity to focus, persist with assignments, reduce impulsive behavior, and problem-solve challenging social situations. Comprehensive treatment strategies that involve significant parent training have been found to be effective in mitigating the symptoms of attention-deficit hyperactivity disorder in children.

In the anxiety disorders, most research has focused on individual or group treatment with children, but behavioral family therapy has been found to augment direct child therapy (Wood et al., 2006). Recently, parent-based approaches to the treatment of childhood anxiety and obsessive-compulsive disorder have emerged. Supportive Parenting for Anxious Childhood Emotions (SPACE) is a completely parent-based treatment for childhood and adolescent anxiety and obsessive-compulsive disorder. Parents in SPACE learn to respond to their child's anxiety-related symptoms and distress in supportive manners that convey to the child both acceptance of the child's genuine distress as well as confidence in the child's ability to cope with and tolerate the distress. A central component of SPACE is the systematic reduction of family accommodation of the child's symptoms, and its replacement with supportive, but not accommodating, responses. SPACE has been found to be as effective as child-based cognitive behavioral therapy for the treatment of anxiety disorders (Lebowitz et al., 2020).

OUTCOME RESEARCH IN FAMILY THERAPY

Clinical trial research into the efficacy of family-based approaches for the treatment of childhood and adolescent problems has increased significantly over the past decades (Markus et al., 1990; Shadish et al., 1995). Much of the research has focused on cognitive-behaviorally–oriented interventions. The largest body of knowledge pertains to the treatment of externalizing disorders such as oppositional defiant disorder, conduct disorder, and delinquency. In this domain, parent-based approaches such as PMT have garnered significant empirical support and can be considered evidence-based. Research has also focused on substance-related problems, eating disorders (Couturier et al., 2013), and to a lesser extent other areas of psychopathology such as mood and anxiety disorders (Carr et al., 2009; Diamond & Siqueland, 1995). In these areas, findings are promising but more research is required to better ascertain the efficacy of family-based treatment and to identify specific interventions that are most efficacious for particular patients and subgroups.

SUMMARY

Family therapy has a long and storied history and encompasses a wide range of therapeutic approaches with a variety of theoretical foundations and correspondingly varied applications. From its early focus on adults and on severe psychopathology, in particular schizophrenia, family therapy has developed in scope and in depth, and now includes treatment modalities centered on the issues of adults, couples, children, and adolescents. It also now includes treatments for a wide range of problems and symptoms. The evidence base for family-based therapies continues to grow and much of the research has supported the efficacy of cognitive behavioral implementations of family-based therapy. Questions remain around the evidence for many of the other family-based therapies, the most active ingredients in treatment and mediators of clinical change, the integration of family-based therapy with other psychosocial and pharmacologic interventions, and the expansion of the family-based approach to even more areas of psychopathology.

References

*Indicates Particularly Recommended

Ackerman, N. W. (1937). *The family as a social and emotional unit* (Vol. 12, pp. 1–3, 7, 8). Kansas Mental Hygiene Society.

Ackerman, N. W. (1958). *The psychodynamics of family life* (xvi, 379 pp.). Basic Books.

Bateson, G., Jackson, D. D., Haley, J., & Weakland, J. (1956). Toward a theory of schizophrenia. *Behavioral Science*, 1(4), 251–264. https://doi.org/10.1002/bs.3830010402

Beck, A. T. (1970). Cognitive therapy: Nature and relation to behavior therapy. *Behavior Therapy*, 1(2), 184–200. https://doi.org/10.1016/S0005-7894(70)80030-2

Bowen, M. (1966). The use of family theory in clinical practice. *Comprehensive Psychiatry*, 7(5), 345–374. https://doi.org/10.1016/S0010-440X(66)80065-2

Bowen, M. (1972). Family therapy and family group therapy. In H. I. Kaplan, B. J. Sadock (Eds.), *Group treatment of mental illness* (xii, 213 pp.). E. P. Dutton.

*Carr, A. (2009). The effectiveness of family therapy and systemic interventions for child-focused problems. *Journal of Family Therapy*, 31(1), 3–45. https://doi.org/10.1111/j.1467-6427.2008.00451.x

*Couturier, J., Kimber, M., & Szatmari, P. (2013). Efficacy of family-based treatment for adolescents with eating disorders: A systematic review and meta-analysis. *International Journal of Eating Disorders*, 46(1), 3–11. https://doi.org/10.1002/eat.22042

*Daley, D., Van Der Oord, S., Ferrin, M., Cortese, S., Danckaerts, M., Doepfner, M., Van den Hoofdakker, B. J., Coghill, D., Thompson, M., Asherson, P., Banaschewski, T., Brandeis, D., Buitelaar, J., Dittmann, R. W., Hollis, C., Holtmann, M., Konofal, E., Lecendreux, M., Rothenberger, A.,... Sonuga-Barke, E. J. (2018). Practitioner review: Current best practice in the use of parent training and other behavioural interventions in the treatment of children and adolescents with attention deficit hyperactivity disorder. *Journal of Child Psychology and Psychiatry*, 59(9), 932–947. https://doi.org/10.1111/jcpp.12825

Diamond, G., & Siqueland, L. (1995). Family therapy for the treatment of depressed adolescents. *Psychotherapy: Theory, Research, Practice, Training*, 32(1), 77–90. https://doi.org/10.1037/0033-3204.32.1.77

Ellis, A. (1969). Rational-emotive therapy. *Journal of Contemporary Psychotherapy*, 1(2), 82–90. https://doi.org/10.1007/BF02110062

Fromm-Reichmann, F. (1948). Notes on the development of treatment of schizophrenics by psychoanalytic psychotherapy. *Psychiatry*, 11(3), 263–273. https://doi.org/10.1080/00332747.1948.11022688

Haley, J. (1963). *Strategies of psychotherapy*. Grune & Stratton.

Jacobson, N. S., Christensen, A., Prince, S. E., Cordova, J., & Eldridge, K. (2000). Integrative behavioral couple therapy: An acceptance-based, promising new treatment for couple discord. *Journal of Consulting and Clinical Psychology*, 68(2), 351–355. https://doi.org/10.1037/0022-006X.68.2.351

Lebowitz, E. R., Marin, C., Martino, A., Shimshoni, Y., & Silverman, W. K. (2020). Parent-based treatment as efficacious as cognitive-behavioral therapy for childhood anxiety: A randomized noninferiority study of supportive parenting for anxious childhood emotions. *Journal of the American Academy of Child and Adolescent Psychiatry*, 59(3), 362–372. https://doi.org/10.1016/j.jaac.2019.02.014

*Liberman, R. P. (1972). Behavioral methods in group and family therapy. *Seminars in Psychiatry*, 4(2), 145–156.

Markus, E., Lange, A., & Pettigrew, T. F. (1990). Effectiveness of family therapy: A meta-analysis. *Journal of Family Therapy*, 12(3), 205–221. https://doi.org/10.1046/j..1990.00388.x

Michelson, D., Davenport, C., Dretzke, J., Barlow, J., & Day, C. (2013). Do evidence-based interventions work when tested in the "real world?" A systematic review and meta-analysis of parent management training for the treatment of child disruptive behavior. *Clinical Child and Family Psychology Review*, 16(1), 18–34. https://doi.org/10.1007/s10567-013-0128-0

*Minuchin, S. (1974). *Families & family therapy*. Harvard University Press.

Minuchin, S., & Fishman, H. C. (1981). *Family therapy techniques*. Harvard University Press.

Minuchin, S., & Nichols, M. P. (1998). Structural family therapy. In F. M. Dattilio (Ed.), *Case studies in couple and family therapy: Systemic and cognitive perspectives* (pp. 108–131). Guilford Press.

Reyno, S. M., & McGrath, P. J. (2006). Predictors of parent training efficacy for child externalizing behavior problem—A meta-analytic review. *Journal of Child Psychology and Psychiatry, 47*(1), 99–111. https://doi.org/10.1111/j.1469-7610.2005.01544.x

Scharff, J. S. (Ed.). (1989). The development of object relations family therapy ideas. *Foundations of object relations family therapy* (pp. 3–10). Jason Aronson.

Selvini-Palazzoli, M., & Viaro, M. (1988). The anorectic process in the family: A six-stage model as a guide for individual therapy. *Family process, 27*(2):129-48. doi: 10.1111/j.1545-5300.1988.00129.x

*Shadish, W. R., Ragsdale, K., Glaser, R. R., & Montgomery, L. M. (1995). The efficacy and effectiveness of marital and family therapy: A perspective from meta-analysis. *Journal of Marital and Family Therapy, 21*(4), 345–360. https://doi.org/10.1111/j.1752-0606.1995.tb00170.x

Stuart, R. B. (1969). Operant-interpersonal treatment for marital discord. *Journal of Consulting and Clinical Psychology, 33*(6), 675–682. https://doi.org/10.1037/h0028475

West, C. (2013). Behavioral marital therapy, third wave. In A. Rambo, C. West, A. L. Schooley, T. V. Boyd (Eds.), *Family therapy review: Contrasting contemporary models* (pp. 221–226). Routledge/Taylor & Francis Group.

West, J. D., & Zarski, J. J. (1983). Paradoxical interventions used during systemic family therapy: Considerations for practitioners. *Family Therapy, 10*(2), 125–134.

Wood, J. J., Piacentini, J. C., Southam-Gerow, M., Chu, B. C., & Sigman, M. (2006). Family cognitive behavioral therapy for child anxiety disorders. *Journal of the American Academy of Child and Adolescent Psychiatry, 45*(3), 314–321. https://doi.org/10.1097/01.chi.0000196425.88341.b0 16540816

Suggested Readings

Bitter, J. R. (2020). *Theory and practice of couples and family counseling (Revised ed.).* American Counseling Association.

Dattilio, F. M. (2010). *Cognitive-behavioral therapy with couples and families: A comprehensive guide for clinicians.* Guilford Press.

Goldenberg, I., Stanton, M., & Goldenberg, H. (2017). *Family therapy an overview.* Cengage Learning.

Minuchin, S., Reiter, M. D., Borda, C., Walker, S. A., Pascale, R., & Reynolds, H. T. M. (2014). *The craft of family therapy: Challenging certainties.* Routledge/Taylor & Francis Group.

Nichols, M. P. (1984). *Family therapy, concepts and methods.* Gardner Press.

Nichols, M. P., & Davis, S. D. (2020). *The essentials of family therapy* (7th ed.). Pearson Education.

■ INDEX

Note: Page numbers followed by *b*, *f* and *t* indicate material in boxes, figures and tables respectively.